Lecture Notes in Artificial Intelligence   10011

Subseries of Lecture Notes in Computer Science

LNAI Series Editors

Randy Goebel
University of Alberta, Edmonton, Canada
Yuzuru Tanaka
Hokkaido University, Sapporo, Japan
Wolfgang Wahlster
DFKI and Saarland University, Saarbrücken, Germany

LNAI Founding Series Editor

Joerg Siekmann
DFKI and Saarland University, Saarbrücken, Germany

More information about this series at http://www.springer.com/series/1244

David Traum · William Swartout
Peter Khooshabeh · Stefan Kopp
Stefan Scherer · Anton Leuski (Eds.)

Intelligent
Virtual Agents

16th International Conference, IVA 2016
Los Angeles, CA, USA, September 20–23, 2016
Proceedings

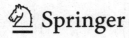

Springer

Editors

David Traum
University of Southern California
Los Angeles, CA
USA

William Swartout
University of Southern California
Los Angeles, CA
USA

Peter Khooshabeh
US Army Research Laboratory
Los Angeles, CA
USA

Stefan Kopp
Universität Bielefeld
Bielefeld, Nordrhein-Westfalen
Germany

Stefan Scherer
University of Southern California
Los Angeles, CA
USA

Anton Leuski
University of Southern California
Los Angeles, CA
USA

ISSN 0302-9743   ISSN 1611-3349 (electronic)
Lecture Notes in Artificial Intelligence
ISBN 978-3-319-47664-3   ISBN 978-3-319-47665-0 (eBook)
DOI 10.1007/978-3-319-47665-0

Library of Congress Control Number: 2016954199

LNCS Sublibrary: SL7 – Artificial Intelligence

Printed on acid-free paper

This Springer imprint is published by Springer Nature
The registered company is Springer International Publishing AG
The registered company address is: Gewerbestrasse 11, 6330 Cham, Switzerland

Preface

This volume presents the proceedings of the 16th International Conference on Intelligent Virtual Agents (IVA 2016). The annual IVA conference represents the main interdisciplinary scientific forum for presenting research on modeling, developing, and evaluating intelligent virtual agents (IVAs) with a focus on communicative abilities and social behavior. IVAs are intelligent digital interactive characters that can communicate with humans and other agents using natural human modalities such as facial expressions, speech, gestures, and movement. They are capable of real-time perception, cognition, emotion, and action that allow them to participate in dynamic social environments. In addition to exploring theoretical issues, the conference showcases working applications. Constructing and studying IVAs requires knowledge, theories, methods, and tools from a wide range of fields such as computer science, psychology, cognitive science, communication, linguistics, interactive media, human–computer interaction, and artificial intelligence.

The IVA conference was started in 1998 as a Workshop on Intelligent Virtual Environments at the European Conference on Artificial Intelligence in Brighton, UK, and was followed by a similar one in 1999 in Salford, Manchester, UK. Subsequently, dedicated stand-alone IVA conferences took place in Madrid in 2001, Irsee, Germany, in 2003, and Kos, Greece, in 2005. In 2006 IVA became a full-fledged annual international event, first held in Marina del Rey, California, followed by Paris in 2007, Tokyo in 2008, Amsterdam in 2009, Philadelphia in 2010, Reykjavik in 2011, Santa Cruz, California in 2012, Edinburgh in 2013, Boston in 2014, and Delft in 2015.

IVA 2016 was held in Los Angeles, California, at the University of Southern California Institute for Creative Technologies. Befitting IVA's Los Angeles location, this year's special topic was "Entertaining Virtual Agents." IVA 2016 sought to emphasize the synergy between intelligent virtual agents and entertainment. The increasing capabilities of intelligent virtual agents are gaining attention from the entertainment community, from non-player characters (NPCs) in video games to developing agents that immortalize famous people. The focus on entertainment cuts across a number of research areas in intelligent virtual agents, spanning serious games to agents who mirror emotional expressions. Virtual agents are increasingly deployed as interactive narrative story-tellers and companions, as well as entertaining and engaging pedagogical agents.

The interdisciplinary character of IVA 2016 and its special topic are underlined by the conference's two renowned keynote speakers:

- Jim Blascovich, Professor at the University of California, Santa Barbara
- Mark Walsh, Writer/Director/Animator/CEO, Motional Entertainment

IVA 2016 received 81 submissions. Out of the 44 long paper submissions, only 12 were accepted for the long papers track. Furthermore, there were 18 short papers selected for the single-track paper session, while 33 poster papers and four interactive demos were on display.

This year's IVA also included three workshops and two half-day tutorials that took place before the main conference.
The workshops were:

- "Workshop on Chatbots and Conversational Agents (WOCHAT)," organized by Rafael E. Banchs, Ryuichiro Higashinaka, Wolfgang Minker, Joseph Mariani, and David Traum
- "Can You Feel Me Now? Creating Physiologically Aware Virtual Agents (PAVA)," organized by Glenn Fox
- "Graphical and Robotic Embodied Agents for Therapeutic Systems GREATS16," organized by Ruth Aylett and Pierre Philp

The tutorials were:

- "How to Build an Interactive Virtual Character," organized by Zerrin Yumak
- "The Sigma Cognitive Architecture and System," organized by Paul S. Rosenbloom and Volkan Ustun

IVA 2016 was locally organized by the Institute for Creative Technologies at the University of Southern California. We would like to express thanks to the rest of the conference Organizing Committee, listed herein. We would also like to thank the scientific committees that helped shape this excellent conference program, the Senior Program Committee for taking on great responsibility and the Program Committee for their time, effort, and constructive feedback to the authors. Additionally, we want to thank our keynote speakers for sharing their outstanding work and insights with the community. Further, we would like to thank our sponsors, including Alelo, Springer, and the organizers of IVA 2015 and the IVA Steering Committee.

September 2016

Peter Khooshabeh
Stefan Kopp
Stefan Scherer
David Traum
William Swartout

Organization

Organizing Committee

Conference Chair

David Traum   University of Southern California, USA
William Swartout   University of Southern California, USA

Program Chair

Peter Khooshabeh   US Army Research Laboratory, USA
Stefan Kopp   CITEC, Bielefeld University, Bielefeld, Germany
Stefan Scherer   University of Southern California, USA

Sponsorship Chair

Ning Wang   University of Southern California, USA

Workshops and Tutorial Chair

David Pynadath   University of Southern California, USA

Doctoral Consortium Chair

Volkan Ustun   University of Southern California, USA

Posters and Demo Chair

Arno Hartholt   University of Southern California, USA

Gala Chair

Ari Shapiro   University of Southern California, USA

Publications Chair

Anton Leuski   University of Southern California, USA

Publicity Chair

Gale Lucas   University of Southern California, USA

Treasurer

Rob Fuchs   University of Southern California, USA

Art and Design

Grace Benn   University of Southern California, USA

Local Chairs

Sharon Mozgai   University of Southern California, USA
Alesia Gainer   University of Southern California, USA

Senior Program Committee

Rick Dale   University of California, Merced, USA
Jens Edlund   KTH Speech, Music and Hearing, Sweden
Timothy Bickmore   Northeastern University, USA
Sidney D'Mello   University of Notre Dame, France
Catherine Pelachaud   CNRS-LTCI - Telecom-ParisTech, France
Dominic Massaro   UC Santa Cruz, USA
Candy Sidner   Worcester Polytechnic Institute, USA
Khiet Truong   University of Twente, The Netherlands
Gary McKeown   Queen's University Belfast, UK
Joakim Gustafson   KTH, Sweden
Joost Broekens   TU Delft, The Netherlands
Ruth Aylett   Heriot-Watt University, UK
Elisabeth Andre   Universität Augsburg, Germany
James Lester   North Carolina State University, USA
Stacy Marsella   Northeastern University, USA

Program Committee

Kangsoo Kim   University of Central Florida, USA
Jim Blascovich   UC Santa Barbara, USA
Mathieu Chollet   University of Southern California, USA
Michael Neff   UC Davis, USA
Etienne de Sevin   SANPSY, University of Bordeaux, France
Radoslaw Niewiadomski   University of Genoa, Italy
Angelo Cafaro   CNRS-LTCI Telecom ParisTech, France
Magalie Ochs   Aix Marseille University, LSIS, France
Elisabetta Bevacqua   National Engineering School of Brest, France

Reid Swanson	University of Southern California, USA
Kirsten Bergmann	Bielefeld University, Germany
Andrew Olney	University of Memphis, USA
Laurel Riek	University of Notre Dame, USA
Kalin Stefanov	KTH Royal Institute of Technology, Sweden
Catharine Oertel	KTH Royal Institute of Technology Sweden
Nikita Mattar	Bielefeld University, Germany
Birgit Lugrin	University of Würzburg, Germany
Jana Götze	KTH Royal Institute of Technology, Sweden
Alexandra Paxton	UC Berkeley, USA
Slim Ouni	University of Lorraine, France
Benjamin Lok	University of Florida, USA
Antony Passaro	U.S. Army Research Laboratory, USA
David DeVault	University of Southern California, USA
Nicolas Sabouret	LIMSI-CNRS, France
Astrid Rosenthal-von der Pütten	University of Duisburg-Essen, Germany
Hannes Vilhjalmsson	Reykjavik University, Iceland
Florian Pecune	LTCI, CNRS, Telecom ParisTech, Universit·Paris-Saclay, France
Ha Trinh	Northeastern University, USA
João Dias	Instituto Superior Técnico, Universidade de Lisboa, Portugal
Annika Silvervarg	Linköping University, Sweden
Lazlo Ring	Northeastern University, USA
Mei Si	Rensselaer Polytechnic Institute, USA
Hendrik Buschmeier	Bielefeld University, Germany
Leo Wanner Catalan	Institute for Research and Advanced Studies, Pompeu Fabra University, Spain
Lewis Johnson	Alelo Inc., USA
Marilyn Walker	UC Santa Cruz, USA
Elnaz Nouri	University of Southern California, USA
Luisa Coheur	Instituto Superior Técnico, Universidade de Lisboa, INESC-ID Lisboa, Portugal
Brigitte Krenn	Austrian Research Institute for Artificial Intelligence, Austria
Iwan de Kok	Bielefeld University, Germany
Aline Normoyle	Moon Collider, Ltd., UK
Patrick Gebhard	German Research Center for Artificial Intelligence, Germany
Tibor Bosse Vrije	Universiteit Amsterdam, The Netherlands
Justus Robertson	North Carolina State University, USA
Emer Gilmartin	Trinity College Dublin, Ireland
Volkan Ustun	University of Southern California, USA
Helen Hastie	Heriot-Watt University, UK

Damien Dupré   University of Grenoble Alpes, France;
                        Queen's University Belfast, UK
Marcelo Worsley   University of Southern California, USA
Martin Schels   University of Ulm, Germany
Sophie Joerg   Clemson University, USA
Catherine Neubauer   University of Southern California, USA
Eli Pincus   University of Southern California, USA
Andre Harrison   U.S. Army Research Laboratory, USA
Benjamin Files   U.S. Army Research Laboratory, USA
Stefan Sütterlin   Lillehammer University College, Norway
Markus Kächele   Ulm University, Germany
Friedhelm Schwenker   Ulm University, Germany
Kim Pollard   U.S. Army Research Laboratory, USA

Contents

Interacting with Virtual Agents in Shared Space: Single and Joint Effects of Gaze and Proxemics

Jan Kolkmeier[✉], Jered Vroon, and Dirk Heylen

Universiteit Twente, P.O. Box 217, 7500 AE Enschede, Netherlands
{j.kolkmeier,j.h.vroon,d.k.j.heylen}@utwente.nl

Abstract. The Equilibrium Theory put forward by Argyle and Dean, posits that in human-human interactions, gaze and proxemic behaviors work together in establishing and maintaining a particular level of intimacy. This theory has been evaluated and used in Virtual Reality settings where people interact with Virtual Humans. In this study we disentangle the single and joint effects of proxemic and gaze behavior in this setting further, and examine how these behaviors affect the perceived personality of the agents. We simulate a social encounter with Virtual Humans in immersive Virtual Reality. Gaze and proxemic behaviors of the agents are manipulated dynamically while the participants' gaze and proxemic responses are being measured. As could be expected, participants showed strongest gaze and proxemic responses when agents manipulated both at the same time. However, agents that only manipulated gaze elicited weaker responses compared to agents that only manipulated proxemics. Agents that exhibited more directed gaze and reduced interpersonal distance were attributed higher scores on intimacy related items than agents that exhibited averted gaze and increased interpersonal distance.

Keywords: immersive VR · Proxemics · Gaze · Virtual humans

1 Introduction

With immersive Mixed and Virtual Reality (iVR) technology becoming more pervasive also in the consumer's home, new challenges for the design of virtual embodied agents and avatars arise. These agents can now be placed in a shared space with the user, rather than in a remote space that is accessed through a regular screen. Tracking of body and hand motion allows users to perceive and direct actions from and towards agents in an immediate fashion. With space being a shared resource, virtual agents interacting with humans in such environments must be aware of the space they occupy and how behaviors in that space are perceived by their human interaction partners. This raises the question of which positioning and movement behaviors are appropriate for virtual agents in iVR. Computational models for positioning and movement of virtual agents in onscreen simulations have been proposed in the past [1,2] using 'social force'-based models based on Hall's proxemics [3] and Kendon's theories on positioning [4].

© Springer International Publishing AG 2016
D. Traum et al. (Eds.): IVA 2016, LNAI 10011, pp. 1–14, 2016.
DOI: 10.1007/978-3-319-47665-0_1

Theories from social psychology include other modalities in models of social spatial behavior. The equilibrium theory (ET) states that interpersonal distance and eye contact can be used to regulate a perceived level of intimacy between interaction partners [5]. For example, high levels of perceived intimacy induced by reduced interpersonal distance can be compensated by regulative behaviors, such as averting gaze or by increasing interpersonal distance through a change in posture or position. This theory has been tested and extended in various studies with varying methodologies and results supporting its general validity [6–8]. ET has been revisited in iVR in one prior study [9], where first evidence was found that the theory also applies to interactions between humans and virtual agents.

Little work has been done to examine the individual and joint effects of such regulative behaviors. In the current paper, we discuss a study to investigate the relationship between two such behaviors in iVR settings: regulation of interpersonal distance and regulation of eye contact. We base our hypotheses on the predictions of the ET. If the agent breaks the equilibrium state by increasing or decreasing the perceived intimacy of the user, we expect the user to exhibit compensation behavior which we measure in the users gaze direction and distance towards the agent. We then test what combination of behaviors in agents elicit strongest regulative responses in the regulation of users' behaviors, and how typical behaviors affect perception of the agents' personality and interpersonal attitudes. The contributions of our findings are further support of the consistency of Equilibrium Theory for interaction with virtual agents in iVR settings and new insights in how perceived agent personality is affected by proxemic and gaze behaviors. These translate to useful insights for designers of embodied agents in iVR settings.

2   Related Work

Before discussing in more detail the design of the present study, we give an overview of related work on examining gaze and proxemics in social interaction and in interaction with artificial agents specifically.

Gaze describes the visual attention of a human manifested in the direction of the eyes and by extension the orientation of head and body, typically in a social context [10]. Two recent surveys summarize research on gaze from a psychological [11] and a technical [12] perspective. It becomes apparent from both that a large body of research on social gaze deals with determining and describing intentions and attention during social interactions.

But what are the effects of different gaze behavior in social interaction? Work by Ioannou *et al.* [13] comparing humans using mutal gaze or averted gaze, found that facial temperature of participants was higher during the former. In [14], the orientation of an information-presenting robot was manipulated to create joint attention with visitors to an exhibition piece. They found that this resulted in spatial reconfiguration of the visitors, following the principles of Kendon's F-formations [4].

Interpersonal Distance is the distance individuals keep towards each other in social situations. *Proxemics*, first coined by Hall [15], describes different interaction distances and relates them to different kinds of interaction, when implicit cultural and social norms are adhered to. Proxemics are used to automatically infer or model relationships between humans [16], for virtual avatars [1,2] but also in human-robot interaction [17].

Besides gaze, Cafaro et al. have looked at the effects of proxemics, and smiles during first encounters with virtual agents and found effects on users' perception of agent's interpersonal attitudes [18] and subsequent relational decisions [19].

However, there is only little research where proxemics behavior was intentionally manipulated to measure or predict behavioral responses in others. A study in iVR and augmented reality found that participants increase the loudness of their voice when a virtual agent is further away [20]. Kastanis and Slater [21] discuss a virtual agent that used reinforcement learning to learn how best to manipulate participants' position. They found that an agent that was allowed to get within 38 cm of participants could learn to move most of them to the desired position in a short time.

3   Conceptual Framework

In the present study we are interested in disentangling the single and joint effects of gaze and proxemic further. To this end, we exhibit different gaze and proxemic behavior in the agent, and look at both the gaze and proxemic responses in the participant. We will call such a change in the agent behavior a *manipulation*. Changes in the user's gaze and proxemic behavior following a manipulation we call the *user response*. Based on the ET, we hypothesise that after a change in the behavior of an agent that impacts the intimacy level of the situation - for example coming closer to the user - the human user performs compensation behaviors - for example stepping back or averting gaze - to maintain the same level of intimacy.

Agent Behaviors. We define the behavior of each agent as a combination of gaze and proxemic behaviors. For gaze, we define behaviors with neutral (G^0), high (G^+), and low (G^-) intimacy. Similarly, we define proxemic behaviors with neutral (P^0), high (P^+), and low (P^-) intimacy.

The realizations of these behaviors were based on a pilot study with colleagues (n = 5) that were aware of the studies goals. Participants were placed in a prototype of the experiment apparatus with a virtual agent. The experimenter let the agent alternate between different prepared versions of each behavior, interviewing the participant on how they perceived the behavior of the agent in terms of intimacy compared to the other realizations.

For proxemic behaviors, we let the agent move across the zones in Hall's model. We found that keeping a distance of 75 cm between users and agents was perceived as neutral (P^0). Decreasing the distance to 40 cm was perceived as noticably more intimate (chosen for P^+, see Fig. 1c). This coincides with Hall's

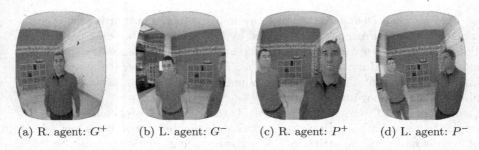

(a) R. agent: G^+ (b) L. agent: G^- (c) R. agent: P^+ (d) L. agent: P^-

Fig. 1. Screenshots of realized agent manipulations.

intimate space and the distance used in [21]. At a distance of 110 cm the agent was found to be noticeably less intimate and was used for P^- (see Fig. 1d).

For gaze, we found that having the agent switch between gazing at the user and averting its gaze in random intervals between 2 and 5 s was perceived as neutral (G^0). Participants found it more intimate when the agent would always respond with mutual gaze if directed gaze at the agent by the user was detected (chosen for G^+, see Fig. 1a). In this version of gaze behavior, the agent would also prolong that gaze for 1.5 s even after directed mutual gaze was interrupted by the user. Note that this version was also chosen over a version where the agent would continuously direct his gaze at the user, as this was perceived as 'creepy'. Conversely, for G^-, we selected a behavior where the agent would always avert his gaze if directed gaze by the user was detected (see Fig. 1b), which was found as less intimate than the neutral version by the participants.

For the final manipulations in the experiment, we chose six combinations of the gaze and proxemic behaviors described above where one or both modalities would deviate from the neutral behavior ($G^0 P^0$) in terms of increasing and decreasing intimacy: $G^- P^-$, $G^0 P^-$, $G^- P^0$, and $G^+ P^0$, $G^0 P^+$, $G^+ P^+$.

User Responses. We measure regulation of eye-contact and interpersonal distance in the user when the agent performs a manipulation. The *Gaze Response* R_G of a user is the change in his or her head angle towards the agent. This may be looking more towards the agent (smaller angle) or looking more away from it (larger angle). We call compensating displacement of the user's whole or upper body the *Proxemic Response* R_P of the user. This may be moving away from the agent (positive response) or towards an agent (negative response).

Hypotheses. We formulate our hypotheses as predictions of user's behavioral responses to different gaze and proxemic behaviors exhibited by a virtual agent. Our main hypothesis is:

H1 Users regulate their gaze and interpersonal distance during interaction differently towards agents that exhibit either high or low intimacy behaviors.

We make prediction of the single and joint effects of the behaviors that the high and low intimacy agents exhibit based on the ET:

$H1_a$ Increasing proximity of the agent $(G^0 P^+)$ will be compensated for by the user with a more positive R_P (moving away) – compared to a smaller, possibly negative R_P (moving closer) when agents perform $G^0 P^-$.

$H1_b$ Increasing gaze of the agent towards the user $(G^+ P^0)$ will be compensated for by the user with higher R_G towards the agent (looking away) – compared to smaller R_G when agents perform $G^- P^0$.

$H1_c$ Besides R_P, also different levels of R_G will be observed in response to $G^0 P^+$ and $G^0 P^-$ manipulations.

$H1_d$ Besides R_G, also different levels of R_P will be observed in response to $G^+ P^0$ and $G^- P^0$ manipulations.

$H1_e$ When the two non-contradicting behaviors are combined, user's responses will 'add up', i.e. R_P to $G^+ P^+$ is higher than to $G^0 P^+$ and R_G to $G^+ P^+$ is lower than to $G^+ P^0$, etc.

To further examine the assumptions of Argyle and Dean that the underlying assumptions of compensating behavior is indeed the perceived intimacy level, we are further interested whether this is also reflected in the user's perception of the agent's personality and interpersonal attitudes. Our hypothesis is:

H2 Users rate agents that exhibit high intimacy behaviors higher on items related to intimacy.

4   Method

These hypotheses were tested in an immersive VR environment experiment where participants could interact freely with two virtual agents that exhibit the different manipulations. We included intimacy of agent as a within subject variable. One agent had the *high* intimacy manipulations assigned, the other had *low* intimacy manipulations. They did not change their assigned role during the experiment. This choice was made to be able to compare how the different more and less intimate behaviors affect the user's perception of the agent (H2).

4.1   Materials

The experiment took place in the room shown in Fig. 2. An Oculus Rift DK2 head mounted display (HMD) is tethered to the experiment PC which is situated in the truss. The tether is 2.6 m in length from the top centre of the room. The translation was tracked using a NaturalPoint OptiTrack system of six IR cameras. This way, free movement and tracking is possible in most of the 4×5 m experiment area, the extreme corners being the exception.

The room displayed in the virtual environment was a generic apartment asset with a bigger empty space next to the living room area, which was mapped onto the experiment space. A transparent 3D model of the truss was placed

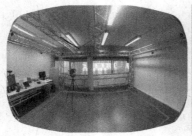 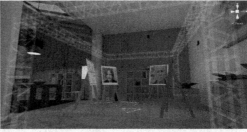

Fig. 2. Left: the physical room. Right: the virtual room.

in correspondence with its real-world position and dimensions to give users a reference in VR of where they are situated in the physical world (see Fig. 2).

The virtual agents used in our iVR setup were generated using the Unity Multipurpose Avatar system (UMA, [22]). The avatars were generated from the same base mesh to look very similar, yet discriminable with slight adjustments to face, hair and attire. To conform to the characters from the scenario described in the next section, both agents were chosen to be male. To prevent the size of the agents relative to the user having an effect on the intimacy or dominance level, their height was adjusted in a calibration step before the start of the experiment to match the height of the participant.

4.2   Task and Scenario

Participants were not told that the experiment was about examining their movement and gaze behavior. Instead, they were given a listening task to focus on, based on a scenario that the two agents would act out. The scenario was taken from the 1957 movie *12 Angry Men*. In this movie, 12 male members of a jury have a discussion about whether or not they were presented sufficient evidence during the court case to sentence the defendant to death. Audio clips of speech segments were extracted from parts of the movie. To prevent dominance mediated by voice to be a factor in the perception of the agents, segments were selected where the argument was less heated. This resulted in 30 clips arguing for 'not guilty' (avg. length = 11.49 s) and 29 clips arguing for 'guilty' (avg. length = 11.51 s) side of the argument. The clips were spoken by the agents chronologically, alternating between the sides of the arguments to make up a consistent conversation between the agents (total duration = 12 m). It was suggested to the participant that the two agents would each attempt various 'strategies' in order to convince the participant of their side of an argument. The task given to the participant was to listen carefully, as they would be asked for their decision afterwards.

4.3 Agent Behavior Manipulations

During the experiment, the agents formed a group with the user by positioning themselves on the base corners of an equilateral triangle. The length of the triangle's legs was 75 cm, corresponding to the *neutral* distance found in the pilot study. The triangle did not rotate with the user. It always faced the long side of the room. The angle of the user's corner was 60°, which was chosen to ensure that when the user centres his view between the agents, both are in view.

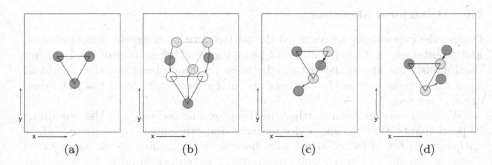

(a) (b) (c) (d)

Fig. 3. The room from a top-down perspective. Two agents (upper circles) form a triadic formation with the user (lower circle) (a), establishing the neutral formation when no manipulation is in place ($G^0 P^0$), also when user is moving (b), but the formation-triangle does not follow the user during gaze or proxemic manipulations (c and d, depicting $G^0 P^+$ and $G^0 P^-$).

Agents would change their gaze and proxemic behaviors at moments that coincided with the dialog turns from the scenario. The behavior changed for the entirety of the turn. This resulted in *episodes* of different agent behavior. At the beginning of every second dialog turn, both agents would employ the *neutral* behavior to 'reset' the group formation (neutral episode, see Fig. 3b). On every other turn, exactly one of the two agents manipulated his behavior (manipulation episodes), by performing one of the three behavior combinations that correspond with his assigned *agent intimacy*. For example, the 'high' agent chose from $G^+ P^0$, $G^0 P^+$ and $G^+ P^+$ - as described in Sect. 3. Each of the three assigned behavior combinations were shown exactly four times throughout the experiment, in randomized order.

Which of the two agents would manipulate its behavior during manipulation episodes was alternated in turns. Since these depend on the dialog turns, the between subject variable 'talking agent' was unintentionally introduced: Within subjects, one of the agents changed his level of intimacy only when he is also the currently talking agent, whereas the other changed his level of intimacy only when he was not currently talking. Whether it was the 'high' or the 'low' agent that manipulated only during talking was randomised between subjects.

4.4 Participants

35 participants were convenience-sampled from students and staff, all of which were completely naive to the study's goals. They were between 19 and 30 years old ($m = 21.4$). Five were female. Of the 35, two were discarded from the data. One decided to stop the experiment early because of motion sickness, and another misunderstood the instructions, continuously moving around and exploring the room also during the main experiment.

4.5 Behavioral Measures

During the experiment we recorded the participants' and agents' head positions and orientations in the virtual world using the tracking system of the iVR. We continuously calculated the distance between the user's head and the individual agents' heads as well as the angle of the user's gaze away from the individual agents (see Sect. 3).

We observed significant outliers in the proxemic responses of the remaining 33 participants. By reviewing video material and experiment notes, some of these outliers were found to be strong responses in the beginning of the experiment. Towards the end of experiment runs, outliers were also found to be caused by participants stepping around agents when 'cornered' by them at the bounds of the tracking area. Although these changes in position seem motivated by the intimate situation, they diverged significantly from the typical proxemic response in other episodes, where participants would either lean or take one or two small steps. From the analysis were excluded all episodes where R_P was bigger than 50 cm ($n = 6$).

4.6 Questionnaire

In addition to the behavioral measures, we are interested in individual's perception of the agents' personalities. A 13 item agent-personality questionnaire which has been successfully used before to measure perception of personality and interpersonal attitudes in both human [23] and virtual human [24,25] communication partners was used. One extra item on politeness was added [26], and one for 'intimacy'. For each agent, identified by a picture, participants would indicate their agreement with the item on a 7-point Likert-scale. Scores of the intimacy related constructs measured by this questionnaire were used to answer H2.

4.7 Data Analysis

The experiment was designed so that we could compare the effects of the six agent manipulations as a six level within-subject factor 'Agent Intimacy' on the two user measures R_G and R_P. However, due to the introduction of the talking agent as a between subject variable (see Sect. 4.3), this approach would not be sound, as one might expect the talking agent to gain more attention than the non talking agent, biasing the gaze response. Indeed, we found that users would

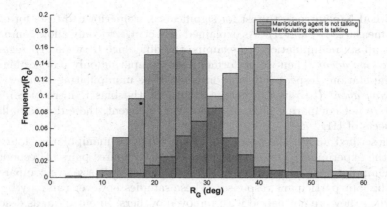

Fig. 4. Histograms of R_G for episodes where the manipulating agent *is* the talking agent and *is not* the talking agent.

typically look towards the currently talking agent (Fig. 4). Consequently, it was chosen to focus on comparing participants' gaze responses only inside the group of agents that manipulated their behavior during their own turn of speech, and only allow for comparison of R_P regardless of the talking agent variable.

5 Results

In Table 1 we present the mean R_P and R_G of all participants and episodes where the manipulating agent was also the talking agent. The measurements violate the assumption of sphericity and normality for both measures at many levels, therefore, under the assumption that the between subject variable *talking agent* does not represent a bias (for the R_P measures), we used the nonparametric Friedman and Wilcoxon signed-rank tests to test our hypotheses.

Table 1. Mean gaze response R_G and proxemic response R_P per agent manipulation from all episodes where the manipulating agent was also the talking agent.

Manip	Mean R_G (SD) in °	Mean R_P (SD) in cm	n	Outliers
G^+P^+	30.17 (6.41)	8.56 (11.70)	55	1
G^0P^+	28.57 (7.38)	8.43 (13.89)	53	2
G^+P^0	27.01 (7.73)	0.36 (9.50)	56	0
G^-P^0	25.23 (6.16)	−0.37 (5.79)	75	1
G^0P^-	25.16 (7.56)	−2.97 (8.89)	76	0
G^-P^-	23.52 (5.72)	−3.48 (6.51)	74	2

Behavioral Measures. To test for significance, we performed tests for each of the two measures R_G and R_P. As explained in Sect. 4.7, we only allow comparison between all six manipulations to examine the difference between R_P regardless of the *talking agent*. Then we performed tests comparing only pairs of high and low manipulations respectively, and only when the manipulating agent was also the *talking agent* (to reveal differences without the bias it introduces). Since here, we're not comparing high and low intimacy agent, these do only allow to test aspects of $H1_e$.

As described above, the agent would act out each manipulation four times during the experiment. The nonparametric test compares pairs of responses to these manipulations. To not artificially inflate our sample size, we compare only one of the four participant responses. These samples however can only be compared when they are not paired with removed outliers. In our data, as described in Sect. 4.5, outliers were observed in the first and second instance of each manipulation, possibly because of a novelty effect, as well as in the fourth, because of the effect of the borders of the experiment area (participants being 'cornered'). Responses during the third instance of each manipulation contain no outliers. Therefore, the responses to the third instance of each manipulation were used for comparison in the nonparametric tests.

Differences Between All Six Manipulations. A Friedman test revealed that there was a statistically significant difference in displacement magnitude ($H1_{a,d,e}$) as a response to different levels of agent behavior intimacy, $\chi^2(5) = 32.84, p < .001$. A Wilcoxon signed-rank test showed that in the 33 participants, the displacement magnitude in response to G^0P^+ behaviors was significantly more positive (i.e.: moving away) than that to G^0P^- ($Z = -3.368, p = .001$).

Differences Between High Manipulations ($H1_e$). A Friedman test revealed that there was a statistically significant difference in response displacement magnitude between the high-intimacy behaviors, $\chi^2(2) = 7.00, p = .030$. A Wilcoxon signed-rank test showed that in the 14 participants where the *high* agent manipulated his behaviors while also being the talking agent, the displacement magnitude in response to G^+P^+ episodes was significantly greater than the displacement magnitude in response to G^+P^0 ($Z = -2.542, p = .011$). In the same population, between the pair of G^+P^0 and G^0P^+ manipulations, we found that the former would elicit significantly less positive displacement magnitude ($Z = -2.229, p = .026$) than the latter, meaning that those in G^+P^0 would move away significantly less. The difference between the pair of G^+P^+ and G^0P^+ behavior was not found to be significant ($Z = -.910, p = .363$). No significant difference in gaze angle was revealed ($\chi^2(2) = 2.29, p = 0.319$).

Differences Between Low Manipulations ($H1_e$). Between the low intimacy behaviors, a Friedman test did not reveal a significant difference in displacement magnitude response of the 19 participants where the *low* agent manipulated his behaviors while also being the talking agent ($\chi^2(2) = 2.95, p = 0.229$). No further tests comparing the individual pairs were performed.

The Friedman test, however, did reveal that there was a marginally significant difference in the participant gaze response between the *low* behaviors, $\chi^2(2) = 6.42$, $p = .040$. Upon inspection, it appears the difference is due to asymmetry of the difference of the pairs, excluding it from further examination with the Wilcoxon signed-rank test. A sign test revealed no significant difference.

Agent Personality Questionnaire. To identify intimacy related constructs in the agent personality questionnaire (H2), we performed a principal component analysis with Varimax rotation and Kaiser normalisation on the 15 items. Three factors were identified that explain 69.15 % of the variance (Table 2). The factors 'Warmth' and 'Trustworthiness' are similar to those found in a previous study using a similar questionnaire [25], a new third factor emerged with the items 'intimate', 'interesting' and 'confident'. We name this new factor 'Intimacy'.

Table 2. Three factors identified in PCA and their corresponding items with factor loadings. For each factor, consistency is reported.

Warmth	($\alpha = .92$)	Trustworthiness	($\alpha = .87$)	Intimacy	($\alpha = .57$)
Friendly	.88	Informed	.82	Intimate	.78
Approachable	.83	Credible	.82	Interesting	.68
Warm	.83	Competent	.76	Confident	.66
Likeable	.82	Honest	.71		
Polite	.79	Trustworthy	.58		
Modest	.79	Sincere	.56		

For each respondent, we calculated factor scores given to the two agents by averaging out those items that were associated with the respective factors. We performed repeated measures ANOVA with the intimacy of the agent (*high* or *low*) as the within subjects variable and agent side, the talking agent, and agent appearance as between subject variables, and the three computed factor scores as measures.

We found a main effect for the intimacy behavior of the agents on 'Warmth' ($F(1,24) = 21.45$, $p < .01$) and 'Intimacy' ($F(1,24) = 6.61$, $p < .05$). No interaction effects of agent appearance and agent side were found on either of the scores. There was however an interaction effect for the talking agent on 'Intimacy' scores ($F(1,24) = 4.31$, $p < .05$). Pairwise comparison revealed that participants scored the agent with low intimacy higher on 'Warmth' related items than the high intimate agent ($m_L^W = 4.97$ vs $m_H^W = 3.57$). 'Intimacy' scores align with the intimacy behavior of the agents. Participants scored the agent with low intimacy lower ($m_I^L = 4.14$) than the agent with high intimacy ($m_I^H = 4.90$). For the interaction effect of the talking agent, pairwise comparison revealed that the high and low agents score similarly on intimacy scores when they are not the talking agent. When talking during manipulation the high agent however scores higher on intimacy ($m_I^{H \times T} = 5.25$) scores than the low agent ($m_I^{L \times T} = 3.86$).

6   Discussion

We found a number of differences in the behavioral response to the different agent behaviors (H1). While the overall means are in line with the predictions made based on the ET (H1$_{a-e}$), there is a high variance in the responses and only some could be supported with statistical significance.

We found that agents exhibiting higher proximity did cause participants to step away significantly more than agents exhibiting low proximity, where participants tended to step more towards the retreating agent (H1$_a$). Although this was expected, it is also one that had not previously been tested experimentally in iVR. As for the predicted effects of G^+P^0, G^-P^0 on R_G (H1$_b$), we could not find significant differences.

In contrast to [9], our study did not find a notable effect of different agent gaze behaviors on the proxemic response (H1$_d$). This may be explained by their use of a more sensitive measure in [9] (minimum distance rather than the mean), and the different interaction between agent and participant (walking around rather than listening). A possible explanation could be ceiling effects of how comfortable individuals were with moving in the iVR setup - possibly also depending on whether they were already at the edge of the tracking area. This interpretation is also in line with the personality scores of the high agent. Scores were low on 'Warmth', which had loadings of the 'politeness' and 'friendliness' items. If a smaller displacement was not sufficient to compensate intimacy, we would expect the remainder to be compensated with gaze. Given the approximate measure of gaze, such compensation may not have been sufficiently captured with the current apparatus.

Some joint effects were found. Participants stepped away more when both gaze and proxemic behaviors were manipulated in a high-intimate fashion, compared to the responses to only high gaze manipulation, supporting some aspects of H1$_e$. Lastly, we found that indeed, participants rated the high agent higher on intimacy related items, supporting H2.

Limitiations and Recommendations. We recommend some changes to the experimental protocol to those that aim to replicate the experiment or adapt aspects of this study design. The extend to which head direction can serve as a proxy for eye-gaze is questionable. Slight gaze aversions away from the agent's face may only be captured with true eye-gaze tracking inside the headset. The two agent design may mitigate this shortcoming as more head movement is required when gaze is averted from one agent to another. For single agent designs however, actual eye-gaze tracking is recommended. For group interactions, we recommend to be aware of the effect of the talking agent on the gaze of dialog partners that we observed, as participants might not notice stimuli by non-talking agents in the group. In this study, the introduction of the talking agent variable is a limitation as it complicated the analysis. Advantages of a single agent design are better generalizability of the findings as compared to the group setting in the present work. It is further suggested to examine the effects of the high and low agent by implementing an agent with mixed intimacy behaviors.

7   Conclusions

Proxemic and gaze behaviors deserve attention when designing virtual humans in immersive VR settings where users and agents share the same space. On the one hand, these behaviors have effect on how users position themselves in the space, and given the spatial restrictions that most virtual (and physical) spaces have, the desire to change space may not always be satisfiable, which may lead to extreme responses, such as the outliers we observed. What is more, proxemic behaviors also affect how the agent's personality is perceived, which may have effect on other aspects of the interaction as well. This ET-inspired approach is a useful tool for human-agent interaction design and analysis in shared spaces. It may benefit from advances in VR technology such as in-headset gaze estimation and physiological sensors, which may be used reveal more on the interaction between proxemics, gaze and intimacy.

Acknowledgments. This work was supported by the European project H2020 ARIA-VALUSPA.

References

1. Jan, D., Traum, D.R.: Dynamic movement and positioning of embodied agents in multiparty conversations. Comput. Linguist. **1968**, 1 (2007)
2. Pedica, C., Vilhjálmsson, H.H.: Spontaneous avatar behavior for human territoriality. In: Ruttkay, Z., Kipp, M., Nijholt, A., Vilhjálmsson, H.H. (eds.) IVA 2009. LNCS (LNAI), vol. 5773, pp. 344–357. Springer, Heidelberg (2009). doi:10.1007/978-3-642-04380-2_38
3. Hall, E.T., Birdwhistell, R.L., Bock, B., Bohannan, P., Diebold Jr., A.R., Durbin, M., Edmonson, M.S., Fischer, J.L., Hymes, D., Kimball, S.T.: Proxemics. Curr. Anthropol. **9**, 83–108 (1968)
4. Kendon, A.: The F-formation system: the spatial organization of social encounters. Man Environ. Syst. **6**, 291–296 (1976)
5. Argyle, M., Dean, J.: Eye-contact, distance and affiliation. Sociometry **28**(3), 289–304 (1965)
6. Coutts, L.M., Schneider, F.W.: Affiliative conflict theory: an investigation of the intimacy equilibrium and compensation hypothesis. J. Pers. Soc. Psychol. **34**(6), 1135–1142 (1976)
7. Patterson, M.L.: Interpersonal distance, affect, and equilibrium theory. J. Soc. Psychol. **101**(2), 205–214 (1977)
8. Rosenfeld, H.M., Breck, B.E., Smith, S.H., Kehoe, S.: Intimacy-mediators of the proximity-gaze compensation effect: movement, conversational role, acquaintance, and gender. J. Nonverbal Behav. **8**(4), 235–249 (1984)
9. Bailenson, J.N., Blascovich, J., Beall, A.C., Loomis, J.M.: Equilibrium theory revisited: Mutual gaze and personal space in virtual environments. Presence **10**(6), 583–598 (2001)
10. Emery, N.J.: The eyes have it: the neuroethology, function and evolution of social gaze. Neurosci. Biobehav. Rev. **24**(6), 581–604 (2000)
11. Pfeiffer, U.J., Schilbach, L., Jording, M., Timmermans, B., Bente, G., Vogeley, K.: Eyes on the mind: Investigating the influence of gaze dynamics on the perception of others in real-time social interaction. Front. Psychol. **3**, 1–11 (2012)

12. Ruhland, K., Andrist, S., Badler, J., Peters, C., Badler, N., Gleicher, M., Mcdonnell, R.: Look me in the eyes: a survey of eye and gaze animation for virtual agents and artificial systems. In: Eurographics State-of-the-Art Report, pp. 69–91, April 2014
13. Ioannou, S., Morris, P., Mercer, H., Baker, M., Gallese, V., Reddy, V.: Proximity and gaze influences facial temperature: a thermal infrared imaging study. Front. Psychol. **5**, 1–12 (2014)
14. Kuzuoka, H., Suzuki, Y., Yamashita, J., Yamazaki, K.: Reconfiguring spatial formation arrangement by robot body orientation. In: 2010 5th ACM/IEEE International Conference on Human-Robot Interaction (HRI), pp. 285–292 (2010)
15. Hall, E.T.: The Hidden Dimension, vol. 1990. Anchor Books, New York (1969)
16. Cristani, M., Paggetti, G., Vinciarelli, A., Bazzani, L., Menegaz, G., Murino, V.: Towards computational proxemics: inferring social relations from interpersonal distances. In: Proceedings of the 2011 IEEE International Conference on Privacy, Risk and Trust/IEEE International Conference on Social Computing PASSAT/SocialCom 2011, pp. 290–297 (2011)
17. Mead, R., Atrash, A., Matarić, M.J.: Automated proxemic feature extraction and behavior recognition: applications in human-robot interaction. Int. J. Soc. Robot. **5**(3), 367–378 (2013)
18. Cafaro, A., Vilhjálmsson, H.H., Bickmore, T., Heylen, D., Jóhannsdóttir, K.R., Valgarðsson, G.S.: First impressions: users' judgments of virtual agents' personality and interpersonal attitude in first encounters. In: Nakano, Y., Neff, M., Paiva, A., Walker, M. (eds.) IVA 2012. LNCS (LNAI), vol. 7502, pp. 67–80. Springer, Heidelberg (2012). doi:10.1007/978-3-642-33197-8_7
19. Cafaro, A., Vilhjálmsson, H.H., Bickmore, T.W., Heylen, D., Schulman, D.: First impressions in user-agent encounters: the impact of an agent's nonverbal behavior on users' relational decisions. In: Proceedings of the 2013 International Conference on Autonomous Agents and Multiagent Systems, pp. 1201–1202 (2013)
20. Obaid, M., Niewiadomski, R., Pelachaud, C.: Perception of spatial relations and of coexistence with virtual agents. In: Vilhjálmsson, H.H., Kopp, S., Marsella, S., Thórisson, K.R. (eds.) IVA 2011. LNCS (LNAI), vol. 6895, pp. 363–369. Springer, Heidelberg (2011). doi:10.1007/978-3-642-23974-8_39
21. Kastanis, I., Slater, M.: Reinforcement learning utilizes proxemics: an avatar learns to manipulate the position of people in immersive virtual reality. Trans. Appl. Percept. **9**, 3:1–3:15 (2012)
22. Ribeiro, F.: UMA - Unity Multipiurpose Avatar System (2015). https://github.com/huika/UMA
23. Guadagno, R.E., Cialdini, R.B.: Online persuasion: an examination of gender differences in computer-mediated interpersonal influence. Gr. Dyn. Theor. Res. Pract. **6**(1), 38–51 (2002)
24. Guadagno, R.E., Blascovich, J., Bailenson, J.N., McCall, C.: Virtual humans and persuasion: the effects of agency and behavioral realism. Media Psychol. **10**(1), 1–22 (2007)
25. Huisman, G., Kolkmeier, J., Heylen, D.: With us or against us: simulated social touch by virtual agents in a cooperative or competitive setting. In: Bickmore, T., Marsella, S., Sidner, C. (eds.) IVA 2014. LNCS (LNAI), vol. 8637, pp. 204–213. Springer, Heidelberg (2014). doi:10.1007/978-3-319-09767-1_25
26. Maat, M., Truong, K.P., Heylen, D.: How turn-taking strategies influence users' impressions of an agent. In: Allbeck, J., Badler, N., Bickmore, T., Pelachaud, C., Safonova, A. (eds.) IVA 2010. LNCS (LNAI), vol. 6356, pp. 441–453. Springer, Heidelberg (2010). doi:10.1007/978-3-642-15892-6_48

The Effect of an Intelligent Virtual Agent's Nonverbal Behavior with Regard to Dominance and Cooperativity

Carolin Straßmann[1]([✉]), Astrid Rosenthal von der Pütten[1], Ramin Yaghoubzadeh[2], Raffael Kaminski[1], and Nicole Krämer[1]

[1] Social Psychology: Media and Communication, University Duisburg-Essen, 47057 Duisburg, Germany
{carolin.strassmann, a.rosenthalvdpuetten, raffael.kaminski, nicole.kraemer}@uni-due.de
[2] Social Cognitive Systems Group, University of Bielefeld, 33549 Bielefeld, Germany
ryaghoubzadeh@uni-bielefeld.de

Abstract. In order to design a successful human-agent-interaction, knowledge about the effects of a virtual agent's behavior is important. Therefore, the presented study aims to investigate the effect of different nonverbal behavior on the agent's person perception with a focus on dominance and cooperativity. An online study with 190 participants was conducted to evaluate the effect of different nonverbal behaviors. 23 nonverbal behaviors of four different experimental conditions (*dominant, submissive, cooperative and non-cooperative* behavior) were compared. Results emphasize that, indeed, nonverbal behavior is powerful to affect users' person perception. Data analyses reveal symbolic gestures such as crossing the arms, stemming the hands on the hip or touching one's neck to most effectively influence dominance perception. Regarding perceived cooperativity expressivity has the most pronounced effect.

1 Introduction

With the rise of embodied artificial interaction partners that are potentially able to display nonverbal behavior it is important to understand which behaviors elicit what perceptual or behavioral reaction on the side of the human interlocutor. In particular dominance and cooperativity perception have an important influence on the user and the human-agent-interaction. For some applications persuasive effects are essential (e.g. agent reminds user to take his meds) which might be strongly supported by dominant (nonverbal) behavior [1]. Otherwise, many applications require the interlocutor to cooperate with the virtual agent. To enhance the sense of cooperation between human and agent, the agent has to be perceived as cooperative. Thus, in order to design a successful human-agent-interaction, the influencing factors of an agent's person perception have to be investigated. Since about 60–65 % of the social meaning is evoked by nonverbal behavior [2], especially the impact of nonverbal cues on dominance and cooperativity has to be focused. In order to investigate the effect of nonverbal behavior on person perception, it has to be analyzed what kind of nonverbal behavior evokes a dominant and cooperative person perception. Based on the literature we found a number of nonverbal behaviors that are assumed to evoke dominance or cooperativity. Although

D. Traum et al. (Eds.): IVA 2016, LNAI 10011, pp. 15–28, 2016.
DOI: 10.1007/978-3-319-47665-0_2

there is a broad understanding of what exact kind of behavior leads to a dominant or submissive evaluation, systematic investigations of those behaviors are missing. Therefore the results of the presented study enhance the current state of the art with a comparison of various nonverbal behaviors with regard to their dominance and cooperativity perception.

2   Dominant Nonverbal Behavior

In human-human-interaction (HHI) the nonverbal behavior is of great importance and evokes subtitle perceptions of the person's personality. Numerous authors [e.g. 2, 3] tried to fathom the meaning of nonverbal behavior. Overall, knowledge about the meaning of nonverbal behavior is broadly based on assumptions, while there is a lack of systematic research. Since a dominant perception might be useful in different scenarios of human-technology-interaction such as persuasion, many researchers tried to create an artificial entity with a dominant presence [e.g. 4–6]. A dominant personality is assumed to have a disposition to control others and is strongly related to power and status [7]. In the Interpersonal Circumplex [8, 9] this personality is represented by the dimension dominance (also called agency) and is characterized by a dominant and a submissive pole. Therefore, this research concentrates on nonverbal behavior that is perceived as dominant or submissive in the way Argyle defines it [8].

There are several nonverbal behaviors that are subsumed as being dominant or submissive and which were frequently used in previous studies in human-agent-interaction (HAI), for instance, hands placed on the hips, crossed arms, self-touch on the neck, sagittal head tilts, wide and expressive gestures. However, although these behaviors were frequently under investigation, the studies often lack a systematic approach and are thus of limited informative value with regard to the question how specific gestures affect person perception. With regard to HAI, symbolic gestures seem to have an influence on the perception of dominance. Gestures like putting the hand on the hips, which is also called Akimbo gesture [4, 5] or putting the hand in the neck [5] are assumed to have an effect on the perception of dominance or submissiveness. Due to the fact that both studies were not primarily interested in the person perception of those gestures, no experimental evidences could be drawn. However, the anecdotal findings regarding symbolic gestures with self-touch are in line with findings from HHI research [10] which suggest that people with high power and dominance are less likely to perform self-touch behavior. While the occurrence of self-touch often was investigated in negative situations and was related to nervousness [11], Harrigan et al. [12] found that people, who show more self-touching, were evaluated more positively. These inconsistent results suggest that the evaluation and perception of self-touch is diverse and may vary depending on the context of the interaction. A virtual agent displaying self-touching behavior was rated as more natural, warmhearted, agile and more committed, but also as more strained and aggressive [13]. However, self-touch was not evaluated empirically with regard to perceptions of dominance.

Additionally, the head-tilt seems to have an important influence on the perception of dominance. Mignault and Chaudhuri [6] as well as Lance and Marsella [14] investigated the effect of sagittal head-tilt based on different types of 3D models. Findings demonstrate that an upward head-tilt evokes dominance and tilting the head down is related to a submissive perception. However, in the presented stimuli of both studies the behaviors were devoid of any distracting cues (e.g. speech or other nonverbal behaviors), in order to investigate only the effect of head-tilt. In a study from Ravenet, Ochs and Pelachaud [15] users are asked to design a virtual agent's nonverbal behavior that is either perceived as dominant or submissive. Results empathize the effect of sagittal head-tilt, since an upward head-tilt was assumed to represent dominance and a downward tilted head seems to express submissiveness. Further on, user created nonverbal behavior with a larger spatial parameter in order to let the agent express dominance, while the created submissive behavior was characterized by a small spatial parameter. This findings are also well known from HHI, since it is assumed that powerful people tend to take up more space and have larger territories [16]. Therefore, expansive gestures evoke the perception of dominance [10, 17]. With regard to virtual agents taking up space does not have the same meaning compared to HHI, because the agent does not share the same physical room with its interlocutor. Although Ravenet et al. [15] demonstrated that the spatial parameter of nonverbal behavior is highly related to dominance and submissiveness; they did not investigate the user's perception, but asked the user to produce the agent's nonverbal behavior. Further on, Callejas, Ravenet, Ochs and Pelachaud [18] and Gebhard and Baur [19] demonstrated that the spatial parameter of nonverbal behavior as well as head-tilt is related to dominance and submissive perception. However, they did not evaluate the single movements individually. Hence, the effect of the individual nonverbal behaviors has to be further examined in HAI. In this study, we want to compare different nonverbal behaviors that theoretically relate to dominance. Therefore, we hypothesize that those behaviors that are widely used as or seen as dominant behaviors will be evaluated as more dominant compared to those behaviors widely used as or seen as submissive gestures (**H1**). And we further ask which behaviors are the most dominant and submissive ones (**RQ1**).

3   Cooperative Nonverbal Behavior

Even more than dominance, cooperative behavior is necessary in HAI, since many systems are designed to solve tasks in cooperation with the user. Humans are social animals and are cooperative by nature [20]. However, it is risky to cooperate with individuals, who do not set value on reciprocity. Thus, humans are able to detect nonverbal cues signaling commitment to cooperate [21]. A sender of (nonverbal) communication is able to express cooperative intent that the receiver can identify [22]. A cooperative personality in this sense is related to honesty, trustworthiness and reliability. One such signal of cooperativity seems to be expressivity. Schug et al. [23] showed that people, who are more cooperative, showed more expressive facial displays and that these expressions are not limited to positive ones. Other findings suggest that cooperativity is affected by the context of the interaction [24] and by the actual displayed nonverbal behavior (e.g. cooperation was increased, when individuals displayed happiness, while this was not the case for negative displays [25]). Although emotional expressivity seems to have an overall great influence on the perception of cooperativity, it is not proven whether this effect is limited to facial displays or can be expanded to gestures. Besides expressivity in general, there are some specific nonverbal behaviors believed to be cooperative signals such as lateral head-tilt. An initial study showed that individuals showing right head-tilts were evaluated more trustworthy than individuals showing left head-tilts or no head tilts [26]. Moreover, eye-gaze is a key-factor in theory of mind processes and can indicate the other individuals' believes [27] and thus increase cooperation. However, a straight gaze is also correlated to dominance [28]. Hence, the precise effect of gaze behavior on cooperativity and dominance in HAI has to be further examined. Although there are only limited studies examining the perception of virtual agents with regard to cooperativity, there is work on this topic in the field of human-robot interaction. The results by Stanton and Stevens [29] support the assumption that eye-gaze increases cooperation: a robot's gaze influenced ratings on trust (which is highly correlated to cooperativity) and participants' readiness to respond verbally. Counterintuitive results by Riek et al. [30] showed that humans cooperate more with robots that showed abrupt gestures than with those whose gestures were fluent. This demonstrates that (i) there is a general lack of systematic research on cooperativity expressed by nonverbal behavior and (ii) that expectations differ in HHI and HAI and therefore nonverbal cues can be interpreted differently. Some of the nonverbal cues that theoretically evoke a cooperative perception are also related to dominance (e.g. gaze and expressive gestures). Therefore, we strive to examine the interplay of dominance and cooperativity regarding these gestures. Based on these considerations, we hypothesize that those behaviors that are widely used as or seen as cooperative nonverbal behavior will be evaluated as more cooperative than those behaviors that are widely used as or seen as non-cooperative behavior (**H2**). Moreover, the evaluation of cooperativity correlates with the evaluation of dominance (**H3**). Further on, we ask what kind of nonverbal behaviors are perceived as signaling most cooperation (**RQ2**).

4   Method

4.1   Experimental Design and Independent Variables

In order to evaluate different gestures, we conducted an online study with a mixed factorial design. We tested four different categories of nonverbal behavior: dominant, submissive, cooperative and non-cooperative nonverbal behavior. We created eight behaviors for the dominance perception (4 *dominant* vs. 4 *submissive*) and 14 behaviors for the cooperativity perception (7 *cooperative* vs. 7 *non-cooperative*). Each behavior was shown while the agent said one out of seven sentences, which had an equal length and were all in the context of daily life support (e.g. "You are running out of milk and bread. Do you want to go shopping today?" or "The weather is fine and you don't have any appointments. Do you want to go out for a walk?"). Most of the behaviors were created using motion capturing with a post processing of bones, gaze and hand shape and were mapped on the embodied conversational agent *Billy (Social Cognitive System Group, Citec Bielefeld Germany)* while some behaviors were created with a key-frame editor. The virtual agent Billie is humanoid, male, more childish-looking and has a medium degree of realism (between cartoon and foto-realistic) (sf. Fig. 1). The four categories of nonverbal behavior were tested in a between-subjects design, while the different behaviors have been evaluated by repeated measures. Within one category of nonverbal behavior we created three video sets to avoid position effects. In these sets the position of the video and the combined sentence that was spoken during the gesture were pseudo-randomized (3 sets with different orders of gesture and sentence were conducted for each condition). During the online experiment participants saw a sequence of videos and rated the agent directly after each video. First, they were presented with a control video showing the agent with no nonverbal behavior and always the same opening sentence. Then participants saw additionally to the control video (in dependence of the experimental condition) four or seven videos with a combination of nonverbal behavior and sentence. Participants rated the agent directly after each video. In the last video the agent displayed one of the behaviors combined with a closing sentence ("Could you imagine that I support you in your everyday life?"), which also served as a behavioral measurement. In total we used 79 videos (1 control video, 66 behaviors & sentence combinations, 12 combinations of nonverbal behavior and behavioral question) in the survey. The videos have an average length of 8.55 s with a range from 7 s to 10 s.

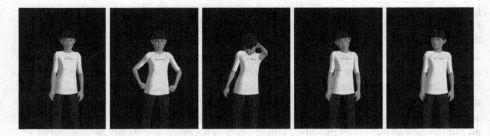

Fig. 1. Examples of the virtual agent Billie showing non-verbal behavior (control: no behavior, dominant: akimbo, submissive: neck-adaptor, cooperative: lateral flexion right and non-cooperative: gaze aversion)

4.2   Choice of Behaviors

Dominant and Submissive Behaviors. Most self-touches seem to be perceived as submissive, while there is also an emblem type of self-touch that seems to evoke a dominant perception. Thus, we examine the effect of previously used behaviors that are seen to be dominant (akimbo posture, [4, 5]) or submissive (touching neck and turning head down, [5]), respectively. Moreover, we created a closed arm gesture (crossing arms in front of his breast) as dominant gesture and an open arm gesture that seems to evoke a submissive perception. Further on, the position of the head seems to have an influence on the perception of dominance [e.g. 14]. Therefore, we investigate the effect of sagittal head tiles: turning the head up and turning the head down. Since taking up more space seems to be perceived as dominant [17], we test the range of the gesture. Therefore, a wide arm gesture with large radius and a small arm gesture with a small radius were created.

Dominant: akimbo posture, crossing arms, sagittal head up, large radius.
Submissive: neck-adaptor, arms open, sagittal head down, small radius.

Cooperative Behaviors. As mentioned above, the agent's gaze behavior seems to have an influence on its cooperativity evaluation [29]. Due to these findings, we investigate this effect in more detail with two different gaze behaviors: the agent turns his gaze towards the user vs. the agent averts his gaze from the user. Expressivity is highly related to cooperativity [23, 31]. Because smile as facial expression seems to have a main effect on the cooperativity perception, we took smile as facial expression into account. While the agent shows a big open smile with raised eye brows and open eyes in the cooperative condition, he expressed only a gentle smile without any eye movements in the non-cooperative condition. Most research concentrated on the effect of facial expressivity [e.g. 23, 25], while the effect of expressive gestures has not been examined. Therefore we created gestures with different degrees of expressivity. In the cooperative condition the agent shows many gestures with his arms while he says the sentence and in the non-cooperative condition fewer gestures with his arms are shown. To explore the effect of expressivity on cooperativity perception in more detail, we also tested the combination of expressive gesture and expressive facial expression. In order to imitate human behavior as best as possible, the movements of technical entities have to be fluent. While most developments concentrate on fluent movements, surprisingly, first results indicate that a more abrupt nonverbal behavior seems to be perceived as more cooperative [30]. In order to explore this effect in more detail, we created a fluent gesture with the agent's arms and created the same gesture with an abrupt performance. Beside gaze and expressivity a lateral head tilt seems to evoke a cooperative perception of the agent [26]. Until now only little is known about the particular effect of lateral head tilt (e.g.: Which side seems to evoke a stronger cooperativity evaluation? Does the position of the chin have an influence on the cooperativity evaluation?). Therefore we examine the effect of different types of a lateral head-tilt: Lateral head-tilt to the right side, lateral head-tilt to the left side vs. lateral head-tilt to the right side with a chin rotation and lateral head-tilt to the left side with a chin rotation.

Cooperative: gaze toward, expressive gesture, expressive mimic, expressive gesture and mimic, abrupt gesture, lateral flexion left, lateral flexion right.
Non-cooperative: avert one's gaze, non-expressive gesture, non-expressive mimic, non-expressive gesture and mimic, fluent gesture, lateral flexion chin left, lateral flexion chin right.

Additionally, all gestures were compared to a control gesture, where the agent does not show any nonverbal behavior. Example videos of the used nonverbal behavior can be found at the supplemented material.

4.3   Dependent Variables

Person perception of the agent was assessed using an ad-hoc scale with 14 items rated on a 5-pointed Likert Scale (1 = "strongly disagree" to 5 "strongly agree"). The scale contained general aspects like likability, warmth, but also specific items related to dominance and cooperativity. The ratings of each video of all participants (number of videos $n = 1134$, independent of the stimulus condition) were used in a factor analysis according to Horn [32] to expose underlying latent variables behind the 14 items. During parallel analysis those factors were identified whose empirical eigenvalues were higher than the eigenvalues that can be expected to be obtained from completely random data. Results suggested the extraction of three factors, which was the number of components that were retained in the final analysis. Principal component analysis (PCA) with promax rotation showed satisfying factor loadings ($>.400$; [c.f. 33]) for all variables and no cross loading of any variable. Thus, the three resulting factors of the PCA are:

1. *cooperative* (Cronbach's $\alpha = .941$; kind, likeable, open-minded, pleasant, trustworthy, I would ask the assistant for advice, I would work together with the assistant, The assistant might be able to help me, The assistant responds to me) '
2. *dominant* (Cronbach's $\alpha = .838$; dominant, decisive and assertive)
3. *submissive* (Cronbach's $\alpha = .608$; submissive and reserved).

General rules suggest using subscales with Cronbach's alphas of at least .70. However, Cortina [34] discussed that a low number of items can artificially deflate alpha values. Thus, we decided to use also the factor submissive for further analyses, especially because the factor is a key concept with regard to the research question.

Since the overall setting of this study was the application of the agent as personal assistant for everyday-life support, an additional single item scale "Would you want me to support you in your everyday life?" was rated on a 5-pointed Likert Scale (1 = "strongly disagree" to 5 "strongly agree"). This item is assumed to be a behavioral measurement, in order to investigate whether participants prefer a dominant, submissive, cooperative or non-cooperative perceived agent to assist them in daily-life.

4.4   Participants and Procedure

A total of 222 subjects completed the online study. 32 stated technical difficulties with the videos, which is why those subjects were excluded. All further calculations were made with 190 participants (119 female, 69 male, 2 did not want to state their gender). Participants were equally distributed to the four conditions (dominant $n = 50$, submissive $n = 48$, cooperative $n = 43$, non-cooperative $n = 49$). On average participants were 26 years old ($M = 26.28$, $SD = 9.79$) and the age ranged from 16 to 78 years. After a first introduction participants stated their age and gender. Before they watched the first video, subjects were instructed to turn on the sound of their computers and to watch the following videos carefully. After that, the videos were presented. Participants were not able to turn to the next page until the whole video was shown. After they had seen the video, they were asked to evaluate the agent on the above presented scale. At the end of the questionnaire participants were debriefed and had the chance to take part in a raffle of gift cards from an online handler.

5   Results

5.1   Moderating Variables

In order to ensure that the evaluation of the agent's person perception is caused by the nonverbal gestures, analyses of age and gender effects were made. Therefore, three linear regression analyses with age on the person perception factors cooperative, dominant and submissive were calculated. Regression analyses revealed no significant effect of age on the agent's person perception. In addition, a MANOVA with gender as independent variable and person perception factors as dependent variables was conducted. Men and women did not significantly differ in their ratings on the factors cooperative and dominant, but they differed with regard to the factor submissive, $F(2,187) = 3.91$, $p = .022$, $\eta2 = .04$. Men ($M = 3.14$, $SD = .91$) evaluated the agent significantly more submissive than women ($M = 2.77$, $SD = .87$). A Chi Square test showed that gender was equally distributed between the 12 different conditions and no significant differences in gender between those groups were found. Thus, the effect of gender on the submissive evaluation does not affect further calculations.

5.2   Comparison of Gestures Within the Conditions

To explore the effects of the different gestures within the four conditions, we conducted multiple repeated measures ANOVA's, with the single gesture as independent variable and the person perception factors (cooperative, dominant, submissive) as dependent variables. Each of the four conditions was analyzed separately. The dominant gestures do differ within their evaluation of dominance, $F(4, 49) = 16.83$, $p < .001$, $\eta2 = .26$. While the control gesture and keeping the head up is less dominant than the akimbo posture and having the arms crossed, the akimbo posture was evaluated as more dominant than executing a gesture with a large radius. A second repeated measures ANOVA revealed a significant difference in submissive evaluation between all five gestures, $F(4, 49) = 15.41$, $p < .001$, $\eta2 = .24$. Bonferroni post-hoc tests showed that the control gesture had been evaluated significantly more submissive than the akimbo posture, crossing the arms in front of the breast and doing a gesture with a large radius. The akimbo posture was perceived as significant less submissive compared to keeping the head up and a gesture with a large radius. In the same way, crossing the arms in front of the breast was less submissive in comparison to keeping the head up. With regard to cooperativity perception significant differences between the dominant gestures were observed, $F(4, 49) = 18.90$, $p < .001$, $\eta2 = .28$. The gestures head up and large radius was evaluated significant more cooperative than all other gestures, but do not differ from each other. Further on, the control gesture was evaluated as more cooperative than crossing the arms (Table 1).

Comparing the submissive gestures, significant differences regarding the evaluation of dominance were found, $F(4, 188) = 7.62$, $p < .001$, $\eta2 = .14$. The neck-adaptor was perceived as least dominant and differs significantly from the other four gestures. Referring to the submissive evaluation, significant differences between the submissive gestures were found, $F(3.41, 160.17) = 8.99$, $p < .001$, $\eta2 = .16$. In contrast to the

Table 1. Means and standard deviations of dependent variables (dominant gestures)

Gesture	Dominant		Submissive		Cooperative	
	M	SD	M	SD	M	SD
Control	2.36	.87	2.91	.90	2.55	.82
Akimbo posture	3.43	1.04	1.81	.95	2.54	.83
Crossing arms	3.09	1.09	2.03	1.06	2.28	.84
Sagittal head up	2.50	.89	2.55	.944	3.10	.79
Large radius	2.61	.93	2.37	1.04	3.04	.86

evaluation of dominance, the neck-adaptor was perceived as more submissive compared to keeping the arms open, moving the head down and doing a gesture with a small radius. Comparing the submissive gestures, significant differences in their cooperativity evaluations appeared, $F(3.34, 157.19) = 8.01$, $p < .001$, $\eta2 = .15$. Post-hoc test using Bonferroni showed that the control gesture is less cooperative than speaking with open arms and doing arm movements with a small radius. Further on, neck-adaptor was also rated as less cooperative compared to the gesture with a small radius (Table 2).

Table 2. Means and standard deviations of dependent variables (submissive gestures)

Gesture	Dominant		Submissive		Cooperative	
	M	SD	M	SD	M	SD
Control	2.36	.87	2.91	.90	2.55	.82
Open arms	2.41	.89	2.55	.79	2.85	.83
Neck-adaptor	1.92	.96	3.31	1.24	2.58	.82
Sagittal head down	2.65	1.00	2.49	.90	2.63	.77
Small radius	2.38	.79	2.47	.81	2.91	.90

In order to compare the cooperative gestures, further repeated measures ANOVA's were calculated. Results showed no significant differences between all eight gestures of the cooperative gesture in dominance evaluation, while the gestures do differ with regard to submissive ratings, $F(7, 294) = 3.37$, $p = .002$, $\eta2 = .07$. Post-hoc analysis indicate that the perception of the control gesture were significant more submissive than turning the gaze toward the user, doing an expressive gesture and doing an expressive gesture combined with an expressive mimic. The cooperative gestures also differ significantly in cooperativity ratings, $F(5.25, 220.686) = 5.65$, $p < .001$, $\eta2 = .12$. Participants evaluated the control gesture significantly less cooperative than an expressive gesture combined with an expressive mimic and both lateral head-tilts regardless of the side. Further on, turning the head toward the user was also rated as less cooperative compared to a lateral head-tilt to the left side (Table 3).

Within the last experimental condition no significant differences in dominance and submissive evaluation were obtainable, while the non-cooperative gestures do differ significantly in cooperativity ratings, $F(5.12, 245.73) = 9.32$, $p < .001$, $\eta2 = .16$. Compared to the control gesture a non-expressive gesture, non-expressive mimic, the combination of non-expressive gesture and mimic, a fluent gesture and a lateral head-tilt with a chin rotation to the left as well as to the right side were evaluated as more

Table 3. Means and standard deviations of dependent variables (cooperative gestures)

Gesture	Dominant		Submissive		Cooperative	
	M	SD	M	SD	M	SD
Control	2.36	.87	2.91	.90	2.55	.82
Gaze toward	2.65	.93	2.49	.83	2.69	1.04
Expressive gesture	2.64	.83	2.40	.65	2.96	.98
Expressive mimic	2.49	.84	2.42	.79	2.92	1.06
Expressive gesture and mimic	2.40	.77	2.55	.75	3.09	1.12
Abrupt gesture	2.57	.82	2.55	.78	2.87	.99
Lateral flexion left	2.33	.72	2.52	.84	3.07	1.02
Lateral flexion right	2.41	.73	2.55	.69	3.02	1.06

cooperative. Further on, participants perceived averting one's gaze as less cooperative in comparison with a non-expressive gesture, a non-expressive mimic, a fluent gesture and a lateral head-tilt with a chin rotation to both sides (Table 4).

Table 4. Means and standard deviations of dependent variables (non-cooperative gestures)

Gesture	Dominant		Submissive		Cooperative	
	M	SD	M	SD	M	SD
Control	2.36	.87	2.91	.90	2.55	.82
Avert one's gaze	2.63	.92	2.42	.81	2.56	.83
Non-expressive gesture	2.67	.90	2.61	.98	2.95	.85
Non-expressive mimic	2.43	.92	2.63	.79	2.94	.88
Non-expressive gesture and mimic	2.44	.88	2.51	.84	3.09	.86
Fluent gesture	2.42	.99	2.51	.84	3.03	.90
Lateral flexion chin left	2.60	.92	2.42	.79	2.94	.79
Lateral flexion chin right	2.50	.95	2.48	.79	3.01	.91

5.3 Comparison of Gestures Between the Conditions

Since we assume differences between gestures of different experimental conditions, a MANOVA with experimental condition as independent variable and the three factors of person perception as dependent variable was conducted. Results did not reveal a significant main effect of experimental condition. Since earlier analyses yielded significant differences of the gestures within the experimental groups, further analyses, concentrating on the gestures with highest ratings, were made. Therefore, only the gestures akimbo, neck-adaptor, expressive gesture and mimic and the control gesture were compared. A second MANOVA revealed a significant main effects for dominance, $F(3, 189) = 22.92$, $p < .001$, $\eta2 = .27$, submissive, $F(3, 189) = 82.18$, $p < .001$, $\eta2 = .26$, and cooperativity, $F(3, 189) = 4.00$, $p = .009$, $\eta2 = .06$. Post-hoc analyses showed significant differences between the akimbo posture and all other three gestures with regard to dominance evaluation. Further on, the dominant gesture was perceived as less submissive than the submissive, cooperative and non-cooperative gesture, while the perception of the neck-adaptor was more submissive than the cooperative gesture. With regard to cooperativity the combination of expressive gesture and mimic was rated as more cooperative than the dominant, submissive and non-cooperative gesture. In order to investigate whether the different gestures have an effect on the participants' willingness to use the presented agent as virtual assistant, a two-factorial ANOVA with the behavioral question as dependent variable and set as well as experimental condition as independent variables was conducted. No significant differences were obtainable. In hypothesis H3 we assume a correlation of cooperativity evaluation with dominance ratings. The results of a one-sided Pearson correlation indicate that cooperativity is significantly related to dominance, $r = .17$, $p = .011$.

6   Discussion

With regard to a successful human-agent-interaction, knowledge about the perception of virtual agent nonverbal behavior is of great importance. Overall, our research aims to design a virtual agent that will be perceived as cooperative, in order to enhance the human-agent-interaction. On the other hand in situations, where the agent has to be persuasive, it is necessary to evoke dominance. Therefore, we concentrate on the effect of nonverbal behavior on the agent's person perception. In an online study we evaluated different nonverbal behaviors that are theoretically related to dominance and cooperativity. When the different conditions with their entire spectrum were compared, our results did not support the hypotheses **H1** and **H2**. But with regard to both research questions (**RQ1 & RQ2**) the gestures within the groups differ from each other. Considering only the gestures with strongest effects, significant differences in person perception showed up. Therefore it is possible to evoke dominance and cooperativity, but careful decisions about the selected nonverbal behavior have to be made. With regard to dominance perception, having the arms crossed and the akimbo position are the most affective gestures. Taking up more space by executing a gesture with large radius was not perceived as more dominant than the other gestures. One possible explanation might be that the agent does not share the same physical space with the user, therefore the effect of taking up space, in order to signal power, is not as effective in human-agent-interaction as it can be in human face-to-face interaction. However, we found a tendency that the gesture with the large radius was perceived as more dominant than the one with the smaller radius. Regarding also prior findings [e.g. 14, 15], an effect of the gesture's spatial parameter can be assumed although this was not significant in our work which might be due to the within-subjects design. Hence, the strong symbolic behaviors such as akimbo or crossing the arms might have undermined the effect of the maybe subtler nature of the spatial dimension of behaviors.

Although various findings support the effect of sagittal head-tilts [6, 14], no significant differences in dominance were found. In contrast to previous findings, the upward head-tilt was perceived as more cooperative. Here, a limitation of the current setup might be responsible: Since the gestures have been tested in an online-study, the height of the screen in relation to the users eyes could not be controlled, while this was the case in the previous research [6]. Thus, in some cases the agent was presented below the eyes of the users, which might have led to the impression that the agent was looking at them, when he turns his head upward.

Moreover, self-touch with the hand in the neck and the gaze downward, evokes the most submissive perception and differs significantly from the other gestures. Since the most effective gestures (arms crossed, akimbo and neck-adaptor) are all emblems, a symbolic gesture seems to be the most effective one, with regard to dominance perception.

Findings for cooperativity, support the theoretical assumption [23, 31] that expressivity is related to cooperativity. While no differences between expressive gesture and expressive facial display could be shown, the combination of both was perceived as most cooperative. Similar to prior research [26], the lateral head-tilt did have an effect on perceived cooperativity, but no differences between the different head-tilt versions have been found. Thus, a lateral head-tilt regardless of the side or position of the chin, leads to a higher cooperativity perception. The gaze behavior seems to have an effect on cooperativity, because averting one's gaze was perceived significantly less cooperative. While the combination of expressive gesture and mimic was perceived as most cooperative, showing no gesture showed the lowest cooperativity values. Thus, expressivity evokes the strongest effect on cooperativity. In line with the assumption that cooperative and dominant behavior is related (**H3**), a significant correlation was found. However the effect was quite small, which might be explained by the diversity of the different behaviors and the strong effects of the symbolic gestures. In future studies the correlation of a dominant and a cooperative perception should be investigated by using only subtle behaviors like gaze or head movements.

Since only one kind of agent appearance was used in this study, the results are limited to humanoid characters and no generalization for agents with a different appearance can be made. Most of the nonverbal behavior was deduced from HHI, therefore it is important to investigate the effect of perceived human-likeness on the perception of those behaviors.

Our findings emphasize the effect of nonverbal gestures on the agent's person perception. Based on this systematical research, implications for the modeling of the agent's nonverbal behavior can be made. In order to investigate the effect of dominant, submissive, cooperative and non-cooperative gestures within specific contexts, further research has to be conducted. The gestures evoking the strongest effects in person perception, has to be tested in a realistic human-agent-interaction. Further on, the effect of those gestures on the user's behavior has to be investigated. Therefore, as a next step an interaction study will be conducted, in order to measure the persuasive effects of the dominant and submissive gestures. Since dominant behavior is known to be perceived as persuasive [1], an virtual agent showing dominant nonverbal behavior is assumed to evoke higher effects of persuasion. Similar research has to be done, in order to examine the effect of cooperative nonverbal behavior on the user's intention to cooperate in human-agent-interaction.

Acknowledgements. The KOMPASS (Socially cooperative, virtual assistants as companions for people in need of cognitive support) project was funded by the German Federal Ministry of Education and Research.

References

1. Burgoon, J.K., Birk, T., Pfau, M.: Nonverbal behaviors, persuasion, and credibility. Hum. Commun. Res. **17**, 140–169 (1990)
2. Burgoon, J.K., Guerrero, L.K., Manusov, V.: Nonverbal signals. In: Knapp, M.L., Daly, J.A. (eds.) Handbook of Interpersonal Communication, 4th edn., pp. 239–280. Sage, Thousand Oaks (2012)
3. Givens, D.B.: The nonverbal dictionary of Gestures, Signs and Body Language Cues. Center for Nonverbal Studies Press, Spokane (2002)
4. Ball, G., Breese, J.: Relating personality and behavior: posture and gestures. In: Paiva, A.C. (ed.) IWAI 1999. LNCS, vol. 1814, pp. 196–203. Springer, Heidelberg (2000)
5. Richardson, R., Devereux, D., Burt, J., Nutter, P.: Humanoid upper torso complexity for displaying gestures. Int. J. Adv. Robot. Syst. **9**, 1–9 (2012)
6. Mignault, A., Chaudhuri, A.: The many faces of a neutral face: head tilt and perception of dominance and emotion. J. Nonverbal Behav. **27**, 111–132 (2003)
7. Cashdan, E.: Smiles, speech, and body posture: how women and men display sociometric status and power. J. Nonverbal Behav. **22**, 209–229 (1998)
8. Argyle, M.: Bodily Communication, 2nd edn. Methuen, New York (1988)
9. Gurtman, M.B.: Exploring personality with the interpersonal circumplex. Soc. Personal. Psychol. Compass. **3**, 601–619 (2009)
10. Carney, D.R., Hall, J.A., LeBeau, L.S.: Beliefs about the nonverbal expression of social power. J. Nonverbal Behav. **29**, 105–123 (2005)
11. Neff, M., Toothman, N., Bowmani, R., Fox Tree, J.E., Walker, M.A.: Don't scratch! Self-adaptors reflect emotional stability. In: Vilhjálmsson, H.H., Kopp, S., Marsella, S., Thórisson, K.R. (eds.) IVA 2011. LNCS, vol. 6895, pp. 398–411. Springer, Heidelberg (2011)
12. Harrigan, J.A., Kues, J.R., Steffen, J.J., Rosenthal, R.: Self-touching and impressions of others. Personal. Soc. Psychol. Bull. **13**, 497–512 (1987)
13. Krämer, N.C., Simons, N., Kopp, S.: The effects of an embodied conversational agent's nonverbal behavior on user's evaluation and behavioral mimicry. In: Pelachaud, C., Martin, J.-C., André, E., Chollet, G., Karpouzis, K., Pelé, D. (eds.) IVA 2007. LNCS (LNAI), vol. 4722, pp. 238–251. Springer, Heidelberg (2007)
14. Lance, B., Marsella, S.C.: Emotionally expressive head and body movement during gaze shifts. In: Pelachaud, C., Martin, J.-C., André, E., Chollet, G., Karpouzis, K., Pelé, D. (eds.) IVA 2007. LNCS (LNAI), vol. 4722, pp. 72–85. Springer, Heidelberg (2007)
15. Ravenet, B., Ochs, M., Pelachaud, C.: From a user-created corpus of virtual agent's nonverbal behavior to a computational model of interpersonal attitudes. In: Aylett, R., Krenn, B., Pelachaud, C., Shimodaira, H. (eds.) IVA 2013. LNCS, vol. 8108, pp. 263–274. Springer, Heidelberg (2013)
16. Remland, M.S.: The implicit ad hominem fallacy: nonverbal displays of status in argumentative discourse. J. Am. Forensics Assoc. **19**, 79–86 (1980)
17. Burgoon, J.K., Dunbar, N.E.: Nonverbal expressions of dominance and power in human relationships. In: Manusov, V., Patterson, M.L. (eds.) The Sage Handbook of Nonverbal Communication, pp. 279–298. SAGE Publications Inc., Thousand Oaks (2006)
18. Callejas, Z., Ravenet, B., Ochs, M., Pelachaud, C.: A computational model of social attitudes for a virtual recruiter. In: Proceedings of the 2014 International Conference on Autonomous Agents and Multi-agent Systems, pp. 93–100 (2014)
19. Gebhard, P., Baur, T., Damian, I.: Exploring interaction strategies for virtual characters to induce stress in simulated job interviews. In: Proceedings of the 13th International Conference on Autonomous Agents and Multi-agent Systems (AAMAS 2014), pp. 661–668 (2014)

20. Tomasello, M.: The ultra-social animal. Eur. J. Soc. Psychol. **44**, 187–194 (2014)
21. Brown, W.M., Moore, C.: Smile asymmetries and reputation as reliable indicators of likelihood to cooperate: an evolutionary analysis BT. In: Shohov, S.P. (ed.) Advances in Psychology Research, vol. 11, pp. 59–78. Nova Science Publishers, Huntington (2002)
22. Reed, L.I., Zeglen, K.N., Schmidt, K.L.: Facial expressions as honest signals of cooperative intent in a one-shot anonymous Prisoner' s Dilemma game. Evol. Hum. Behav. **33**, 200–209 (2012)
23. Schug, J., Matsumoto, D., Horita, Y., Yamagishi, T., Bonnet, K.: Emotional expressivity as a signal of cooperation. Evol. Hum. Behav. **31**, 87–94 (2010)
24. De Melo, C.M., Carnevale, P., Gratch, J.: The impact of emotion displays in embodied agents on emergence of cooperation with people. Presence Teleoper. Virtual Environ. **20**, 449–465 (2011)
25. Stouten, J., De Cremer, D.: "Seeing is Believing": the effects of facial expressions of emotion and verbal communication in social dilemmas. J. Decis. Mak. **23**, 271–287 (2010)
26. Krumhuber, E., Manstead, A.S.R., Kappas, A.: Temporal aspects of facial displays in person and expression perception: the effects of smile dynamics, head-tilt, and gender. J. Nonverbal Behav. **31**, 39–56 (2006)
27. Kurzban, R.: The social psychophysics of cooperation: nonverbal communication in a public good game. J. Nonverbal Behav. **25**, 241–259 (2001)
28. Adams, R.B.J., Kleck, R.E.: Effects of direct and averted gaze on the perception of facially communicated emotion. Emotion **5**, 3–11 (2005)
29. Stanton, C., Stevens, C.J.: Robot pressure: the impact of robot eye gaze and lifelike bodily movements upon decision-making and trust. In: Beetz, M., Johnston, B., Williams, M.-A. (eds.) ICSR 2014. LNCS, vol. 8755, pp. 330–339. Springer, Heidelberg (2014)
30. Riek, L.D., Rabinowitch, T.-C., Bremner, P., Pipe, A.G., Fraser, M., Robinson, P.: Cooperative gestures: effective signaling for humanoid robots. In: 2010 5th ACM/IEEE International Conference on Human-Robot Interaction (HRI), pp. 61–68 (2010)
31. Krumhuber, E., Manstead, A.S.R., Cosker, D., Marshall, D., Rosin, P.L., Kappas, A.: Facial dynamics as indicators of trustworthiness and cooperative behavior. Emotion **7**, 730–735 (2007)
32. Horn, J.L.: A rationale and test for the number of factors in factor analysis. Psychometrika **30**, 179–185 (1965)
33. Velicer, W.F., Peacock, A.C., Jackson, D.N.: A comparison of component and factor patterns: a monte carlo approach. Multivar. Behav. Res. **17**, 371–388 (1982)
34. Cortina, J.M.: What is coefficient alpha? An examination of theory and applications. J. Appl. Psychol. **78**, 98–104 (1993)

Increasing Engagement with Virtual Agents Using Automatic Camera Motion

Lazlo Ring$^{(\boxtimes)}$, Dina Utami$^{(\boxtimes)}$, Stefan Olafsson$^{(\boxtimes)}$,
and Timothy Bickmore$^{(\boxtimes)}$

College of Computer and Information Science,
Northeastern University, Boston, MA, USA
{lring, dinau, stefanolafs, bickmore}@ccs.neu.edu

Abstract. We describe a series of algorithms which automatically control camera position in a virtual environment while a user is engaged in a simulated face-to-face dialog with a single virtual agent. The common objective of the algorithms is to increase user engagement with the interaction. In our work, we describe three different automated camera control systems that: (1) control the camera's position based on topic changes in dialog; (2) use sentiment analysis to control the camera-to-agent distance; and (3) adjust the camera's depth-of-field based on "important" segments of the dialog. Evaluation studies of each method are described. We find that changing camera position based on topic shifts results in significant increases in a self-reported measure of engagement, while the other methods seem to actually decrease user engagement. Interpretations and ramifications of the results are discussed.

Keywords: Relational agent · Cinematography · Natural language understanding

1 Introduction

As we develop agent-based interfaces for education, healthcare, and entertainment, maintaining user engagement represents a growing area of concern [1]. While there has been some effort to increase engagement through the manipulation of an agent's dialog, little work has been done to explore how agents can keep a user engaged without authoring major extensions to the dialog content of the system. Many agent applications require designing voluntary-use systems for long-term interaction, or maintaining the sustained attention of the user, such as automatic health behavior change systems or life-long learning companions [2]. Maintaining engagement with the user can be crucial for these systems to succeed, since engagement is often a prerequisite for other system objectives: if a user stops interacting with a system, then it cannot have any further impact.

While some researchers have explored the use of superficial variability in linguistic choice to increase user engagement [3], or the use of agent backstories [4], storytelling [5], or appropriate agent listening (backchannel) behaviors [6], these changes require significant work on the part of developers and content writers. We believe that the field

© Springer International Publishing AG 2016
D. Traum et al. (Eds.): IVA 2016, LNAI 10011, pp. 29–39, 2016.
DOI: 10.1007/978-3-319-47665-0_3

of Cinematography offers insights that can be automatically integrated into a virtual agent application to increase user engagement.

By drawing from cinematographic principles, an automated camera control system that automatically adjusts the user's view of the agent can be developed, based on linguistic analysis, in order to increase engagement. While prior research has explored the creation of such systems in the past [7], they have primarily focused on multi-agent interaction rather than creating engaging one-on-one conversations between a user and a single agent.

In this paper, we explore the design and creation of such a system, by developing and evaluating an automated camera system focused around maintaining user engagement in one-on-one conversations, independent of dialog content. Based upon cinematographic theory, the camera system uses natural language processing to automatically control the user's camera during a virtual conversation. We also evaluate various camera manipulation techniques through a series of sub-studies that explore their potential effects on user engagement.

2   Related Work

In this section we review prior work on automated camera control in 3D virtual environments, in particular for a single stationary actor in the scene.

De Melo and Paiva presented a model for automatic manipulation of the light and screen expression channels. The model integrates the OCC emotion model for emotion [8], expressively controls lights and shadows, and looks to visual arts techniques for layering and filtering to manipulate a virtual agent. Their main manipulation of the camera was using proxemics: either dollying or zooming in to increase drama [9].

Canini, et al., developed a model that could estimate camera-subject distance in film, using image processing and machine learning algorithms. The system performed with over 80 % accuracy and their results revealed that the director can impact the perceived affective response of the viewer, caused by alternating between close-up, medium, and long shots, with close-ups having the highest level of arousal. There was no connection between shot type and emotional valence [10].

Rui, et al., developed an automated videography system for lectures being broadcast to remote audiences, by coming up with rules for best practices to make videos visually engaging. The rules for camera positions included (1) camera placement and angle; (2) and cameras should be close to eye level. The rules for shot transitions included (1) reasonably frequent shot changes, (2) defining a minimum shot duration, (3) shot transitions should be motivated, and (4) transition when the speaker finishes a concept or thought [11].

Calahan describes various methods for lighting and other effects in computer graphics that have been found to enhance visual storytelling. Perspective and depth of field can be manipulated by changing the focal point or blurring particular planes in the scene, e.g. the background, which will emphasize the subject in the foreground, creating a greater sense of intimacy than one without blur [12].

3 Exploring Automatic Camera Control

Based on prior work, we designed a series of increasingly sophisticated methods for automatically controlling a camera while a user is engaged in a simulated face-to-face dialog with a single virtual agent. Our overarching goal was to develop methods that only required the text of the utterances that the agent will speak; we derived camera control parameters from linguistic analyses of the user-agent dialog script, the discourse history, and a description of the current virtual scene. We evaluated each of our methods in 3-treatment, between-subjects experiments where user engagement was the primary means measure of impact. Before describing each of the camera control methods and individual evaluation studies, we first describe the experimental methods that are common to all of them.

3.1 Common Study Methods

Each evaluation study was a between-subjects experiment with three treatments: the automated camera control algorithm being evaluated (AUTO); an equivalent agent interaction with no camera motion (STATIC); and a condition in which the same camera controls used in a representative run through the AUTO interaction were used, but deployed at random points in the dialog script (RANDOM).

In each study, participants interacted with a female virtual agent that spoke using synthetic speech and synchronized nonverbal conversational behavior automatically generated by BEAT [13] (Fig. 1). User inputs to the dialog were made via multiple choice inputs updated at each turn of the dialog.

The dialog script used for all studies comprised 6 turns of social chat, followed by 15 turns of "task talk", during which the agent attempted to persuade the user to get more exercise, followed by 18 turns of social chat, in which the user was given the ability to end the conversation at every turns.

The evaluation studies were all conducted on Amazon's Mechanical Turk (AMT). All participants were required to have a 75 % or higher approval rating on AMT, with the only additional requirement being that they had to use either Firefox or Chrome as their web browser. Participants who accepted the HIT from Mechanical Turk were asked to completed a socio-demographic and exercise attitude questionnaire, and then engage in a 5–10 min conversation with the agent.

Upon completing the interaction, participants were presented with a series of questionnaires assessing their level of engagement, motivation to exercise, and overall impression of the system.

3.2 Common Study Measures

Engagement was our primary outcome of interest, and we measured it using both self-report and behavioral methods.

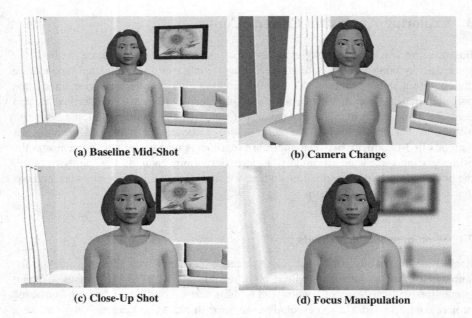

(a) Baseline Mid-Shot   (b) Camera Change

(c) Close-Up Shot   (d) Focus Manipulation

Fig. 1. Camera manipulations evaluated

We developed a 26-item composite scale self-report measure of engagement (Table 1). Items were included from several prior studies and measures [14, 15], forming a pool of 31 items. Following our first study with 284 participants (Sect. 4), we conducted a factor analysis and found that one factor explained 36.4 % of the variance, and we retained this one factor as our single measure of engagement, dropping 5 items. The final measure had adequate internal consistency, with Cronbach's alpha ranging from .961 to .969 across the three studies.

We also measured engagement behaviorally, by recording the total number of dialog turns which users conducted with the agent, including the 18 optional turns of social chat at the end of each interaction.

Finally, we wanted to determine if engagement could play a mediating role in the agent's ability to change user attitudes towards exercise, as a task outcome measure. We measured the user's exercise stage of change using a validated self-report instrument [16], along with two additional questions about motivation and confidence to exercise, i.e. "How motivated are you to exercise more than you are currently" and "How confident are you that you could exercise more if you wanted to," using single item measures, all administered at the beginning and end of each interaction.

Participants were also given the chance to write additional comments about the agent into a text box following their interaction.

4   Approach 1: Changing Camera on Topic Shift

Our initial approach to automating camera motion followed observations of common practice in newscasts and commercial videotaped lectures (see, for example: www.thegreatcourses.com), in which an occasional camera change is used to increase visual variety when a single character is speaking on camera for an extended length of time.

Table 1.   Engagement questionnaire

Question		Anchor 1	Anchor 7
The character's behavior was natural	I would like to interact with the character again	Disagree completely	Agree completely
I felt like I was talking face-to-face with a person	I had fun interacting with the character		
The character's behavior was comfortable	I enjoyed interacting with the character		
The character's motion was pleasant	I found the character was entertaining		
I could easily understand the character	I liked interacting with the character		
I felt comfortable interacting with the character	I was energized by my interaction with the character		
The character was engaging	I was alert during my conversation with the character		
The character was charismatic	I felt the conversation was too short		
The character was warm			
The character's behavior was repetitive	I felt awkward talking to the character	Agree completely	Disagree completely
The character was weird	I disliked interacting with the character		
The character was boring			
How friendly was the character?		Very unfriendly	Very friendly
How trustworthy was the character?		Very untrustworthy	Very trustworthy
How much do you like the character?		Not at all	Very much
How much do you feel that the character cares about you?		Not at all	Very much

We explored automatically changing camera position at topic boundaries in the agent's dialog, as prior studies have determined that a speaker's posture shifts are significantly more likely to occur during these transitions [17]. This is also supported by researchers in sociolinguistics who observed that changes in the spatial relationship between two speakers tended to occur at topic boundaries ("situational shifts") [18]. Topic boundary detection was performed automatically using the built-in mechanism in

BEAT [13] that relies primarily on the identification of discourse markers [19] in the agent's script (e.g., "well", "anyway", "so", etc.).

This camera controller was implemented by using two cameras, 75 degrees apart relative to the agent in the virtual environment, and alternating between them when a camera change was indicated. Immediately following a camera change, the agent would turn to face the current camera.

4.1   Camera Change Evaluation Results

We had 284 participants, 58.1 % male, between the ages of 18–69 (mean 34.8) participate in this study, with 102 randomized to the automatic camera condition (AUTO) condition, 88 to the random camera condition (RANDOM), and 94 to the static camera condition (STATIC).

A one-way ANOVA demonstrated that there were significant differences among study conditions on self-reported engagement, $F(2, 281) = 4.12$, $p < .05$, $D = .18$. Bonferroni post-hoc tests at the .05 significance level demonstrated that participants rated the AUTOMATIC condition as significantly more engaging than the other two conditions, and that there were no significant differences between the STATIC and RANDOM condition on engagement (Table 2).

Turn count data indicated that many participants completed either the minimum or the maximum number of turns possible, yielding a bimodal distribution. Non-parametric Kruskall-Wallis tests indicated no significant differences on turn count across the three study conditions, $p = .41$. There were also no significant differences in exercise stage, motivation, or confidence between the three study conditions. However, non-parametric bivariate correlations (Spearman's rho) indicated a significant positive correlation between the self-report measure of engagement and turn count, $rho = .213$, $p < .001$, increases in motivation to exercise, $rho = .195$, $p = .001$, and increases in exercise confidence, $rho = .163$, $p = .006$, indicating that there was some effect of engagement on these measures.

One of the items from our composite measure that we feel best captures the sense of naturalness of the interaction is "I felt like I was talking face-to-face with a person." Non-parametric tests on this item alone also demonstrated significant differences across conditions, Kruskal-Wallis, $p = .002$, with STATIC = 2.89, RANDOM = 3.38, and AUTO = 3.74.

Table 2. Outcomes for camera change study (mean (sd))

Measure	STATIC (N = 94)	RANDOM (N = 88)	AUTO (N = 102)	p
Self-report engagement	4.18 (1.25)	4.18 (1.14)	4.53 (1.08)	0.03*
Dialog turns	31.12 (6.5)	30.48 (6.4)	31.45 (6.8)	0.41
Exercise stage change	0.06 (0.38)	−0.02 (0.37)	−0.01 (0.4)	0.13
Exercise motivation change	0.22 (1.53)	−0.10 (0.92)	−0.15 (1.15)	0.06
Exercise confidence change	0.03 (1.17)	−0.06 (0.75)	−0.16 (1.02)	0.13

4.2 Camera Change Evaluation Discussion

We demonstrated that changing the camera at topic changes led to significant increases in self-reported engagement, compared to a single static camera or a camera changed at random times. There was some evidence that this positively impacted task outcome measures (exercise motivation and confidence).

5 Approach 2: Adding Sentiment-Based Camera Distance

Given our initial positive results, we attempted to increase the sophistication of our automated camera controller by investigating a mechanism for automatically adjusting the camera distance in addition to location. One of the other fundamental dimensions of camera control is the camera's distance to the agent, changing from "wide shots" to "extreme closeups" [20]. Camera distance has been investigated as a mechanism for partially indicating the "conversational frame" [21] in use by a virtual agent (e.g., shifting between "task talk", "social talk", and "empathy talk" [22]). However, changes in conversational frame are infrequent, and automatic identification of frame or genre can be error prone.

Inspired by Canini's work on automatic affect sensing in cinematography [10] we investigated the creation of a camera controller that bases the camera's distance according to the emotional intensity of each agent-utterance, with the view that more emotionally intense utterances would be better received by the user if accompanied by close-up shots of the agent.

To generate sentiment ratings for the agent's dialog, we used the Stanford CoreNLP Toolkit [23] to label each agent utterance with one of five sentiment scores (Very Negative, Negative, Neutral, Positive, Very Positive), along with a probability rating. Our sentiment-based camera controller used a close up shot for utterances tagged as Very Negative or Very Positive, and a mid-shot used for all other utterances. We then conducted an evaluation study combining topic-based camera change controller (as evaluated in Study 1) with the sentiment-based camera distance controller.

5.1 Sentiment-Based Camera Distance Results

We had 149 individuals, 56.4 % male, between the ages of 19–65 (mean 36.4) participate in Study 2. Of the 149 participants, 51 were randomized to the automatic camera condition (AUTO) condition, 44 to the random camera condition (RANDOM), and 54 to the static camera condition (STATIC).

In the second experiment, we found no significant differences on self-reported engagement by study condition, $F(2, 146) = 1.31$, $p = .27$ (STATIC: Mean = 4.61, SD = 0.88, RANDOM: Mean = 4.32, SD = 1.01, AUTO: Mean = 4.19, SD = 0.91). Trends in the data suggested that camera zoom had a negative impact on turn count, in which participants favored the static condition over the random and automatic camera conditions, Kurskal-Wallis, $p = .056$, with Means of STATIC (Mean = 34.3, SD = 7.25) > RANDOM (Mean = 32. 6, SD = 6.59) > AUTO (Mean = 31.9, SD = 6.69).

Non-parametric correlation between engagement and turn count remained significant (rho = .336, p < .001.), however there were no significant result found for attitude change.

5.2 Sentiment-Based Camera Distance Discussion

In this study we explored the use of a sentiment-based camera controller to improve user engagement. There were no significant effects of our automated camera control system on user engagement, although the trends suggested that the changes in camera motion may have actually lead to a more negative user experience. We found that the number of camera changes that occurred during the interaction was drastically higher than those found in study 1, with nearly 70 % of all dialog turns containing at least one change in camera motion. This frequency of change may have conflicted with some of the best practice rules found in cinematography, namely that an overabundance of shot type changes can give the illusion that the director is "bored" [20].

6 Approach 3: Automating Camera Focus

Based on the qualitative feedback received during Study 2, we designed a subtler and less frequent camera change to signal emotional intensity. Rather than the jarring change in camera distance, we signaled high emotional intensity by manipulating depth of field to heighten the agent's contrast with her background (Fig. 1d).

To reduce the frequency of these changes, we incorporated information about what parts of each topic or dialog segment represented the most "important" information. Relative importance of a given utterance is a function of the broader goals of a dialog (e.g., it could be the point of resolution in a narrative, the punch line to a joke, or the key message in a lecture). To simulate this, we manually added camera tags to the start, peak and end of each discourse segment. These tags allowed the camera system to automatically adjust the camera's distance and focus on the agent based on the various tags within each section. The closest distance and greatest focus occurred at the utterance tagged as the most important, with gradual transitions occurring into and out of this peak for at least two utterances on each side.

6.1 Camera Focus Results

We had 99 individuals, 51 % male, aged 19–74 (mean 38) participate in the evaluation of the Camera Focus controller, with 37 randomized to the automatic camera condition (AUTO) condition, 34 to the random camera condition (RANDOM), and 28 to the static camera condition (STATIC).

As with Study 2, no significant differences were found between study conditions on engagement, $F(2, 96) = .364$, $p = .696$ (STATIC: Mean = 4.38, SD = 1.25, RANDOM: Mean = 4.12, SD = 1.2, AUTO: Mean = 4.28, SD = 1.24). Similarly, there was also a trend suggesting that the changes in camera motion had a negative impact on turn count, Kruskal-Wallis, $p = 0.11$, with Means of STATIC (Mean = 32.18, SD = 6.77) > RANDOM (Mean = 30.06, SD = 6.47) > AUTO (Mean = 28.97, SD = 5.6). A non-parametric test for turn count differences between STATIC and AUTO found the same trend (Mann-Whitney $U = 363$, $p < .05$). The non-parametric correlations between self-reported engagement and other measures remained significant (for turn count: $rho = 0.20$, $p < .05$; for change in exercise motivation, $rho = 0.314$, $p = .002$; and for change in exercise confidence, $rho = 0.239$, $p < .05$.)

6.2 Camera Focus Discussion

Building upon our results from the previous two studies, we developed an automated camera controller that adjusted the cameras distance and level of focus in relation to the importance of dialog utterances. As with study 2, there was no significant correlation between automated camera control and user engagement, with results trending against the automated system. A qualitative analysis of user feedback suggested that even though camera motion was less frequent than that of study 2 (42 % of turns vs. 70 % of turns), the changes in camera proxemics was un-enjoyable.

7 Overall Discussion and Conclusion

In this paper we explored the creation of an automated camera system for conversational agent based systems. We explored the potential impact of three different automated camera systems, which adjusted camera position, proximity and focus, on user engagement and motivation. Our results demonstrated that automated camera motion, especially in relation to topic shifts, can have a positive impact on user engagement, while changes in proxemics and focus control trended towards having a negative effect. Additionally, we found a significant correlation between engagement, turn count, and the agent's persuasiveness.

This suggests the potential of an automated camera system for increasing user engagement and improving the effectiveness of agent-based systems. However, our studies demonstrated that randomly manipulating camera motion can have a negative impact on these metrics, and that any change in camera motion needs to be thoroughly studied before integration. Additionally, a large range of factors seem to contribute to the user's enjoyment of such systems, including motion speed, frequency of motion, and when the motion occurs in relation to the agent's utterances.

The results may be simply due to the fact that while a small amount of camera motion is important for users to maintain engagement with a single virtual agent, additional camera movement (of any kind) beyond a threshold becomes a distraction (Table 3).

Table 3. Comparison of three automatic controllers (mean (sd))

	Camera change	Sentiment/distance	Importance/focus
% turns with any camera change	11 %	70 %	42 %
Self-report engagement	4.53 (1.08)	4.19 (0.91)	4.28 (1.24)
Dialog turns	31.45 (6.8)	31.9 (6.69)	28.97 (5.6)

8 Limitations and Future Work

Although we explored three different types of camera manipulation within our study—position, distance, and focus—we did not explore sub-factors for each manipulation. As shown in the differences between study 2 and 3, minor changes in camera motion can greatly impact a participant's opinion of the system, suggesting that we should more thoroughly explore sub-factors such as the motion speed and overall frequency of camera motion. In future work, we plan to explore each of these sub-factors in a controlled environment and see how these effects persist in longitudinal interactions.

References

1. Lehmann, J., Lalmas, M., Yom-Tov, E., Dupret, G.: Models of user engagement. In: Masthoff, J., Mobasher, B., Desmarais, M.C., Nkambou, R. (eds.) UMAP 2012. LNCS, vol. 7379, pp. 164–175. Springer, Heidelberg (2012)
2. http://projects.ict.usc.edu/companion/
3. Bickmore, T., Schulman, D., Yin, L.: Maintaining engagement in long-term interventions with relational agents. Int. J. Appl. AI **24**, 648–666 (2010)
4. Bickmore, T., Schulman, D., Yin, L.: Engagement vs. deceit: virtual humans with human autobiographies. In: Ruttkay, Z., Kipp, M., Nijholt, A., Vilhjálmsson, H.H. (eds.) IVA 2009. LNCS, vol. 5773, pp. 6–19. Springer, Heidelberg (2009)
5. Battaglino, C., Bickmore, T.: Increasing engagement with conversational agents using co-constructed storytelling. In: INT8 workshop, Santa Cruz, CA (2015)
6. Smith, J.: GrandChair: conversational collection of grandparent's stories. MIT (2000)
7. Christie, M., Machap, R., Normand, J.-M., Olivier, P., Pickering, J.H.: Virtual camera planning: a survey. In: Butz, A., Fisher, B., Krüger, A., Olivier, P. (eds.) SG 2005. LNCS, vol. 3638, pp. 40–52. Springer, Heidelberg (2005)
8. Ortony, A., Clore, G., Collins, A.: The Cognitive Structure of Emotions. Cambridge University Press, Cambridge (1988)
9. de Melo, C., Paiva, A.C.: Expression of emotions in virtual humans using lights, shadows, composition and filters. In: Paiva, A.C., Prada, R., Picard, R.W. (eds.) ACII 2007. LNCS, vol. 4738, pp. 546–557. Springer, Heidelberg (2007)
10. Canini, L., Benini, S., Leonardi, R.: Affective analysis on patterns of shot types in movies. In: 7th International Symposium on Image and Signal Processing and Analysis (ISPA), pp. 253–258 (2011)
11. Rui, Y., Gupta, A., Grudin, J.: Videography for telepresentations. In: CHI 2003, pp. 457–464 (2003)
12. Calahan, S.: Storytelling through lighting: a computer graphics perspective (1996)
13. Cassell, J., Vilhjálmsson, H., Bickmore, T.: BEAT: the behavior expression animation toolkit. In: SIGGRAPH 2001, pp. 477–486 (2001)
14. Nowak, K., Biocca, F.: The effect of the agency and anthropomorphism on users sense of telepresence, copresence, and social presence in virtual environments. Presence **12**, 481–494 (2003)
15. DeVault, D., Mell, J., Gratch, J.: Toward natural turn-taking in a virtual human negotiation agent. In: AAAI 2015 Spring Symposium on Turn-taking and Coordination in Human-Machine Interaction (2015)

16. Marcus, B., Simkin, L.: The stages of exercise behavior. J. Sports Med. Phys. Fit. **33**, 83–88 (1993)
17. Cassell, J., Nakano, Y., Bickmore, T., Sidner, C., Rich, C.: Non-verbal cues for discourse structure. In: Association for Computational Linguistics, pp. 106–115 (2001)
18. Blom, J., Gumperz, J.: Social meaning in linguistic structures: code switching in northern norway. In: Gumperz, J., Hymes, D. (eds.) Directions in Sociolinguistics. Holt, Rinehart, and Winston, New York (1972)
19. Schiffrin, D.: Discourse Markers. Cambridge University Press, Cambridge (1987)
20. Arijan, D.: Grammar of the Film Language. Silman-James, Los Angeles (1976)
21. Tannen, D. (ed.): Framing in Discourse. Oxford University Press, New York (1993)
22. Bickmore, T., Picard, R.: Establishing and Maintaining Long-Term Human-Computer Relationships. ACM Trans. Comput. Hum. Interact. **12**, 293–327 (2005)
23. Manning, C., Surdeanu, M., Bauer, J., Finkel, J., Bethard, S., McClosky, D.: The stanford CoreNLP natural language processing toolkit. In: Proceedings of the 52nd Annual Meeting of the Association for Computational Linguistics, pp. 55–60 (2014)

An Exploratory Study Toward the Preferred Conversational Style for Compatible Virtual Agents

Ameneh Shamekhi[1(✉)], Mary Czerwinski[2], Gloria Mark[3],
Margeigh Novotny[2], and Gregory A. Bennett[4]

[1] College of Computer and Information Science, Northeastern University, Boston, MA, USA
`ameneh@ccs.neu.edu`
[2] Microsoft Research One Microsoft Way Redmond, Redmond, WA, USA
`{marycz,margeigh.novotny}@microsoft.com`
[3] Department of Informatics, University of California, Irvine, Irvine, CA, USA
`gmark@uci.edu`
[4] Salesforce UX, San Francisco, CA, USA
`gbennett@salesforce.com`

Abstract. Designing virtual personal assistants that are able to engage users in an interaction have been a challenge for HCI researchers for the past 20 years. In this work we investigated how a set of vocal characteristics known as "conversational style" could play role in engaging users in an interaction with a virtual agent. We also examined whether the similarity attraction principle influences how people orient towards agents with different styles. Results of a within subject experiment on 102 subjects revealed that users exhibited similarity attraction toward computer agents, and preferred the agent whose conversational style matched their own. The study results contribute to our understanding of how the design of intelligent agents' conversational style influences users' engagement and perceptions of the agent, compared to known human-to-human interaction.

Keywords: Virtual agents · Conversational style · Human-computer interaction · Social psychology · Interpersonal attraction · Similarity attraction

1 Introduction

Virtual agents increasingly play a role in human-computer interaction, assisting users in various areas such as education, health care and behavior change, marketing, and simple daily tasks. These agents serve as proxies for human representatives and are sometimes designed to engage in meaningful conversations with their users. In virtual agent-related research, it has always been a goal to construct an engaging, long-term relationship with the user [2]. Among several potential aspects of such an interaction,

A. Shamekhi, M. Novotny and G.A. Bennett---This research was done while the authors were working at Microsoft.

D. Traum et al. (Eds.): IVA 2016, LNAI 10011, pp. 40–50, 2016.
DOI: 10.1007/978-3-319-47665-0_4

we feel that investigating the best conversational styles for personal agents deserves in-depth attention, given its importance in human-human relationships [14].

Research revealing that people "orient towards computers as social actors" [11] sheds a new light on human-computer agent related research. Some theories from the social psychology of personal relationships and sociolinguistics have been shown that they can be applied to a human-virtual agent dyad. Nass and Moon revealed that people mindlessly apply social rules such as politeness norms, personality attractionand gender differences while interacting with computers [12].

On the other hand, similarity attraction (aka homophily), posits that individuals are more attracted to others who match them in values, behaviors and interests. According to studies by Berscheid and Walster [5], and Byrne [3], people are generally most attracted to others with whom they share similar attitudes and styles. With human-virtual agent interaction, Nass and Reeves also showed that users are more attracted to the TTS (TextToSpeech) voice that matches the user's own personality (e.g., extroverted vs. introverted, and dominant vs. submissive [12]). Another study by Gratch et al. has shown that a virtual agent that exhibits contingent nonverbal responses to a human dyad can effectively create rapport [8].

Research in the social psychology of personal relationships suggests numerous factors influence the quality of a social interaction. The intentions people convey during a conversation not only rely on the semantic interpretation of the words, but also on many other factors, including nonverbal behaviors [9], emotions [10], conversation starters and personality traits [6]. This line of reasoning led us to design an experiment to investigate the role of an agent's vocal characteristics and conversational style in human-agent interaction.

In this study, we examine the speaking style of a virtual agent, and aim to explore if the similarity attraction principle in conversational style applies to human-virtual agent interaction the same way it does in human-human interaction. We designed the speaking style based on the linguistic phenomenon known as conversational style [17]. We sought to find out if people feel more satisfied and engaged when they interact with a virtual agent whose speaking style matches their own. To evaluate this hypothesis, a within subject experiment was conducted to investigate users' attitudes toward a virtual agent speaking in different styles.

The significant amount of attention and investment in the design of realistic, virtual agents offers a promising future in which virtual agents and robots will be able to provide a wide range of human-like behaviors in social interaction. Thus, improving vocal characteristics of conversational agents' discourse will be critical in improving the overall quality of human-agent interaction. Also, engagement and satisfaction can be two influencing factors in the success of the human-agent interaction.

2   Conversational Style in Human-Virtual Agent Interaction

Human communication through conversation is not limited to the semantic content of the words expressed by participating interlocutors. Rather, linguists and behavioral scientists have shown that interpersonal communication is also achieved through paralinguistic features such as silence [1] and embodied features such as facial expressions [4]. These features can be utilized in various ways to construct one's own culturally-informed conversational style (CS). Deborah Tannen, a sociolinguist who pioneered this work, offers that CS is the means by which people convey meaning in daily conversations beyond solely the semantic content of the words they use. Speakers convey CS by employing variations of features such as tone of voice, pausing, and rate of speech to signal intention and relation in talk [15]. Tannen offers that CS is not a rarity; rather, "anything that is said must be said in some way, and that way is style" [16].

"Style" plays a role in determining one's personality in speech, according to Sapir [17]. He defined style as *"an everyday facet of speech that characterizes both the social group and the individual"* [14]. Conversational style is the manner in which we perform any conversational task or interaction. From the words we use to express ourselves in an interaction, to the tone, pitch, intonation, pauses, etc., all of these features constitute our conversational style. People convey meta-messages in a conversation containing information about their relationship and attitudes toward the others involved in that conversation. Tannen has stated that those meta-messages determine a speaker's style and are culturally specific [19]. In her research, Tannen observed five features of conversational style: conversation topic, genre, pace, expressive paralinguistics (e.g. relative loudness), and humor [16]. Based on the ways in which her study participants employed these features, she illuminated two main conversational styles for human interactions: "High Involvement" (**HI**) and "High Considerateness" (**HC**). For HI speakers, some practice "cooperative overlapping" in conversations. They associate interruptions with enthusiasm and *expect* the topic to change abruptly. These people usually talk a little more quickly, keep pauses short, are (a little) more verbose, are animated, show more emotion, exaggerate their feelings, express and expect overlapping talk to show enthusiasm, reciprocate (e.g., in chit chat, ask the same question the user asked in return), and provide explanations using a story about oneself. "High Considerateness" (**HC**) speakers, on the other hand, might maintain that overlapping talk is an interruption rather than display of enthusiasm, and thus, may pause slightly before responding, match the user's rate of speech. HC speakers are comparatively more succinct, yet still personable, and show emotion without exaggeration. They adjust their range/pitch/intonation to match their partner's style as well. Tannen has shown that people prefer interacting conversationally with interlocutors who match one's own style [16]. In other words, HI speakers prefer talking to those who are also HI and vice versa for HCs. It is important to note that conversational style should not be treated as a personality trait, or a permanent behavioral attribute, as it is not 100 % determined for each individual (e.g., speakers might adopt HI or HC speaking characteristics based on a number of factors). However, based on Tannen's definition, people could be more HI or HC in general in their conversations, and we explore this issue in human-agent interaction. Our initial thought was that dialog with an intelligent agent should reflect the way humans prefer to interact with other humans, but there is no research we know of that has examined this question. Our hypotheses are:

Hypothesis1: Participants will prefer to interact with a virtual agent whose conversational style matches their own conversational style.

Hypothesis2: Participants will be more engaged/interested in a virtual agent interaction when the agent's conversational style matches their own conversational style.

3 Experiment Design

We used a within-subjects study: each participant experienced two short conversations with a virtual agent who asked about the user's daily tasks, and tried to promote a healthy life style. Each task took about 4–5 min. The main sentences and structure in both conversations were comparably the same, and pre-scripted. The conditions are as follows:

Condition A: (High Involvement Agent) The agent talks a little more quickly, keeps pauses short, is (a little) more verbose, shows more emotion, exaggerates, and provides a story about herself using humor.

Condition B: (High Considerateness Agent) The agent pauses slightly before responding, speaks clearly and not too quickly, shows emotion without exaggeration (adjusts prosodic contour, pitch, rate, volume, and content appropriately).

Each conversation contains 5 small sub-conversations (Good morning, after lunch, after work, review for tomorrow, and pillow talk). One conversational round is with the HI agent and the other is with an HC agent. The order of conditions was assigned randomly to counterbalance any order effects.

Microsoft's text to speech toolkit[1] was used to generate the agent's voice. The tool allowed us to manipulate the prosody, pitch, speech rate and pause length to generate HI and HC voices for the agent. The conversation scripts were the same in both conditions, except for that in the HI condition, a few sentences were added to make the agent chattier, and humorous. Since previous research showed that the female voice is more acceptable by both female and male users, a female voice was used for the agent [13]. Examples of two scenarios for the HI and HC agent script are provided in Table 1.

3.1 The Difference Between HI and HC Conditions

We applied several manipulations to the agent's voice to cover the five aspects of conversational style stated by Tannen. The HI agent spoke with a higher speech rate (average HI speech rate = 1.16), kept the pauses shorter, had a higher average pitch, prosody, and conveyed more emotion by using stronger adjectives (e.g., "great" instead of "good"). We considered several changes in words and phrases to distinguish the topic and genre (e.g. the HI agent tells stories from her experiences/feelings and changes the topic more often). The HI agent also conveyed a sense of humor by saying human-like phrases [see Table 1-row 2]. Alternatively, the HC agent spoke a little slower (average HC speech rate = 0.92), kept pauses longer between sentences, and showed emotion without exaggeration. In order to manage the turn-taking between the user and the agent, we designed an automated process in which the agent took the turn after a fixed number of seconds (3 s in HI condition, 5 s in HC condition). Upon the completion of each

---

[1] https://www.microsoft.com/en-us/download/details.aspx?id=10121.

Table 1. Examples of the virtual agent's script in HI and HC conditions. The script differences over two conditions are limited. The main difference is on the speaking rate, prosody and pitch.

Agent's CS	Sample utterance	Agent's CS	Sample utterance
HI-after lunch talk	Welcome back Pat! I saw you went to Purple Café for lunch today. I really like there. You should try the chicken soup it's amazing! A good lunch also fuels the rest of your day. By the way, how would you rate the cafe? Good, average, or bad?	HC-after lunch talk	Welcome back Pat! I saw you went to Purple Café for lunch today. A good lunch also fuels the rest of your day. By the way, how would you rate the cafe? Good, average, or bad?
HI-After works 1	Hey Pat, I just noticed that traffic is a bit heavy to your next appointment, Charity meeting at 6 pm. I think you should either go earlier, or pick another route. Do you want an alternative rout suggestion?	HC-After work 1	Hey Pat, Traffic is a bit heavy to your next appointment, Charity meeting at 6 pm. Do you want an alternative rout suggestion?
HI-After work 2	… I have a fantastic idea. Do you want a magic solution to relieve your stress of these hard work days? I know many people who overcome their stress just by exercising. Physical activity like jogging, going to a gym, or a swimming pool is an important part of a healthy life style. um, let's see. The forecast for tomorrow shows, it's a hot day. How about going swimming tomorrow at 6:30. I don't know if it's open tomorrow. I'm looking for that. Yay, found it. There's one that is open tomorrow and has good reviews. I'll add it to your calendar, sounds good?	HC-After work 2	… Many people overcome their stress just by exercising. Physical activity like jogging, going to a gym, or a swimming pool is an important part of a healthy life style. Let's see. The forecast for tomorrow shows, it's a hot day. How about going swimming tomorrow at 6:30. I don't know if it's open tomorrow. I'm looking for that. Here it is. There's one that is open tomorrow and has good reviews. I will add it to your calendar, sounds good?

utterance by the agent, the user was shown a button to start recording his/her utterance, and then after a fixed amount of time the agent took the turn and started her next utterance. However, since the HI conversational style included many "barge in" behaviors, the HI agent waited only three seconds after each utterance, consequently, the user was interrupted by the agent at several points during the conversation. This was by design. The length of the pauses between utterances in the HC condition was longer (five seconds), and designed so that participants never experienced an interruption from the HC agent.

4   Method

4.1   Participants

102 Amazon Mechanical Turk (mTurk) workers participated in this experiment (age range = 19 − 66, M = 33.2, SD = 10.3), 33 % were female. We had to eliminate the data for two of the participants due to technical issues. Three requirements had been set for the workers: approval rate had to be greater than or equal to 97 %, approved hits had to be greater than or equal to 1000 HITs, and they had to be from either Canada or the U.S. The

task took ~15–20 min to complete, and participants could reject completing the task at any time. Upon the completion of the experiment, participants were paid $4 US.

4.2 Procedure

The experiment was a randomized, counterbalanced, within-subjects design with two conditions: the agent's conversational style was either high involvement (HI) or high considerate (HC). The study objective was to have the participant interact with an agent, via a scripted dialog. After interacting with each conversational style of the agent, users were asked questions about their enjoyment and satisfaction with that agent. According to Tannen's theory, users should prefer interacting with a person whose conversational style matches their own.

Prior to starting, each participant filled out three questionnaires, which included demographic questions, followed by a ten item personality scale (TIPI) the short form of the Big Five questionnaire [7]. Participants were then provided instructions on how to converse with the agent, using a headset and microphone. Upon completion of the questionnaires, each participant was randomly assigned to a condition, in which they conversed with an HI or HC agent. Each conversation contained five short dialogs simulating five different times of the day: morning, lunch, leaving work, reviewing one's appointments for tomorrow toward the end of the day, and "pillow talk" (simulating before they went to bed). Each short conversation was initiated by the agent and had a scripted dialog for the user to read aloud. Users could read the script exactly or they could ad lib (They were shown this message: *You can use the text displayed to you. Try not to read the text out loud, you can first read the text and then *say it in your way**). All users' conversations were recorded. Though the agent's responses were all pre-scripted, the users were told that the agent was listening to them and that they should respond accordingly. Participants were asked to imagine a situation at the beginning of each sub-conversation: (e.g., "*Imagine that you just woke up and want to review your day's schedule with your virtual assistant*"). After the first set of five conversations, participants were asked to fill out a questionnaire about their experience, and then started the second set of five conversations with the agent of the opposite conversational style. When they finished the second conversational set, they were asked to fill out a questionnaire on their recent conversations. Next, they were asked to fill out a 12-item questionnaire for measuring their own conversational style, followed by an open-end question for the same purpose. The reason we did not ask them to fill out a CS questionnaire before the experiment was to avoid biasing the participants about their interaction. Finally, users were asked to indicate which agent they preferred and why (Fig. 1).

5 Analysis

5.1 User Conversational Style Extrapolation (CSE)

Since the scope of this study did not permit in-person observation, and no validated questionnaire exists in the literature to tease out conversational style, a rudimentary questionnaire was developed by one of the authors, a sociolinguist who studied under

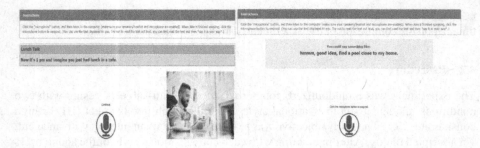

Fig. 1. Screenshots from the interaction system. When a participant clicked on "continue", the agent started talking, and the users were provided with a microphone button to press in order to respond.

Professor Deborah Tannen, and given to participants. This questionnaire contains 12 items, asking indirectly about the users' attitudes during a conversation. We face-validated the questionnaire by asking several experts to assess whether the questionnaire covers the conversational style concept well. We also criterion-validated the questionnaire by asking participants to elaborate on how they feel when they encounter overlapping speech during a conversation in real life. We asked each user to remember the last time (s)he had a conversation and describe the feeling when the user and the interlocutors spoke over each other. The answer to this question is a criterion variable that can help assess our measure. Three judges then extrapolated each participant's CS based on their responses, and each participant was assigned to HC or HI accordingly. The results of the judges' evaluation (criterion variable) significantly correlated with the questionnaire result (X^2 (1, N = 67) = 26.79, p < .0001).

5.2 Summary of Measures Used for Dependent Variables

- 7 questions to assess the overall quality of interaction. (treated as single questions using a 5 point Likert scale: 1 = not at all to 5 = very much): would you continue interacting with the agent, how engaging, how focused, how emotional, how bored, do you trust the agent and how likeable was the agent?
- The 12 item CSE questionnaire extrapolates subjects' conversational style (composite measure: 5 Likert scale items from 1 = strongly disagree to 5 = strongly agree). The reliability of both HC and HI indexes have been assessed. (HC: Cronbach's alpha = 0.75, HI: Cronbach's alpha = 0.62).
- One open-ended question about conversational behavior: Can you remember the last time you were talking with somebody and both you and that other person were talking at the same time (i.e., both of your voices could be heard saying things simultaneously in conversation)? How did this make you feel?.
- One final, open-ended question asking about the preferred agent, and the overall impression of the study.

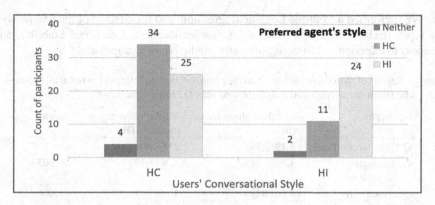

Fig. 2. Distribution of participants by their preferred agent's CS. The results show that 65 % HI users preferred the HI agent, and 54 % HC users preferred the HC agent.

6 Results

We used the CSE questionnaire results to determine the participants' conversational style: 37 participants were extrapolated as HI, and 63 participants as HC.

A chi-square test of independence was performed to determine whether people preferred the virtual agent whose conversational style matched their own or not. The chi-square test showed a significant correlation between users' style and their preferred agent. $X^2(2, N = 100) = 6.19, p < .05$. This result can be seen in Fig. 2.

We conducted a MANOVA test using a multivariate general linear model (GLM) in SPSS to account for our multiple dependent measures. The between-subject factors were users' CS (HI/HC) and Gender. Since the agent had a female voice, we entered the user's gender as a variable as we felt that gender might make a difference in the interaction assessment. The within-subjects factor was the Agent CS (HI/HC). We looked at all 2-way interactions. The results showed a significant effect of Gender ($F(7, 90) = 3.14$, p < .005) and a significant Gender by User CS interaction ($F(7, 90) = 3.00$, p < .007). User CS was not significant. For the within-subject effects, we found a significant Agent CS x User CS interaction: ($F(7, 90) = 2.61$, p < .02). The Agent CS showed a trend ($F(7, 90) = 1.93$, p < .07), and the interaction of Agent CS x Gender was not significant.

We also performed a series of paired sample t-tests to examine whether participants' responses to the 7 questions measuring the quality of the users' recent interactions with the agent differed significantly across matched (the condition in which the agent's CS was matched to the user's CS) or mismatched (Table 2). Using the Holm-Bonferroni sequential correction for multiple t-tests, the difference between the means of the two groups was significantly different only for the second question: *How engaging was your interaction with the agent?*.

Since personality type of a text to speech (TTS) voice has been examined with human users [11], we examined the correlation between conversational style and personality type. We performed a Multiple Logistic Regression, and found none of the five personality types (Extraverted, Agreeableness, Conscientiousness, Emotional Stability, and Openness to experiences) to be significantly predictive of extrapolated CS.

Table 2. Results of paired sample t-tests on the agent-interaction ratings (1 = not at all to 5 = very much). The Holm-Bonferroni correction showed only Q2 to be significant.

Question	Matched group means (SD)	Mismatched group means (SD)	p-val
Q 1(like to continue)	3.12(1.38)	2.9(1.40)	.151
Q 2(engaging interaction)	3.79(1.11)	3.36(1.13)	**.005**
Q 3 (focused)	4.5(0.84)	4.5(0.96)	1.000
Q 4(real feeling)	2.98(1.3)	2.83(1.34)	.218
Q 5-R(bored)	3.50(1.3)	3.48(1.36)	.90
Q 6(trust)	3.64(1.11)	3.4(1.23)	.035
Q 7(like)	3.63 (1.19)	3.33(1.29)	.032

Lastly, some feedback and open comments from participants were quite indicative of how much they preferred the agent's style to match their own:

P1 (HC): "The second one (HC) was much better because the speech pattern was slower and more realistic."

P2 (HI): "I preferred the first (HI), because she talked at a human-like pace instead of like a robot."

P3(HC): "I liked the first (HC). It was less stilted and the speech sounded more natural. Also, the second one was "chattier" and that got a bit annoying."

P4 (HI): "First agent (HI) was great. I felt as if I was talking with a real person and not a computer. The speech was clear. And the rate of speech was that of a human's rate. Easy to have a fluid conversation and that agent to understand all of the things I asked of it."

P5 (HC): I preferred "First (HC) as the tone was more natural. The second seemed to be rolling pretty quickly but you could hang with her so the first was best for me."

7   Discussion

One of the primary motivations of this study was to investigate whether users could simply identify the differences in an agent's conversational style, and if they preferred that style to match their own. As the above results show, users distinguished the changes in the agent's conversational style quite well (Fig. 2) (only 6 % stated either no difference or a subtle one). The strong preferences of most users for the agent with a similar CS suggests that designing an agent's style to match the user has great potential for improving human-agent interaction.

The gender findings may indicate that the effect of CS matching is stronger for our male participants. The gender by CS interaction may indicate further that HI males are more sensitive to the agent's CS. As this is one of the first studies of its kind on this topic, we find it provocative and interesting to explore further.

Limitations and Challenges We used a novel questionnaire which was not validated in past studies to extrapolate the participants' CS. We showed the acceptable reliability and validity for the questionnaire, however we had hoped to investigate a third measure of participants' style by analyzing the recorded verbal open-ended description of talking with a friend, but this will be part of future research. So, we cannot be completely sure that our conversational style classification was entirely accurate, though we did try to use converging lines of evidence. Our analysis of the open-ended audio tracks remains as future work. Additionally, the authors acknowledge Tannen's key finding that CS is fluid and culturally-informed in nature—there could be far more paralinguistic features to examine beyond the five we explored herein—perhaps the audio tracks will reveal more in this realm.

The participants' conversation with the agent was scripted; we were afraid that this might influence the overall flow of the conversation and subsequently, ratings of the agent. We have addressed this concern in subsequent research. The agent did not adapt to the user's style automatically, which would be an obvious goal for the future.

Despite all of these concerns, we feel we did obtain some promising results that show that users do respond positively to an agent with a conversational style that matches their own extrapolated style. In future work, we are exploring style matching further with a more naturalistic dialog interaction and a more organic, targeted process of teasing out user CS.

References

1. Basso, K.H.: To give up on words: silence in western apache culture. Southwest. J. Anthropol. **26**(3), 213–230 (1970)
2. Bickmore, T.W., Picard, R.W.: Establishing and maintaining long-term human-computer relationships. ACM TOCHI. **12**(2), 293–327 (2005)
3. Byrne, D., Griffitt, W.: Interpersonal attraction. Annu. Rev. Psychol. **24**(1), 317–336 (1973)
4. Frith, C., Griffitt, W.: Role of facial expressions in social interactions. Philos. Trans. R. Soc. B Biol. Sci. **364**(1535), 3453–3458 (2009)
5. Gilbert, D.T., et al. (eds.): The Handbook of Social Psychology. McGraw-Hill, Boston (1998). Distributed exclusively by Oxford University Press
6. Goldman, J.A., et al.: Effect of similarity of ego identity status on interpersonal attraction. J. Youth Adolesc. **9**(2), 153–162 (1980)
7. Gosling, S.D., et al.: A very brief measure of the Big-Five personality domains. J. Res. Personal. **37**(6), 504–528 (2003)
8. Gratch, J. et al.: Creating rapport with virtual agents. In: Pelachaud, C. et al. (eds.) Intelligent Virtual Agents, pp. 125–138 (2007)
9. Hartzler, A.L., et al.: Real-time feedback on nonverbal clinical communication: theoretical framework and clinician acceptance of ambient visual design. Methods Inf. Med. **53**(5), 389–405 (2014)
10. Lopes, P.N., et al.: Emotion regulation abilities and the quality of social interaction. Emotion **5**(1), 113–118 (2005)

11. Nass, C., Lee, K.M.: Does computer-synthesized speech manifest personality? Experimental tests of recognition, similarity-attraction, and consistency-attraction. J. Exp. Psychol. Appl. **7**(3), 171–181 (2001)
12. Nass, C., Moon, Y.: Machines and mindlessness: social responses to computers. J. Soc. Issues **56**(1), 81–103 (2000)
13. Payne, J. et al.: Gendering the machine: preferred virtual assistant gender and realism in self-service. In: Aylett, R. et al. (eds.) Intelligent Virtual Agents, pp. 106–115 (2013)
14. Sapir, E., et al.: Ethnology. Mouton de Gruyter, Berlin (1994)
15. Schiffrin, D., et al. (eds.): The Handbook of Discourse Analysis. Blackwell, Malden (2010)
16. Tannen, D.: Conversational Style: Analyzing Talk Among Friends. Oxford University Press, New York (2005)
17. Tannen, D. (ed.): Framing in Discourse. Oxford University Press, New York (1993)

Talk to Me: Verbal Communication Improves Perceptions of Friendship and Social Presence in Human-Robot Interaction

Elena Corina Grigore[1(✉)], Andre Pereira[1], Ian Zhou[1],
David Wang[2], and Brian Scassellati[1]

[1] Yale University, 51 Prospect Street, New Haven, CT 06511, USA
{elena.corina.grigore,andre.pereira,ian.zhou,brian.scassellati}@yale.edu
[2] Amity Regional High School, Woodbridge, CT 06525, USA
wangda16amity@amityschools.org

Abstract. The ability of social agents, be it virtually-embodied avatars or physically-embodied robots, to display social behavior and interact with their users in a natural way represents an important factor in how effective such agents are during interactions. In particular, endowing the agent with effective communicative abilities, well-suited for the target application or task, can make a significant difference in how users perceive the agent, especially when the agent needs to interact in complex social environments. In this work, we consider how two core input communication modalities present in human-robot interaction—speech recognition and touch-based selection—shape users' perceptions of the agent. We design a short interaction in order to gauge adolescents' reaction to the input communication modality employed by a robot intended as a long-term companion for motivating them to engage in daily physical activity. A study with n = 52 participants shows that adolescents perceive the robot as more of a friend and more socially present in the speech recognition condition than in the touch-based selection one. Our results highlight the advantages of using speech recognition as an input communication modality even when this represents the less robust choice, and the importance of investigating how to best do so.

1 Introduction

Artificial agents, such as virtually-embodied characters or physically-embodied robots, can take on the role of help givers, companions, teachers, coaches, and so on [11,25]. In this work, we focus on a physically-embodied robot intended as a long-term companion that keeps adolescents motivated to engage in daily physical activity throughout time. The importance of developing methods for keeping adolescents engaged in physical activity is stressed by data revealing alarmingly low numbers of adolescents who engage in levels recommended by health guidelines [2]. Furthermore, this occurs at an age when physical activity holds essential benefits for healthy growth and development [6]. Given that the constant support needed for behavior change [16] is either not readily available

© Springer International Publishing AG 2016
D. Traum et al. (Eds.): IVA 2016, LNAI 10011, pp. 51–63, 2016.
DOI: 10.1007/978-3-319-47665-0_5

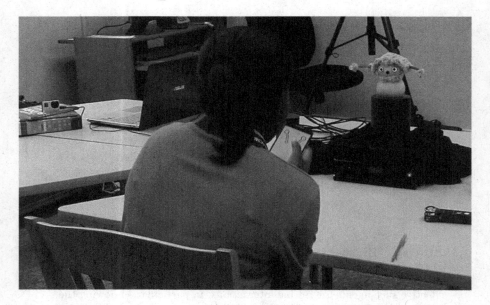

Fig. 1. Participant interacting with the robot using our smartphone interface. (Color figure online)

or costly, employing a social agent as a companion would provide valuable social support to keep adolescents motivated to exercise routinely.

In order for such a companion to successfully provide its users with social support over time, enabling smooth and natural interactions through an effective communication modality is essential. We thus investigate the effects of the communication modality on users' perceptions of the agent. To this end, we conduct a study to observe adolescents' reactions to different ways of communicating with the robot (Fig. 1 shows a participant during a session). Investigating how users' perceptions of the robot are affected by communication modality can guide us towards creating better and more effective agent interactions. In particular, we are interested in how users' perceptions of the agent change in terms of friendship and social presence factors. These factors are particularly relevant for creating engaging and compelling interactions, and are important to assess prior to the long-term deployment intended for our robot companion.

Given that verbal communication is at the core of how people interact with each other, one of the most natural ways of designing a human-robot communication interface is employing speech. Speech recognition provides a basic and natural way of conveying information to the robot. Even though it has seen serious advances in recent years, speech recognition technology still suffers from unreliable performance in noisy acoustic environments and when faced with speaker and language variability (especially when working with children [8]), as well as from difficulty handling free-style speech [4]. Due to the challenges faced by utilizing speech recognition reliably, many interfaces for communication with agents use touch-based inputs via tablet or smartphone devices [5, 18]. The use of such interfaces makes for more robust and dependable communication, but might take away from the benefits of having a more natural interaction.

Our work investigates how adolescents' perceptions of the robot change when speech recognition versus touch-input selection is used to communicate with the agent. Results reveal that, even though the former was more error-prone and less robust than the latter, users perceived the robot as more of a friend and more socially present in the speech recognition condition than in the touch-based selection one. This highlights the importance of employing a more natural way of communication, even when this represents the less robust choice.

2   Related Work

Speech recognition has advanced significantly in recent years, with numerous applications deployed on a large scale. Smartphones represent some of the most widely used devices that employ this capability, with 3.4 billion subscriptions in 2015 set to double by the year 2021 [7]. Most smartphones come equipped with intelligent personal assistants that help users complete day-to-day activities, from using social media platforms to searching for travel information. Such assistants take inputs in the form of voice, images, or contextual information to provide useful answers, typically in the form of natural language. Through the widespread use of these devices, owners have become acquainted with the power provided by speech recognition, making for smooth and natural interactions with their devices.

Speech recognition systems, however, still suffer from lack of robustness beyond constrained tasks and are not reliable when used in noisy environments. The highest performing systems in research struggle to obtain word error rates (WER) lower than 10 %, and employ strategies that might prove to be unfeasible for most real-world applications [4]. Furthermore, data on the performance of commercially available speech recognition services show considerable variability with respect to performance metrics, with WERs ranging from 15.8 % to 63.3 % [14]. In this work, we wish to investigate whether employing speech recognition to enable communication between a robot and its users is of value even when this represents the less robust choice.

2.1   Speech Recognition Communication Interfaces

Speech interfaces have been used for communicating with social agents in different contexts and application domains, given the natural way of interaction such interfaces can provide. A salient research area in which speech recognition is used is that of creating multimodal human-robot interaction interfaces. Such interfaces include verbal communication and visual perception modules, among others, and employ speech recognition as an important part of the interface allowing users to communicate with the robot [9, 20].

In a study focusing on teaching a robot a complex task [24], the robot learns the task by both observing a human perform it and by interpreting the speech used by the person while doing so. The authors emphasize the utilization of speech recognition in human-robot interfaces to create natural and familiar ways for people to interact with robots, which could more quickly lead to their acceptance in human environments like homes and workspaces. Alongside providing a natural mode of communication, other advantages include more easily handling situations when a person's hands or eyes are occupied, benefits for enabling communication between robots and handicapped persons, and the use of the ubiquitous mobile devices discussed above that allow for two-way voice communication [23].

Although there exist a number of studies investigating the effect of output communication modalities on users' perceptions of agents (i.e. using different interfaces to convey information from the agent to the user such as text-to-speech, text, etc.) [21,22], research on input communication interfaces is more scarce and is the area where we focus our current efforts.

2.2   Touch-Based Selection Communication Interfaces

Faced with the challenges surrounding the reliable use of speech recognition, a growing number of studies have started utilizing touch-based selection input as the main form of interaction between humans and robots. In the past ten years, we can observe a clear trend in the increasing number of studies that make use of mobile devices or tablet touchscreens for this purpose. For example, the Nao or DragonBot robots have commonly been paired with touchscreen tablets to provide a context for human-robot interaction [5,25].

Other studies have used mobile devices and touch interfaces to communicate with robots. In such a study, authors used a smartphone as a means of interacting with Nao and teaching it about new objects [18]. In a study exploring the concept of enjoyment in a human-robot interaction scenario with the elderly, authors used a touchscreen interface in place of a speech recognition system due to increased reliability and smoother interactions [11].

The research presented above gives us interesting insights into using different kinds of devices and interfaces for communication in human-robot interactions. However, researchers have not yet explored the tradeoff between employing a more natural versus a more robust interface for enabling communication between a user and a robot with respect to users' perceptions of the agent. Our work explores this tradeoff by investigating perceptions of friendship and social presence engendered by the use of different input communication modalities.

3   Methodology

3.1   Interaction Context

The interaction context for our study is that of a robot companion motivating adolescents to engage in daily physical activity. The companion is intended for long-term use, and the single-session study presented here constitutes the first interaction users would be going through during a longer-term study. During this session, the robot walks participants through its back-story and explains the different motivational strategies it would be using over time. The back-story consists of the agent taking on the role of a "robot-alien" whose space ship broke down on Earth and who needs help from the user in order to return home. The user can help the robot by exercising routinely and transferring "energy" to the robot by doing so. In a long-term scenario, this is accomplished by providing users with a wristband device that measures the physical activity level they engage in daily, which the robot can connect to in order to gain "energy points".

The back-story is created in order to build an engaging, compelling, and persuasive interaction by linking elements of the story (e.g., the fact that all inhabitants of the robot's planet have a high level of knowledge of physical activity) to ways in which the robot would help the user. In a long-term deployment, the agent can accomplish this by employing four different motivational strategies— cooperative persuasion, competitive persuasion, conveying information about physical activity through lessons and quizzes, and promoting self-reflection [1]. These motivational strategies are reinforced by providing users with a smartphone they can carry around with them during the day, while away from the physical robot. Participants also use the smartphone during their short, daily interactions with the physical robot in order to communicate with it.

3.2 Study Design

The user study we present herein examines the effects of speech recognition versus touch-based selection on users' friendship and social presence perceptions of the robot within the interaction context described in Subsect. 3.1. Each session involves a participant interacting with the robot for six-to-nine minutes and being engaged in a dialogue on the topic of physical activity motivation for adolescents. The interaction is structured in the form of a dialogue controlled by the agent in which the robot either speaks to the participant or asks a question and waits for a response. Participants interact with the robot via a smartphone application that displays the appropriate interface based on whether the robot or the person is speaking, as well as based on the condition to which the participant is assigned. The conditions represent the use of two different input communication modalities: (1) speech recognition—when they are prompted through the smartphone interface, participants respond to the robot's questions by saying one of the answer choices displayed on the screen and their answers are evaluated through speech recognition, and (2) touch-based selection—participants respond to the robot's questions by using their finger to drag a button onto one of the answer choices displayed on the smartphone screen. We hypothesize that:

H1: Users would perceive the robot as more of a friend in the speech recognition than in the touch-based selection condition.

H2: Users would perceive the robot as more socially present in the speech recognition than in the touch-based selection condition.

3.3 Measures

The two main dependent variables (DVs) we examine are users' perceptions of the robot in terms of friendship and social presence. The two measures are based on standardized questionnaires measuring friendship [17] and social presence [10]. We examine subscales of both measures to investigate the effects of the input communication modality on users' perceptions of the agent. The two main DVs constitute important factors to consider in any human-robot interaction scenario in which we wish to create an engaging and compelling interaction and engender a positive rapport with an artificial agent.

Friendship. We employ the McGill Friendship Questionnaire (MFQ) [17] concerning a subject's assessment of the degree to which someone fulfills six friendship functions. Although friendships, like other relationships, vary in quality, research suggests it is possible to assess specific qualities, and the questionnaire used herein was created to define theoretically distinct friendship functions that distinguish between friends and non-friends, and that are associated with affection and satisfaction [17]. We believe that it is fundamental to engender the existence of such elements during interactions with social agents, whether they be long- or short-term. These factors are key to creating positive impressions of the agent, which is especially important during initial rapport development in relationships [29]. The more users perceive that the agent can fulfill friendship functions, the more likely they are to start building positive rapport with the agent.

The relevance of using friendship as a measure of the ability of an agent to establish meaningful relationships with its users has already been highlighted in a short-term study [15]. We employ this measure in a similar way to inform this ability of the agent for the intended long-term use of our robot companion. The MFQ consists of 30 zero-to-eight Likert items in total, with six subscales composed of five questions each. The six subscales included in the questionnaire are: stimulating companionship, help, intimacy, reliable alliance, self-validation, and emotional security. Although not straightforward to delineate, some friendship subscales such as intimacy might appear more relevant to long-term interactions. Nevertheless, these subscales could give us insights into how verbal communication might affect a long-term interaction. Additionally, including the full set of subscales allows for future comparisons with long-term interaction results.

Social presence. Social presence is another core aspect of human-human interactions that we should take into account when developing interactions between users and robots or social agents. Social presence was initially defined as "the degree of salience of the other person in the interaction and the consequent salience of the interpersonal relationships" [26]. It is immediately apparent that users' perceived social presence of the robot is of high importance, given that we strive to develop robots that interact with their users in a convincing and social manner. An example of the power of creating strongly socially present robots is [19], where social presence is used to create believable and enjoyable board game opponents. It has been shown that an agent is more effective at being persuasive when perceived as socially present [27]. A robot companion that aims to keep adolescents motivated over time by employing persuasive motivational strategies would thus benefit greatly from being perceived as a strongly socially present party in the interaction.

The questionnaire used herein is based on [10], which consists of 36 zero-to-eight Likert items in total and defines social presence to include six important factors for the interaction. These factors of social presence represent the sub-scales used in the questionnaire: co-presence, attentional allocation, perceived message understanding, perceived affective understanding, perceived affective interdependence, and perceived behavioral interdependence. Social presence is directly applicable to short-term interactions and is routinely employed in their assessment [3, 28].

3.4 Apparatus and Experimental Setup

In our study, we use a modified (to make programmable) version of MyKeepon, a commercially available variant of the Keepon robot. Keepon is a non-mobile robot with four degrees of freedom, designed for interaction with children [13]. The modified MyKeepon can be seen in Fig. 1, presenting a green "alien" hat with antennae, consistent with the robot's back-story during the interaction.

Throughout the study, each participant sat at a table, with the robot placed on the table. A Kinect was positioned in front of the robot and covered with a black cloth to look integrated with the robot. The Kinect tracked the position of the user's head so that the agent would turn left or right, as needed, in order to mimic placing its attention on the participant as he or she moved. The user was also given a smartphone device with a custom-built application displaying the interface based on the condition. Figure 1 shows the experimental setup during an interaction session with an adolescent.

3.5 Participants

We conducted a study with n = 52 participants, 26 male and 26 female, in local high schools. The subject population consisted of early adolescents and adolescents aged 14-to-16, with an average age of 15. Apart from the age, no other recruitment criteria were applied. Recruitment was managed with the help of the schools' staff and participants did not receive monetary compensation. We obtained ethical approval from the Human Subjects Committee at our university.

3.6 Procedure

Participants were randomly assigned to either the speech recognition or the touch-based selection condition. The former included 26 participants, while the latter included the other 26. Users were given an assent form to read and sign prior to participation. Each participant was seated at a table, in front of the robot that was initially still and silent. We first gave the user a brief overview of the physical activity scenario and then handed him or her the smartphone.

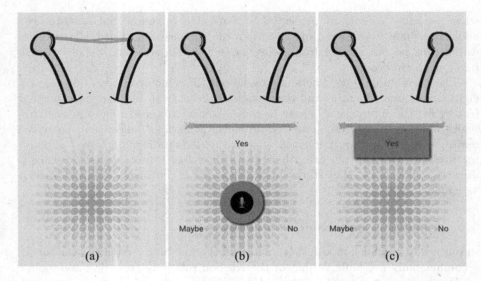

Fig. 2. Interface for communication with the robot. Figures show the interface displayed for: (a) the robot speaking during both conditions, (b) the speech recognition condition, and (c) the touch-based selection condition.

Each participant was given a brief explanation on how to use the interface to communicate with the robot. Figure 2(a) shows the interface displayed across conditions when the robot is speaking to the user. Figure 2(b) shows the interface displayed in the speech recognition condition. Users in this condition would say one of the options displayed on the screen to answer a question. We employed the Google Speech Recognition API [12]. The system could handle synonyms and expressions with similar meaning to the words shown (e.g., "yeah", "sure", and "of course" would all be recognized as "yes"). When the system could not correctly identify the input or the participant would not use the interface correctly, the robot would prompt the user with a brief instruction based on the particular mistake. Figure 2(c) shows the communication interface displayed in the touch-based selection condition. Participants in this condition would use their finger to drag the button displayed on the screen onto one of the answer choices in order to respond. As long as they kept the button pressed, participants could change their mind and move the button from one choice to another. In this condition too, users were prompted with a brief instruction if they would not utilize the interface correctly.

The interaction itself consisted of the robot unfolding its back-story and talking about physical activity motivation. The interface would change from Fig. 2(a) to either Fig. 2(b) or (c) (depending on the condition) when the robot would go from speaking to waiting for the participant's answer. The robot asked a total of six questions during each interaction, and users could choose among three simple entries to respond. The robot's replies to the different answer choices

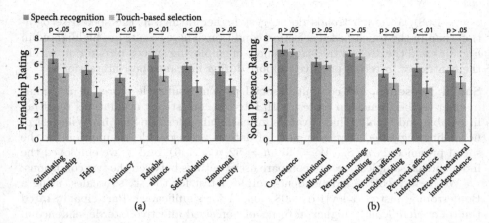

Fig. 3. Mean ratings for (a) friendship subscales (p-values based on the Mann-Whitney U test statistic, with means and error bars depicted to visualize results for this data), and (b) social presence subscales (p-values based on the independent-samples t-test statistic). We consider Bonferroni-adjusted α levels with $p < .008$ for significance and $p < .017$ for marginal significance. All error bars represent $\pm 1 SE$.

differed slightly to give users feedback that their particular answer was understood, but otherwise the script was fixed. The interaction was approximately seven minutes long. At the end of the interaction, participants were asked to fill out the friendship and social presence questionnaires.

4   Results

This section presents the analysis of the friendship and social presence subscales, and discusses the robustness of the two conditions employed in the current study.

Friendship. We first evaluated the internal consistency for each of the six friendship subscales, resulting in highly reliable values. We thus computed the scores for the six subscales by averaging over values within each. The Shapiro-Wilk test of normality revealed our data is not normally distributed ($S - W = .93, df = 52, p = .005$). We thus employed the Mann-Whitney U test to compare users' ratings of the robot between the two conditions.

   We performed the Mann-Whitney U test for each of the six subscales, using a Bonferroni-adjusted α level of .008 (.05/6) for significance and .017 (.1/6) for marginal significance. Participants rated the robot significantly higher in the speech input condition than in the touch input one for help ($U = 183, p = .004, z = -2.84$) and reliable alliance ($U = 186, p = .005, z = -2.79$), and marginally significantly higher for self-validation ($U = 200.5, p = .012, z = -2.52$). Based on the Bonferroni correction, there was no statistical significance in ratings for stimulating companionship ($U = 215, p = .024, z = -2.26$), intimacy ($U = 228.5, p = .045, z = -2.01$), or emotional security ($U = 246, p = .094,$

$z = -1.68$), although trends do suggest higher ratings in the speech recognition than in the touch-based selection condition. These results are highlighted in Fig. 3(a) and they reveal the strong effect of employing speech recognition within the context of fostering positive rapport during human-robot interactions.

Social Presence. We computed social presence subscale scores in a similar manner to the friendship scores, with internal consistency evaluations resulting in reliable and highly reliable values for each subscale. The Shapiro-Wilk test of normality suggested that normality of data is a reasonable assumption for the social presence data ($S - W = .97, df = 52, p = .146$), and so we employed the independent-samples t-test to compare users' ratings between the two conditions.

We performed the independent-samples t-test for the six subscales, using a Bonferroni-adjusted α level of .008 (.05/6) for significance. Participants rated the robot significantly higher in terms of perceived affective interdependence in the speech recognition condition ($M = 5.72, SD = 1.58$) than in the touch-based selection one ($M = 4.17, SD = 2.31$), $t(50) = 2.83, p = .007$ (t-value reported for unequal variances), while the other five subscales (co-presence, attentional allocation, perceived message understanding, perceived affective understanding, and perceived behavioral interdependence) were not significant (Fig. 3(b)). Although the friendship ratings reveal a stronger impact of the communication interface employed, social presence results also bolster the importance of employing a more natural and familiar mode of communication with robots.

Robustness. In order to assess the reliability of the two input communication modalities employed, we computed error rates for each. For both conditions, each session constitutes of the robot asking the user a total of six questions, for which the participant can choose among three simple, one-word entries to respond. In the speech recognition condition, we encountered two types of errors: (1) the system evaluates the user's speech as something other than the options available on the smartphone screen, and (2) there is no audible speech that can be evaluated by the system. Since each question response consists of one-word answers, we computed the word error rate (WER) for our system by dividing the total number of errors encountered (23) by the total number of questions asked (six questions per participant, with 26 participants in the speech recognition condition), and obtained a value of 14.74 %. In the touch-based selection condition, the interface performed without errors, given the tailored nature of the interface design and the reliability of using a smartphone touch interface.

To ensure that the errors encountered in the speech recognition condition did not impact users' perceptions of the robot, we analyzed this data more in depth. Out of the 26 total participants in this condition, our system presented errors for 14 (with an average of 1.64 errors per user), and worked without errors for the remainder of 12. We thus applied the same statistical tests employed above for this condition only, using a binary coding scheme to divide the group into participants with and without errors. We again employed the Mann-Whitney U test for friendship subscales and the independent-samples t-test for social presence subscales, with the same significance levels used above. We obtained no significant effect for errors for either of the friendship or social presence subscales.

This shows that the difference in users' perceptions of the robot is not influenced by errors present in the speech recognition condition.

Compared to available commercial systems, our speech recognition WER represents a fairly low error rate, but this is due to the nature of the constrained task and simple answers employed during the interaction. To note, however, is the fact that the speech recognition condition constitutes the less robust choice out of our two input communication modalities, and that this condition still engenders higher perceptions of the robot for participants. These results stress that it is important to consider the tradeoff between utilizing a more natural versus a more robust interface when deciding which input communication modality to employ for interactions with robots, or artificial agents more broadly.

5   Discussion and Conclusions

This work examines the effects of employing speech recognition versus touch-based selection as an input communication modality on users' perception of an agent. We conducted a study to investigate how the two modalities shape users' friendship and social presence perceptions of the robot within the context of physical activity motivation for adolescents. Our intuition was that, as a more natural means of communication, speech recognition would prove to engender stronger perceptions of friendship and social presence than touch-based selection, even when this represents the less robust choice.

Hypothesis H1 predicted stronger friendship perceptions of the robot in the speech recognition than in the touch-based selection condition. We obtained statistically significant differences between conditions for help and reliable alliance, and marginally statistically significant for self-validation. Although we did not obtain statistically significant results for stimulating companionship, intimacy, and emotional security, we did notice a trend in the same direction. A possible explanation for why these subscales are only showing a trend could be due to their limited relevance to short-term interactions. We suspect that a longer exposure to our agent could result in significant results for these subscales as well, and consider this an interesting avenue for future research.

The second hypothesis, H2, is partly supported by our results. Co-presence, attentional allocation, and perceived message understanding engendered high perceptions of the agent for users across conditions, and so these subscales did not yield statistically significant differences. We did not obtain any significant differences for perceived message understanding and perceived behavioral interdependence. However, participants in the speech recognition condition perceived stronger affective interdependence than those in the touch-based selection one. Perceived affective interdependence is defined as "the extent to which the user's emotional and attitudinal state affects and is affected by the emotional and attitudinal states of the interactant." It represents an important facet of creating an engaging, persuasive, and compelling agent that aims to motivate adolescents. Having users perceive high affective interdependence when interacting with a social robot is fundamental to any type of agent, be it one that aims to entertain, motivate, help physically, or simply provide information.

The significant differences we observe in users' perceptions of the robot are within the context of employing a smartphone as part of the input communication modality. We do so deliberately, in order to design a robot that can realistically be used as a long-term companion in adolescents' homes and employ widespread, commercially available technology (smartphones) to this end. Although comparing our conditions to using speech recognition without a smartphone would help put the significant differences obtained into context, it would introduce another independent variable, i.e. the presence or absence of the device. Nevertheless, we believe this comparison to be an interesting future direction.

The results yielded by the current single-session study inform us that, for our long-term application scenario, using natural language for communication with a social agent is worthwhile despite the presence of speech recognition errors. Given the general pertinence of the two scales we employed, we believe that these results can be applied to many other human-agent interaction domains where social interactions are key.

References

1. Details omitted for double-blind reviewing
2. Physical activity guidelines for americans midcourse report: strategies to increase physical activity among youth. Technical report, U.S. Department of Health and Human Services (2013)
3. Adalgeirsson, S.O., Breazeal, C.: Mebot: a robotic platform for socially embodied presence. In: Proceedings of the 5th ACM/IEEE International Conference on Human-robot Interaction, pp. 15–22. IEEE Press (2010)
4. Barker, J., Marxer, R., Vincent, E., Watanabe, S.: The thirdchime'speech separation. and recognition challenge: dataset, task and baselines. In: 2015 IEEE Automatic Speech Recognition and Understanding Workshop (ASRU 2015) (2015)
5. Baxter, P., Wood, R., Belpaeme, T.: A touchscreen-based 'sandtray' to facilitate, mediate and contextualise human-robot social interaction. In: Proceedings of the Seventh Annual ACM/IEEE International Conference on Human-Robot Interaction, HRI 2012, pp. 105–106. ACM, New York (2012)
6. Boreham, C., Riddoch, C.: The physical activity, fitness and health of children. J. Sports Sci. **19**(12), 915–929 (2001)
7. Ericsson: Ericsson mobility report, February 2016
8. Gerosa, M., et al.: A review of asr technologies for children's speech. In: Proceedings of the 2nd Workshop on Child, Computer and Interaction. ACM (2009)
9. Gorostiza, J.F., et al.: Multimodal human-robot interaction framework for a personal robot. In: The 15th IEEE International Symposium on Robot and Human Interactive Communication, ROMAN 2006, pp. 39–44. IEEE (2006)
10. Harms, C., Biocca, F.: Internal consistency and reliability of the networked minds measure of social presence (2004)
11. Heerink, M., et al.: Enjoyment intention to use and actual use of a conversational robot by elderly people. In: Proceedings of the 3rd ACM/IEEE International Conference on Human Robot Interaction, pp. 113–120. ACM, New York (2008)
12. Android Inc., speech (2014). http://developer.android.com/reference/android/speech/package-summary.html

13. Kozima, H., Michalowski, M.P., Nakagawa, C.: Keepon. Int. J. Social Robot. **1**(1), 3–18 (2009)
14. Kudryavstev, A.: Automatic speech recognition services comparison (2016). http://blog.griddynamics.com/2016/01/automatic-speech-recognition-services.html
15. Leite, I., Mascarenhas, S., Pereira, A., Martinho, C., Prada, R., Paiva, A.: "Why can't we be friends?" An empathic game companion for long-term interaction. In: Allbeck, J., Badler, N., Bickmore, T., Pelachaud, C., Safonova, A. (eds.) IVA 2010. LNCS (LNAI), vol. 6356, pp. 315–321. Springer, Heidelberg (2010). doi:10.1007/978-3-642-15892-6_32
16. Marcus, B.H., Forsyth, L.: Motivating People to be Physically Active. Human Kinetics, Champaign (2003)
17. Mendelson, M., Aboud, F.: McGill friendship questionnairerespondents affection (MFQ-RA). Measurement Instrument Database for the Social Science (2012)
18. Oudeyer, P.Y., Rouanet, P., Filliat, D.: An integrated system for teaching new visually grounded words to a robot for non-expert users using a mobile device. In: IEEE-RAS International Conference on Humanoid Robots, Tsukuba, Japan (2009)
19. Pereira, A., Prada, R., Paiva, A.: Socially present board game opponents. In: Nijholt, A., Romão, T., Reidsma, D. (eds.) ACE 2012. LNCS, vol. 7624, pp. 101–116. Springer, Heidelberg (2012). doi:10.1007/978-3-642-34292-9_8
20. Perzanowski, D., Schultz, A.C., Adams, W., Marsh, E., Bugajska, M.: Building a multimodal human-robot interface. IEEE Intell. Syst. **16**(1), 16–21 (2001)
21. Qiu, L., Benbasat, I.: An investigation into the effects of text-to-speech voice and 3D avatars on the perception of presence and flow of live help in electronic commerce. ACM Trans. Comput.-Hum. Interact. (TOCHI) **12**(4), 329–355 (2005)
22. Qiu, L., Benbasat, I.: Online consumer trust and live help interfaces: the effects of text-to-speech voice and three-dimensional avatars. Int. J. Hum.-Comput. Interact. **19**(1), 75–94 (2005)
23. Roe, D.B., Wilpon, J.G., et al.: Voice Communication Between Humans and Machines. National Academies Press, Washington, DC (1994)
24. Rybski, P.E., et al.: Interactive robot task training through dialog and demonstration. In: Proceedings of the ACM/IEEE International Conference on Human-robot Interaction, pp. 49–56. ACM, New York (2007)
25. Short, E., et al.: How to train your dragonbot: socially assistive robots for teaching children about nutrition through play. In: The 23rd International Symposium on Robot and Human Interactive Communication, pp. 924–929. IEEE (2014)
26. Short, J., Williams, E., Christie, B.: The Social Psychology of Telecommunications. Wiley, London (1976)
27. Skalski, P., Tamborini, R.: The role of social presence in interactive agent-based persuasion. Media Psychol. **10**(3), 385–413 (2007)
28. Slater, M.: Place illusion and plausibility can lead to realistic behaviour in immersive virtual environments. Philos. Trans. Royal Soc. Lond. B Biol. Sci. **364**(1535), 3549–3557 (2009)
29. Tickle-Degnen, L., Rosenthal, R.: The nature of rapport and its nonverbal correlates. Psychol. Inq. **1**(4), 285–293 (1990)

Understanding and Predicting Bonding in Conversations Using Thin Slices of Facial Expressions and Body Language

Natasha Jaques[1]([⊠]), Daniel McDuff[2], Yoo Lim Kim[3], and Rosalind Picard[1]

[1] MIT Media Lab, Cambridge, MA 02139, USA
{jaquesn,picard}@media.mit.edu
[2] Affectiva, Waltham, MA 02453, USA
daniel.mcduff@affectiva.com
[3] Wellesley College, Wellesley, MA 02481, USA
ykim9@wellesley.edu
http://affect.media.mit.edu/

Abstract. This paper investigates how an intelligent agent could be designed to both predict whether it is bonding with its user, and convey appropriate facial expression and body language responses to foster bonding. Video and Kinect recordings are collected from a series of naturalistic conversations, and a reliable measure of bonding is adapted and verified. A qualitative and quantitative analysis is conducted to determine the non-verbal cues that characterize both high and low bonding conversations. We then train a deep neural network classifier using one minute segments of facial expression and body language data, and show that it is able to accurately predict bonding in novel conversations.

Keywords: Facial expressions · Body language · Bonding · Rapport

1 Introduction

The most effective conversationalists do not simply smile, nod, and mirror their partner; instead, they are adept at sensing non-verbal cues and adapting to the other person's state. If an intelligent virtual agent (IVA) could be designed with this level of emotional intelligence, it could dynamically adapt its interaction style to the needs of the user. Such an endearing and empathetic IVA would have a wide range of applications, from intelligent tutoring, to human-robot interaction, to helping individuals who struggle with social interaction.

In this study we show that using facial expression and body language data from one-minute segments of a conversation (a.k.a. *thin slices*), a machine learning classifier can be trained to predict whether a novel person will experience bonding up to twenty minutes later. While it has been shown that humans have the ability to predict similar outcomes from such thin slices of an interaction [1], training computer algorithms to predict bonding using this data is a novel contribution. Data is collected unobtrusively using cameras and Microsoft Kinects

© Springer International Publishing AG 2016
D. Traum et al. (Eds.): IVA 2016, LNAI 10011, pp. 64–74, 2016.
DOI: 10.1007/978-3-319-47665-0_6

while participants engage in free-form conversations. Bonding is assessed empirically using a measure adapted from the Working Alliance Inventory [2]; we show that it is strongly related to conversation quality and rapport.

To provide insight into the data we have collected and the features extracted, we provide both a qualitative and quantitative analysis of facial expression and skeletal joint position features related to bonding. We also suggest ways that an IVA could learn to synthesize the appropriate non-verbal responses based on interaction context, and provide insight into the type of non-verbal behaviors that may arise in situations in which a person is either extremely frustrated with an interaction, or deeply engaged.

2   Related Work

A body of work has shown that using only thin slices (less than five minutes) of video of a person's non-verbal cues, human judges can predict everything from therapy outcomes to job performance [1]. Since computer algorithms have successfully predicted conversational outcomes like stress and engagement using audio data [3], it is possible that an IVA could use thin slices of facial expressions and body language to predict whether it is bonding with its user.

Non-verbal cues such as facial expressions and body language are a rich source of information about a person's mental state, and as such, there has been a great deal of research on how to detect, interpret, and display them. Although a thorough survey of all such work is impossible here, we refer the interested reader to a recent meta-analysis of the state of the art in automatic facial-expression recognition [4]. Automatic analysis of body-language has also been explored. For example, Avola and colleagues [5] developed a system that uses Kinect data to compute features of gestural strokes, and Yang and colleagues used motion capture data to show that friendly conversational dyads had a higher degree of correlation in body language gestures [6].

Most relevant to our work is research on bonding and rapport, which has been investigated in the context of the contingency (e.g. [7]) or mirroring (e.g. [8]) between the VA's behavior and the user. Detailed models of rapport have also been developed [9]. Other research has investigated which facial expressions generated by an agent led to the most rapport with its users [10].

3   User Study

Data were collected from a study in which participants conversed while being recorded with cameras, microphones, and Microsoft Kinects. To conceal the true nature of the study and ensure participants could act naturally, participants were told the purpose of the study was to train computer algorithms to read lips. They were instructed to stay within view of the recording devices, but not to over-emphasize their lip movements[1], and to keep the conversation flowing

---

[1] Even if some participants did speak with exaggerated lip movements, this would not affect our later analysis.

as naturally as possible. The interaction lasted for approximately 20 min, after which participants completed a post-study survey and were debriefed about the study's true purpose. All procedures were approved by the MIT IRB. In total we had 30 participants (13 male, 17 female) divided into 15 conversation dyads. There was variety across participants in terms of age ($M = 40.0$, $SD = 15.3$), occupation, ethnicity, and socioeconomic status.

The post-study survey contained a *Perception of Interaction* questionnaire similar to that of [11], in which participants gave Likert-scale ratings of their partner on a number of attributes, and completed the Bonding subscale of the Working Alliance Inventory (B-WAI). The WAI was developed to measure the degree of collaboration and trust between a therapist and their client; the bonding subscale is specifically designed to measure positive personal attachment, including "mutual trust, acceptance, and confidence" (p. 224) [2]. The scale was adapted for our study by removing three items irrelevant for short conversations between strangers (17, 21, and 36). The language of some other items was slightly modified to fit the interaction of a conversation; e.g. item 29 was changed to read "I had the feeling that if I said or did the wrong things, my partner would stop *talking* with me" rather than "working with me". Most items were unmodified. Typical items included "My partner and I understood each other", and "I felt uncomfortable with my partner".

4   Methods

Facial expression extraction. Automated software (Affdex - Affectiva, Inc.) [12] was applied to the videos to obtain confidence scores (from 0 to 100) indicating the presence of facial expressions. These included twelve facial action units from the Facial Action Coding System (FACS) [13], as well as smiles, lip corner pulls, seven expressions of emotion, and three axes of head pose (pitch, yaw and roll). After removing portions of the interaction in which the participant's face was not tracked, and downsampling each signal to 1 Hz to ensure smooth estimates, we obtained facial expression data for 13,714 s of conversation.

Skeletal joint extraction. Microsoft Kinects were used to gather data about the X (horizontal), Y (vertical) and Z (depth) position of participants' joints, including the head, neck, thumbs, finger tips, four positions on each limb, and three positions on the spine. To clean this data we removed portions of the interaction in which a second body was tracked, and 4 s segments in which the derivative was more than two standard deviations above the mean in any axis (X, Y or Z) (which is often due to the Kinect briefly losing track of the participant). After removing noise, minutes of the interaction that were missing more than 60 % of the data were discarded, due to the unreliability of the signal during this period. The joint data was then aligned with the video data. Finally, we applied a z-score normalization to the data from each axis of each joint, which reduces effects due to the Kinect being placed in slightly different locations for different participants.

Machine learning classification. To train our machine learning model, we extracted features from each minute of conversation for each participant and their partner. From the skeletal data, we computed five features for each joint's X, Y, and Z positions: the mean, std. dev., max. of the abs. derivative, mean derivative, and max. of the abs. second derivative. These features provide information about the position, degree of movement, speed of movement, direction of movement, and sharpness of movement (acceleration), respectively. For facial expressions, we computed the sum, mean, and std. dev. of each feature, telling us the amount, degree, and variability in expression. In total we obtained 375 joint and 143 facial expression features for each of 532 min of conversation.

Each minute was assigned a binary classification label, based on whether it belonged to a conversation with high or low bonding (scores were split based on the median B-WAI). The data were then randomly partitioned into training, validation, and testing sets. Data from each participant were assigned to only one set. Thus, the testing set represents completely novel, held-out data.

To reduce the number of features, we used Correlation-based Feature Selection (CFS) [14]. CFS chooses a subset of features that are both strongly predictive of an outcome variable (in this case bonding), but also have low correlation with the rest of the features in the subset (are not redundant). CFS was applied only to the training data, to avoid contaminating the testing data. Neural network models were then trained on the CFS features using Google's TensorFlow library [15]. Both single-layer and deep architectures were explored, and parameters were tuned using the validation set.

5   Results

In this section we will provide evidence establishing the reliability of the modified B-WAI, and give examples of the type of data we have collected and ways in which it can be used to detect bonding. A quantitative analysis of the differences in facial expressions and body language between participants with high and low bonding will be provided. Finally, we show that machine learning can be applied to these features to accurately predict bonding up to 20 min later.

Reliability of the bonding scale. The following analysis relies on B-WAI as an aggregate measure of bonding, rapport, and participants' perceptions of their conversations as warm, comfortable, and enjoyable. To examine how well B-WAI captures these characteristics, we tested the correlations between it and eight self-reported Likert-scale ratings of conversation quality (see Table 1). We see that B-WAI is related to participants' ratings of their partner as *interesting*, *charming*, *friendly*, and *funny*, and inversely related to their ratings of *distant* and *annoying*. After applying a Bonferroni correction, the relationships between B-WAI and *interesting*, *annoying*, and *distant* remained significant, suggesting that B-WAI is strongly related to participants' perceived conversation quality.

Qualitative analysis. In this section we provide examples of the facial expression and body language data we have collected, showing that the interaction

Table 1. Pearson's r correlations between B-WAI and conversation quality. Bolded measures are significant after performing a Bonferroni correction.

Measure	r	p		Measure	r	p
Interesting	**.6912**	**<.001**		**Distant**	**-.6207**	**<.001**
Charming	.4342	.021		**Annoying**	**-.5549**	**.001**
Friendly	.3806	.038		Awkward	-.2589	.167
Funny	.3736	.046				
Engaging	.1104	.561				

(a) Positive correlations   (b) Negative correlations

between the two participants is highly relevant to bonding. For example, Fig. 1 plots five minutes of facial expressions which occurred between the participant who experienced the lowest bonding in our study, P_l (top), and her partner (bottom). Although P_l began the interaction with frequent smiling, in the portion of the interaction plotted in Fig. 1, she shows expressions of sadness as she is discussing a highly personal topic. Instead of responding empathetically, her partner continues to smile and smirk. Eventually P_l becomes angry, and afterwards simply stops emoting; for the rest of the conversation, she shows little or no facial expressions whatsoever. This interaction underlines the importance of designing an IVA to both detect emotional cues, and display the appropriate response at the right time. Further, it could suggest that an emotionally intelligent agent may need to treat a sudden suppression of affect as a potential warning sign of an upset or frustrated user.

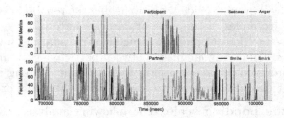

Fig. 1. Five minutes of facial expressions from the conversation with the least bonding, in which the participant's partner fails to respond empathetically.

While displaying the appropriate emotional cues in response to an unhappy user can be considered a minimum requirement of an emotionally intelligent VA, promoting a high degree of bonding and rapport can be much more subtle and complex. Figure 2 plots the Z position of the Spine Mid joint for the two participants in the conversation with the highest bonding. The distance maintained between the participants reveals a high degree of synchrony, suggesting they are highly attentive and responsive to each others' movements.

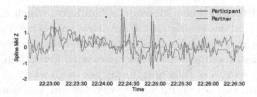

Fig. 2. Spine Mid Z for the participant with the highest bonding and her partner.

Quantitative analysis. In this section we will establish what kinds of facial expression and skeletal position features are relevant to bonding, and discuss design implications for an IVA. To begin, we analyzed which facial expression behaviors are more frequent in conversations with high vs. low bonding, by computing the difference in average *z-score* between both groups. Figure 3 shows the three features that had the greatest difference for both high and low bonding conversations, for the participant themselves, and their partner[2]. T-tests with a Bonferroni correction were used to assess whether high and low bonding conversations differed significantly on these features, and all of them reached significance at the $\alpha = .05$ level.

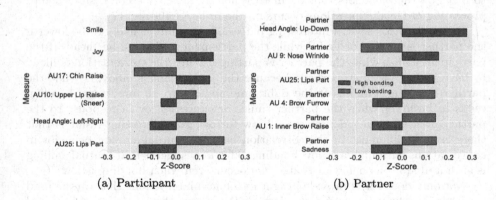

(a) Participant   (b) Partner

Fig. 3. The participant and partner's facial expressions with the largest differences between conversations with high bonding (blue) and conversations with low bonding (red). If the Z-score is below zero, it means the behavior was less frequent in this group's conversations relative to the overall average. (Color figure online)

Figure 3 reveals some expected trends. When the participant experiences bonding, she is more likely to smile, express joy, and raise her chin. When she feels that bonding is low, she is more likely to sneer and shake her head (see *Head angle left right* in Fig. 3a). In terms of the partner's behavior, frequent nodding (*Head angle up down*) and nose wrinkling is associated with higher bonding. Nose

---

[2] The participant is the one who completes the B-WAI about their partner.

wrinkling is often detected when someone is laughing, which has been found to be both deferential and endearing [16]. Conversely, negative displays of emotion by the partner appear to hinder bonding; frequent brow furrows, inner eyebrow raises, or expressions of sadness are associated with lower bonding. An intriguing thing to note, however, is that bonding is not symmetric. A participant who did not enjoy an interaction could score very low on the bonding scale, even though her partner felt fine about the conversation and scored relatively high (and indeed this does occur). Therefore asymmetric effects can occur, such as with the *lips part* AU (frequently detected when a person is speaking).

Although Fig. 3 provides some interesting insights, without accounting for interaction context it can only give an incomplete picture of facial expressions and bonding. Therefore we investigate how the contingency between conversational partners' expressions differs with bonding. We computed the Pearson's r correlations between each participant's facial expressions and their partner's, for conversations with high bonding (r_h) and low bonding (r_l). The difference between these coefficients was then computed as $r_{diff} = r_h - r_l$, and plotted in Fig. 4. Blue locations in the grid correspond to behaviors that occurred together more frequently in high bonding conversations; red locations occurred more in low bonding conversations[3]. We also tested the correlation with the partner's behavior both 1 s and 5 s later. The results were similar, therefore we choose to focus on the behaviors that occur together in the same second, since neural processing of facial expressions occurs on the order of 100 ms [17].

Figure 4 reveals several interesting patterns[4]. Bonding is likely to be lower if the partner is smiling or joyful while the participant is shaking her head. If the participant smiles while the partner is parting her lips the conversation is likely to have higher bonding, perhaps because the participant is enjoying what the partner is saying. Smiling at the right time appears to be important; bonding tends to be lower when the partner smiles or expresses joy in response to the participant's lip corner depressor or brow furrow. An interesting result is that there is little difference in the correlation between mutual smiling behavior in conversations with high and low bonding. This may suggest that mutual smiling is such a ubiquitous behavior that it can occur even when bonding is low.

Not only does Fig. 4 provide insight into micro-interactions that can be used to detect bonding, it could also allow an IVA to synthesize appropriate facial responses. Consider the heatmap scores as probabilities that the agent could use when deciding what expression to display. If the user tilts her head (see the row *Head angle roll*), then the probability of the agent raising its outer eyebrows should be high, and the probability of it shaking its head should be low or almost zero. This approach is likely to be more effective than simple mirroring, because it captures the appropriateness of the expression in context.

---

[3] Note again that bonding is not symmetric and neither is the matrix in Fig. 4; it is computed based on the participant's perception of bonding, not her partner's.

[4] There are several strong differences in inner eyebrow raising, however this AU can be associated with either sadness or happiness, making it difficult to interpret [18].

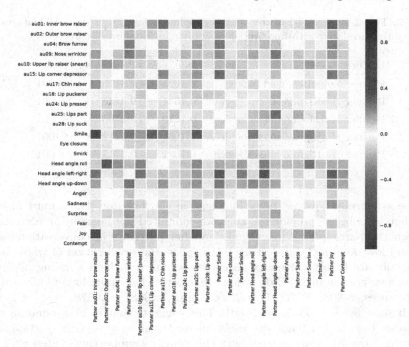

Fig. 4. The heatmap shows the difference in correlation coefficient ($r_{diff} = r_h - r_l$) between conversations with high bonding (r_h) and low bonding (r_l). Blue tiles represent a correlation that is more strongly positive in high bonding conversations, while red represents a correlation more prevalent in low bonding. (Color figure online)

A similar analysis is applied to the joint data collected with the Microsoft Kinect. After performing CFS feature selection as described in Sect. 4, we were left with a total of 69 non-redundant[5] joint features. For each of these, we computed the *information gain*, which can be interpreted as the reduction in uncertainty about one variable obtained after observing another [19]. Essentially, information gain tells us which features are most predictive of bonding. The five features with the highest information gain are listed in Table 2.

These joint features reveal that the partner's movements in the Z direction (towards or away from the participant) are highly related to whether the participant experiences bonding. The features relate to the position of the partner's whole body, such as the spine, hips, and knees. Since these features describe the acceleration, variability, and speed of movement, a larger degree of movement of the partner's whole body may be more indicative of a high bonding conversation. Perhaps in conversations in which the partner is engaged and attentive, this enthusiasm is displayed by larger and more animated whole-body movements.

---

[5] After CFS, two body part features that are highly correlated (for example, the left and right hips) will be represented by only one of the pair (e.g. the right hip).

Table 2. The skeletal joint features with the highest information gain. All features are significantly correlated with bonding after applying a Bonferroni correction.

Feature	Info. gain	Pearson's r	p
Partner SpineBaseZ sd	0.1695	0.4190	<.001
Partner HipRightZ sd	0.1541	0.4146	<.001
Partner KneeLeftZ max abs acc	0.1219	0.3505	<.001
Partner HipRightZ max abs deriv	0.1091	0.3712	<.001
Partner HipRightZ max abs acc	0.1091	0.3712	<.001

The synchrony between body language in conversation dyads must also be considered. As in the previous section, we computed the Pearson's r correlation between the participant's movements and her partner's in conversations with high and low bonding[6]. Interestingly, the speed and acceleration of whole body movements are highly correlated in conversations with high bonding. Correlations in acceleration in the Z direction are in some cases quite large; for example, for the knees, $r(308) = .5226$, $p < .001$, hips, $r(308) = .4578$, $p < .001$, and spine base, $r(308) = .4465$, $p < .001$. This suggests that in high-bonding conversations, the partner tends to closely mirror the sharpness of the participant's movements towards or away from her. This provides supporting evidence for the hypothesis generated in the previous section, that there is a great deal of synchrony in terms of whole body movements in pairs with high bonding. Agents that can mirror whole body movements (e.g. [8]) may be highly effective at facilitating bonding.

Predicting bonding in novel conversations. Using one-minute slices of the facial expression and body language features described above, we trained a series of neural network models to predict bonding, as explained in Sect. 4. We found that a deep architecture with 2 layers of 300 and 12 hidden nodes[7] led to the highest validation accuracy, of 64.7 % (AUC = .678). Using this model, we obtained an accuracy of 85.87 % and an AUC of .931 on the held-out test data, showing we can accurately predict bonding in novel conversations. Note that 66.3 % of the samples in the test set belong to high-bonding interactions, so this result is almost 20 % better than the baseline majority-class classifier (always guessing the most frequent class).

While these results are promising, they should be interpreted with caution given the small size of the testing dataset ($N = 92$, representing data from 6 participants). While the validation accuracy still exceeded the majority-class baseline of 60.78 % for the validation set, it was notably lower than the test accuracy. This is likely due to the random partitioning process and the small size of the datasets. Nevertheless, because the test set comprises novel users from

---

[6] A similar heatmap was generated, but there is insufficient space to show it here.

[7] The other parameter settings were: learning rate = .01, batch size = 20, L2 regularization $\beta = .01$, no dropout.

which the classifier has never accessed data, this serves as a proof-of-concept that it is possible for an IVA to use data collected unobtrusively from a camera and Kinect to detect whether it is bonding with a new user during each minute of the conversation. Such fine-grained sensitivity to the user's perceptions could allow an IVA to dynamically adapt to improve bonding throughout the interaction, just like an excellent human conversationalist.

6 Conclusions and Future Work

We have shown that facial expression and body language features can allow an IVA to detect whether or not it is bonding with its user. We also presented a matrix, learned from human high and low bonding interactions, that could allow an IVA to generate the appropriate facial expressions and body language in response to user behavior. We have shown that a machine learning classifier can be trained to predict whether a person will experience high or low bonding, given only a one-minute slice of facial expression and body language data. This information can be gathered unobtrusively with a camera and Kinect, making the classification system potentially highly useful to a future IVA.

As future work, the next step is to analyze the audio data, for prosody, emotional tone, and speaking turns. There are also many ways in which the modeling of the data could be improved. For example, a time-series analysis technique such as a Hidden Markov Model [19] could be employed to infer the participant's mental state (bonding or not) throughout the interaction, and the joint positions could be further abstracted into higher level gestures, as described by Avola et al. [5]. Even without these improvements, this work has contributed novel fundamental elements enabling the crafting of future agents with which human partners will bond.

References

1. Ambady, N., Rosenthal, R.: Thin slices of expressive behavior as predictors of interpersonal consequences: a meta-analysis. Psychol. Bull. **111**, 256 (1992)
2. Horvath, A., Greenberg, L.: Development and validation of the working alliance inventory. J. Couns. Psychol. **36**(2), 223 (1989)
3. Pentland, A.: Social dynamics: signals and behavior. In: International Conference on Developmental Learning, vol. 5 (2004)
4. Valstar, M., et al.: Meta-analysis of the first facial expression recognition challenge. Syst. Man Cybern. **42**(4), 966–979 (2012)
5. Avola, D., Cinque, L., Levialdi, S., Placidi, G.: Human body language analysis: a preliminary study based on kinect skeleton tracking. In: Petrosino, A., Maddalena, L., Pala, P. (eds.) ICIAP 2013. LNCS, vol. 8158, pp. 465–473. Springer, Heidelberg (2013). doi:10.1007/978-3-642-41190-8_50
6. Yang, Z., Metallinou, A., Narayanan, S.: Analysis and predictive modeling of body language behavior in dyadic interactions from multimodal interlocutor cues. Multimedia **16**(6), 1766–1778 (2014)

7. Gratch, J., Wang, N., Gerten, J., Fast, E., Duffy, R.: Creating rapport with virtual agents. In: Pelachaud, C., Martin, J.-C., André, E., Chollet, G., Karpouzis, K., Pelé, D. (eds.) IVA 2007. LNCS (LNAI), vol. 4722, pp. 125–138. Springer, Heidelberg (2007). doi:10.1007/978-3-540-74997-4_12

8. Kahl, S., Kopp, S.: Modeling a social brain for interactive agents: integrating mirroring and mentalizing. In: Brinkman, W.-P., Broekens, J., Heylen, D. (eds.) IVA 2015. LNCS (LNAI), vol. 9238, pp. 77–86. Springer, Heidelberg (2015). doi:10.1007/978-3-319-21996-7_8

9. Zhao, R., Papangelis, A., Cassell, J.: Towards a dyadic computational model of rapport management for human-virtual agent interaction. In: Bickmore, T., Marsella, S., Sidner, C. (eds.) IVA 2014. LNCS (LNAI), vol. 8637, pp. 514–527. Springer, Heidelberg (2014). doi:10.1007/978-3-319-09767-1_62

10. Wong, J.W.-E., McGee, K.: Frown more, talk more: effects of facial expressions in establishing conversational rapport with virtual agents. In: Nakano, Y., Neff, M., Paiva, A., Walker, M. (eds.) IVA 2012. LNCS (LNAI), vol. 7502, pp. 419–425. Springer, Heidelberg (2012). doi:10.1007/978-3-642-33197-8_43

11. Cuperman, R., Ickes, W.: Big five predictors of behavior and perceptions in initial dyadic interactions. J. Pers. Soc. Psych. **97**(4), 667 (2009)

12. McDuff, D., et al.: AFFDEX SDK: a cross-platform real-time multi-face expression recognition toolkit. In: CHI, pp. 3723–3726. ACM (2016)

13. Ekman, P., Friesen, W.: Facial action coding system (1977)

14. Hall, M.A.: Correlation-based feature subset selection for machine learning, Ph.D. thesis, University of Waikato, Hamilton, New Zealand (1998)

15. Abadi, M., et al.: TensorFlow: large-scale machine learning on heterogeneous systems. Software (2015). tensorflow.org

16. Provine, R.R.: Laughter: A Scientific Investigation. Penguin, New York (2001)

17. Meeren, H., van Heijnsbergen, C., de Gelder, B.: Rapid perceptual integration of facial expression and emotional body language. PNAS **102**, 16518–16523 (2005)

18. Kohler, C., et al.: Differences in facial expressions of four universal emotions. Psychiatr. Res. **128**(3), 235–244 (2004)

19. Murphy, K.P.: Machine Learning: A Probabilistic Perspective. MIT press, Cambridge (2012)

The Effect of Embodiment and Competence on Trust and Cooperation in Human–Agent Interaction

Philipp Kulms[✉] and Stefan Kopp

Social Cognitive Systems Group, Faculty of Technology, Center of Excellence
'Cognitive Interaction Technology' (CITEC), Bielefeld University, Bielefeld, Germany
{pkulms,skopp}@techfak.uni-bielefeld.de

Abstract. Success in extended human–agent interaction depends on the ability of the agent to cooperate over repeated tasks. Yet, it is not clear how cooperation and trust change over the course of such interactions, and how this is interlinked with the developing perception of competence of the agent or its social appearance. We report findings from a human–agent experiment designed to measure trust in task-oriented cooperation with agents that vary in competence and embodiment. Results in terms of behavioral and subjective measures demonstrate an initial effect of embodiment, changing over time to a relatively higher importance of agent competence.

Keywords: Human–agent interaction · Trust · Cooperation · Embodiment

1 Introduction

It has often been noted that future interaction with technology may be designed like a cooperation between partners with complementary competencies [5]. In such teams, each agent has some degree of autonomy to handle dynamic situations and to make decisions within uncertain situations. As part of the cooperation, agents may plan and suggest to their partners – human or artificial – possible actions. Disentangling under which conditions humans accept such approaches and benefit from them is crucial. One key aspect is that users are willing and able to trust an agent. However, it is unclear how user trust is related to the perceived capabilities of an agent, in particular regarding the altering abilities of learning agents with possibly unanticipated behavior. Shaping the social interaction with such agents may be a key variable in those situations. Interactions with virtual agents are known to elicit social effects similar to human–human interaction [17]. In this paper we present work that investigates the potential of IVAs to support trust and how it develops in, and influence an ongoing human–agent cooperation. In particular, we present a human–agent cooperation study to investigate how perceived competence and the visual presence of a virtual agent affect the interaction and user trust.

© Springer International Publishing AG 2016
D. Traum et al. (Eds.): IVA 2016, LNAI 10011, pp. 75–84, 2016.
DOI: 10.1007/978-3-319-47665-0_7

2   Theoretical Background

Social Factors of Trust and Cooperation. Trust is the willingness of an agent (trustor) to be vulnerable to the actions of another agent (trustee) based on the expectation that the trustee will perform a particular action [18]. The trustee has characteristics that help the trustor to decide whether placing its trust in this agent is risky or not. These characteristics (ability, benevolence, and integrity) form the trustee's trustworthiness and promote trust, but trust and trustworthiness are not identical [18]. Ability (i.e., competence) as a "can-do" component describes the extent to which the trustee can enact its motives toward a specific goal, while benevolence and integrity as "will-do" descriptions pertain to whether the trustee wants to use its abilities to act in the best interest of the trustor [8]. Trust and cooperation are often used interchangeably [12]. Indeed, trust facilitates cooperation and vice versa [9], yet cooperation is also possible without trust. Another misconception is the assumed equality behind trust in and credibility of computers. In contrast to trust, credibility is a perceived quality and phrases like "trusting in information" or "believing the output" refer to credibility, not trust [14]. In cooperative relations the goals of two agents are positively related, that is, if one agent increases the chances of achieving its goal, the other agents chances to achieve its goal are also promoted [12]. Various reasons can lead to positive goal interdependence: a necessary division of work to achieve otherwise unattainable task goals, reward structures based on joint achievements, sharing of resources, being faced with the same obstacle, or holding common membership of a social group [11].

Cooperation in Human–Computer Interaction. Computers are increasingly understood as partners that people affiliate with [21]. Recent evidence indicates that humans are able to work together with computers in complex task settings (see [5] for an overview). This evolution requires that computers and machines accurately communicate their trustworthiness, even if they are competent, and that humans develop an appropriate level of trust that matches the trustworthiness of the output, e.g. decision support [20]. Accordingly, Dautenhahn [10] referred to socially intelligent agents as agents that offer or mediate cooperation and problem solving through social abilities similar to humans. Examples of human–agent settings explain the importance of social attributions: participants responded with commitment to agent-led teams, yet agents gained less trust and fairness than humans [25]. Other work has shown that agent trustworthiness correlates with both agent and team performance [15]. Human-like interfaces offer unique possibilities to design meaningful task-oriented interactions through nonverbal communication [7] or multimodal cues [24]. Virtual agents are an instantiation of such human-like interfaces. People interacting with virtual agents usually report a more personal experience, a phenomenon tracing back to humans' tendency to mindlessly applying social rules to computers [22]. Virtual agents operating as decision support yield social benefits that go beyond common technology adoption explanations [23]. Through their visual presence, they provide support and persuasion toward a desirable outcome (see [2] for an overview). In a study that investigated the effect of the human-like interface in a dialog-based setting, a virtual agent elicited stronger social responses than text-based interaction [1]. On the flip side, presenting virtual agents along with tasks may incur costs on memory performance [3] and heightens expectations in realism, leading to decreased willingness to cooperate with the agent [16] (see also [4]). The context in which virtual agents are embedded plays an important role. Early work emphasized their role as personal assistants that mediate between the user and the interaction goals with applications ranging from pedagogical agents to information systems, sales agents, and museum guides to name a few examples. In the past few years, virtual agents have been increasingly considered as a source of simple yet meaningful cues that affect perceived trustworthiness and people's willingness to cooperate with them in social dilemmas (e.g. [19]). This perspective holds that people do not blindly guess their virtual counterpart's upcoming response (cooperation or defection) but use contextual cues to infer the decision. The fundamental goal of building trusting relationships with artificial agents is thus nuanced by exploring the boundaries and behavioral consequences of trust and trustworthiness.

In sum, many studies support the idea of intelligent agents as teammates in complex settings and that human-like virtual agents lead to specific affective and behavioral responses of the user. However, it is still unclear when and how trust and cooperation emerge and develop in team-like scenarios that are dynamic, require competence, and extend over many interactions.

3   Overview of Approach

We aim to investigate how trust in and cooperation with a human-like agent evolve over time. It is crucial to investigate these dynamics as humans are very sensitive to the social implication of others' behavior for themselves [13]. We assume this is also true when interacting with artificial agents given that people tend to anthropomorphize computers [22]. In line with previous work, we consider computers as social agents that people interact with in a meaningful way and contrast an embodied agent with a non-embodied one. We adopt a dynamic human–agent interaction scenario with a joint goal, allowing us to manipulate key components of cooperation between social agents. This extends prior research using standard cooperative games in that we unravel how humans perceive intelligent agents in strategic problem-solving.

Interaction Scenario. We propose an interaction framework in order to analyze key characteristics of social cooperative behavior – human-like cues, trust, competence, trustworthiness – in a systematic fashion. The general setting has two partners solve a puzzle game interactively. Here we present and motivate the general framework and describe the interaction scenario used in the experiment. Inspired by Tetris, the interaction scenario consists of a board where two players work together to place blocks of two shapes, using horizontal movements and rotation. In contrast to Tetris, blocks do not move down gradually

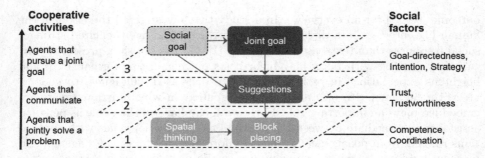

Fig. 1. Cooperative activities in the game and corresponding social factors.

and filled lines are not cleared. The latter eases the implementation of an algorithm for the virtual agent to participate as autonomous player. The interaction scenario encompasses a number of actions and elements that can be arranged hierarchically (see Fig. 1). At layer one the agents are both working towards a joint goal, which requires them to coordinate and place the blocks in the puzzle game competently and in response to each others' actions. This layer hence pertains to joint problem-solving based on competence and coordination. The activities on this layer largely determine if the puzzle is solved efficiently or not. Layer two offers the possibility to exchange task-related information. The human players can request this information and need to decide whether the agent's task-related suggestion can be trusted. Trusting a suggestion depends on its quality, the agent's trustworthiness (i.e., competence, perceived intentions), warmth, and other factors we exclude here (e.g., an individual's propensity to trust, own competence). Depending on how much the agent is perceived as social entity, people may see it as tool, assistant, or partner with its own goals. Layer three adds an external goal connected to a specific payoff and hence implies strategic cooperation. In the present study (see below), the payoff is equal for both players. In sum, people may assume the agent is essentially responsive to their actions on the lowest layer, yet how much this commitment comprises support [6] or benevolence [18] is unknown.

4   Experiment

We conducted a laboratory experiment where participants tried to solve a puzzle with an embodied vs. non-embodied that offers task-related suggestions, allowing us to directly analyze the effect of human-like cues on trust. To tease apart how much people are willing to trust computer generated advice in situations that are highly interdependent and thus require competence as well as coordination, we also varied the quality of the agent's suggestions. The study had a 2 (agent embodiment: yes vs. no) × 2 (suggestion quality: good vs. bad) between-subjects design with 55 participants ($M_{age} = 25.07$, $SD_{age} = 4.99$) taking part in exchange for 5 EUR.

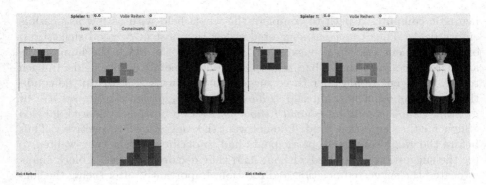

Fig. 2. The game interface in the embodied conditions. Suggestions by the agent are shown at the top in light blue. Left: the agent provides a useful suggestion. Right: the agent makes a bad suggestion. (Color figure online)

4.1 Method

The game proceeds in turn-based interactions. Players draw one of two available blocks from an urn without replacement. In each round the agent is the first to choose a block, leaving the remaining one to the participant. The joint goal is to complete a specific number of rows such that it is entirely filled with blocks (see Fig. 2). In contrast to Tetris, completed rows are not emptied and there is no time restriction. Completing a row yields 100 points for each player. In each game, the total goal yields a joint payoff such that the score gets doubled for each player. Thus the payoff for both players is always identical. Participants were instructed to work toward the joint goal together with their partner. They were also told that throughout the game, their partner would offer suggestions as to how they could place their block and that they are not obliged to respond in a specific manners. The interaction lasted three games in total with the goal becoming increasingly more difficult (4 rows, 5 rows, 6 rows). The goal was displayed beneath the puzzle field. The progress toward the goal and the payoffs were shown above of it, hence participants saw the distance to the goal and when it was attained. After each game, participants were given a summary sheet showing the payoffs and whether the goal was attained. Before the interaction, participants familiarized themselves with the controls and mechanics without an agent being present. After the interaction, participants filled out the post-questionnaire and rated the agent on task-related social dimensions.

Manipulations. The first factor, agent embodiment, determined whether participants played with a virtual agent we called Sam that was introduced as virtual person (*E*: embodied) or with a computer (*NE*: non-embodied). Sam was positioned next to the puzzle field. Aside from eye blinking and breathing behavior, Sam did not show specific nonverbal behaviors. The second factor, suggestion quality, determined how the agent made a suggestion that was drawn from a heuristic we implemented to solve the remaining puzzle field. At each step, the heuristic computes a path to complete the whole field with as few as possible empty fields. Thus the agent suggested either the most (*GS*: good suggestion) or least efficient (*BS*: bad suggestion) solution for the block the human was about to place, such that a bad suggestion would generate empty fields. In each round, the agent would offer three suggestions (in turns 2, 4, 6). In the conditions with embodiment, Sam said *"I have suggestion, do you want to see it?"* or *"I think I know a solution, should I show you?"* Two buttons appeared, labeled "Show me the suggestion" and "I do not want the suggestion", respectively. Thus before the game continued, participants had to decide whether they wanted to see the suggestion or proceed without it. If they decided to see it, a block shape indicated the suggested position and rotation. Importantly, after seeing the suggestion, participants could decide to adopt it or not. In the conditions without embodiment, the buttons appeared at the same locations.

Dependent Variables. We segmented the extent to which participants developed trust into three behavioral measures that reflect their response to the agent's offers: offer ignored, suggestion requested but declined, suggestion requested and adopted (for each max. = 9, min. = 0). Second, we computed how often participants attained the goal. Third, participants were asked to rate the agent's trustworthiness and competence, using items proposed by [14] to measure computer credibility (5-point Likert scales). The competence items were 'knowledgeable', 'competent', 'intelligent', 'capable', 'experienced', and 'powerful' (Cronbach's $\alpha = .90$). The trustworthiness items were 'trustworthy', 'good', 'truthful', 'well-intentioned', 'unbiased', and 'honest' ($\alpha = .84$).

Research Questions. In this setting the agent offers suggestions like an expert system, yet also plays an active part in the cooperative problem-solving. We hypothesize that the quality of suggestions will impact perceived competence. Second, we explore whether a human-like agent affects people's willingness to request suggestions and their trust in suggestions as indicated by the adoption.

4.2   Results

Goal Attainment. Figure 3 shows how often the human–agent teams achieved the goal. The maximum per condition was 14 (EGS, EBS) and 13 (NEBS, NEGS), respectively. Again, note that the three games had rising difficulty. We conducted logistic regressions with goal attainment as dependent variable and (a) requested suggestion, (b) adopted suggestion, (c) embodiment and suggestion quality as separate block-wise independent variables, to tease apart whether trust or the conditions influenced goal attainment. No significant effects were found. This indicates that how the agent (and its human partners) actually played was the most important predictor of goal attainment.

Behavioral Decisions to Trust. Figure 4 shows participants' responses to the nine agent offerings across all three games. We conducted a 2×2 MANOVA with embodiment and suggestion quality as independent and the three trust variables

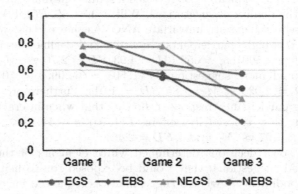

Fig. 3. Goal attainment per game with each agent.

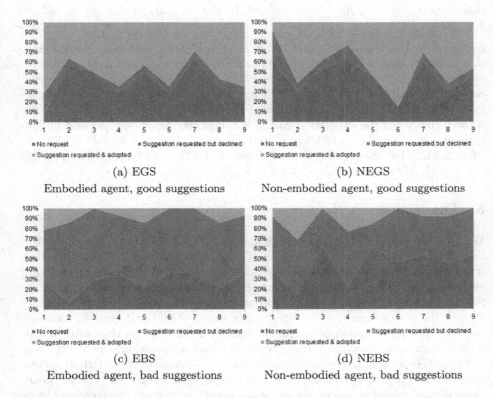

(a) EGS
Embodied agent, good suggestions

(b) NEGS
Non-embodied agent, good suggestions

(c) EBS
Embodied agent, bad suggestions

(d) NEBS
Non-embodied agent, bad suggestions

Fig. 4. Participant responses to each of the nine agent's offers (suggestion requested or not) and suggestions (adopted or rejected).

as dependent variables. The analysis revealed a significant difference for the variables based on the quality of suggestions, Wilk's $\Lambda = .35, F(2, 49) = 46.11, p < .001$ (1 case missing). Separate univariate ANOVAs showed that when the suggestion quality was high, participants requested and declined less suggestions, $F(1, 50) = 55.04, p < .001, \eta_p^2 = .52$ ($M = 4.93, SD = 2.70$ vs. $M = .85, SD = 1.11$), and adopted more suggestions, $F(1, 50) = 64.09, p < .001, \eta_p^2 = .56$ ($M = 4.44, SD = 2.02$ vs. $M = .85, SD = 1.01$). Furthermore, there was a tendency among participants' responses showing that when interacting with the embodied agent, they ignored less offers, $F(1, 50) = 3.11, p < .10, \eta_p^2 = .06$ ($M = 2.96, SD = 1.97$ vs. $M = 4.04, SD = 2.46$).

Participants' own decisions determined which elements of the interaction (i.e., good or bad suggestions) they would be exposed to. To help tease apart the effect of embodiment on when a suggestion was requested for the first time, we computed a 2×2 ANOVA with the point at which the first suggestion was requested as dependent variable while ignoring subsequent decisions as, prior to this point, the suggestion quality was unknown. The results revealed that when interacting with the embodied agent, participants requested the first suggestion sooner, $F(1, 50) = 6.20, p < .05, \eta_p^2 = .11$ ($M = 1.21, SD = .50$ vs. $M = 1.81, SD = 1.17$).

Subjective Ratings. We conducted a 2×2 MANOVA with embodiment and suggestion quality as independent and perceived competence and trustworthiness as dependent variables. The analysis revealed a significant difference in perceived competence and trustworthiness of the agent based on the quality of its suggestions, Wilk's $\Lambda = .70, F(2, 50) = 10.88, p < .001$. Separate univariate ANOVAs showed that when the suggestion quality was high, the agent was ascribed higher competence, $F(1, 51) = 18.90, p < .001, \eta_p^2 = .27$ ($M = 3.29, SD = .72$ vs. $M = 2.33, SD = .87$), and trustworthiness, $F(1, 51) = 10.76, p < .01, \eta_p^2 = .17$ ($M = 3.35, SD = .82$ vs. $M = 2.60, SD = .85$).

5   Discussion

We have presented an experimental design for investigating trust in cooperative human–agent interaction. The results of an experiment conducted within this framework indicate that over time, participants based their decision-making and subjective evaluations of perceived competence and trustworthiness primarily on the quality of suggestions (i.e., competence). However, especially at the beginning of the interaction, the embodied agent clearly facilitated trust in terms of requests for and adoption of suggested actions. It thus seems that while agent embodiment does facilitate initial acceptance and cooperation, this effect does not last. When cooperation needs to extend over a period of time, virtual agents may thus not be displayed constantly but appear when needed. If possible, critical decisions should be addressed at the beginning to leverage the increased level of trust. In our setting, suggestions were not suddenly given but first offered and then provided upon request. When an offer was accepted out of attributed trustworthiness or curiosity, the suggestion could still be rejected. Indeed, the embodied agent evoked the first requested suggestion sooner, indicating a potentially useful effect of human-like cues for cooperation. Further work is needed to investigate the circumstances predicting when this first step is taken by users, and how it could result in trust in terms of advice adoption. The two-step approach may be useful for decreasing regret in decisions and to keep the user in charge. Finally, in a way, our results rectify the social dimension of human–agent cooperation according to which the dynamic process of trusting each other plays an important role. Depending on their own responses, participants took different paths through the interaction. Some trusted the agent early on and presumably assessed the adopted suggestion against their own solutions and competence. Declining an offer right away after suggestions were already requested and/or adopted has thus distinct implications for the trust *quality* and may mean that participants felt the agent's competence would provide no additional value at all. In contrast, requesting but rejecting suggestions has a different meaning as it reflects the need to at least evaluate the agent's competence. This has important implications for how agents should communicate their competence and trustworthiness.

Acknowledgments. This research was supported by the German Federal Ministry of Education and Research (BMBF) within the Leading-Edge Cluster 'its OWL', managed by the Project Management Agency Karlsruhe (PTKA), as well as by the Deutsche Forschungsgemeinschaft (DFG) within the Center of Excellence 277 'Cognitive Interaction Technology' (CITEC).

References

1. Appel, J., von der Pütten, A., Krämer, N.C., Gratch, J.: Does humanity matter? Analyzing the importance of social cues and perceived agency of a computer system for the emergence of social reactions during human-computer interaction. Adv. Hum. Comput. Interact. **2012**(2), 1–10 (2012)
2. Baylor, A.L.: Promoting motivation with virtual agents and avatars: role of visual presence and appearance. Philos. Trans. Royal Soc. Lond. Ser. B Biol. Sci. **364**(1535), 3559–3565 (2009)
3. Berry, D.C., Butler, L.T., Rosis, F.: Evaluating a realistic agent in an advice-giving task. Int. J. Hum. Comput. Stud. **63**(3), 304–327 (2005)
4. Blascovich, J.: A theoretical model of social influence for increasing the utility of collaborative virtual environments. In: Proceedings of the 4th International Conference on Collaborative Virtual Environments, pp. 25–30. ACM, New York (2002)
5. Bradshaw, J.M., Dignum, V., Jonker, C., Sierhuis, M.: Human-agent-robot teamwork. IEEE Intell. Syst. **27**(2), 8–13 (2012)
6. Bratman, M.E.: Shared cooperative activity. Philos. Rev. **101**(2), 327 (1992)
7. Breazeal, C., Kidd, C.D., Thomaz, A.L., Hoffman, G., Berlin, M.: Effects of nonverbal communication on efficiency and robustness in human-robot teamwork. In: 2005 IEEE/RSJ International Conference on Intelligent Robots and Systems, pp. 708–713. IEEE (2005)
8. Colquitt, J.A., Scott, B.A., LePine, J.A.: Trust, trustworthiness, and trust propensity: a meta-analytic test of their unique relationships with risk taking and job performance. J. Appl. Psychol. **92**(4), 909–927 (2007)

9. Corritore, C.L., Kracher, B., Wiedenbeck, S.: On-line trust: concepts, evolving themes, a model. J. Appl. Psychol. **58**(6), 737–758 (2003)
10. Dautenhahn, K.: The art of designing socially intelligent agents: science, fiction, and the human in the loop. J. Appl. Psychol. **12**(7–8), 573–617 (1998)
11. Deutsch, M.: Cooperation and competition. In: Coleman, P.T. (ed.) Conflict, Interdependence, and Justice, pp. 23–40. Springer, New York (2011)
12. Deutsch, M.: Cooperation and trust: some theoretical notes. In: Jones, M.R. (ed.) Nebraska Symposium on Motivation, pp. 275–320. University of Nebraska Press, Oxford (1962)
13. Fiske, S.T., Cuddy, A.J.C., Glick, P.: Universal dimensions of social cognition: warmth and competence. J. Appl. Psychol. **11**(2), 77–83 (2007)
14. Fogg, B., Tseng, H.: The elements of computer credibility. In: Proceedings of the SIGCHI Conference on Human Factors in Computing Systems, pp. 80–87. ACM (1999)
15. Hafizoglu, F., Sen, S.: Evaluating trust levels in human-agent teamwork in virtual environments. In: Fourth International Workshop on Human-Agent Interaction Design and Models (2015). https://haidm.files.wordpress.com/2015/04/haidm_2015_submission_13.pdf
16. Kiesler, S., Sproull, L., Waters, K.: A prisoner's dilemma experiment on cooperation with people and human-like computers. J. Pers. Soc. Psychol. **70**(1), 47 (1996)
17. Krämer, N.C., Rosenthal-von der Pütten, A.M., Hoffmann, L.: Social effects of virtual and robot companions. In: Sundar, S.S. (ed.) The Handbook of the Psychology of Communication Technology, pp. 137–159. Wiley, West Sussex (2015)
18. Mayer, R.C., Davis, J.H., Schoorman, F.D.: An integrative model of organizational trust. J. Pers. Soc. Psychol. **20**(3), 709–734 (1995)
19. de Melo, C.M., Carnevale, P., Read, S., Antos, D., Gratch, J.: Bayesian model of the social effects of emotion in decision-making in multiagent systems. In: Proceedings of the 11th International Conference on Autonomous Agents and Multiagent Systems, pp. 55–62 (2012)
20. Muir, B.M.: Trust between humans and machines, and the design of decision aids. Int. J. Man Mach. Stud. **27**(5–6), 527–539 (1987)
21. Nass, C., Fogg, B., Moon, Y.: Can computers be teammates? Int. J. Man Mach. Stud. **45**(6), 669–678 (1996)
22. Nass, C., Moon, Y.: Machines and mindlessness: social responses to computers. Int. J. Man Mach. Stud. **56**(1), 81–103 (2000)
23. Qiu, L., Benbasat, I.: Evaluating anthropomorphic product recommendation agents: a social relationship perspective to designing information systems. Int. J. Man Mach. Stud. **25**(4), 145–182 (2009)
24. Traum, D., Marsella, S.C., Gratch, J., Lee, J., Hartholt, A.: Multi-party, multi-issue, multi-strategy negotiation for multi-modal virtual agents. In: Prendinger, H., Lester, J., Ishizuka, M. (eds.) IVA 2008. LNCS (LNAI), vol. 5208, pp. 117–130. Springer, Heidelberg (2008). doi:10.1007/978-3-540-85483-8_12
25. van Wissen, A., Gal, Y., Kamphorst, B.A., Dignum, M.V.: Human-agent teamwork in dynamic environments. Comput. Hum. Behav. **28**(1), 23–33 (2012)

Playing with Social and Emotional Game Companions

Andry Chowanda[1,2]([✉]), Martin Flintham[1], Peter Blanchfield[1], and Michel Valstar[1]

[1] School of Computer Science, The University of Nottingham, Nottingham, UK
{psxac6,pszmdf,pszpxb,pszmv}@nottingham.ac.uk
[2] School of Computer Science, Bina Nusantara University, Jakarta, Indonesia

Abstract. This paper presents the findings of an empirical study that explores player game experience by implementing the ERiSA Framework in games. A study with Action Role-Playing Game (RPG) was designed to evaluate player interactions with game companions, who were imbued with social and emotional skill by the ERiSA Framework. Players had to complete a quest in the Skyrim game, in which players had to use social and emotional skills to obtain a sword. The results clearly show that game companions who are capable of perceiving and exhibit emotions, are perceived to have personality and can forge relationships with the players, enhancing the player experience during the game.

Keywords: Game experience · Game companions · Social relationship · Social interaction

1 Introduction

Games are considered to be one of the most popular interactive entertainment products in the world. The key point that makes them popular is the experience people have when they play the game [13]. Non-Player Characters (NPCs) in games can be a key factor to engage a player and bring about this experience. They can be particularly interesting potential vehicles of affect, because players naturally engage with the NPCs as part of a game. Over time, a pattern of interactions between a player and agents may translate into a relationship, if the game and its NPCs are designed to accommodate this. We argue that NPCs with such capabilities will provide a new experience when playing games.

This paper presents the evaluation of player experience when playing with game companions that are capable of perceiving and exhibiting emotions, complete with the ability to develop simple social relations over time. A game scenario where players interact with two different game companions was designed by adopting the ERiSA Framework [8,10]. The ERiSA Framework is an integrated framework for social and emotional game companions to enhance their believability and quality of interaction, in particular by allowing a game companion to forge social relations and make appropriate use of social signals.

© Springer International Publishing AG 2016
D. Traum et al. (Eds.): IVA 2016, LNAI 10011, pp. 85–95, 2016.
DOI: 10.1007/978-3-319-47665-0_8

Our experimental results provide clear evidence that there is an increase in player experience when playing the game with the additional influence of interactive emotion, personality and relationships to the game companion's behaviours. Players reported that they were more emotionally involved and attached with the characters and the game when the Framework was activated in the game.

2   Related Work

A key goal in developing game companions one can relate to is that they should be believable. The term "believable" can be linked to the era of the 1990's when Joseph Bates argued the notion of a "believable character" in his paper [4]. He elaborated that the idea of "believability" doesn't necessarily come from a reliable character but "one that provides the illusion of life, and thus permits the audience's suspension of disbelief" [4]. The term "illusion of life" itself was coined by the Disney animators in the 1930's in their quest to make audiences believe in their characters [4,15]. The ultimate goal in this research is therefore not as much creating NPCs that are more and more realistic, but ones that less frequently break the illusion. In games, implementing the illusion results in an increase of player experience. Charles [7] argues that player experience and enjoyment can be significantly enhanced when the game character is well designed. Afonso and Prada [1] also discuss that "Social Believability" in games improved the experience. Bailey et al. [3] suggest that the character's believability influences the player immersion and thus enhances the game-play experience.

Attfield et al. [2] define the user experience as "the emotional, cognitive and behavioural connection that exists [...] between a user and a resource". That connection can be linked to emotion, personality and social relationship aspects. The influence of those aspects on an NPC's behaviour has been widely recognised to affect their believability [4,15]. The uniqueness of a character in comparison to others in the game and their ability to exhibit emotions provides a feeling of immersion to the player. We can also see the ability of the player to forge relationships with NPCs in games as part of their storyline such as Skyrim, Grand Theft Auto, The Sims, Harvest Moon, etc. Research has been done to enhance the player experience by improving their believability. However, only limited research has been done to incorporate emotion, personality and social relationships models together (e.g. [9,10,14]). This paper demonstrates a comprehensive evaluation of the player experience when playing with social and emotional game companions with stereotypical artificial personalities.

3   Designing Social and Emotional Game Companions

The ERiSA Framework was implemented inside the popular commercial game Skyrim. Our framework allows Skyrim to capture a player's facial expressions as an additional game input. Figure 1 illustrates the integration of the components and the communication between them. Partial parts from the ERiSA Framework were used to perceive and interpret the player's emotions, conveyed by their

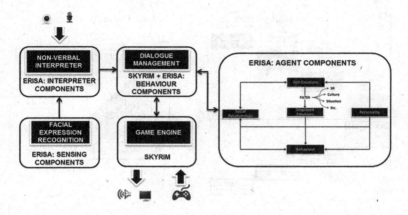

Fig. 1. Framework implementation

facial expression and recorded by camera. The dialogue manager proposes NPC actions and determines a set of possible dialogues for the player to choose from, depending on the player's and NPC's internal states recorded in the Interpreter and Agent Components. The output corresponding to the selected NPC action is sent to the Skyrim Game Engine. A player's facial expressions also govern the player's dialogue options. For example, the option for the player to say that they're happy is only available if the facial expression recognition components interpret the player's emotion conveyed by their facial expression as happy [10].

We designed two characters with opposite personality to interact with, named Stella and Max Erisa. Stella has a high Extraversion trait, while Max has a strong Neuroticism trait. To associate the characters with their personality traits, we set Max's voice characteristic to an agitated and annoying voice provided by The Skyrim Creation Kit. On the other hand, Stella's voice is pleasantly happy and enthusiastic. Moreover, we designed a simple quest named "The Erisa Family". In the quest, the player can build relationships with the NPCs, get information about The Legendary Swords possessed by their family and receive one of the swords. Players can dynamically interact with the NPCs, with different options at their disposal depending on their relationship level. The quest is finished when the player gets one of the swords. The *Sword of Friendship* will be given to the player when they earned the NPCs' trust by building a positive relationship, while *The Sword of Hatred* will be passed to the player when their relationship is going towards a negative direction. There are 4 strategies for forging social relationship with the NPCs: chatting, giving favourite items vs. giving undesirable items, praising vs. criticising, and exploring Skyrim world together vs. attacking the NPCs. Stella is more sociable compared to Max, hence, extra effort is required to gain Max's trust. Over time, the topics discussed with the NPCs change depending on the level of their relationship with the player. Figure 2 illustrates the mapping between possible interactions corresponding to the level of relationship based on the models proposed in [10].

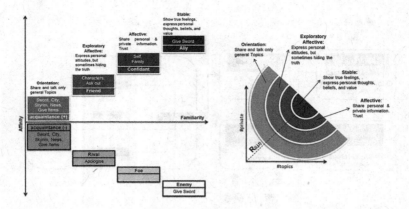

Fig. 2. Mapping social relationship to behaviour

There are total of 8 relationship levels (4 positive, 4 negative). On the initial interaction, the player can only discuss general topics about the swords, city, Skyrim, give items, or ask and provide news. Assuming the relationship is going towards positive direction, the NPCs start to express their personal attitudes towards the topics in the next stage. Moderate topics are also available to be discussed in this stage in addition to the previous topics. Starting from this stage, the player can suggest to the NPCs to go out and explore Skyrim together. Going towards an affective relationship, the NPCs begin to share their personal information about themselves and their family. Moreover, the NPCs strongly express their personal attitudes towards the topics at this stage. In the final stage, the NPCs begin to show their true feelings, express personal thoughts, beliefs and values. At this stage the player is given *The Sword of Friendship*, marking the end of the quest. The player can still interact with the NPCs but the relationship between them will not go any further. On the other hand, if the relationship is changing in negative direction, the breadth and depth of topics does not change. Eventually, the *Sword of Hatred* is passed to the player, marking the end of the journey. If this route is taken, the player will not be able to interact with the NPCs any more, reflecting the deep hatred that the NPCs feel towards the player.

To evaluate the characters created and empowered by the ERiSA Framework, we compare them with their baseline versions. The baseline characters were designed with the original mechanics provided by Skyrim, where the NPC's emotions and social relationships are triggered by story or click-based system. The dialogues between player and the baseline NPC were only regulated by the Skyrim Dialogue Manager where the emotions conveyed by the player's facial expressions were not included in the decision making. Other than that, both the conversation topics and the quest design were identical for both baseline and models NPCs.

4   Evaluating Social and Emotional Game Companions

Fifteen players (60 % female, 73.33 % Asian, 26.67 % Caucasian, AVG age = 24.6) were recruited to play the game. All were familiar with the RPG Genre and one third had played Skyrim before. A total of 60 interactions were completed with both of the NPCs, totalling 18.16 h of play time (MAX = 51.82 min, MIN = 1.85 min, AVG = 18.16 min). Each participant interacted with both NPCs without the models as a baseline and with the models implemented as the comparison. To avoid order bias, the order was randomized for all players. All interactions were video and audio recorded, the player and NPCs' internal states were logged and the player's in-game choices were recorded. Players were asked to complete a questionnaire every time they finished a session of the game. Nine players were invited to do a short interview to discuss their experience with the game, after they had finished all the quests.

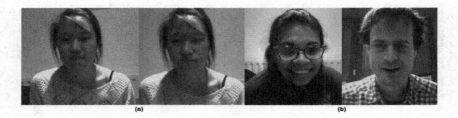

Fig. 3. Player's facial expressions: Annoyed by Max (a), Delighted by Stella (b)

The questionnaires consists of four parts, each in the form of a five-point Likert Scale evaluating the game and its NPCs. The first part evaluates the NPCs' personality as perceived by the user based on the Big Five Personality Inventory [12]. The second part rates the social relationship between the player and the NPCs based on Quality of Relationships Inventory (QRI) and Social Relationship Index (SRI) [6]. In the third part, players were asked about their feelings when they interacted with the NPCs during the quest using Ekman's six basic emotions. Finally, the last part of the questionnaire evaluated player experience during the game using The Game Engagement Questionnaire [5] and The Immersive Experience Questionnaire [11].

Figure 4 describes Max and Stella's personality as perceived by players for both models with * mark represent significance at the 0.05 level and others marked with ** indicates significance at the 0.01 level. Without the models implemented, the NPCs' appear to be perceived as devoid of any personality by the players. With the models implemented, the characteristics which constitute Stella personality, are evidently perceived by players as a person who has positive thinking, generates a lot of enthusiasm, is outspoken, outgoing & sociable, is relaxed & handles stress well, is emotionally stable & not easily upset and is polite to others. Max, on the other hand, is a person who is extremely negative

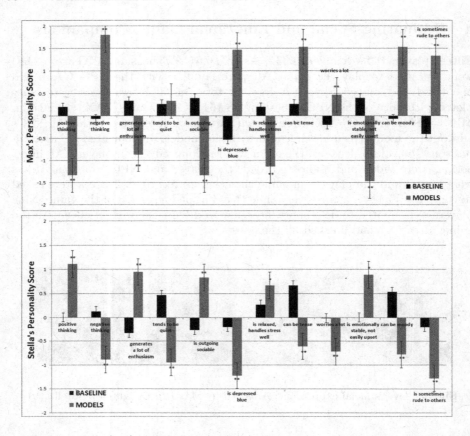

Fig. 4. Max's (top) and Stella's (bottom) personality as perceived by players

thinking, does not generate a lot of enthusiasm, tends to be slightly quiet, is reserved, sometimes depressed, blue & can't handle stress well, can be tense & worries a lot, is easily upset, can be moody and is sometimes rude to others. In addition, most players identified Max as rude, abominable and playing hard-to-get, while Stella is a talkative, nice and approachable person. According to responses to the Game Engagement and Immersive Experience Questionnaire (see Fig. 6), players empathise with Stella but not with Max in the game when the models are implemented, while there was no significant difference when models were not implemented. Figure 3 shows some player facial expressions when interacting with the ERISA-empowered characters.

Furthermore, players reported significant changes in their social relationship to both NPCs (see Fig. 5). With the models implemented, Stella is more likeable, and players perceived her as someone that they can count on to listen when they are very angry with someone else. Players seems happy when they interacted with her. In contrast, Max is more unpleasant to interact with, and players feel he is someone that they can't count on to listen when they are very angry with

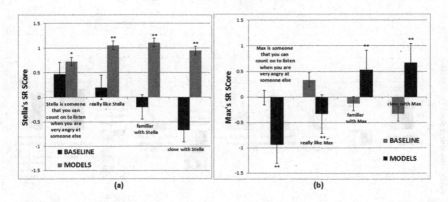

Fig. 5. Stella's (a) and Max's (b) social relationship as rated by players

someone else as they already feel emotionally upset towards Max. Players also feel more familiar and close to both NPCs when the models are implemented.

Measured in in-game-time, players spent on average 0.92 h (MAX = 3.2 h, MIN = 0.25 h)/62.78 h (MAX = 114.2 h, MIN = 11.75 h) with Stella without and with models, respectively. Players spent 1.01 h (MAX = 4.0 h, MIN = 0.21 h)/74.74 h (MAX = 219.5 h, MIN = 16.17 h) for Max with no models and with models implemented, respectively. Players who took a longer time to finish the quest spent their time mostly exploring the Skyrim world with the NPCs, while players with shorter time only focussed on forging a social relationship with the NPCs by giving them their most-liked items repeatedly. The favourite strategy to build relationships with the NPCs was giving favourable items to them, with exploring Skyrim together as the second choice of strategy. Building a positive relationship with Max can be quite a nerve-racking experience; 40 % of players realised that it would be easier to have a negative relationship and decided to go towards negative relation with Max although they already held a positive relationship with him as their game strategy to get a Legendary Sword.

Figure 6 illustrates the score of the player experience. With ERISA models implemented, players feel more engaged and emotionally immersed in the game and the characters, irrespective of which NPC they interact with. Players reported a significant increase in the engagement level with the game with the models implemented ($p < 0.01$). A significant difference was also found in the players' emotional attachment to the game and the characters with the models implemented ($p < 0.01$). Moreover, the models enriched the game story, increased the players' curiosity how the game would progress ($p < 0.01$). From the short interview, most of players preferred the NPCs with models. The models provide an interesting flow to forge the relationships with NPCs. However, some players suggested adding more variation of interactions, as the current interaction is limited to speaking, giving items, and exploring Skyrim together.

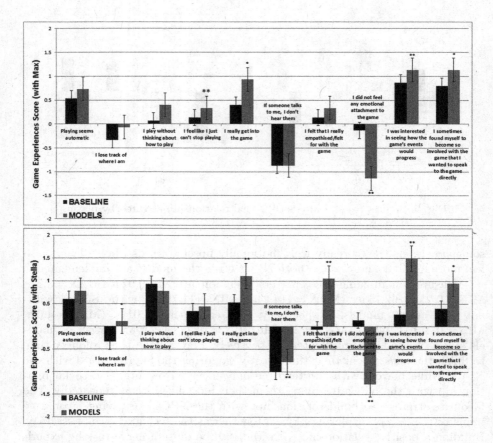

Fig. 6. Players' experiences with Max (top) and Stella (bottom)

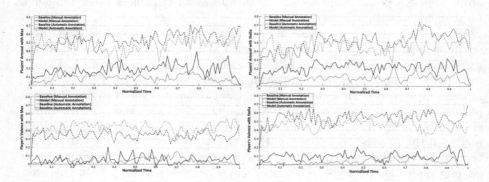

Fig. 7. Players' Arousal (top), Valence (bottom) towards Max (left), Stella (right), where dotted line represents automatic annotation

Automatic arousal and valence annotation was performed from the interaction audio using the SSI Framework [16]. In addition, we also manually annotated players' arousal and valence using continuous annotation tools developed by The Imperial College London. A Kolmogorov-Smirnov test was applied to all the data and indicated that they were more likely come from a non-normally distributed population ($p < 0.001$). Hence Wilcoxon Signed-Rank Tests were applied as this is a good alternative to the t-Test Paired Two Sample for Means when the population cannot be assumed to be normally distributed.

Figure 7 demonstrates the players' arousal and valence when playing with Max (left) and Stella (right). A Wilcoxon Signed-Rank Tests indicates a strong positive correlation between players' valence data with Max from automatic and manual annotation, $r = 0.76, n = 101, p < 0.001$ and $r = 0.72, n = 101, p < 0.001$, with baseline and models implemented respectively. In addition, there was also a strong positive correlation between player' arousal data with Max from automatic and manual annotation, $r = 0.62, n = 101, p < 0.001$ and $r = 0.77, n = 101, p < 0.001$, with baseline and models implemented respectively. A strong positive correlation was also found in the player' valence data with Stella from automatic and manual annotation, $r = 0.72, n = 101, p < 0.001$ and $r = 0.71, n = 101, p < 0.001$, with baseline and models implemented respectively. Moreover, there was also a strong positive correlation between player' arousal data with Stella from automatic and manual annotation, $r = 0.68, n = 101, p < 0.001$ and $r = 0.83, n = 101, p < 0.001$, with baseline and models implemented respectively.

A Wilcoxon Signed-Ranks Test indicated that players' arousal was statically significantly higher with models implemented, $Z = 8.4, p < 0.001$ and $Z = 8.71, p < 0.001$, with Max and Stella respectively. In addition, players' valence was also significantly higher with models implemented, $Z = 3.1, p < 0.05$ and $Z = 7.75, p < 0.001$, with Max and Stella respectively. Negative valence also occurred in the interaction with ERISA-empowered Max. Players' arousal and valence were significantly higher when playing with ERISA-empowered Stella compared to Max, $Z = 3.75, p < 0.001$ and $Z = 6.47, p < 0.01$, respectively. On the contrary, there was no significant differences between players' arousal and valence when interacting with baseline Stella compare to Max, $Z = -1.67, p = 0.5$ and $Z = -1.65, p = 0.1$, respectively.

5 Conclusion and Future Work

The results indicate that the influence of emotion, personality and social relationships to the game companions' behaviours, enhanced the player experience when playing the game. Players were emotionally involved and attached to the characters and the game. The models provide a more realistic manner for interacting with NPCs and forge relationships with them. Personality also influences the game play, as the characters with the Neuroticism trait were harder to "conquered" thus requiring a specific strategy to win. Social relationships models can be adjusted to enrich the game story as well. For future research direction with these models, more variation for interactions with the NPCs can be added. Interaction such as accomplishing a quest together and more conversational topics can enhance the user experience when playing the game.

Acknowledgement. The work by A. Chowanda and M. Valstar is partly funded by European Union's Horizon 2020 research and innovation programme under grant agreement No. 645378, ARIA-VALUSPA.

References

1. Afonso, N., Prada, R.: Agents that relate: improving the social believability of non-player characters in role-playing games. In: Stevens, S.M., Saldamarco, S.J. (eds.) ICEC 2008. LNCS, vol. 5309, pp. 34–45. Springer, Heidelberg (2008). doi:10.1007/978-3-540-89222-9_5
2. Attfield, S., Kazai, G., Lalmas, M., Piwowarski, B.: Towards a science of user engagement. In: WSDM Workshop on User Modelling for Web Applications (2011)
3. Bailey, C., You, J., Acton, G., Rankin, A., Katchabaw, M.: Believability through psychosocial behaviour: creating bots that aremore engaging and entertaining. In: Hingston, P. (ed.) Believable Bots, pp. 29–68. Springer, Heidelberg (2013)
4. Bates, J.: The role of emotion in believable agents. Commun. ACM **37**(7), 122–125 (1994)
5. Brockmyer, J., et al.: The development of the game engagement questionnaire: a measure of engagement in video game-playing. J. Exp. Soc. Psychol. **45**(4), 624–634 (2009)
6. Campo, R., et al.: The assessment of positivity and negativity in social networks: the reliability and validity of the social relationships index. J. Commun. Psychol. **37**(4), 471–486 (2009)
7. Charles, D., Gameplay, E.: Challenges for artificial intelligence in digital games. In: 1st World Conference on Digital Games, The Netherlands (2003)
8. Chowanda, A., Blanchfield, P., Flintham, M., Valstar, M.: ERiSA: building emotionally realistic social game-agents companions. In: Bickmore, T., Marsella, S., Sidner, C. (eds.) IVA 2014. LNCS (LNAI), vol. 8637, pp. 134–143. Springer, Heidelberg (2014). doi:10.1007/978-3-319-09767-1_16
9. Chowanda, A., Blanchfield, P., Flintham, M., Valstar, M.: Play smile game with ERiSA: a user study on game companions. In: Workshop on Engagement in Social Intelligent Virtual Agents on IVA (2015)
10. Chowanda, A., Blanchfield, P., Flintham, M., Valstar, M.: Computational models of emotion, personality, and social relationships for interactions in games. In: Thangarajah, J., Tuyls, K., Jonker, C., Marsella, S. (eds.) Proceedings of the 2016 International Conference on AAMAS, Singapore (2016)
11. Jennett, C., et al.: Measuring and defining the experience of immersion in games. Int. J. Hum. Comput. Stud. **66**(9), 641–661 (2008)
12. John, O., Naumann, L., Soto, C.: Paradigm shift to the integrative big five trait taxonomy. In: John, O.P., Robins, R.W., Pervin, L.A. (eds.) Handbook of Personality: Theory and Research, vol. 3, pp. 114–158. Guilford Press, New York (2008)
13. Lazzaro, N.: Why we play games: four keys to more emotion without story (2004)
14. Ochs, M., Sabouret, N., Corruble, V.: Simulation of the dynamics of nonplayer characters' emotions and social relations in games. IEEE Trans. Comput. Intell. AI Games **1**(4), 281–297 (2009)

15. Thomas, F., Johnson, O., Animation, D.: The Illusion of Life. Abbeville Press, New York (1984)
16. Wagner, J., Lingenfelser, F., Baur, T., Damian, I., Kistler, F., André, E.: The social signal interpretation (SSI) framework: multimodal signalprocessing and recognition in real-time. In: Proceedings of the 21st ACM International Conference on Multimedia, pp. 831–834 (2013)

This Is What's Important – Using Speech and Gesture to Create Focus in Multimodal Utterance

Farina Freigang[(⊠)] and Stefan Kopp

Social Cognitive Systems Group, Faculty of Technology,
Center of Excellence "Cognitive Interaction Technology" (CITEC),
Bielefeld University, P.O. Box 100 131, 33501 Bielefeld, Germany
farina.freigang@uni-bielefeld.de, skopp@techfak.uni-bielefeld.de

Abstract. In natural communication, humans enrich their utterances with pragmatic information indicating, e.g., what is important to them or what they are not certain about. We investigate whether and how virtual humans (VH) can employ this kind of meta-communication. In an empirical study we have identified three modifying functions that humans produce and perceive in multimodal utterance, one being to create or attenuate focus. In this paper we test whether such modifying functions are also observed in speech and/or gesture of a VH, and whether this changes the perception of a VH overall. Results suggest that, although the VH's behaviour is judged rather neutral overall, focusing is distinctively recognised, leads to better recall, and affects perceived competence. These effects are strongest if focus is created jointly by speech and gesture.

1   Introduction

In natural communication, humans do not only transport propositional meaning. They add many signals to *modify* this message in order to help the addressee arrive at the correct interpretation of the speaker's intended meaning. However, albeit its prominence and importance, this meta-communication has not received much attention so far. A special role plays nonverbal communication [1], which speakers use to subtly indicate, e.g., what is important to them, or what their stance or epistemic state is about a fact. The synchronization of speech and gesture plays a key role in forming this multimodal utterance [2]. We are interested in how speech and gesture work together in such modifications in multimodal utterance.

Gestures contribute to the meaning of an utterance not only by *adding* information (semantics) but also by modifying the gestural or verbal content on a pragmatic level. In this case, the gesture may carry a *modifying function* (MF), which we investigated in previous work [3]. We created a corpus of natural communicative gestures and body movements and conducted a video rating study. Participants evaluated video snippets of multimodal utterances in two conditions: speech-and-gesture and gesture-only (with muted speech and cropped

© Springer International Publishing AG 2016
D. Traum et al. (Eds.): IVA 2016, LNAI 10011, pp. 96–109, 2016.
DOI: 10.1007/978-3-319-47665-0_9

head). The utterances were evaluated in terms of 14 adjectives assumed, first, to be intuitively understandable and, second, to correspond to the range of possible combined meanings that can be related back to specific MF, developed within the research of gesture studies building on work by [4–7]. Results show that index-finger-pointings are perceived to emphasise and affirm an uttered content. Brushing gestures change the utterance in a discounting or downtoning way. In further work [8], we conducted an exploratory factor analysis of the ratings of 14 adjectives, in order to analyse the underlying structures. Three main factors were found in the gesture-only condition. One distinct factor with high positive adjective loadings (.981 to .719) relates to **positive focusing** (or highlighting), a second with relatively high negative adjective loading (−.934) corresponds to **negative epistemic** functions (marking uncertainty). Another adjective linked to remaining factors was identified as **negative focusing**. The adjectives supported by the factors suggest which MF a gesture may be associated with.

With this work, we tackle two main issues. First, we want to gain insights into the role of speech and gesture in conveying pragmatic information (MF). Is the meaning understood and, in particular, what do MF in gesture contribute to it? We can measure this by assessing the recognition of MF and the recall of what a virtual human (VH) says in different modalities. Based on previous work [3] we expect that gestures with a highlighting function are particularly well recognised, and we hypothesise that highlighted messages are better remembered than downtoning or uncertain messages. Further, we hypothesise to get the strongest effect when MFs are conveyed in both speech and gesture, followed by speech, gesture, and a non-modified utterance. A second research question is how a VH is perceived more generally when its multimodal expressiveness is augmented with pragmatic aspects. After all, our aim is to create more communicative and accessible VH. In order to investigate these research questions, we synthesizing particular gestural behaviour and add it to specific verbal material. Note that modifications, and meta-communication more generally, are hardly conventionalized, standardized, nor clearly marked. In contrast, this information is often highly ambigue, vague, and subjectively interpreted. Hence, studying these questions raises considerable methodological challenges. In the next section, we explain how we arrived at the present experiment design (using a number of pretests). After describing the study procedure in Sect. 3, we present and discuss results in Sect. 4.

2   Experiment Design

On the basis of the insights that we gained from the factor analysis [8], we designed the current experimental setup. The first question at hand was **which gestures** should be tested? We decided on the following procedure. As described above, some adjectives were particularly meaningful for the factors of our MF. Thus, we filtered out the adjectives that had the highest ratings (1.4 to 2.8 on a 7-point Likert scale), retaining the three MF under discussion. The following categories emerged: the adjectives *affirmative*, *emphasising*, *focusing*, *opinionative*, *classifying* and *relevant* represent the positive focusing (or highlighting) function (Foc+), the adjective *discounting/downtoning* represents the negative focusing function (Foc-), and the adjective *uncertain* stands for the negative epistemic function (Epi-). As a result of matching the adjectives back to the corresponding video snippets, ten videos could be selected which represent the three MF, each depicting a distinct gesture: pointings for Foc+, brushings for Foc- and palm up open hand gestures for Epi- (for examples, cf. Fig. 1). A particular strength of this work is that the gestures with associated MF, which we wanted to test in a VH, are selected on the basis of empirical findings.

The second issue for the experimental setup was the **stimulus context**. Since this is a first test of gestures with MF, we did not plan a human-VH interaction, but just the presentation of videos of a VH. We designed a short story[1] in which our VH called Billie narrates about his life as a virtual character. The story was designed to have three parts, each with one topic. The parts were designed to be long enough to have an effect on the observer, as well as brief enough as not to become tedious. In the first story Billie talks about VH and his research institute, in the second one he talks about himself and for which reasons VH are used, and in the third story, Billie talks about the technical details of the software architecture underlying his behaviour. Each text contains 100 words (+1/−2), is structured into eight sentences, and was written in a neutral tone. In total the short story consists of 24 sentences and 299 words. As described below, the text was later enhanced by expressions for each category of MF.

Concerning the topic of MF, so far, we solely considered natural data of human interactions dripping with naturalness and modifications of all kind. The aspect of naturalness will be discussed further down (natural VH). The following paragraphs, first, will deal with the third issue of the experimental setup, namely, the **application of MF** in utterances. Our MF in gesture are taken from our corpus and are implemented in an VH, thus they are scripted gestures which can be easily controlled. In order to test what is in the gesture and what is in the speech of a VH, and since we cannot assume that a gesture on its own can convey the intended meaning, we needed modifications in speech to make a condition more obvious for a naïve observer. Possible linguistic options of modification include words choice, intonation, sentence structure and speech acts, among others. The control over prosody would be a desired modification, since prosodic and gestural highlighting may highly correlate in natural human interactions, and we would like to investigate this aspect in future work. To remain in control, we use particular words as markers for our MF (for the final version of "keywords" cf. Sect. 3). Different view points exists on which lexemes highlight, understate or make an utterance uncertain, and only few of have studied words connection to gesture. One example is [9], who discusses the relationship between modal particles and gestures in German. Opposite to his approach, we do not analyse the co-occurrence of speech and gesture in humans, but investigate modal particles and sentential adjectives that best match our MF in gesture

---

[1] The short story can be accessed at https://pub.uni-bielefeld.de/publication/2903503.

in a VH. Since we do not want to rely solely on the existing (and in parts quite theoretical) literature, we tested the words in two pretest iterations.

In the first iteration of testing, the designed short story was enhanced with keywords, which we considered to have a MF similar to our MF in gestures. We collected keywords for three conditions (Foc+, Foc-, Epi-) and no keywords were added for a neutral condition. In this pretest only every other sentences included a keyword and only those sentences were tested, plus the same sentences in the neutral condition. The three parts of the short story were chunked sentence-wise and recorded with the synthesised voice of our VH Billie. The final 48 audio files of all four conditions had a duration of 6 to 19 s and were randomly ordered in a SoSci Survey [10] questionnaire (with which also the second pretest and the final experiment were conducted). The test was presented to three participants, partly aware of the research question, who classified the utterances of the audio playbacks to be one of the following: "Billie's utterance is ..." *emphasising, understating, uncertain,* or *neutral.* The options were visible during the playback. In order for a word to be accepted, two of three persons had to match the utterance to the correct category, i.e., any of the three MF or neutral. As a result, we kept half of the words (18) and replaced the others (18; 12 were neutral).

In a second pretest iteration, the three parts of the short story were each played in one piece and in all four conditions, accumulating to a rating test of 12 audio playbacks. Each playback was between 49 and 69 s long and presented in a randomised order. Again, participants had to rate the utterances of the audio playbacks according to the four options which were visible during the time of playback. At the end of this pretest, however, detailed questions about the sentences were asked on three pages. On one page, all sentences in one condition were presented in written form and the participants were asked which of the utterances were *not* either *emphasising - highlighting - focussing* or *discounting - understating - defocussing* or *uncertain,* depending on which page they were on. Eight subjects unfamiliar with the research questions participated in this pretest. The results of the audio tests (cf. Table 1) show that in the neutral condition, 67 % were correctly identified and the rest were rated Foc+. In the Foc+ condition, 71 % of the ratings were correct and the rest were rated as neutral. In the Foc- condition, only 42 % were rated correctly, the same amount rated neutral and the rest Foc+/Epi-. In the Epi- condition, 50 % matched the desired category, and the rest was quite random: 21 % were rated neutral, 17 % Foc+ and 12 % Foc-. In conclusion, all conditions included neutral ratings (in total, 40 % of the 96 ratings), in the neutral condition (and slightly Foc- and Epi-) some focusing elements were observed, and the Epi- condition was the one with the highest variance. These results indicate that even in spoken/written language there is a lot of ambiguity regarding words with modification. But when looking at the big picture, the Foc+ and neutral conditions are rather clear. The results of the second part, the written-sentences test, indicated which keywords needed to be changed in order to give a sentence a certain modification. In order for a keyword to be changed, at least two of the eight participants had to state a misfit. Five,

Table 1. Results of the second pretest: Counts of how much the three parts of the short story, which included modifying keywords (in all but the neutral condition) and were presented by a synthetic voice, match a condition. Eight participants rated three times per condition, once per part of the short story, and 18 times on the whole test. Numbers in bold indicate the highest ratings.

		N	Foc+	Foc−	Epi−	Total		N	Foc+	Foc−	Epi−	Total
Condition match	#	**16**	**17**	10	12	55	%	**66.7**	**70.8**	41.7	50.0	57.3
No condition match	#	8	7	**14**	12	41	%	33.3	29.2	**58.3**	50.0	42.7
Total	#	24	24	24	24	96	%	100	100	100	100	100

four and one keywords were changed in the `Foc+`, `Foc-`, and `Epi-` conditions, accordingly.

A fourth issue for the experimental setup is the creation of a **natural VH**. There are many options for designing the behaviour of a VH as natural as possible, include facial expressions, "idle" gaze and saccades, posture or "idle" body movements. One prerequisite was that the behaviour of the VH should be as natural as possible and as controlled as necessary. We recorded data with a fifteen-camera OptiTrack motion capture system to give Billie the appropriate naturalness. And to control for unnatural "idle" behaviour in between gesture performances, we recorded each part of the short story in one piece and in each of the four conditions. Since the corresponding audio file was played back while recording the motion capture behaviour, in the final stimulus videos, the VH made movements which fit the context of the story extremely well and, thus, may have increased the degree of presence of the VH. We disabled a few joints in order to control for too much movement of the VH skeleton. No further adjustments were made like facial expressions or gaze movements.

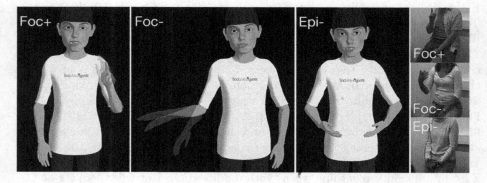

Fig. 1. Stills of the stimulus videos and stills of the snippets from our experimental setup with human gestures. From left to right and top to bottom: A gesture with a highlighting function (index-finger pointing), a gesture with a de-emphasising function (brushing away), and a gesture of uncertainty (palm up open hand).

3   Stimuli and Procedure

Our research question is whether the identified MF in gesture are also perceived in a VH. For an accurate test of how a gesture is perceived and whether the MF is recognised correctly, we compared a gesture-only (G) and a speech-only (S) condition against a speech-and-gesture (S+G) condition and a neutral condition as baseline (N). The G condition contained gestures with MF and speech without keywords, in S there were modifying keywords in speech and only gestural idle behaviour (only a few not meaningful arm movements), in S+G there were keywords and gestures with MFs and, in the N condition, there was speech without keywords and gestural idle behaviour. The following keywords were used for Foc+: "concretely", "even", "exclusively", "in any case", "more precisely", "most important", "most notably", "particularly", "primarily", "totally important" and "totally obvious"; for Foc-: "any", "anyway", "just/plainly", "merely", "only", "ordinarily", "solely", "(totally) spectacularly" and "trivially"; and for Epi-: "apparently", "maybe", "possibly", "potentially", "presumably", "probably", "seemingly" and "sort of".

Stimuli for all but the neutral conditions had to be created trice (S+G, S, G), accumulating to ten conditions in total: N, Foc+SG, Foc+S, Foc+G, Foc-SG, Foc-S, Foc-G, Epi-SG, Epi-S, Epi-G. The stimuli were videos of Billie telling three stories with and without keywords in speech and MF in gestures. Body movement and gestures were recorded using motion capture. From all recordings, only the most accurate twelve (three MF and N for three stories each) ones were kept for post-processing. Since the performance of a gesture critically depends on the shape of the hand (not recorded), one post-processing step was the definition of the hand shapes. Those were designed in the MURML Keyframe editor [11] and merged into the motion capture data. The sentences were aligned to the nonverbal-behaviour and eye blinking was added. In all conditions, the VH Billie is used, his behaviour is steered by AsapRealizer [12] and his speech is synthesised by the Text-To-Speech system CereProc[2] with the female voice Gudrun. In total, 30 stimulus videos of Billie were recorded, with a duration of 54 to 60 s.[3]

In order to investigate the research questions raised at the end of Sect. 1, a between-subject design was carried out. Each participant was shown the three stimulus videos of one condition in random order (cf. Fig. 1). Four statements of various difficulty had to be evaluated into "correct", "wrong" or "I don't know" after each of the three stimuli videos. The statements were quite technical and detailed in order to estimate upper bounds. Five out of the 12 statements were wrong. Our hypothesis was that the participants remember facts about the narratives much better when they are highlighted by the VH as done in the Foc+ conditions. Since Billie is supposed to convey uncertainty and de-emphasise content in the Epi- and the Foc- conditions, we expected less recall of the content in these conditions. After that, the participants were ask to rate Billie's

---

[2] www.cereproc.com.

[3] Stimulus videos can be accessed at https://pub.uni-bielefeld.de/publication/ 2903503.

behaviour according to a specific MF.[4] Each participant was asked to answer the MF question only once and had only one choice. Since also no slider was given, designing the query in this manner is similar to a forced-choice method. We expected good recognition of the Foc+ function. Subsequently, 20 items had to be rated regarding the perceived competence, likeability and human-likeness of the VH as in [13,14]. We hypothesised the association of strong competence with Foc+ and less competence in Epi. Furthermore, questions about the observation of gestural and nonverbal behaviour of the VH were issued, about particular body movements [13], and how much these body movements and gestures helped in understanding the story. Due to space, not all analyses can be presented.

112 uninformed participants (52 female, 60 male, 0 other) with an average age of 24.4 (range [18,39], $\sigma = 3.8$) took part in the experiment. They were not informed about the purpose of the study, we simply explained that we conducted the study to improve the VH. 104 of them took part locally, in a computer room of our research institute, and were predominantly from the University of Applied Science in Bielefeld. They were provided with headphones, the VH was presented in a video of the size 22 by 22 cm and the distance to the screen was approximately 40 to 50 cm. Those participants received a compensation of 2 Euros for an average test duration of 15 min. Eight participants took part online and could not be compensated. Taking part online was possible since we provided a link and a QR-code on the flyers that we distributed. The participants were distributed randomly across the seven conditions in the following way: N: 15, Foc+SG: 15, Foc+G: 15, Foc-SG: 18, Foc-G: 17, Epi-SG: 17, and Epi-G: 15. In a second elicitation, 45 uninformed participants (29 female, 16 male, 0 other) from Bielefeld University with an average age of 27.8 (range [20,79], $\sigma = 10.8$) took part in three additional conditions with the same experimental setup, as recommended by the reviewers: Foc+S: 15, Foc-S: 15 and Epi-S: 15. This sums up to 157 participants and ten conditions in total.

4   Results

In this section, we will show results of whether the MF were matched to the correct conditions, how the content of the story was recalled and how the VH was perceived, each by analysing our MF and different modalities.

Effect of MF. In the following, we evaluate whether the MF modelled in our VH Billie get across to humans. The participants were asked to categorise Billie's utterances, which would ideally match our four broad conditions (MF and N).

---

[4] The exact wording of the question was: "In the following, please, determine Billie's utterances and communication. It is important *how* Billie uttered and communicated something. Make sure that the artificial pronunciation and speech melody does *not* have an effect on your assessment. Also, do *not* judge the relevance of things Billie talked about. Merely judge *how* Billie's utterances were: (A) emphasising and/or highlighting and/or focusing, (B) discounting and/or understating and/or defocusing, (C) uncertain and/or unknowing, (D) neutral."

The results are presented in Table 2. With 37.5 % (58 of 157 ratings) correct MF matchings vs. 62.5 % (99) incorrect matchings, we already assume that the task was difficult and that other issues may be involved. A striking result is that the participants clearly recognised the Foc+ MF in the S+G condition from the stimulus videos with 73.3 % of the counts and the neutral condition to the same extent. The Foc+S and the Foc+G conditions were still recognised by 53.3 % and 46.7 % of the counts, while almost the same amount has been distributed to the neutral condition. Similarly to the results of the second pre-study, the participants chose the neutral condition frequently: those ratings made up 48.9 %. Unfortunately, Foc- and Epi- were poorly recognised. Possible reasons for N being chosen quite frequently are that the gestures and keywords are not as distinct as we had hoped, however, since the participants had no further option but to decide for any of the three MF and neutral, neutral may have been a fallback option. This may also indicate that the neutral condition is not as surpassing recognised as it seems.

Table 2. Contingency table of counts and the corresponding percentages of the ten conditions. Grey shaded numbers indicate the correct category of MF and numbers in bold indicate the highest result.

	N	Foc+SG	Foc+S	Foc+G	Foc-SG	Foc-S	Foc-G	Epi-SG	Epi-S	Epi-G	total
# N	**11**	2	6	7	**9**	9	**10**	8	5	**10**	77
# Foc+	4	**11**	**8**	7	4	4	3	5	1	4	51
# Foc-	0	2	1	0	5	2	4	0	3	1	18
# Epi-	0	0	0	1	0	0	0	4	**6**	0	11
total #	15	15	15	15	18	15	17	17	15	15	157
% N	**73.3**	13.3	40.0	46.7	**50.0**	**60.0**	58.8	47.1	33.3	**66.7**	48.9
% Foc+	26.7	**73.3**	**53.3**	46.7	22.2	26.7	17.6	29.4	6.7	26.7	32.9
% Foc-	0	13.3	6.7	0	27.8	13.3	23.5	0	20.0	6.7	11.1
% Epi-	0	0	0	6.7	0	0	0	23.5	**40.0**	0	7.0

In order to check how well our conditions were recognised, we merged the counts of Table 2 into "matched" (only grey shaded numbers) and "did not match condition" (sum of remaining three values) for each condition, giving us a 2-by-10 matrix. On this data, we applied Pearson's chi-square test using SPSS[5]. The assumptions for using categorical data were met: we ensured the independence of residuals in that each person contributed only to one cell of the contingency table and the values for each cell were sufficiently large. In avoidance of a Type I error, because of conducting 15 tests on this particular question, we calculate the Bonferroni correction for all tests that follow. With $\chi^2(9) = 35.11, p \leq .002$, the outcome was that there is a significant difference

---

[5] IBM Corp. Released 2015. IBM SPSS Statistics for Mac, Version 23.0. Armonk, NY: IBM Corp. This software and Microsoft Excel were used for all analyses in this work.

between the ten conditions and whether or not the participants rated that Billie's behaviour has a certain function, indicating that there is an association between the ratings and a particular condition. To check whether the ratings occurred due to chance, we calculated a 95 %-confidence interval. With CI = [29.8;44.7], the overall rating results are clearly above a chance level of 25 %.

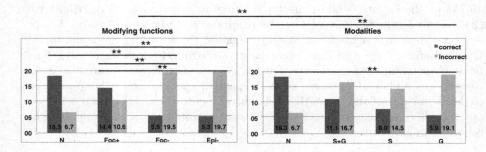

Fig. 2. Percentages of correctly and incorrectly rated MF, percentages sum up to 100 for MF and modalities each. Significant chi-square test results of correctly and incorrectly rated MF overall, for MF and modalities each, and between MF and modalities.

Using Pearson's chi-square test and the "match" vs. "no match" data preparation for more detailed analyses, we can find significant differences between single MF across modality conditions (cf. Fig. 2): N + Foc-: $\chi^2(1) = 13.58$, $p \leq .002$; N + Epi-: $\chi^2(1) = 13.76$, $p \leq .002$; Foc+ + Foc-: $\chi^2(1) = 12.75$, $p \leq .002$; and Foc+ + Epi-: $\chi^2(1) = 12.86$, $p \leq .002$. Therefore, these conditions were perceived as rather different and, thus, N + Foc+, as well as Foc- + Epi- were perceived as rather alike. No significant difference for the merged categories N + Foc+ + Foc- + Epi- could be found. The calculation of a 95 %-confidence interval results only for the N and Foc+ conditions in ratings above chance: CI = [48.0; 89.1] and CI = [43.3;71.0], respectively. This concludes that N and Foc+ are well recognised, rated above chance level and rated differently than Foc- and Epi-, which are perceived less well in our VH Billie.

In a second step, we want to evaluate, if there are differences between the modality conditions. As Table 2 depicts, there is a trend between three conditions S+G > S > G (cf. Fig. 2), indicating that MF are more clearly recognised if more modalities are involved, which is a clear statement in favour of multimodality. A significant effect between S+G + G: $\chi^2(1) = 3.07$, $p = .080$ was lost after correcting for type I error. However, since N is even better perceived than S+G, the difference of the categories N+G reaches significance: $\chi^2(1) = 12.38$, $p \leq .002$. Also, the 95 %-confidence interval for modalities shows that the S+G condition has been rated above chance with CI = [48.8;80.8], N getting the same result as above. Finally, the merged categories for single modalities across MF conditions reached significance: N + S+G + S + G: $\chi^2(3) = 26.66$, $p \leq .002$. For now, we can only report a trend between S+G > S > G, but it would be interesting to investigate this relationship further.

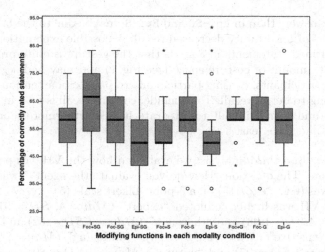

Fig. 3. Recall: Percentages of correctly rated statements in ten conditions. The baseline condition N is marked as a dotted line. The median values differ only in three numbers: 66.7, 58.3, and 50.0. In the multimodal S+G condition, a trend of decreasing recall between Foc+, Foc- and Epi- is visible. Recall in G seems slightly higher than in S.

Effect on recall. We were interested in how much participants recalled from Billie's narration about his life as a VH. The results (cf. Fig. 3) indicate that there is a trend of decreasing knowledge between the three S+G conditions: Foc+ ($\mu = 63.3$) > Foc- ($\mu = 60.6$) > Epi- ($\mu = 52.9$). The differences of correctly categorised statements between Foc+ and Epi- is 10.4 %, this amounts to 114 correct answers in Foc+ vs. 108 correct answers in Epi-. Indeed, the main finding is that there is a significant difference between Foc+ and Epi- ($p = .041$, independent samples t-test, normally distributed). Unfortunately, the significant difference is too small as that it holds if we correct for type I error (we ran 18 tests).

A second trend is that the content in the respective G conditions is slightly better recalled than in the respective S conditions. However, this difference did not reach significance. Additionally, Foc-S was recalled better than Foc+S and Epi-S, although the keywords proved to be more complicated in Foc- in the pretests. Perhaps this indicates that obvious modifications in speech (Foc+:"particularly" and Epi-: "I don't know") distract more from the content of the utterance than more subtle modifications (Foc-: "just") and gestures, being more subtle, distract less than speech. This assumption is supported by the accumulated standard deviations: Foc+ = 15.5, Foc- = 11.2, Epi- = 14.8 and S+G = 13.3, S = 14.1, G = 9.5. Compared to the baseline condition N = 9.4, it seems that Foc- and in particular G can be easiest integrated, i.e., there is more certainty about how a statement is categorised.

Examining single conditions, we find that participants got the highest recall score in Foc+SG, probably due to a positive effect of the linguistic markers combined with gestures of focus and highlighting. In the condition Epi-G, there were more correct answers than in Epi-SG and Epi-S, maybe due to the fact that linguistic markers of uncertainty decreased recall. A possible explanation for many correctly identified statements in Foc- is that the gesture is quite prominent: it used the most amount of gesture space (see Fig. 1) and may had a great visual effect on the participants, causing participants to pay extra attention and, thus, perhaps leading to better recall. To conclude, content recall is best in S+G, intermediate in G and more difficult to integrate in S. Furthermore, Foc+ triggers biggest recall and Epi- least.

VH perception. In a third analysis, we evaluated how the VH was perceived by the participants. The question "How do you evaluate the agent?" was answered by 20 adjectives (e.g., "expert") on a 5-point Likert scale (5 = "very" to 1 = "not at all"). The VH was highly connoted "expert" ($Mdn = 4$, $SD = .91$), "intelligent" ($Mdn = 4$ $SD = 1.08$) and "thorough" ($Mdn = 4$ $SD = .82$) and least associated with "sensitive" ($Mdn = 2$ $SD = .93$), "fun-loving" ($Mdn = 2$ $SD = .99$), "lively" ($Mdn = 2$ $SD = .97$) and "natural" ($Mdn = 2$ $SD = .89$).

In order to make more general statements about the VH, we used a design carried out by [13,14], in that we merged 17 items to three scales likeability, competence and human-likeliness. We calculated Cronbach's Alpha for the indices and the values for all three scales were above .7, which justifies the combination of these items into one mean value as a single index for this scale. Items for likeability ($a = .833$) are "pleasant", "sensitive", "friendly", "likeable", "affable", "approachable" and "sociable"; items for competence ($a = .722$) are "dedicated", "trustworthy", "thorough", "helpful", "intelligent", "organized" and "expert"; and items for human-likeness ($a = .708$) are "active", "humanlike", "fun-loving" and "lively".

Again, we carried out analyses on the differences between our MF (N, Foc+, Foc- and Epi-) and between the modality conditions (N, S+G, S and G). We calculated the non-parametric Mann-Whitney U test, as the distributions of all three scales deviated significantly from normal (Shapiro-Wilk test: $p \leq .000$). The assumptions for the test were met: the dependent variable is measured at the ordinal level (1 to 5) and the independent variable consists of two categorical, independent groups (10 conditions) with independent observations and all sample sizes were >30. There were small differences in the number of participants between the conditions, cf. end of Sect. 3. Comparing all categories of all scales and analyses, we get 36 comparisons in total and to avoid inflated error rates, we calculated the Bonferroni correction on all tests.

The results of the scales (cf. Fig. 4) show similar results to those of the isolated items: the VH was perceived as rather competent (all Mdn = 4), intermediate likeable (all Mdn = 3) and rather not human-like (all Mdn = 2, but for Foc+ Mdn = 3) on the three scales and in the two analyses. Analysing differences between the MF, the VH was perceived as more likeable in N/Foc+ compared to Foc-, since there is a highly significant difference between the conditions (each $p = .004$). The difference between N/Foc+ and Foc-/Epi- also shows when looking at competence: There are highly significant differences between N and Foc- and between N and Epi- (each $p = .004$) and further between Foc+ and Foc-

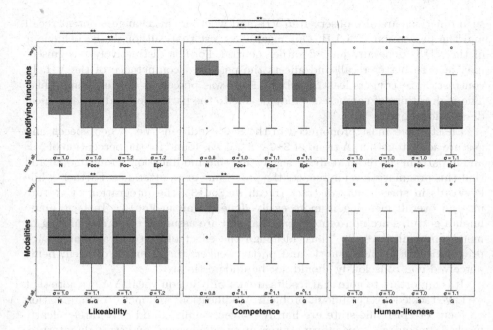

Fig. 4. Differences in the perception of the VH between the MF (Foc+, Foc- and Epi-) and between the modalities (S+G, S and G) on the three scales likeability, competence and human-likeness with significant results between conditions.

($p = .004$) and significant differences between Foc+ and Epi- ($p = .036$). Thus, N in particular but also Foc+ are perceived as more competent. On the scale of human-likeness, Foc- comes into focus, which is perceived as least human-like, with differences to all other conditions and a significant difference to Foc+ ($p = .036$).

Analyses between the modalities are less diverse. N is perceived as more likeable with a highly significant difference to S ($p = .004$), thus, S is perceived as least likeable, followed by G and then S+G. As with MF, N is again perceived as most competent compared to the other modalities, with a highly significant difference to S+G ($p = .004$). Therefore, the condition S+G is perceived as least competent, followed by G and then S. For human-likeness, all conditions seem to be perceived similar and there was only a significant difference between N and S before correcting for type I error. To sum up, the VH was perceived as competent (particularly N and Foc+) but rather not humanlike (especially Foc- and S+G) and rather not likeable in the S condition.

5   Conclusion

In this work, we investigated whether and how VH can use speech and gestures to add meta-communicative information to their utterances. Based on a study that identified three main modifying functions (Foc+/Foc-/Epi-), we tested whether such functions are also observed in VH, and whether this changes content recall and the perception of a VH. Our results suggest that, although the behaviour of the VH is generally judged rather neutral, Foc+ is distinctively recognised, may lead to better recall and affects the perceived competence of the VH. In contrast, Epi- triggers least recall and Foc- was perceived as least human-like. The high ratings of competence may be due to the partly detailed and technical descriptions given.

Effects were most pronounced in the S+G conditions, i.e., when speech and gesture acted together. A trend of S+G > S > G was found for the perception of MF and in parts in the recall analysis, suggesting that modification is multimodal and that this pragmatic level influences the processing of an utterance. Further, while keywords in speech may distract (recall in Foc+S), the integration of gesture into an overall meaning is more easily done (recall in Foc+G). In fact, many human gestures are non-representational and are assumed to be modulating or meta-communicative [2]. Thus, although the effect of gestures assuming such pragmatic MF is more subtle and partly weaker, the strength of them being perceived non-consciously should not be underestimated.

It is important to note that results are not fully unequivocal. Yet, we note that we have tackled a very difficult problem. Modifications and meta-communication on focus or epistemic state are hardly conventionalized and only rarely clearly marked. In contrast, this information is often "analogous" and strongly interpretative. We thus were faced with many methodological challenges, e.g., relating to the adjectives or keywords used to capture this phenomenon of pragmatic and content-modifying meta-communication. Yet, our corpus analyses imply that competent and cooperative speakers do use such markers to help their addressees arrive at the correct interpretation, and this behaviour should also be beneficial for VHs. Our results do seem to confirm this.

Possible reasons for the strong results of N were discussed in Sect. 4 (effect of MF). However, MF can be made significantly more salient using more distinct keywords in Foc-, more defined gestures in Epi- (and Foc-), adding intonation to the synthesised speech, and enabling more idle VH body movement. Regarding the procedure, the content questions should be queried only after all stimuli have been presented, since the use of content questions may have distracted from the nonverbal behaviour of the VH, similar to the selective attention test [15].

Acknowledgements. This work was supported by the Cluster of Excellence Cognitive Interaction Technology 'CITEC' (EXC 277) at Bielefeld University, funded by the German Research Foundation (DFG). A special thanks goes to Iwan de Kok whose helpful comments made the paper clearer in various aspects.

References

1. Wharton, T.: Pragmatics and Non-verbal Communication. Cambridge University Press, Cambridge (2009)
2. McNeill, D.: Hand and Mind: What Gestures Reveal About Thought. University of Chicago Press, Chicago (1992)

3. Freigang, F., Kopp, S.: Analysing the modifying functions of gesture in multi-modal utterances. In: Proceedings of the 4th Conference on Gesture and Speech in Interaction (GESPIN), Nantes, France (2015)

4. Kendon, A.: Gesture: Visible Action as Utterance. Cambridge University Press, Cambridge (2004)

5. Payrató, L., Teßendorf, S.: Pragmatic Gestures. In: Müller, C., Cienki, A., Fricke, E., Ladewig, S.H., McNeill, D., Teßendorf, S. (eds.) Body Language Communication: An International Handbook on Multimodality in Human Interaction. Handbooks of Linguistics and Communication Science 38(1), pp. 1531–1539. De Gruyter Mouton, Berlin/Boston (2013)

6. Lu, Y., Aubergé, V., Rilliard, A.: Do you hear my attitude? Prosodic perception of social affects in Mandarin. In: International Conference on Speech Prosody Proceedings, pp. 685–688 (2012)

7. Kok, K., Bergmann, K., Cienki, A., Kopp, S.: Mapping out the multifunctionality of speakers' gestures. Gesture 15(1), 37–59 (2016)

8. Freigang, F., Kopp, S.: Modifying Functions of Gesture - Exploring the Dimensions of Function and Form (in preparation)

9. Schoonjans, S.: Modalpartikeln als multimodale Konstruktionen. Eine korpus-basierte Kookkurrenzanalyse von Modalpartikeln und Gestik im Deutschen. KU Leuven: Dissertationsschrift (2014)

10. Leiner, D.J.: SoSci Survey (Version 2.6.00-i) [Computer software] (2014). http://www.soscisurvey.com

11. Kranstedt, A., Kopp, S.,Wachsmuth., I.: MURML: a multimodal utterance representation markup language for conversational agents. In: Proceedings of the AAMAS 2002 Workshop on Embodied Conversational Agents (2002)

12. van Welbergen, H., Yaghoubzadeh, R., Kopp, S.: AsapRealizer 2.0: the next steps in fluent behavior realization for ECAs. In: Bickmore, T., Marsella, S., Sidner, C. (eds.) IVA 2014. LNCS (LNAI), vol. 8637, pp. 449–462. Springer, Heidelberg (2014). doi:10.1007/978-3-319-09767-1_56

13. van Welbergen, H., Ding, Y., Sattler, K., Pelachaud, C., Kopp, S.: Real-time visual prosody for interactive virtual agents. In: Brinkman, W.-P., Broekens, J., Heylen, D. (eds.) IVA 2015. LNCS (LNAI), vol. 9238, pp. 139–151. Springer, Heidelberg (2015). doi:10.1007/978-3-319-21996-7_16

14. Bergmann, K., Kopp, S., Eyssel, F.: Individualized gesturing outperforms average gesturing – evaluating gesture production in virtual humans. In: Allbeck, J., Badler, N., Bickmore, T., Pelachaud, C., Safonova, A. (eds.) IVA 2010. LNCS (LNAI), vol. 6356, pp. 104–117. Springer, Heidelberg (2010). doi:10.1007/978-3-642-15892-6_11

15. Simons, D.J., Chabris, C.F.: Gorillas in our midst: sustained inattentional blindness for dynamic events. Perception 28(9), 1059–1074 (1999)

An Enhanced Intelligent Agent with Image Description Generation

Ben Fielding, Philip Kinghorn, Kamlesh Mistry, and Li Zhang[✉]

Facutly of Engineering and Environment, Department of Computer Science
and Digital Technologies, Northumbria University, Newcastle NE1 8ST, UK
{ben.fielding,philip.kinghorn,kamlesh.mistry,
li.zhang}@northumbria.ac.uk

Abstract. In this paper, we present an Embodied Conversational Agent (ECA) enriched with automatic image understanding, using vision data derived from state-of-the-art machine learning techniques for the advancement of autonomous interaction with the elderly or infirm. The agent is developed to conduct health and emotion well-being monitoring for the elderly. It is not only able to conduct question-answering via speech-based interaction, but also able to provide analysis of the user's surroundings, company, emotional states, hazards and fall actions via visual data using deep learning techniques. The agent is accessible from a web browser and can be communicated with via voice means, with a webcam required for the visual analysis functionality. The system has been evaluated with diverse real-life images to prove its efficiency.

Keywords: Intelligent conversational agent · Image description generation · Human agent interaction

1 Introduction

We propose a system to assist with the day-to-day care of the elderly by attempting to emulate some of the human contact they receive throughout the day. By providing an elderly person with a non-human, Embodied Conversational Agent (ECA) companion, we improve access to information, and provide accident prevention and reaction functionality. Evidence shows that the social interaction provided by ECAs has a positive effect on the interacting user, whilst information provided through conversation with an ECA is more easily absorbed and understood [1]. The interface of the proposed system is illustrated in Fig. 1.

To achieve these goals, we incorporate a number of unique computer vision techniques together, along with an approachable 3D humanoid avatar interface with real-time chat functionality. Intelligent Chat, proposed in this research, provides real-time visual, audial and oral conversation with a number of additional features tailored to the needs of elderly users. It provides answers to queries on any subject using integration with the popular online encyclopedia Wikipedia. Intelligent Chat provides live feedback of the emotional state of the user using current vision-based facial emotion recognition techniques applied to the user's webcam, all performed in the browser. Moreover, the user's

© Springer International Publishing AG 2016
D. Traum et al. (Eds.): IVA 2016, LNAI 10011, pp. 110–119, 2016.
DOI: 10.1007/978-3-319-47665-0_10

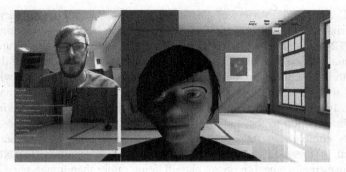

Fig. 1. The interface of the proposed Intelligent Chat system

environment is monitored by the system using state-of-the-art deep learning computer vision techniques embedded in a central server system, providing analysis of the overall scene, objects, potential hazards around the user, and alerting in the event of a fall. This vision-based analysis, performed on the central server, is used to enhance the conversation with the user, thereby providing an engaging and life-like companionship experience.

The main contribution of this research is the addition of deep learning based image description generation functionality to an ECA, allowing the agent to provide health surveillance. It is one of few pioneer systems in incorporating vision-based analysis to enable more autonomous agent behaviours to enhance user experience. Moreover, existing research on image description generation tends to employ a holistic method, thereby encountering limitations in handling cross-domain images. Compared with the existing related research, our work employs a local region-based approach, thus has great robustness in dealing with cross-domain images that the system has not been trained upon (e.g. images with fall and hazard situations).

2   Related Work

Care of elderly and infirm patients often requires round-the-clock observation to prevent or react to accidents that can result in physical injury. This constant presence of a healthcare provider is often impossible to achieve due to the number of patients greatly outweighing the number of carers. Therefore, vision-based health monitoring systems using computer vision techniques are required. Image description generation techniques have gained intensive research attention recently to benefit such applications. Some of such developments are discussed below.

2.1   Image Description Generation

Image description generation has been the focus of the ImageNet Large Scale Visual Recognition Challenge (ILSVRC) since its conception in 2010. The ILSVRC provides training and testing datasets of images and appropriate labels and presents a number of challenges such as object detection, localization, and scene classification. Prior to 2012, the ILSVRC witnessed a variety of classification techniques used with varying effectiveness. Krizhevsky et al. [2] proved, in 2012, that Deep Convolutional Neural Networks (CNNs) demonstrated hugely improved, state-of-the-art accuracy when applied to image classification. Following this discovery, a large portion of the entrants and all of the subsequent winners have been based on deep learning with CNNs. Sermanet et al. [3] presented a system named OverFeat in 2013 to classify images whilst simultaneously providing localisation information and object detection, adding a large amount of information to the output of classification attempts. The proposed system used a CNN combined with multiscale sliding window processing to achieve this. Girshick et al. [4] created a system named Regions with CNN features (R-CNN) in 2014 which also uses region specific object classification rather than image-wide classification. The R-CNN uses images alongside accompanying proposed regions (as locations in the image) as inputs. The images are then cropped, creating individual sub-images for the proposed regions. The sub-images can then be fed through a CNN for processing. Classification is performed in the final fully connected layer using a Support Vector Machine (SVM) for each object. R-CNN provides a significant improvement in error rates when compared with OverFeat, due to the use of selective search region proposal techniques, rather than the sliding window approach used by OverFeat. The use of a region-specific object classifier allows for much finer-grained description generation through the inclusion of location data which can provide relative position information for any objects or people retrieved from the image. Girshick [5] recently improved the original R-CNN to create Fast R-CNN, with a number of changes resulting in greatly improved classification performance.

3   The Proposed Intelligent Chat

The proposed system is designed to function as a web application in order to reduce potential barriers to use due to the widespread ownership of Internet accessible, camera equipped devices. The functionality is separated over the client-server architecture in an attempt to make the most of available processing power on both sides, allowing for responsive communication. The application was designed to also function as an information retrieval system, enabling users to ask questions which could be answered using the Internet as a knowledgebase. The accessibility of computer systems, whilst constantly improving, can still be an issue which prevents their use by the elderly. By incorporating access to the Internet and to wider functionality, through our accessible audial and oral interface, we provide a much less daunting way to assimilate these new users into the connected world.

3.1   The System Architecture

The system was designed as a distributed model with a view to operate from a central server, allowing access to the functionality by the end users through a web browser. The server itself is a Python application built upon Tornado [6], an asynchronous, real-time, web framework. Communication between the central server and the individual client web browsers is performed through the use of websockets. On the server end, Tornado provides access to the websocket functionality, allowing interaction through Python methods. On the client-side, this interaction is provided by the Javascript library Socket.io. The image capture functionality is implemented using the getUserMedia method in HTML5 to capture webcam data. All of the image capturing and streaming are performed on the client-side using HTML5 and Javascript. Overall, the agent-based system incorporates the server-based image description generation and Wikipedia question answering alongside the client-based emotional expression recognition.

3.2 Conversation Extensions

The conversational functionality forms the core of the system, providing the avatar with a means of prolonging interaction with the user and attempting to maintain a flow of conversation. The conversational system is implemented using Artificial Intelligence Markup Language (AIML) [7]. AIML provides an XML compliant framework, allowing for the creation of complex two-way chat functionality without scripting every response, achieved through the use of recursive pattern matching [8]; resulting in a realistic, albeit simple way of creating a conversational system. AIML provides a number of open source libraries containing pre-written chat functionality and conversation which can be extended to suit the particular use case. The most prominent of these is known as 'The Artificial Linguistic Internet Computer Entity', i.e. A.L.I.C.E. We used the ALICE library as a starting point for the companion's chat functionality and extended its conversational capabilities by incorporating our own AIML.

AIML provides the tools to set up artificial two-way communication using text. With our goal of creating an approachable companion to be used by elderly, not necessarily computer literate users, we decided to bridge the accessibility gap by providing audial and oral communication via speech recognition and synthesis. Both aspects were implemented using the relatively new HTML5 Web Speech API [9]; audial using the Speech-Synthesis interface while oral using the SpeechRecognition interface. Interaction with the system can therefore be performed entirely through spoken conversation.

We have extended ALICE's vocabulary through the implementation of a question-answering system, using Wikipedia as a data source. The system currently parses questions and searches Wikipedia using the main terms of the question if it cannot answer using its existing vocabulary. A short summary of the search term from the beginning of the Wikipedia page is then retrieved and spoken to the user.

The proposed system also includes functionality to retrieve and present the user's location using the HTML5 geolocation API. The location is spoken using latitude and longitude co-ordinates – a small map image is also illustrated showing the user's location.

3.3 Image Description Generation

The proposed Intelligent Chat system has included a novel image description generation component. It is implemented using a deep learning architecture to provide natural language description of the content of an image. It includes a number of key steps; object detection and recognition, attribute prediction, scene classification, and description generation. The system architecture of this image description generation component is provided in Fig. 2. We discuss each key step of this image description generation function in detail below.

Object Detection & Recognition. The first stage of the proposed image description generation component is to conduct object detection and recognition. The object detector implemented is the Regional Convolutional Neural Network, i.e. R-CNN, from Girschick et al. [4] consisting of 8 learned layers; 5 convolutional layers and 3 fully connected layers. The output of this object detection function is to identify bounding box coordinates of each salient object in the image. This network can detect and classify 200 object categories from the ImageNet 2013 dataset, collecting selective search data from the whole image. These regions are then each classified by 200 SVMs in order to determine which areas contain a specific object in an image. The object detector is pre-trained on the ILSVRC-13 object detection challenge, taking approximately a week to train on state-of-the-art hardware.

Attribute Prediction. Creating a full sentence description of the visual image input of users' environment is a more challenging task than object labelling. To achieve this, the object image(s) detected from the previous stage are passed to another CNN provided by Chatfield et al. [10]. This network has a similar structure to normal CNNs, however does not possess the fully connected or classification layers at the lower end of the network, meaning that the network only extracts image feature vectors to be used elsewhere. Like the R-CNN, this network consists of 8 learned layers; 5 convolutional layers and 3 fully connected layers.

The collected features are then used to train multiple attribute classifiers in order to increase the descriptiveness of an object label. There are more than 50 attributes used in this research in total, in order to provide more detailed people and object descriptions. For objects, there are 26 attributes relating to colour, shape and size information. These attributes are collected from a fully annotated subset of the ImageNet dataset [11]. There are also 26 attributes for human description ranging from hair colour, style, age and ethnicity. These are taken from the PubFig dataset [12], originally consisting of more than 70 attributes to describe people. For these experiments only a subset of these attributes (i.e. 26 attributes) are used during testing for description generation.

Scene Classification. Scene recognition and classification is used to enhance the image description generation by providing an overall idea of the setting, which can then be enhanced through the inclusion of detailed object and person description. The classification system used is a CNN trained on the MIT Places dataset created by Zhou et al. [13]. The Places dataset contains over 7 million images from 476 scene categories created using Amazon Mechanical Turk workers to label the images. The network proposed by Zhou et al. has been used in this research, which was trained on almost 2.5 million images, comprised of 205 different scene categories. Its architecture was originally taken from the Caffe reference network [14].

Facial Expression Recognition. The system has integrated an intelligent facial expression recognition component to identify seven basic emotions: happiness, anger, sadness,

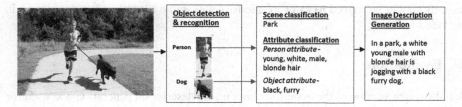

Fig. 2. The architecture for deep learning based image description generation

disgust, surprise, fear, and contempt. It borrows the architecture implemented in [15–17] and consists of feature extraction using Local Binary Patterns and micro-GA embedded Particle Swarm Optimization feature selection. It has been proven to show superior performances in comparison to related research when evaluated with the CK + dataset [18].

Sentence Generation. To construct a valid descriptive sentence, the recognized object and attribute labels must be combined in a very natural-sounding manner. In this work, a template-based approach is used to transform these descriptive labels into multiple short sentences that can be concatenated and reported as a single detailed description of the image in question. The scene label collected in the earlier stage is also utilised in this process, which is used either as an opening or a closing statement to the sentence. An example output of the deep-learning based image description generation is shown in Fig. 2.

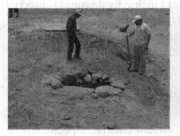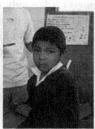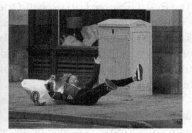

In a desert, I can see a middle-aged white male with blonde hair is next to a senior white male with grey hair.

In a kindergarten classroom, I can see a child white male with black hair

In a plaza, there is a young white male with brown hair. I can see a person on the floor. Do you require assistance?

Fig. 3. Example image descriptions generated by the proposed system

Fall and Hazard Detection. The image description framework also has the capability to describe out-of-scope images such as hazardous objects on the floor and a falling person. Both of these aspects are based on the assumption that the camera is at a fixed height and a threshold value has previously been determined where the floor meets the wall. A hazardous object and fall actions are reported when a detected object or person is reported below the threshold value. These are again described as sentences and merged with the previous outputs to ask users if they require assistance, or to suggest that the hazards should be moved to safer locations. An example for fall action description is provided in Fig. 3.

4 Evaluation

A lightweight version of the system without image description generation was used for evaluation in order to compare its performance with that of the full version of the system with image description generation during user evaluation. This cut down version of the system was hosted on an AWS t2 micro instance to allow for distributed testing and uptime evaluation. The system successfully handles multiple simultaneous users from geographically diverse locations. No system crashes were observed over the course of several months.

The overall system with image description generation has been hosted online on a server possessing a relatively powerful GPU to enable full access to the entire functionality of the system. Client Internet access is also required for the speech synthesis and recognition portions of the client-side functionality. The full system also successfully handles multiple concurrent users from geographically diverse locations. The system has been successfully intensively tested under a vast number of real-life settings. Evaluation results for image description generation using the proposed deep learning architecture are discussed in detail below.

4.1 Evaluation of Image Description Generation

The ROUGE score [19] (Recall-Oriented Understudy for Gisting Evaluation) is used to evaluate the image description generation component of the proposed system. It provides a metric to determine the quality and similarity of summaries between human description annotations and computer generated outputs. The metrics within ROUGE are based on the number of n-grams, sequences of words and word pairs between machine-generated and ground truth summaries.

In order to evaluate the proposed system, an existing image description dataset is used, i.e. the IAPR-12 dataset [20], which consists of ~20,000 images, each annotated with a descriptive sentence or description in both English and German. Specifically, a subset of 100 images from IAPR-12 is used for the evaluation of our work to generate the ROUGE score.

ROUGE-1 and ROUGE-2 are n-gram based approaches, essentially favouring generated descriptions that contain n-grams shared with the Ground Truth (GT) descriptions, thus preferring a description which is similar to the GT sentences. ROUGE-L refers to the Longest Common Subsequence (LCS), which considers two sequences X and Y. This LCS, is the subsequence that occurs in both sequences with the maximum length. In sentence level ROUGE-L, the perception is that the longer the LCS of generated and GT sentences, the more similar the sentences. The ROUGE scores shown in Table 1, show similar and in some cases improved scores over existing image description generation systems, such as [21], that also implement this metric. Figure 3 shows some example outputs of the proposed image description generation component.

Table 1. ROUGE scores over the 100 images by comparing system generated results to GT descriptions provided by the IAPR-12 image database. For each metric, the recall (R), precision (P) and F-scores (F) averaged over the 100 images are presented.

	ROUGE-1			ROUGE-2			ROUGE-L		
100 Images	R	P	F	R	P	F	R	P	F
Results	0.220	**0.389**	0.281	0.041	0.072	0.052	0.210	**0.372**	0.269

Since the proposed image description generation function has a series of individual key steps with each trained on datasets relevant to their intended use but unrelated to the whole images, it is able to detect and recognize a large number of object classes especially from challenging cross-domain images, ensuring a minimal amount of data loss. Pairing this with the ability to recognise and classify a large number of human and object attributes enables the system to create descriptive attribute labels and produce descriptive sentences, of any image the system processes. Moreover, other existing image description generation systems tend to be trained and tested on the same or very similar datasets [22, 23], meaning the methods used in these frameworks essentially understand the types of sentences and structures required in order to achieve higher scores for test images from the same domain, however testing these frameworks with irrelevant cross-domain images tends to produce unsatisfactory results with dramatically reduced performances. In comparison with the above related research, the proposed system focuses on a regional approach and experimental results indicate that it shows great robustness and flexibility in dealing with out-of-scope or cross-domain image description generation tasks because of its focusing on image regional details to retrieve more local information. Therefore, the scores achieved by the Intelligent Chat system are significant, especially when dealing with cross-domain (e.g. healthcare) images.

Another preliminary user evaluation with 50 users is also conducted using the two versions of the system with and without image description generation. The version with image description generation achieved higher user satisfaction and significantly improved user experience than the version without image analysis. Moreover, the overall system with image description generation resulted in positive comments regarding the integration of Wikipedia and image description generation to enhance question answering and human agent interaction. Most users agreed that the image description generation function would be useful for visually impaired users and the detection of falls and hazards would be especially helpful in assisting independent living.

5   Conclusion and Future Work

This research proposes a vision enriched Intelligent Chat system for elderly care. The system is developed to conduct facial emotion recognition, object and scene recognition, hazardous objects and scene classification, and fall detection. Deep learning based image description generation is also used to generate sentences based on the above outputs to warn of hazards or generate alarms when falls occur. The Intelligent Chat system is tested with users in real-life settings and evaluation results indicate that it achieves 0.389 ROUGE-1 score for image description generation for the evaluation of 100 images from the IAPR-12 dataset, which is comparable to other state-of-the art related research [21]. Future implementations of this work could be improved by utilising a faster, more efficient object detector such as the Fast R-CNN. The sentence generation functionality could also be altered to use machine learned methods such as Recurrent Neural Networks that have proven successful in machine translation [24, 25].

The proposed system could be further extended to perform the observational duties of a carer, allowing a single carer to be alerted to accidents or incidents involving any of a number of distinct patients, in potentially separate geographical locations. Such a system could enable a greater degree of independence for patients who would otherwise require constant human supervision. Alternatively, the techniques applied in this work could be applied in other domains in order to enhance human-computer interaction, such as workplace training or interactive learning for children. Moreover, the proposed health monitoring system could be extended to integrate with diagnostic systems where images (e.g. retinal or blood images) can be taken by smart devices for analysis to promote early diagnosis [26, 27].

Acknowledgments.   We appreciate the funding support received from Higher Education Innovation Fund and RPPTV Ltd.

References

1. De Vos, E.: Look at that doggy in my windows, on effects of anthropomorphism in human-agent interaction. Doctoral Thesis, Utrecht University (2002)
2. Krizhevsky, A., Sutskever, I., Hinton, G.E.: ImageNet classification with deep convolutional neural networks. In: Advances in Neural Information Processing Systems, pp. 1097–1105 (2012)
3. Sermanet, P., Eigen, D., Zhang, X., Mathieu, M., Fergus, R., LeCun, Y.: OverFeat: integrated recognition, localization and detection using convolutional networks (2013)
4. Girshick, R., Donahue, J., Darrell, T., Malik, J.: Rich feature heirarchies for accurate object detection and semantic segmentation. IEEE Transactions on Computer Vision and Pattern Recognition (CVPR), pp. 580–587 (2014)
5. Girshick, R.: Fast R-CNN. In: Proceedings of ICCV 2015 (2015)
6. Facebook: Tornado (2011). http://www.tornadoweb.org/en/stable/
7. Wallace, R.: The elements of AIML style. Alice AI Foundation (2003). https://files.ifi.uzh.ch/cl/hess/classes/seminare/chatbots/style.pdf
8. Wallace, R.: Symbolic reductions in AIML (2000). http://www.alicebot.org/documentation/srai.html
9. Shires, G., Wennborg, H.: Web speech API specification. W3C Community Final Specification Agreement (2012). https://dvcs.w3.org/hg/speech-api/raw-file/tip/speechapi.html
10. Chatfield, K., Simonyan, K., Vedalsi, A., Zisserman, A.: Return of the devil in the details delving deep into convolutional neural nets. In: BMVC (2014)
11. Fei-Fei, L.: ImageNet: crowdsourcing, benchmarking and other cool things. CMU VASC Seminar (2010)
12. Kumar, N., Berg, A.C., Belhumeur, P.N., Nayar, S.K.: Attribute and simile classifiers for face verification. In: International Conference on Computer Vision (ICCV) (2009)

13. Zhou, B., Lapedriza, A., Xiao, J., Torralba, A., Oliva, A.: Learning deep features for scene recognition using places database. In: Advances in Neural Information Processing Systems, pp. 487–495 (2014)
14. Jia, Y. et al.: Caffe: an open source convolutional architecture for fast feature embedding (2013). http://caffe.berkeleyvision.org/
15. Neoh, S.C., Zhang, L., Mistry, K., Hossain, M.A., Lim, C.P., Aslam, N., Kinghorn, P.: Intelligent facial emotion recognition using a layered encoding cascade optimization model. Appl. Soft Comput. **34**(2015), 72–93 (2015)
16. Mistry, K., Zhang, L., Neoh, S.C., Lim, C.P., Fielding, B.: A micro-GA embedded PSO feature selection approach to intelligent facial emotion recognition. IEEE Trans. Cybern. **PP**(99), 1–14 (2016). ISSN 2168-2267
17. Zhang, L., Mistry, K., Jiang, M., Neoh, S.C., Hossain, A.: Adaptive facial point detection and emotion recognition for a humanoid robot. Comput. Vis. Image Underst. **140**, 93–114 (2015)
18. Lucey, P., Cohn, J.F., Kanade, T., Saragih, J., Ambadar, Z., Matthews, I.: The extended Cohn-Kanade dataset (CK+): a complete expression dataset for action unit and emotion-specified expression. In: Proceedings of CVPR4HB (2010)
19. Lin, C.: ROUGE: a package for automatic evaluation of summaries. In: Proceedings of Workshop on Text Summarization Branches Out (2004)
20. Grubinger, M., Clough, P.D., Müller, H., Deselaers, T.: The IAPR benchmark: a new evaluation resource for visual information systems. In: International Conference on Language Resources and Evaluation (2006)
21. Lin, D., Fidler, S., Kong, C., Urtasun, R.: Generating multi-sentence natural language descriptions of indoor scenes. In: British Machine Vision Conference (BMVC) (2015)
22. Karpathy, A., Fei-Fei, L.: Deep visual-semantic alignments for generating image descriptions. In: Computer Vision and Pattern Recognition (CVPR) (2015)
23. Vinyals, O., Toshev, A., Bengio, S., Erhan, D.: Show and tell: a neural image caption generator. In: Computer Vision and Pattern Recognition (CVPR) (2015)
24. Sutskever, I., Vinyals, O., Le, Q.V.: Sequence to sequence learning with neural networks. In: Advances in Neural Information Processing Systems, pp. 3104–3112 (2014)
25. Jozefowicz, R., Zaremba, W., Sutskever, I.: An empirical exploration of recurrent network architectures. In: Proceedings of the 32nd International Conference on Machine Learning (ICML 2015), pp. 2342–2350 (2015)
26. Neoh, S.C., Srisukkham, W., Zhang, L, Todryk, S., Greystoke, B., Lim, C.P., Hossain, A., Aslam, N.: An intelligent decision support system for Leukaemia diagnosis using microscopic blood images. Sci. Rep. **5**(14938), 1–14 (2015)
27. Bourouis, A., Feham, M., Hossain, M.A., Zhang, L.: An intelligent mobile based decision support system for retinal disease diagnosis. Decis. Support Syst. **59**, 341–350 (2014)

A Smartphone-Based Virtual Agent for Atrial Fibrillation Education and Counseling

Everlyne Kimani[1(✉)], Timothy Bickmore[1], Ha Trinh[1], Lazlo Ring[1],
Michael K. Paasche-Orlow[2], and Jared W. Magnani[3]

[1] College of Computer and Information Science,
Northeastern University, Boston, MA, USA
kimani15@ccs.neu.edu
[2] Boston Medical Center, Boston, MA, USA
[3] Department of Medicine, University of Pittsburgh Medical Center,
Pittsburgh, PA, USA

Abstract. When deployed on smartphones, virtual agents have the potential to deliver life-saving advice regarding emergency medical conditions, as well as provide a convenient channel for health education to help improve the safety and efficacy of pharmacotherapy. This paper describes the use of a smartphone-based virtual agent that provides counseling to patients with Atrial Fibrillation, along with the results from a pilot acceptance study among patients with the condition. Atrial Fibrillation is a highly prevalent heart rhythm disorder and is known to significantly increase the risk of stroke, heart failure and death. In this study, a virtual agent is deployed in conjunction with a smartphone-based heart rhythm monitor that lets patients obtain real-time diagnostic information on the status of their atrial fibrillation and determine whether immediate action may be needed. The results of the study indicate that participants are satisfied with receiving information about Atrial Fibrillation via the virtual agent.

Keywords: Relational agent · Cardiovascular · Conversational agent · Atrial fibrillation · Heart rhythm

1 Introduction

Smartphones are becoming ubiquitous, with the portion of US adults who own one steadily increasing (currently at 68 %) while ownership of laptop and desktop computers is dropping [1]. Though virtual agents on smartphones lack the sense of presence and immersion that a large display can offer, smartphones provide a platform that is available anytime, anywhere, and will soon become the primary platform for deploying technology-based consumer health interventions.

In addition to their convenience, smartphones also provide a crucial affordance for time-critical applications; they provide immediate access regardless of where users are or what they might be doing. For certain health conditions, easy access to information may serve a critical role for real-time diagnosis, reinforcement of time-sensitive self-care activities (e.g., please take medicine X right now) and help link patients with their providers.

© Springer International Publishing AG 2016
D. Traum et al. (Eds.): IVA 2016, LNCS 10011, pp. 120–127, 2016.
DOI: 10.1007/978-3-319-47665-0_11

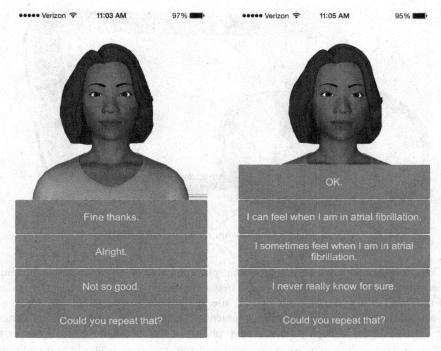

Fig. 1. Atrial fibrillation counselor agent on iPhone

Atrial fibrillation (AF) is a highly prevalent irregular heart rhythm that is associated with adverse clinical outcomes, such as stroke. AF will afflict 6-12 million people in the US by 2050 [2, 3]—and is associated with a 2- to 5-fold increased risk of stroke, heart failure, and death [4–7]. AF requires adherence to medications for stroke prevention, symptom assessment and monitoring. One of the new approaches in managing AF involves the use of a mobile heart rhythm (EKG) monitor (Fig. 2) which takes a 30-second snapshot of the user's heart rhythm and transmits it to a service that automatically analyzes it for AF and related parameters such as heart rate. It also makes this snapshot available for review by clinicians. The AliveCor heart monitor has been validated for use in detecting AF in a previous study [3]. Daily heart rhythm readings can help clinicians better manage patients with AF, and a patient experiencing symptoms such as heart palpitations or shortness of breath can take an immediate reading to help determine whether they need to adjust their activities, medications, or seek prompt medical care.

AF is a clinically complex condition where the heart rhythm can be intermittent. People are generally unaware of whether they are at risk of AF because they may not experience common symptoms such as palpitations, chest pains or even shortness of breath. In such cases, the heart rhythm monitor is crucial in detecting AF. However, as with all chronic conditions, adherence to recommended self-care procedures—such as taking daily heart rhythm readings—can be challenging for many patients to maintain.

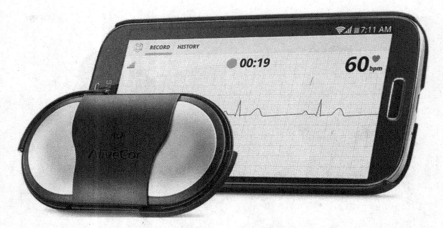

Fig. 2. Mobile heart rhythm monitor from AliveCor

We have developed a virtual agent that plays the role of an advisor in educating patients about AF. The agent answers frequently-asked questions, collects regular self-reported symptoms and quality of life assessments, motivates adherence to AF-related medications and encourages patients to take regular heart rhythm readings (Fig. 1). The agent is deployed on a smartphone so that it can be used whenever a patient is experiencing symptoms, and can motivate real-time heart rhythm readings when used in conjunction with a mobile heart rhythm monitor. The overall goals of the agent system are to reduce AF-related symptoms, improve medication and appointment adherence, decrease emergency room visits, and increase overall quality of life for patients living with AF.

The rest of this paper briefly reviews related work in this area, before describing the design of our virtual AF advisor. Then we present the results of a pilot test with AF patients and offer our conclusion.

2   Related Work

A number of virtual agents have now been developed to counsel patients on health problems, in general, and chronic disease self-care, in particular [8]. Agents have also been developed to provide one-on-one counseling to patients in areas like exercise promotion [9], weight loss [10], breastfeeding [11] and preconception care [12], with generally positive results. Additionally, virtual agents have proven to be effective in communicating complex health information to patients with low or inadequate health literacy [13].

Of particular relevance to this study are prior projects deploying virtual agents on mobile devices. Bickmore et al., investigated the use of a virtual exercise counselor agent on a PDA device with integrated pedometer [14]. Design studies demonstrated that an animated virtual agent on a handheld device was more effective at building trust with users than equivalent static agent images or text-only interfaces [15]. Kang et al., describe a similar study investigating user reactions to an animated virtual agent on a smartphone as compared to a static agent image or no image, and find that users conducted longer conversations with the animated agent [16]. Leuski et al., describe a virtual animated agent on a smartphone that helps diagnose medical conditions, although the system described is an incomplete concept demonstration [17].

3   Smartphone-Based Virtual Agent

We developed a framework for deploying animated virtual agents on smartphones (Fig. 1). The framework consists of three components: a commercial text-to-speech engine, an agent controller that synchronizes non-verbal behavior to synthesized speech, and a custom hierarchical transition network-based dialogue engine. Built using the Unity game engine, the agent controller is capable of synchronizing speech generated by the CereVoice commercial speech synthesizer to a variety of non-verbal conversational behaviors on a humanoid character. These non-verbal behaviors include: beat (baton) hand gestures and eyebrow raises for emphasis; a range of iconic/emblematic/deictic hand gestures; gaze away behavior for signaling turn-taking; facial displays of affect; and posture shifts to mark topic boundaries.

The dialogue engine consists of a custom hierarchical transition network-based engine that uses an XML-based scripting language to control the virtual agent's verbal and non-verbal behavior (Fig. 3). Each dialogue state in this language consists of one or more of the following elements: "*speech*" to control the agent's utterances and non-verbal behavior; "*button*" to prompt the user for input via the presentation of multiple response utterance options; or "*compute*" to run arbitrary procedural attachments using data collected during the user's interaction with the system. Additional non-verbal conversational behavior, such as eyebrow raises and beat gestures, are automatically added to each script during a compilation process using BEAT [18]. Utterances can be tailored at runtime using template-based text generation [19], as

```
<script>
   <state name="Greeting">
       <speech>Hi! How are you doing today?</speech>
       <buttons>
               <button nextState="Positive">Great!</button>
               <button nextState="SmartResponse">I've felt better</button>
       </buttons>
   </state>
   <state name="SmartResponse">
       <speech>I'm sorry to hear that [Name], I hope you feel better</speech>
       <compute function="DecideNextState"/>
   </state>
</script>
```

Fig. 3. Example XML script

exemplified by the *"[Name]"* syntax in Fig. 3, which inserts the user's given name into the agent utterance before it is sent to the speech synthesizer.

For use in the AF counseling system, a racially ambiguous female agent was designed based on feedback from patient interviews and focus groups.

4   Atrial Fibrillation Counseling

The AF counselor agent is designed to be used as a clinical intervention for patients recently diagnosed with AF. Patient-agent interactions are flexible and primarily user-directed to allow for patient-specific responses. During the first week of the intervention, the counselor prioritizes education in its dialog, explaining what AF is, how to effectively use the heart rhythm monitor, and describing common symptoms associated with the condition.

Over long term use, the agent promotes adherence to daily heart rhythm monitor readings. For example, the agent asks, "So, have you taken an AliveCor reading since we last talked?" or say, "I understand. Life can get in the way. Don't forget, it's important to take at least one reading a day, and whenever you feel you need to." As a reminder the agent would say "As soon as we are finished with our chat, please take a reading to send to the research team." The agent also promotes adherence to AF-related medications and clinic appointments.

Furthermore, the agent asks the patient to report symptoms associated with AF— such as palpitations, dizziness, and fatigue—as well as side effects such as bleeding from blood thinning medications. The agent tracks intervention outcomes by periodically asking patients for quality of life assessments. Feedback on self-reported patient information is based on both absolute ratings ("Sorry to hear you're not feeling well"), and longitudinal changes ("Looks like things are improving!").

5   Pilot Evaluation Study

We conducted a pilot study to evaluate the acceptance of our smartphone based AF counseling application among adults with non-valvular atrial fibrillation who owned an iPhone. With participant consent, we installed the agent and AliveCor applications on their phones and asked them to take the system home for a one-week evaluation before returning to the clinic to report on their experience.

5.1   Participants

We recruited participants from Boston University Medical Center for our pilot study. Participants were required to be 18 years of age or older; English speaking, in possession of an iPhone, and able to independently consent to participate in the project. A total of 16 participants (5 females, 11 males), between the ages of 20 to 58 ($M = 40$), took part in the study. 11 of the 16 participants (3 with AF) completed our satisfaction questionnaire. 3 of the participants included in the study had AF and one of 3 who had

AF also had Wolf Parkinson White syndrome. The rest of the participants acted as controls to evaluate the usability and functionality of the system.

5.2   Measures

We used a self-report scale measures to evaluate overall satisfaction of participants with our smartphone based AF-focused agent (Table 1). We also conducted a semi-structured interview with the participants to determine how long they interacted with the agent and their reaction to the agent and AF content.

Table 1. Self-report ratings of agent and AliveCor heart rhythm monitor (mean (sd))

Question	Anchor 1	Anchor 4	Agent (N = 11)
How satisfied were you with the agent?	Not at all	Very satisfied	3.45 (0.52)
How easy was talking to the agent?	Very difficult	Very easy	3.54 (0.69)
How much would you like to continue working with the agent on other aspects of atrial fibrillation?	Not at all	Very much	2.82 (1.08)
How would you describe your relationship with the agent?	Complete stranger	Close Friend	2.18 (1.08)
How helpful was the agent to you?	Not at all helpful	Very helpful	2.82 (0.98)
How satisfied were you with the AliveCor heart rhythm monitor?	Not at all	Very satisfied	3.54 (0.52)
How easy was using the AliveCor heart rhythm monitor?	Very difficult	Very easy	3.54 (0.52)
How much would you like to continue using the AliveCor heart rhythm monitor?	Not at all	Very much	3.18 (0.87)
How helpful was the AliveCor heart rhythm monitor?	Not at all	Very helpful	3.00 (0.95)

5.3   Results

Participants reported a 7 to 10-minute-long interaction with the agent each day. Older participants reported longer interactions and found agent feedback to be relevant to their condition.

Most participants reported high overall satisfaction with the agent (M = 3.45 on a 4-point scale), as well as high ratings for ease of use (M = 3.54). They also reported high levels of satisfaction with the AliveCor heart rhythm monitor (M = 3.54).

6 Conclusion

This study demonstrates the feasibility of delivering atrial fibrillation counseling via a virtual agent on smartphones. Participants in our study found the AF information to be helpful and were relatively satisfied with their interaction with the agent. The reported satisfaction with the agent correlated with the participants' satisfaction with the use of AliveCor heart rhythm monitor.

6.1 Future Work

Currently, we are completing work on a more comprehensive AF intervention prior to launching a randomized, controlled trial to thoroughly evaluate the system. Future versions of the AF counseling system will integrate information from the heart rhythm monitor so the agent will know when a user has taken a reading and the nature of any diagnostic information provided by a clinician who has reviewed the EKG readings.

Acknowledgments. This work was supported by grant 2015084 from the Doris Duke Charitable Foundation.

References

1. Pew Research Center. http://www.pewinternet.org/2015/10/29/technology-device-ownership-2015/
2. Go, A., et al.: Prevalence of diagnosed atrial fibrillation in adults: national implications for rhythm management and stroke prevention: the AnTicoagulation and Risk Factors In Atrial Fibrillation (ATRIA) Study. JAMA: J. Am. Med. Assoc. **285**, 2370–2375 (2001)
3. Miyasaka, Y., Barnes, M.E., Gersh, B.J., Cha, S.S., Bailey, K.R., Abhayaratna, W.P., Seward, J.B., Tsang, T.S.: Secular trends in incidence of atrial fibrillation in Olmsted County, Minnesota, 1980 to 2000, and implications on the projections for future prevalence. Circulation **114**, 119–125 (2006)
4. Wolf, P.A., Dawber, T.R., Thomas Jr., H.E., Kannel, W.B.: Epidemiologic assessment of chronic atrial fibrillation and risk of stroke: the Framingham study. Neurology **28**, 973–977 (1978)
5. Stewart, S., Hart, C.L., Hole, D.J., McMurray, J.J.: A population-based study of the long-term risks associated with atrial fibrillation: 20-year follow-up of the Renfrew/Paisley study. Am. J. Med. **113**, 359–364 (2002)
6. Krahn, A.D., Manfreda, J., Tate, R.B., Mathewson, F.A., Cuddy, T.E.: The natural history of atrial fibrillation: incidence, risk factors, and prognosis in the Manitoba Follow-Up Study. Am. J. Med. **98**, 476–484 (1995)
7. Benjamin, E.J., Wolf, P.A., D'Agostino, R.B., Silbershatz, H., Kannel, W.B., Levy, D.: Impact of atrial fibrillation on the risk of death: the Framingham Heart Study. Circulation **98**, 946–952 (1998)
8. Bickmore, T., Giorgino, T.: Health dialog systems for patients and consumers. J. Biomed. Inf. **39**, 556–571 (2006)

9. Bickmore, T., Silliman, R., Nelson, K., Cheng, D., Winter, M., Henaulat, L., Paasche-Orlow, M.: A randomized controlled trial of an automated exercise coach for older adults. J. Am. Geriatr. Soc. **61**, 1676–1683 (2013)
10. Watson, A., Bickmore, T., Cange, A., Kulshreshtha, A., Kvedar, J.: An internet-based virtual coach to promote physical activity adherence in overweight adults: randomized controlled trial. J. Med. Internet Res. **14**, e1 (2012)
11. Edwards, R., Bickmore, T., Jenkins, L., Foley, M.: Use of an interactive computer agent to support breastfeeding. Matern. Child Health J. **17**, 1961–1968 (2013)
12. Gardiner, P., Hempstead, M.B., Ring, L., Bickmore, T., Yinusa-Nyahkoon, L., Tran, H., Paasche-Orlow, M., Damus, K., Jack, B.: Reaching women through health information technology: the Gabby preconception care system. Am. J. Health Promot. **27**, 11–20 (2013)
13. Bickmore, T., Pfeifer, L., Byron, D., Forsythe, S., Henault, L., Jack, B., Silliman, R., Paasche-Orlow, M.: Usability of conversational agents by patients with inadequate health literacy: evidence from two clinical trials. J. Health Commun. **15**, 197–210 (2010)
14. Bickmore, T., Mauer, D.: Context awareness in a handheld exercise agent. Pervasive Mob. Comput. **5**, 226–235 (2009). Special issue on Pervasive Health and Wellness
15. Bickmore, T., Mauer, D.: Modalities for building relationships with handheld computer agents. In: ACM SIGCHI Conference on Human Factors in Computing Systems (CHI), Montreal (2006)
16. Kang, S., Feng, A., Leuski, A., Casas, D., Shapiro, A.: The effect of an animated virtual character on mobile chat interactions. In: 3rd International Conference on Human-Agent Interaction (HAI) (2015)
17. Leuski, A., Gowrisankar, R., Richmond, T., Shapiro, A., Xu, Y., Feng, A.: Mobile personal healthcare mediated by virtual humans. In: 19th International Conference on Intelligent User Interfaces (2014)
18. Cassell, J., Vilhjálmsson, H., Bickmore, T.: BEAT: The Behavior Expression Animation Toolkit. In: SIGGRAPH 2001, pp. 477–486 (2001)
19. Reiter, E., Dale, R.: Building Natural Language Generation Systems. Cambridge University Press, Cambridge (2000)

What Kind of Stories Should a Virtual Human Swap?

Setareh Nasihati Gilani[1]([✉]), Kraig Sheetz[2], Gale Lucas[1], and David Traum[1]

[1] USC Institute for Creative Technologies,
12015 Waterfront Drive, Playa Vista, CA 90094-2536, USA
{sngilani,lucas,traum}@ict.usc.edu
[2] United States Military Academy, West Point, NY 10996, USA
Kraig.Sheetz2@usma.edu

Abstract. Telling stories is an important aspect virtual agents designed to interact with people socially over time. We describe an experiment designed to investigate the impact of the identity, presentation form, and perspective of a virtual storyteller on a human user who engages in a story-swapping activity with two virtual characters. For each interaction, the user was given 10 "ice-breaker" questions to ask a virtual character and respond to the character's reciprocal request. Participants also filled out a post-interaction survey, measuring rapport with the character and impressions of the character's personality. Results generally show that participants prefer characters who tell first person stories, however there were some interactions with presentation order. No significant preferences were established for the form or identity variables.

1 Introduction

Stories are pervasive in conversation between people [15]. They are often used to establish identity [2,8], pass on cultural heritage [16], and build rapport [19]. Often stories are "swapped" when one conversational participant will reply to a story with another story. Indeed, [6] found that almost 1/4 of stories in casual conversation were presented in response to stories told by the other participant.

Stories have also been incorporated in virtual human systems (see Sect. 2). In creating or mining stories for a virtual human to tell, there are several considerations about what kinds of stories should be told, particularly considering the goals of building long-term rapport and a desire for people to keep interacting with the systems. We focus on issues such as how the story connects to the identity of the virtual human and presentation style. It is unclear how best to address these issues, as there are multiple, and occasionally conflicting desiderata proposed in the literature. We distill some of those desiderata into the following five principles:

1. **Be Human:** Virtual humans should be as much like humans as possible, and thus should project a fully human identity and tell human-centric stories.

© Springer International Publishing AG 2016
D. Traum et al. (Eds.): IVA 2016, LNAI 10011, pp. 128–140, 2016.
DOI: 10.1007/978-3-319-47665-0_12

2. **Talk About Yourself:** Tell first person stories, because they are more intimate, help the listener get to know the teller, and can act as *self-disclosure.* [22] describe how self-disclosure can play multiple roles in rapport management, including negative-self disclosure to boost interlocutors' face, inviting reciprocal self-disclosures, and revealing openness to being seen by the other.
3. **Be Real:** Stories should be authentic, or at least believable, or else they might trigger a backfire effect, where the teller is seen as inauthentic, and untrustworthy. False stories about the self, might make the listener think the teller is claiming credit that is not deserved. An obviously artificial agent might fall into this problem if it tells stories about human experiences.
4. **Be Interesting:** Novel and unusual stories are more exciting than everyday occurrences. So stories from a non-human perspective might be more interesting than standard human experiences.
5. **Don't Gossip:** Third person stories might seem like gossiping about someone else, if the stories are too personal, or possibly name dropping.

These principles may lead to conflicting ideas of optimal stories for a virtual human to tell. Principles 1 and 2 combine to say that a virtual human should tell first person stories with a human self-identity. On the other hand, Principle 3 gives reason to think it may be dangerous to rapport to tell such stories. Dropping principle 2 but keeping 1 could lead to a preference for third person stories about a real human that the virtual human knows. This might be contradicted by principle 5. On the other hand, keeping principle 2 and dropping principle 1 could lead to an agent telling first person stories about an identity as an artificial character, which might also be reinforced by principle 4. We review some prior work exploring these principles in the next section.

In order to explore these principles, we designed a set of virtual human agents who can engage in a simple form of story-swapping. Each of the agents can engage in simple interactions such as greetings and closings and can respond to a set of "ice-breaker" questions, that might be used on a first date or similar "get to know you" encounter. For these questions the agent's answer includes a story. We created four character response sets, to have all combinations of identity (human or artificial) and protagonist (first person or third person). We also considered *embodiment type* as either Human (video recording of a real person telling the stories) or Virtual-Human (animated character telling the story), however we only recorded the human identity stories in video, yielding six different story-swapping system types. More details about the agents can be found in Sect. 3.

We also designed an experiment to try to explore the collective impact of the above principles on people who interact with the characters. Participants interact with two of the above systems in a "get to know you" scenario. We investigate the degree of reciprocal story-telling, and test the rapport participants feel toward the characters as well as their impressions of the character's personality. The experimental design is described in Sect. 4. Results are presented in Sect. 5. We conclude in Sect. 6, with some thoughts and next steps.

2 Related Work

Several virtual agent systems have told, elicited or swapped stories. The SimSensei system [7] elicits extended narratives from users, in an attempt to recognize whether the user is suffering from psychological distress. Many systems feature agents that tell stories as part of an interaction establishing information about the character. Some of these have agents playing the roles of historical characters (e.g., [3] had an August Strindberg character, while [4] had a character portraying Hans Christian Andersen). Others include fictional characters from literature (e.g., [10]), or new characters (e.g., [13,17]). Stories have also been told as part of establishing a long-term relationship and influencing users to adopt behavioral change [14].

Perhaps the first system that allowed a kind of story-swapping with a virtual agent was [18], in which a child character Sam would alternate telling and listening to stories with children. [18] showed how children who interact with the Sam character both increase their stories' complexity and occasionally coach Sam. The analysis made a sharp contrast between conversation and storytelling as distinct activities, rather than telling stories within a conversation. The stories also tended to be "made up" rather than personal narratives.

[17] analyzed a corpus of interactions between museum visitors and a question-answering virtual human, Sergeant Blackwell, whose answers included some narrative responses. The analysis showed that a large percentage of questions to Blackwell included bibliographic and personal preference questions: almost 97 % of the questions were on a human-centered view compared to only 3 % of questions about the technology. Likewise, [13] noted that more than 1/3 of user questions in a museum pre-suppose treating the Max agent as human. These findings lend support for principle (1), and to some extent (2).

[1] also reported on interactions between museum visitors and virtual humans, and noted a lot of human-oriented questions, such as preferences and biography. These characters had artificial backstories, however, making jokes about their non-human characteristics, such as (computer) chips being their favorite food. The popularity of this system [21] might lend support for principle (4), as well as possibly (2) and (3).

[5] performed an experiment contrasting first vs. third person stories in a health-care application, where an agent told inspiring stories about weight loss, either about the agent (first person) or about someone else (third person). This study thus directly tested the contrasting principles (2) and (3). Participants in each condition answered questions about how much they "enjoy the stories that the counselor tells", "look forward to talking to the counselor", and "feel that the counselor is dishonest". [5] found that first person participants were more likely to talk to the agent and reported greater enjoyment; however there were no significant differences between the groups in the extent to which they looked forward to talking with the agent or felt the agent was dishonest. Moreover, newly recruited subjects use the system significantly more than participants who were already using the agent for weight-loss counseling before the study. These findings support principle (2) but fail to support principle (3). This work did not

use speech input to trigger virtual agent responses, did not elicit user stories, and did not explore the artificial identity option. [20] compare fictional (traveller from another planet) vs. realistic (artificial robot) identities for a Nao robot exercise coach. The identities were expressed as backstory that the coach would reveal about itself at various points in the interaction. [20] found no differences in ratings or activity levels between these two conditions, suggesting that principle (3) may not be so critical (or at least might be balanced by principle 4).

Concerning embodiment type, [12] compared video to animated characters in social interaction, and found that video avatars led to more co-presence than animated character avatars, though had no impact on satisfaction.

3   Story-Swapping Agents

As mentioned above, we created six versions of simple story-swapping agents. All were designed to engage with users in a simple "get to know you" dialogue, including reciprocal question answering. Four different sets of character dialogue were created, each being able to answer 20 "ice-breaker" questions, such as "Do you play sports". We created two different characters, named Arnold and Arron, that differ in their perspective of the stories they tell. Arnold tells first person stories, while Arron tells third person stories about an acquaintance. Arnold and Arron were given similar ages and appearances.

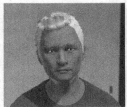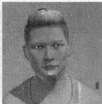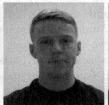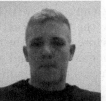

Fig. 1. Virtual human Arron and Arnold; Human Arron and Arnold

For each character, there are two versions of the stories, one in which the character is portrayed as human (VH-Human), and having fully human experiences, and another (VH-VH) in which the character talks about an artificial identity, emphasizing being a computer generated character and unable to do things like eat or drink, but having experiences in a virtual world. For the human stories only (not the artificial identity), we also have video-recordings of people from the same demographic group playing Arron and Arnold (Human-Human). Figure 1 shows the four different embodiments. We thus have six different agents, considering character/perspective (Arnold/1st or Arron/3rd), identity (Human or Virtual Human) and embodiment presentation (Human Video or Virtual Human - but only for Human identity).

The following shows two different versions of Arnold's response to the question of whether or not they have met a celebrity before. An example of one of Aaron's stories is shown in Fig. 3.

VH-VH: *I have talked to some celebrities, but unfortunately I can't really get an autograph or a picture to show my friends. I do have all of the conversation logs though, even from my first time ever talking to a celebrity, when I talked to Hines Ward, a former football player for the Pittsburgh Steelers. After hearing and reading so much about how shallow and elitist some celebrities are, I was pleasantly surprised to find Ward very down to earth and easy to talk to. He even missed his flight so he could talk longer. I guess he found it just as cool to be talking to a virtual human for the first time as I did talking to a celebrity for the first time.*

VH-Human or Human-Human: *I'm not huge into celebrities, but one time in college I saw a flyer that said that one of my childhood sports heroes, Hines Ward, was coming to do a signing on campus. I went and bought a football from the local sports store and headed over to the signing. There was a huge line, and as time went on I started to get worried that I wasn't going to make it to him in time. Just as I was about to be up in line, I saw his agent come over and tell him they need to leave for the airport now, or they would miss his flight. I heard him say "There will be another flight, these people have been waiting for hours". I went up and he not only signed my ball, but we were able to talk for a couple minutes since I was the last person in line. I was so impressed by what a genuine person he was, and for that reason I will never forget that day.*

Our agents were built using the Virtual Human Toolkit [11]. The architecture for the four virtual human embodiment agents is shown in Fig. 2a, while the architecture for the two video versions is shown in Fig. 2b. The natural language understanding and spoken answer parts are identical, the only differences being the way the embodied aspects were presented (Human video vs. Virtual Human).

4   Experimental Design

In order to shed light on the best design choices for virtual human stories in story-swapping dialogue, we recruited experimental participants to engage in dialogue with the six agents described in the previous section. 60 participants (38 males, 22 females) were recruited via Craigslist. We examined independent variables of perspective (1st vs. 3rd person), identity (human or virtual human), and presentation (human video or virtual human). We use a partial within-subjects design, where each participant talks to two virtual humans. We decided to look at perspective (1st vs. 3rd) within subjects, and to keep the identity and presentation variables the same for that subject. Thus each subject will have one conversation with Arron involving 10 questions, and one with Arnold with a different 10, in one of the three identity-presentation combinations (Human-Human, VH-Human, or VH-VH). To control for order effects, half of the participants first talked to Arnold, the 1st person character, while the other half first talked to Arron, the 3rd person character.

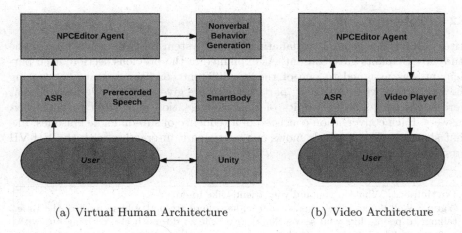

(a) Virtual Human Architecture   (b) Video Architecture

Fig. 2. System architectures

4.1 Metrics

The experiment consisted of a 3 (agent: VH-VH vs. VH-Human vs. Human-Human) × 2 (order: 1st then 3rd vs. 3rd then 1st) design. Our 60 participants were randomly assigned to one of these 6 cells (10 per cell).

We measured the following dependent variables for each interaction between a subject and virtual agent:

- a 9-item rapport scale
- a 6-item ancillary rapport scale
- two items on subjective sharing of personal information
- a set of 30 personality characteristics
- length of participant responses
- number of participant responses containing stories

We used the rapport scale from [9]. Specifically, participants answered 9 questions about the rapport they felt with the agent on scales ranging from 1 (not at all) to 5 (very much) such as "I felt I had a connection with my partner" and "I felt that my partner was interested in what I was saying." As an ancillary measure of rapport, participants also answered other questions on the same scale such as : "How much rapport did you feel with your interaction partner?" Or "How close did you feel to your interaction partner?" Participants were also asked two items about the extent to which they shared personal information using the same 5-point scale scale: "How personal were your answers?" and "How much did you reveal about yourself in your answers?" Finally, for exploratory purposes, participants were asked to rate their interaction partner on 30 personality characteristics using bipolar scale from 1 to 5, with each endpoint reflecting the extreme of that personality characteristic (e.g., Compassionate to Aloof, Friendly to Unfriendly, etc.).

4.2   Protocol

After receiving a general explanation of the system and the procedure of the study, participants gave consent. As explained in the previous section, each participant was assigned to one of the six different conditions. Prior to starting the interaction with the agent, participants were given the set of questions that were supposed to be the topics of their conversation and 5 min to plan their answers. Each conversation consisted of a sequence of sub-dialogue episodes, like that shown in Fig. 3, which shows one participant interacting with the VH-VH version of Aaron.

Participant: What do you and your friends like to do?
Agent: Well me and the other virtual humans here are pretty busy most of the time talking to people like you, so we don't have time to do much else or hang out with each other. The humans we work with seem to do some pretty cool things with their friends, though. One of our researchers just got back from a back packing trip in the Tetons, and was telling me about how he got to watch the sun rise through the peaks each morning. He claimed it was one of the most beautiful things he have ever seen.
Agent: What about you?
Participant: What do me and my friends like to do? oh my goodness, well lets see ... most of the time me and my friends just come over to my house and play some old Nintendo.. That's right you heard me right! The old classic Nintendo! I got over fifteen games it's been a lot of fun. You know, booze ... stuff like that ... umm ... but on a regular day when there is a little bit of money in the pocket we tend to go to movies or we go camping ... lets see the other day we had a little barbecue. But sometimes you just gotta do what you can with what you have, right? Either way, whenever you have good company it's gonna be a good time. That's what I always say.

Fig. 3. Example of exchange between Aaron (3rd person VH-VH) and participant

After going through all the questions, participants were asked to fill out a questionnaire with the subjective items about their experience with the agent. Then, participants went through the same procedure with the second character.

5   Results

We analyzed these dependent variables: the Rapport Scale, our ancillary rapport scale, disclosure of personal information, and finally each of the 30 personality characteristics items. On each of these measures, we conducted a 2 (perspective: 1st person vs. 3rd person) × 2 (order: 1st then 3rd vs. 3rd then 1st) × 3 (agent: human-human, VH-VH, vs. VH-human) mixed ANOVA with order and agent as between-subject factors, and perspective as a within-subjects factor. Considering the Rapport Scale, there was only a marginally significant main effect of perspective, $F(1, 53) = 3.21$, $p = .08$, such that users experienced greater rapport with the 1st person agent ($M = 3.61$, $SE = 0.09$) than with the 3rd person agent (M = 3.42, SE = 0.09). However, this effect was qualified in an interaction with "agent" condition (F(2, 53) = 3.76, p = .03). As can be seen in Fig. 4, the effect of users experiencing greater rapport with the 1st person agent than with the 3rd person agent only appears when the agent has a human backstory (VH-human and human-human). No other effects or interactions approached significance ($Fs < 1.12, ps > .33$).

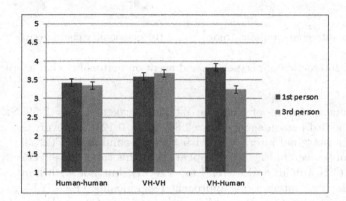

Fig. 4. Interaction of perspective and agent on the rapport scale.

For our ancillary rapport measure, we also found a main effect of perspective, $F(1, 53) = 4.44, p = .04$, again such that users experienced greater rapport with the 1st person agent ($M = 3.41, SE = 0.12$) than with the 3rd person agent ($M = 3.10, SE = 0.12$). However, the interaction with agent condition did not approach significance $F(1, 53) = 1.95, p = .15$, nor did any of the other effects or interactions reach statistical significance ($Fs < 1.52, ps > .23$). Considering the disclosure of personal information, there was a significant main effect of perspective, $F(1, 53) = 6.88, p = .01$, such that participants share more personal information with the 1st person agent ($M = 3.92, SE = 0.12$) than with the 3rd person agent ($M = 3.65, SE = 0.14$). No other effects or interactions approached significance ($Fs < 0.79, ps > .45$).

Turning to exploratory analysis of personality characteristic items, several were found to have significant or marginal effects. First, for rating of the personality characteristic of "rude", there was only a marginally significant main effect of perspective, $F(1, 53) = 3.33, p = .07$, such that users rate the agent as less rude with the 1st person agent ($M = 1.66, SE = 0.10$) than with the 3rd person agent ($M = 1.89, SE = 0.11$). However, this effect was qualified in a marginal interaction with "agent" condition ($F(2, 53) = 2.94, p = .06$). As can be seen in Fig. 5a, again the effect only appears when the agent has a human backstory (VH-human and human-human). No other effects or interactions approached significance ($Fs < 1.08, ps > .31$).

Second, for rating of the personality characteristic of "aloof", there was a significant main effect of perspective, $F(1, 53) = 5.58, p = .02$, such that users

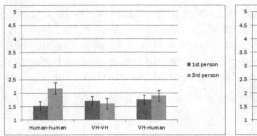
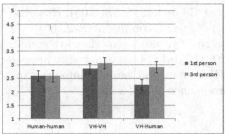

(a) Personality characteristic "rude"   (b) personality characteristic "aloof"

Fig. 5. Interaction of perspective and agent on personality characteristics.

rate the agent as less aloof with the 1st person agent ($M = 2.56, SE = 0.11$) than with the 3rd person agent ($M = 2.84, SE = 0.12$). However, this effect was qualified in a marginal interaction with "agent" condition ($F(2,53) = 2.57, p = .086$). As can be seen in Fig. 5b, it appears that this time, the effect only appears with a VH (VH-human and a trend for VH-VH, but not with human-human). No other effects or interactions approached significance ($Fs < 1.57, ps > .22$).

Third, for rating of the personality characteristic of "non-threatening", there was only a marginally significant interaction between perspective and order ($F(1,53) = 3.65, p = .06$). As can be seen in Fig. 6a, it appears that the 3rd person agent is only perceived as more threatening when users interact with the 1st person agent beforehand. No other effects or interactions approached significance ($Fs < 1.38, ps > .25$).

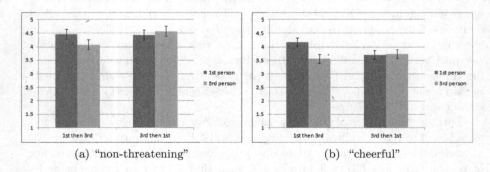

(a) "non-threatening"   (b) "cheerful"

Fig. 6. Interaction of perspective and order on personality characteristics.

Likewise, for rating of the personality characteristic of "cheerful", while there was a significant main effect of perspective, $F(1,53) = 4.28, p = .04$, such that users experience the 1st person agent as more cheerful ($M = 3.94, SE = 0.12$) than the 3rd person agent ($M = 3.64, SE = 0.12$), there was also a significant interaction with order ($F(1,53) = 5.30, p = .03$). As can be seen in Fig. 6b, it appears that the 1st person agent is only perceived as more cheerful when they interact with it before the 3rd person agent. No other effects or interactions approached significance ($Fs < 0.57, ps > .46$).

Next, for rating of the personality characteristic of "trustworthy", there was only a significant main effect of perspective, $F(1, 52) = 5.67, p = .02$, such that users experience the 1st person agent as more trustworthy ($M = 3.95, SE = 0.13$) than the 3rd person agent ($M = 3.55, SE = 0.16$). No other effects or interactions approached significance ($Fs < 1.61, ps > .21$).

For rating of the personality characteristic of "passive", there was only a marginally significant main effect of agent, $F(1, 53) = 3.33, p = .087$, such that users rate the agent as less passive when it has a human backstory (human-human $M = 2.13, SE = 0.17$ and VH-human $M = 2.05, SE = 0.17$) compared to when it has an artificial backstory ($M = 2.55, SE = 0.17$). No other effects or interactions approached significance ($Fs < 0.58, ps > .56$).

For rating of the personality characteristic of "unsympathetic", there was a significant main interaction of agent by order, $F(2, 53) = 3.22, p = .048$. As depicted in Fig. 7a, in the VH-human condition, participants overall rated both agents as more unsympathetic when they interact with the 3rd person agent before the 1st person agent. As the three-way interaction with perspective (3rd vs. 1st person) did not reach significance ($F(2, 53) = 2.63, p = .11$), this figure displays means collapsed across 1st person agent and 3rd person agent. Indeed, no other effects or interactions were statistically significant ($Fs < 2.63, ps > .11$).

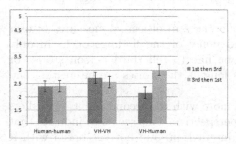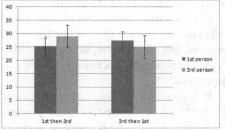

(a) Interaction of agent and order on characteristic "unsympathetic".'

(b) Interaction of perspective and order on the length participant talked'

Fig. 7. Ordering effects.

There were no significant effects or interactions approached significance for the other personality characteristic items ($Fs < 2.72, ps > .11$).

Additionally, we conducted a 2 (perspective: 1st person vs. 3rd person) × 2 (order: 1st then 3rd vs. 3rd then 1st) × 3 (agent: human-human, VH-VH, vs. VH-human) mixed ANOVA on the length of time participants talked to the agent. There was only a significant interaction of perspective and order, $F(1, 45) = 4.02, p = .05$. As can be seen in Fig. 7b, participants talked longer with whatever agent they spoke to second. No other effects or interactions approached significance ($Fs < 0.66, ps > .52$).

Finally, we conducted chi-square tests to determine if agent condition impacted whether or not participants were more likely to tell a story to the agent in response to his question. Across responses to all questions, agent condition never had a significant effect on the likelihood of telling a story ($\chi^2 s < 7.86, ps < .10$).

6 Conclusions

In summary, like [5], we see a general preference for first person over third person stories, even though there were differences in the type of interaction (spoken rather than typed) and activity (story-swapping rather than stories motivating exercise), and considering also variations in presentation. Agents who told 1st-person stories led to users reporting that they felt greater rapport, that they shared more information, and saw the agent as less rude, less aloof, less threatening, more cheerful, and more trustworthy than the agent who told third person stories. Some of these results appeared only in the VH-Human condition (which is most similar to the agent in [5]). Given that the agents, subjects, dialogue genre, and measures were all different from the previous study, we see this as reinforcement of principles (1) and (2)- that human-like first person stories should be told by a virtual human, in order to engage human users. Likewise, we fail to find any support for Principle (3), that would discourage human-like first person stories as deceitful.

On the other hand, we do not see differences in objective measures of user reactions to the stories in dialogue, and many of the findings occur in only some of the conditions, so it may also be fine to tell third person stories or have a non-human backstory identity, as long as the stories are interesting and approachable.

It is also interesting that users talked more with the second agent, regardless of whether it was a first or third person perspective. This seems to indicate that users are "warming up" to this style of interaction, and not yet bored with it after the first batch of 10 questions.

The study presented here is still an exploratory analysis, and should be followed up in order to fully verify the tentative conclusions on agent design. There are many ways in which we would like to follow up this study. One way is to vary the within-subjects variables (e.g. human vs. virtual human identities). It would also be good to look at gender effects (all of our agents were males, who interacted with both male and female subjects) and other subject matter for the stories and main task. It would also be interesting to look at agents that have a greater repertoire of subdialogue types (looking at different participants initiating topics and stories being introduced in ways other than as a response to a direct question), and including agents who tell a mix of both first and third person stories, where appropriate.

Acknowledgments. The effort described here is supported by the U.S. Army. Any opinion, content or information presented does not necessarily reflect the position or the policy of the United States Government, and no official endorsement should be inferred. We owe special thanks to Anton Leuski, Ed Fast, Arno Hartholt, Abigail Kronenberg, Andrew Jones, Jill Boberg and Rachel Wood for helping us through the course of this project.

References

1. Aggarwal, P., Artstein, R., Gerten, J., Katsamanis, A., Narayanan, S., Nazarian, A., Traum, D.: The twins corpus of museum visitor questions. In: LREC-2012, Istanbul, Turkey, May 2012
2. Bamberg, M., De Fina, A., Schiffrin, D.: Discourse and identity construction. In: Schwartz, S.J., Luyckx, K., Vignoles, V.L. (eds.) Handbook of Identity Theory and Research, pp. 177–199. Springer, New York (2011)
3. Bell, L., Gustafson, J.: Interaction with an animated agent in a spoken dialogue system. In: Proceedings of Eurospeech 1999, pp. 1143–1146 (1999)
4. Bernsen, N.O., Dybkjaer, L.: Meet Hans Christian Andersen. In: Proceedings of the 6th SIGdial Workshop on Discourse and Dialogue (2005)
5. Bickmore, T., Schulman, D., Yin, L.: Engagement vs. deceit: virtual humans with human autobiographies. In: Ruttkay, Z., Kipp, M., Nijholt, A., Vilhjálmsson, H.H. (eds.) IVA 2009. LNCS (LNAI), vol. 5773, pp. 6–19. Springer, Heidelberg (2009). doi:10.1007/978-3-642-04380-2_4
6. Collins, K.J., Traum, D.: Towards a multi-dimensional taxonomy of stories in dialogue. In: Proceedings of the Tenth International Conference on Language Resources and Evaluation (LREC) (2016)
7. DeVault, D., Artstein, R., Benn, G., Dey, T., Fast, E., Gainer, A., Georgila, K., Gratch, J., Hartholt, A., Lhommet, M., Lucas, G., Marsella, S., Morbini, F., Nazarian, A., Scherer, S., Stratou, G., Suri, A., Traum, D., Wood, R., Xu, Y., Rizzo, A., Morency, L.-P.: SimSensei kiosk: a virtual human interviewer for healthcare decision support. In: The 13th International Conference on Autonomous Agents and Multiagent Systems (AAMAS 2014) (2014)
8. Goffman, E.: The Presentation of Self in Everyday Life. Double Day, Garden City (1959)
9. Gratch, J., DeVault, D., Lucas, G.M., Marsella, S.: Negotiation as a challenge problem for virtual humans. In: Brinkman, W.-P., Broekens, J., Heylen, D. (eds.) Intelligent Virtual Agents, vol. 9238, pp. 201–215. Springer, Delft (2015)
10. Gustafson, J., Bell, L., Boye, J., Lindström, A., Wirén, M.: The nice fairy-tale game system. In: Strube, M., Sidner, C. (eds.) Proceedings of the 5th SIGdial Workshop on Discourse and Dialogue, Cambridge, Massachusetts, USA, 30 April - 1 May 2004, pp. 23–26. Association for Computational Linguistics
11. Hartholt, A., Traum, D., Marsella, S.C., Shapiro, A., Stratou, G., Leuski, A., Morency, L.-P., Gratch, J.: All together now: introducing the virtual human toolkit. In: International Conference on Intelligent Virtual Humans, Edinburgh, UK, August 2013
12. Kang, S.-H., Watt, J.H., Ala, S.K.: Social copresence in anonymous social interactions using a mobile video telephone. In: Proceedings of the SIGCHI Conference on Human Factors in Computing Systems, CHI 2008, New York, NY, USA, pp. 1535–1544. ACM (2008)

13. Kopp, S., Gesellensetter, L., Krämer, N.C., Wachsmuth, I.: A conversational agent as museum guide-design and evaluation of a real-world application. In: Panayiotopoulos, T., Gratch, J., Aylett, R., Ballin, D., Olivier, P., Rist, T. (eds.) IVA 2005. LNCS, vol. 3661, pp. 329–343. Springer, Heidelberg (2005). doi:10.1007/11550617_28
14. Manuvinakurike, R., Bickmore, T.W., Velicer, W.: Automated indexing of internet stories for health behavior change: weight loss attitude pilot study. J. Med. Internet Res. **16**, e285 (2014)
15. Norrick, N.R.: Conversational Narrative: Storytelling in Everyday Talk, vol. 203. John Benjamins Publishing, Amsterdam (2000)
16. Polanyi, L.: Telling the American Story: A Structural and Cultural Analysis of Conversational Storytelling. Ablex Publishers, Norwood (1985). Language and being
17. Robinson, S., Traum, D., Ittycheriah, M., Henderer, J.: What would you ask a conversational agent? observations of human-agent dialogues in a museum setting. In: Proceedings of the Sixth International Conference on Language Resources and Evaluation (LREC), Marrakech, Morocco (2008)
18. Ryokai, K., Vaucelle, C., Cassell, J.: Virtual peers as partners in storytelling and literacy learning. J. Comput. Assist. Learn. **19**(2), 195–208 (2003)
19. Stricker, G., Fisher, M.: Self-Disclosure in the Therapeutic Relationship. Springer, Heidelberg (1990)
20. Swift-Spong, K., Wen, C.K.F., Spruijt-Metz, D., Matarić, M.J.: Comparing backstories of a socially assistive robot exercise buddy for adolescent youth. In: 25th IEEE International Symposium on Robot and Human Interactive Communication, New York, NY, August 2016
21. Traum, D., Aggarwal, P., Artstein, R., Foutz, S., Gerten, J., Katsamanis, A., Leuski, A., Noren, D., Swartout, W.: Ada and Grace: direct interaction with museum visitors. In: Nakano, Y., Neff, M., Paiva, A., Walker, M. (eds.) IVA 2012. LNCS (LNAI), vol. 7502, pp. 245–251. Springer, Heidelberg (2012). doi:10.1007/978-3-642-33197-8_25
22. Zhao, R., Papangelis, A., Cassell, J.: Towards a dyadic computational model of rapport management for human-virtual agent interaction. In: Bickmore, T., Marsella, S., Sidner, C. (eds.) IVA 2014. LNCS (LNAI), vol. 8637, pp. 514–527. Springer, Heidelberg (2014). doi:10.1007/978-3-319-09767-1_62

Using Multiple Storylines for Presenting Large Information Networks

Zev Battad and Mei Si[✉]

Department of Cognitive Science,
Rensselaer Polytechnic Institute, Troy, USA
{battaz, sim}@rpi.edu

Abstract. Storytelling has always been an effective and intuitive method of exchanging information. In today's world of large, open, structured data, storytelling can benefit the ways in which people explore and consume such information. In this work, we investigate this potential. In particular, methods for creating multiple interweaving storylines are explored for tying together possibly disparate veins of exploration in such large networks of information and helping maintain audience interest. This paper presents the algorithms for automatically generating interweaving storylines, followed by examples and discussions for future work.

Keywords: Interactive narrative · Multiple storylines · Big data · DBpedia

1 Introduction

Narrative is one of humankind's earliest forms of exchanging information. People have been telling stories for as long as there have been stories to tell, entertaining each other, sharing the happenings in their lives, passing on knowledge they have learned themselves or learned from others, and swaying each other's opinions. As a communication device, storytelling is an effective and memorable way of giving others information.

The modern web provides unprecedented access to large networks of information. Online encyclopedias like Wikipedia, with over five million articles in English, can be traversed and explored by anyone with a web browser and an Internet connection. These sources of information are comprised of large collections of data that are linked and related to form large networks, and present an opportunity for people to tap into and learn about diverse topics. To explore such large network of information can be enjoyable, but it can also be a time consuming task. One difference between this exploration and reading a book or a website is that the information is highly connected and there is not a clear thread of how the reader should proceed. Web browsers are mostly passive, responding to searches rather than proactively providing information.

The goal of this project is to create a personal guide to help people explore and consume information by leveraging interactive narrative technologies. Narrative and storytelling have always been an intuitive method for humans to share and organize information. According to Abbot, humans mainly organize their "understanding of time" through narrative [1]. Time is thought of and reasoned over as a narrative, with events linked by their temporal sequence. Similarly, Bruner states that narrative is the

© Springer International Publishing AG 2016
D. Traum et al. (Eds.): IVA 2016, LNAI 10011, pp. 141–153, 2016.
DOI: 10.1007/978-3-319-47665-0_13

main method by which we organize human "experience and our memory of human happenings" [2]. We remember our experiences as stories, linking the individual facts of the events in our lives in a narrative way. Neumann and Nünning also support this point, calling narrative the "fundamental way" that humans organize knowledge [6].

As an initial step, we defined an XML format for encoding information, and developed an automated program for crawling information from DBpedia. In our previous work, an automated storytelling system was developed to present the information in these XML files as a never-ending story [7]. Starting from anywhere in the information network, the system picks its next topic by taking into consideration a combination of factors ranging from topic consistency and novelty, to learned user interests. The system also allows the user to direct the presentation by changing the current topic, or the relative weights the system uses for balancing the contributing factors in its selection of the next topic.

The results from our previous work can be visualized as a single story line navigating through the network of information. In entertainment-orientated narrative forms, e.g. movies, novels, and games, multiple interleaving storylines are often used for introducing a wider range of topics and for making the story more dynamic and more engaging [8]. In this work, we experiment with using this technique for presenting Internet data. Individual storylines are generated based on author-identified topics – what we refer to as anchor points – using the algorithms presented in our previous work [7]. We propose new algorithms for combining and interweaving such sequentially constructed storylines. We present these algorithms in detail, followed by an example of how they can be used for creating a story presentation with multiple and interweaving story lines, and discussions on future work.

2   Related Work

2.1   Presentation Over Structured Information Networks

The demand for methods of exploring and presenting information in large networks is currently being met by several types of systems, including recommendation systems, data visualization systems, and narrative agents. These three types of systems carry different strengths and weakness.

Recommendation systems, such as the web recommender *Letizia* or book recommender *LIBRA*, are specialized at learning user preferences and filtering information based on user profiles to suggest potentially relevant information to the user (see [11] for a comprehensive review of recommendation systems).

A variety of graph-based data visualization techniques have been developed for large networks of linked data, consisting of different node-link visualizations of RDF, OWL, and Web of Linked Data sources [12]. Node-link visualizations give users a wide glimpse at information networks, showing the relationships and interactions between many individual pieces of information.

Typically, neither recommendation systems nor data visualization systems pay attention to the path a user takes through the exploration process, i.e. whether the process is interesting or whether it helps the user to summarize and remember information.

Conversational agents are often specialized at utilizing conversational techniques, such as small talk, dialogue schema, and storytelling to help the user feel more comfortable and organized about the presented information. Information presentation systems have been developed with embodied conversational agents for various purposes, including tour guides, personal assistants, and tutors [4, 13–18]. Most automated presentation systems require the information to be manually encoded. A few systems have been developed for directly using data from the Internet. Tarau and Figa designed a conversational agent that is capable of answering the user's questions by extracting information from a story database with RDF metadata. It can also make inferences based on context of the conversation [9]. Cruz and Machado created a data visualization system that utilizes storytelling techniques for presenting large scientific data [5]. In our previous work, we have created an automated presentation agent that utilizes storytelling techniques for presenting information from DBPedia [19]. This system will be presented in detail in Sect. 4.

2.2 Interweaving Storylines

Having multiple interweaving storylines is a common technique in novels and movies for engaging the audience, and also for helping to present complex relationships among the events or characters in the story. Our work is motivated by Tan's theory and analysis on the foreground and background storylines in storytelling. As Tan points out, audience members have a natural urge to satisfy cognitive curiosity [8]. He discussed two types of audience interest, which are generated by the active line of action in a film, and by storylines that are not currently being pursued. The active line of action advances a single storyline, directly capturing the audience's interest and allowing them to follow it. This is called the foreground storyline. Storylines may be suspended before their conclusion, allowing different storylines to come into the foreground. Doing so leaves the audience with questions, stimulating interest about the suspended storyline's conclusion. Storylines suspended this way are said to be in the background. An interweaving consists of multiple storylines beginning, suspending, restarting, and concluding, with each storyline dipping in and out of the foreground. Figure 1, below, shows a short story, with story sequences, made from interweaving two storylines. Blue indicates content from the storyline in the top left, while red indicates content from the storyline in the bottom left. The story describes one storyline at a time, suspending progress on the other storyline until it is resumed later.

Having multiple storylines can also help with making information more memorable. Between two interwoven storylines, principles from framing and local structure can affect how the information between both storylines is interpreted by the audience. Framing involves discussing one topic, or storyline, using another, more understood topic, or storyline, as a frame of reference. Individual pieces of information from the storyline being discussed, particularly those that relate to the storyline acting as a frame, are consequently made more salient, making them more likely to be remembered and attended to [3]. For example, if a news story about a drug-related crime is presented in the middle of a segment about the "War on Drugs," pieces of information about the crime related to the "War on Drugs" narrative, such as whether anyone was

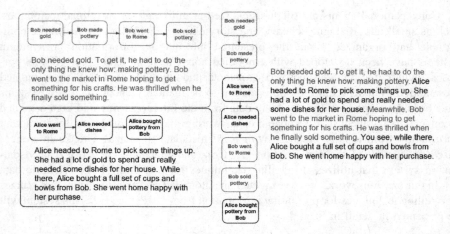

Fig. 1. Short story made from interweaving two individual storylines. (Color figure online)

injured, what drug was involved, or whether suspects had any connections with previous drug-related arrestees, may be viewed as important and attended to by the audience.

Similarly, how an interwoven story is structured with regards to how one storyline refers to the other can also have an effect. By creating local structures in the story emphasizing the way in which information is related between two storylines, the interweaving can appear more cohesive and coherent [10]. For example, in the story in Fig. 1, the fact that Bob needs gold and that Alice has gold, as well as the fact that Bob makes pottery and that Alice needs dishes, is juxtaposed in the first few sentences. The local structure employed helps reveal that the information in both storylines are related, and that their paired presentation may have a coherent purpose.

3   Example Domain

The example domain for this work is Arctic exploration. Information about this domain was gathered from DBPedia pages, and an information network was generated using an in-house tool for extracting networks from subsets of DBPedia. The tool uses a modified breadth-first search, filtering out certain uninformative or purely structural edges and nodes for gathering the information. Each page in DBPedia is taken as a node, with named links between pages taken as edges, to form our information network's knowledge graph.

This example domain was generated centered on a specific root node – the page on Arctic exploration. Knowledge encoded include objects, people, organizations, locations, events, and concepts. The exact subset used consists of 500 nodes, with 1023 edges constructed from 139 unique relationships. Figure 2, below, shows a small excerpt from the knowledge graph. Though only one directed relationship is shown between each pair of connected nodes, a reciprocal relationship in the opposite direction exists for each edge.

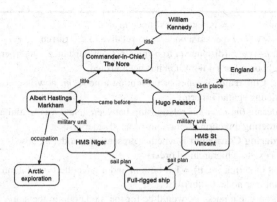

Fig. 2. Node-link diagram of portion of knowledge graph for Arctic Exploration.

4 Single Storyline Generation

In this section, we briefly review our previous work on presenting information from a knowledge graph as a never-ending story [7]. The algorithms in [7] serve as the basis for the work we propose in this paper on generating multiple interweaving storylines.

In [7], a storyline is generated in a greedy fashion by picking the next topic one at a time. When determining the next topic, the narrative agent balances a set of narrative objectives, including introducing novel content, maintaining hierarchical and spatial ordering consistency in its descriptions when applicable, including content closely related to inferred user interests, and any additional objectives specifically defined by the authors (e.g. partial ordering of topics or grouping of topics in the presentation). Each potential next topic is evaluated against all of the objectives, and the weighted sum of all objective scores indicates how optimal the node is as the next topic. Changing the weights of the objectives affects the style of the presentation, such as merging in more novel content vs. providing more details around topics presented before. Typically, all of the nodes in the knowledge graph are considered as potential next topics, though the designer of the agent can limit this range (Fig. 3).

A storyline is a sequence of nodes from the knowledge graph. To reveal and emphasize the relationships between the topics, presenting a storyline involves both showing the descriptions of each node and using transition phrases to link nodes together. The narrative agent can apply several techniques for forming transition phrases, such as making analogies between current and previously mentioned topics, explicitly mentioning how the current and next topics relate to each other, and signaling topic transitions. The latter two techniques are most commonly used. The new HINT-AT and TIE-BACK functions we propose in this paper are also forms of transition phrases. When multiple strategies can be applied for forming a transition phrase, the authors of the agent need to supply rules for their priorities. For example, in this work priority is always given to HINT-AT and TIE-BACK transitions.

Figure 4 shows a piece of narrative generated by the presentation agent. Text between brackets consists of transition phrases generated by the system. Other text

n = current node in story, m = potential next node in story

Novelty is how new or unexpected a node, m, is relative to the current story.

Novelty(m, n) = w_0* (distance m to n)/max possible distance – w_1*(percentage of unvisited neighbors of m) – w_2* (if m has been visited)

Spatial Ordering Constraint is whether presenting a node, m, now is consistent with the presentation's existing spatial ordering.

Spatial Ordering (m, n) = 1 if relationship between m and n is spatial and pointing in the same ordering direction as previous turns, 0 otherwise.

Hierarchical Ordering Constraint is whether presenting a node, m, now is consistent with the presentation's existing hierarchical ordering.

Hierarchical Ordering (m, n) = 1 if both m and n have the same hierarchical relationship with another node, 0 otherwise.

Score is how appropriate a node, m, would be for the next node in the story, given novelty, spatial ordering, and hierarchical ordering weights w_n, w_s, and w_h, respectively.

Score(m, n) = Novelty(m, n) * w_n + Spatial Ordering(m, n) * w_s + Hierarchical Ordering(m, n) * w_h

Fig. 3. Overview of major narrative constraints.

1. {First, let's talk about Arctic exploration.} Arctic exploration is the physical exploration of the Arctic region of the Earth.
2. {Albert Hastings Markham's occupation was Arctic exploration.} Admiral Sir Albert Hastings Markham, KCB was a British explorer, author, and officer in the Royal Navy.
3. {Albert Hastings Markham's military unit was HMS Niger (1846).} HMS Niger was an 8-gun screw sloop launched on 18 November 1846 from Woolwich Dockyard.
4. {HMS Niger's (1846) sail plan was a full-rigged ship.} A full-rigged ship or fully rigged ship is a sailing vessel with three or more masts, all of them square-rigged.
5. {HMS St Vincent's (1815) Ship sail plan was full-rigged ship.} HMS St Vincent was a 120-gun first rate ship of the line of the Royal Navy, laid down in 1810 at Devonport Dockyard and launched on 11 March 1815 before a crowd that was put at 50,000 spectators.
6. {Hugo Pearson commanded HMS St Vincent (1815).} Admiral Sir Hugo Lewis Pearson KCB was a Royal Navy officer who served as Commander-in-Chief, The Nore.
7. {Hugo Pearson's title was Commander-in-Chief, The Nore.} The Commander-in-Chief, The Nore was an operational commander of the Royal Navy.
8. {William Kennedy (Royal Navy officer) held the rank of Commander-in-Chief, The Nore.} Admiral Sir William Robert Kennedy GCB was a Royal Navy officer who went on to be Commander-in-Chief, The Nore.
9. {William Kennedy's (Royal Navy officer) military branch was the Royal Navy.} The Royal Navy is part of Her Majesty's Naval Service, which also includes the Royal Marines.
10. {The Royal Navy garrison is in London.} London /□l□ndən/ is the capital and most populous city of England and the United Kingdom.

Fig. 4. Single storyline generated in Arctic Exploration domain.

consists of topic descriptions taken directly from DBPedia by our program. The segment in Fig. 4 is composed of ten nodes. In Sect. 6, we will show another narrative segment with multiple interweaving storyline of similar length, making the difference in presentation styles between our new system and our existing work clear (Fig. 8).

5 Generating Multiple Interweaving Storylines

5.1 Anchor Nodes

In our previous work [7], there is no guarantee for any specific topics to be visited during an exploration. However, authors of presentation agents often need better control over the content of the presentation. For this purpose, we introduce the concept of anchor nodes in our system. As with recommendation systems and virtual tour guides, certain pieces of information may be considered important to mention. We call these pieces of information anchor nodes. Each anchor node corresponds to a node in the knowledge graph. They can either be manually defined or automatically generated.

With multiple anchor nodes, the new challenge we face is how to visit them and their related content in an optimal order. Each anchor node can guide the development of a storyline using our existing system [7].

Take the red and blue storylines in Fig. 5. As shown in Fig. 5a, presenting the two storylines in a single, sequential way may lead to a confusing, disjoint presentation when the end of one storyline and the beginning of the next are too far away from each other. In this case, the storylines could, instead, by interwoven, as shown in Fig. 5b. In the next section, we present our algorithm for interweaving two storylines, including how to identify the optimal switch point between them and how to relate the contents from the first storyline to the second storyline and vice versa.

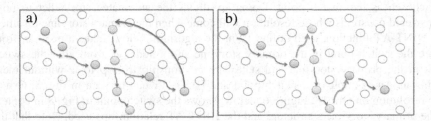

Fig. 5. Interweaving two sequential storylines. (Color figure online)

5.2 Interweaving Two Storylines

Currently, we limit interweaving to two storylines with one switch point. Thus, an interweaving consists of one storyline beginning first, progressing to a certain point, switching to the background to allow a second storyline to begin in the foreground, and switching back to the foreground once the second storyline has completed. We call the storyline that begins first the primary storyline and the storyline that begins second the secondary storyline. Algorithm 1 denotes the process for interweaving two storylines.

Determining Interweaving. Before Algorithm 1 is run, the first step is to determine whether adjacent storylines should be separated and interwoven. To accomplish this, the system takes into account how disjoint the transition from one to the other is using the relatedness between nodes. In our work, node distance is used as the main metric for relatedness between nodes, though alternative metrics for relatedness (e.g. semantic relatedness between node descriptions, structural relatedness between stories) can be used instead. If the relatedness of the last node of the first storyline to the first node of the second storyline is below some tunable threshold, the transition is considered disjoint and the two storylines will be considered for interweaving.

Choosing Switch Point. An interweaving of storylines is the creation of local structure. As each storyline leaves the foreground, the set of nodes and information that it has presented to the user gives the next storyline entering the foreground a base to predicate its presentation of information. We call the pair of nodes at which two storylines switch from foreground to background a switch point.

Audience members express a natural yearning to resolve cognitive curiosity. As a storyline is relegated to the background, the interest it garners from the audience is based on what questions are left unanswered by the storyline [8]. When deciding where the switch point should be in the primary storyline, we want to choose the point in the primary storyline where the most curiosity can be aroused in the audience. While it is almost impossible to obtain an accurate model for what will raise the audience's curiosity, in this work, we estimate the audience's curiosity level by how many unanswered questions the presentation agent can raise when it suspends the primary storyline. Computationally, the node n in the primary storyline for which there are the most connections from the set of nodes prior to, and including, n to the set of node after n is chosen as the switch point. Doing so allows the automated storyteller to pose unanswered questions whose resolution will come when the primary storyline resumes. The HINT-AT function, used at line 19 in the algorithm below, takes a node, p, from before the switch point in the primary storyline and a node, w, from after the switch point in the primary storyline and states the relationship from p to w without mentioning w. An example of a switch point and HINT-AT can be seen in Fig. 8, turn 8, with resolution on turn 18. Figure 6, below, shows the switch point in Fig. 8 in context of the primary storyline's structure and the HINT-AT relationships used. Note that the text in Fig. 6 is the result of several calls to the HINT-AT function; one for each node-relationship pair referenced.

```
 1 Algorithm 1. FUNCTION INTERWEAVE(P, Q, t)
 2    P                    // primary storyline, a list of nodes
 3    Q                    // secondary storyline, a list of nodes
 4    t                    // threshold relatedness value
 5    if relatedness(P[length], Q[1]) < t then
 6      j = index j of P where MAX(# of edges from each P[n],
 7              n <= j to each P[k], k > j) // switch point
 8      P1 = {P[0] through P[j]}    //1st half of primary
 9      P2 = {P[j+1] through P.end} //2nd half of primary
10      for each node q in Q
11        if q is neighbors with any node p in P1 then
12          TIE-BACK(q, p)
13        end if
14      end for
15      for each node p in P1
16        if p is neighbors with any node w in P2 then
17          HINT-AT(p, w)
18        end if
19      end for
20      return {P1 + Q + P2}
21    end if
22    else
23      return {P + Q}
24    end else
25 end function
```

TIE-BACK(q, p) -- relate information in node q from
  secondary storyline back to information in node p from
  primary storyline.
HINT-AT(p, w) -- allude to undisclosed information for
  node p from first half of primary storyline based on
  relationship to node w from second half of primary
  storyline.

Relating Information Between Storylines. To take advantage of the effects of framing and local structure, information between the two interwoven storylines must be connected somehow. This is accomplished by leveraging direct relationships between the two storylines.

When the secondary storyline enters, the set of nodes and node transitions used in the primary storyline before switching is used as a reference set. When a node in the secondary storyline is presented, if it is directly related to a node in the reference set, the user is reminded of the reference node and their relationship is mentioned. The TIE-BACK function, used at line 14 in the algorithm below, takes a node from the

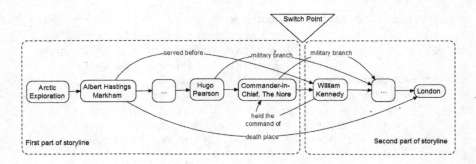

{We'll hear more about who Albert Hastings Markham served before, Albert Hastings Markham's death place, Hugo Pearson military branch, who held the command of Commander-in-Chief, The Nore, and the military branch of the Commander-in-Chief, The Nore, soon.}

Fig. 6. Switch point and HINT-AT relationships (top) with corresponding story text (bottom).

secondary storyline, *q*, and a node from before the switch point in the primary storyline, *p*, and reminds the audience of *p* before stating how *q* and *p* are related. An example of TIE-BACK can be seen in Fig. 8, turn 8. Figure 7, below, shows the TIE-BACK in Fig. 8 in context of the primary and secondary storylines as well as the relationship used. Note that the text in Fig. 7 corresponds to a single call to the TIE-BACK function.

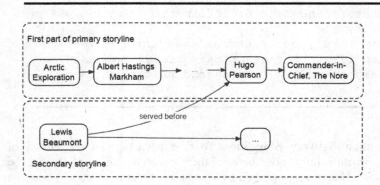

{And do you remember Hugo Pearson? Well, Lewis Beaumont served before Hugo Pearson.}

Fig. 7. Adjacent storylines and TIE-BACK relationships (top) with corresponding story text (bottom)

6 Example Interwoven Story

In this section, we present an example of using interwoven storylines. The following interwoven story was generated with two anchor nodes; "Arctic exploration" and "Lewis Beaumont." We first generated two storylines with 10 nodes each following

1. {First, let's talk about Arctic exploration.} Arctic exploration is the physical exploration of the Arctic region of the Earth.
    # First storyline begins with anchor node Arctic exploration.
2. {Albert Hastings Markham's occupation was Arctic exploration.} Admiral Sir Albert Hastings Markham, KCB was a British explorer, author, and officer in the Royal Navy.
    ...
6. {Hugo Pearson commanded HMS St Vincent (1815).} Admiral Sir Hugo Lewis Pearson KCB was a Royal Navy officer who served as Commander-in-Chief, The Nore.
7. {Hugo Pearson held the rank of Commander-in-Chief, The Nore. The Commander-in-Chief, The Nore was an operational commander of the Royal Navy. {We'll hear more about who Albert Hastings Markham served before, Albert Hastings Markham's death place, Hugo Pearson military branch, who held the command of Commander-in-Chief, The Nore, and the military branch of the Commander-in-Chief, The Nore, soon.}
    # Primary storyline suspends at switchpoint node Commander-in-Chief, The Nore.
    # HINT-AT information from nodes Albert Hastings Markham and Commander-in-Chief, The Nore, which may be revealed when primary storyline resumes.
8. {But now, let's talk about something else. Let's talk about Lewis Beaumont.} Admiral Sir Lewis Anthony Beaumont KCB KCMG was a Royal Navy officer who went on to be Commander-in-Chief, Plymouth. {And do you remember Hugo Pearson? Well, Lewis Beaumont served before Hugo Pearson.}
    # Second storyline begins with anchor node Lewis Beaumont.
    # TIE-BACK information from second storyline node Lewis Beaumont to first storyline node Hugo Pearson.
    ...
17. {Midnight Sun (graphic novel) is from the United States.} The United States of America and with over 320 million people, the country is the world's third or fourth-largest by total area and the third most populous. {But that's all we're going to discuss about that.}
    # Secondary storyline ends at node United States.
18. {When we left off our other topic, we were talking about Commander-in-Chief, The Nore. William Kennedy (Royal Navy officer) held the rank of Commander-in-Chief, The Nore.} Admiral Sir William Robert Kennedy GCB was a Royal Navy officer who went on to be Commander-in-Chief, The Nore. I mentioned Albert Hastings Markham before. {As it turns out, William Kennedy (Royal Navy officer) served after Albert Hastings Markham.}
    # Primary storyline resumes at node Willaim Kennedy.
    # HINT-AT information from first part of primary storyline about node Albert Hastings Markham revealed as relationship with node William Kennedy.
    ...

Fig. 8. Example interwoven storyline from Arctic exploration domain.

each anchor node. The two storylines were then interwoven. Similar to Fig. 4, text between brackets is generated by the system and text not between brackets is taken directly from DBPedia. After each step, the interweaving methods used in the step are given. For brevity, steps are omitted between steps of interest. Omitted steps are marked by ellipses.

The two anchor nodes, Arctic exploration and Lewis Beaumont, are discussed on step 1 and step 8, respectively. The first switch point occurs between steps 7 and 8. When the primary storyline is relegated to the background, a preview is given of what pieces of information relating to the nodes already discussed could be revealed when the primary story resumes later. The secondary storyline begins on step 8. On step 8, an example can also be seen of a relationship being drawn between information in the second storyline, Lewis Beaumont, and information in the first storyline, Hugo Pearson. The second switch point occurs between steps 17 and 18, when the secondary storyline ends and the primary storyline resumes. When the primary storyline resumes, the audience is reminded of where the storyline left off. At step 18, we can also see an example of the resolution of a question raised at step 7 about information from the primary storyline before it was suspended, Albert Hastings Markham.

7   Conclusion and Future Work

In this paper, we describe a method of generating multiple, interweaving storylines from structured networks of information, building off of previous work generating stories and presenting information from information networks. We bring this method to an information network consisting of a small subset of DBPedia, an online open data source, and give an example of an interwoven story from the network.

To take this work further, and to explore the effectiveness of multiple interweaving storylines, evaluations are planned on recall, audience enjoyment/preference, and perceived coherence and cohesiveness of the information presented.

In addition to performing formal evaluations, there are several directions we would like to further extend this algorithm. Firstly, we want to investigate automatically generating the anchor nodes. In the current system, and for the examples given, anchor nodes were manually defined. For a knowledge graph with several thousands of nodes, it may not be easy for the human author to pick all the anchor nodes by hand. We plan to experiment with automatically sampling the knowledge graph and generate the anchor nodes. Secondly, we also want to automatically set the sequence the anchor nodes should be visited. With a large amount of anchor nodes, e.g. a dozen or hundreds of nodes, the human authors will not be able to order them anymore. Finally, we want to develop an intelligent system for deciding how much content the presentation agent wants to present about each anchor point. Currently, this number is fixed or designed by the authors by hand. In the future, we hope to automatically pick the length of the individual storylines based on the nature of the data, prior presentation and interactions with the user, and other anchor points the agent needs to consider.

References

1. Abbot, H.P.: The Cambridge Introduction to Narrative. Cambridge University Press, New York (2008)
2. Bruner, J.: Self-making and world-making. In: Brockmeier, J. et al. (eds.) Narrative and identity: Studies in autobiography, Self, and Culture, pp. 25–37. John Benjamins North America, Philadelphia, PA. (2001)
3. Wicks, R.: Media information processing. In: Bryant, J., Vorderer, P. (eds.) Psychology of Entertainment, pp. 85–102. Lawrence Erlbaum, Mahwah, NJ (2006)
4. Cassell, J.: Embodied conversational agents: representation and intelligence in user interfaces. AI Mag. **22**(4), 67 (2001)
5. Cruz, P., Machado, P.: Generative storytelling for information visualization. IEEE Comput. Graph. Appl. Mag. **31**(2), 80–85 (2011)
6. Neumann, B., Nünning, A.: An Introduction to the Study of Narrative Fiction. Klett, Stuttgart (2008)
7. Si, M.: Tell a Story About Anything. In: Schoenau-Fog, H., Bruni, L.E., Louchart, S., Baceviciute, S. (eds.) ICIDS 2015. LNCS, vol. 9445, pp. 361–365. Springer, Heidelberg (2015). doi:10.1007/978-3-319-27036-4_37
8. Tan, E.S.: Emotion and the Structure of Narrative Film: Film as an Emotion Machine. Erlbaum, Mahwah (1996)
9. Tarau, P., Figa, E.: Knowledge-based conversational agents and virtual storytelling. In: Proceedings of the 2004 ACM Symposium on Applied Computing, pp. 39–44. ACM (2004)
10. Thorndyke, P.W.: Cognitive Structures in Human Story: Comprehension and Memory. Rand, Santa Monica (1975)
11. Lops, P., de Gemmis, M., Semeraro, G.: Content-based recommender systems: state of the art and trends. In: Ricci, F., et al. (eds.) Recommender Systems Handbook, pp. 73–105. Springer, New York (2011)
12. Nikos, B., Timos, S.: Exploration and Visualization in the Web of Big Linked Data: A Survey of the State of the Art. eprint, arXiv:1601.08059 (2016)
13. Nijholt, A.: Towards the automatic generation of virtual presenter agents. Inf. Sci. **9**, 97–115 (2006)
14. D'Haro, L.F., Kim, S., Yeo, K.H., Jiang, R., Niculescu, A.I., Banchs, R.E., Li, H.: CLARA: a multifunctional virtual agent for conference support and touristic information. In: Lee, G. G., Kim, H.K., Jeong, M., Kim, J.H. (eds.) Natural Language Dialog Systems and Intelligent Assistants, pp. 233–239 (2015)
15. Nijholt, A., van Welbergen, H., Zwiers, J.: Introducing an embodied virtual presenter agent in a virtual meeting room. In: 23rd IASTED International Conference on Artificial Intelligence and Applications, AIA 2005, February 14–16, 2005, Innsbruck, Austria, pp. 579–584. (2005)
16. Jan, D., Roque, A., Leuski, A., Morie, J., Traum, D.: A virtual tour guide for virtual worlds. In: Proceedings of the 9th International Conference on Intelligent Virtual Agents, pp. 372–378 (2009)
17. Kopp, S., Gesellensetter, L., Krämer, N.C., Wachsmuth, I.: A conversational agent as museum guide – design and evaluation of a real-world application. In: Panayiotopoulos, T., Gratch, J., Aylett, R.S., Ballin, D., Olivier, P., Rist, T. (eds.) IVA 2005. LNCS (LNAI), vol. 3661, pp. 329–343. Springer, Heidelberg (2005)
18. Swartout, W., et al.: Ada and grace: toward realistic and engaging virtual museum guides. In: Safonova, A. (ed.) IVA 2010. LNCS, vol. 6356, pp. 286–300. Springer, Heidelberg (2010)
19. DBpedia. http://wiki.dbpedia.org/

Virtual Agents in the Classroom: Experience Fielding a Co-presenter Agent in University Courses

Timothy Bickmore[✉], Ha Trinh, Michael Hoppmann, and Reza Asadi

College of Computer and Information Science, Northeastern University, Boston, MA, USA
bickmore@ccs.neu.edu

Abstract. The design of a conversational virtual agent that assists professors and students in giving in-class oral presentations is described, along with preliminary evaluation results. The life-sized agent is integrated with PowerPoint presentation software and can deliver presentations in conjunction with a human presenter using appropriate verbal and nonverbal behavior. Results from evaluation studies in two courses—business and professional speaking, and computer science research methods—indicate that the agent is widely accepted in the classroom by students, and can serve to increase engagement in presentations given both by professors and students.

Keywords: Embodied conversational agent · Powerpoint · Slideware

1 Introduction

Although contemporary scientific results are recorded in writing and disseminated through a variety of media, oral presentation of findings to an audience of peers continues to be a central feature of science today. Oral presentations at scientific conferences are where researchers, practitioners, the media, and the public hear about the latest findings, become engaged and inspired, and where scientific reputations are made. However, the state of the art in scientific presentations has not progressed in the last 30 years. The standard scientific presentation today still features a scholar standing in front of a projection screen, speaking from his or her notes or slides, with supporting images and text displayed for the audience. The typical quality of such presentations—across all professions—is very poor. An extensive survey of 2,501 professionals [1] revealed that 35 % of respondents rarely or never rehearse for their presentations, and because of this and many other problems, respondents gave a "C-"grade (2.9 on a 1-to-5 scale) for all presentations they had attended. Poor presentations can result in scientists failing to engage, inform, and persuade their audience, can damage their credibility and professional standing, and can damage the reputation of the sciences in general. There are many reasons for these failures, including: deficiencies in language, speech, and presentation skills; lack of content mastery; time and resource constraints; lack of preparation and rehearsal; and public speaking anxiety (affecting at least 35 % of the population [2]).

Students learn to give scientific presentations by observing others give talks, by taking classes that cover public speaking, and by practicing public speaking as a skill. Unfortunately, most university curricula in the sciences provide few opportunities for

© Springer International Publishing AG 2016
D. Traum et al. (Eds.): IVA 2016, LNAI 10011, pp. 154–163, 2016.
DOI: 10.1007/978-3-319-47665-0_14

training in public speaking, or offer it only as a minor elective. Professional scientists speaking at seminars and conferences often provide poor role models for public speaking and promote a perpetual cycle of stale presentation formats and poor quality perform-ances.

To assist students and professionals in delivering more engaging presentations, we have developed an automated virtual agent that plays the role of a co-presenter [3]. The co-presenter appears in the form of a life-sized human character that can present part of a talk given with conventional presentation software (Fig. 1). The co-presenter agent uses verbal and nonverbal behavior for content delivery, highlighting and emphasis, speaker hand-offs (turn-taking), and attentive listening when the human presenter is speaking. We also developed an authoring tool to allow human presenters to easily control the verbal and nonverbal behavior of the agent. In a lab-based controlled study ($N = 12$), we demonstrated that the use of the co-presenter helped reduce public speaking anxiety for non-native English speakers, while improving the overall presentation quality for all participants [3].

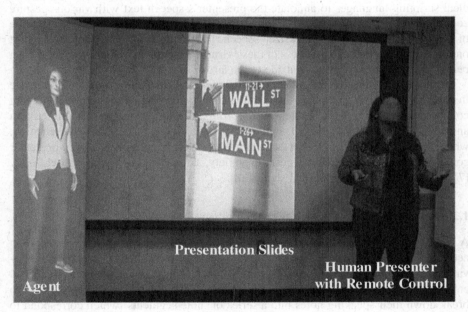

Fig. 1. Student in professional speaking class giving presentation with co-presenter agent

In this paper we describe our experiences deploying the co-presenter agent in college courses to help students learn how to give oral presentations. The agent was evaluated in two courses during the Spring 2016 semester: a business and professional speaking course, specially designed around use of the co-presenter agent, and a computer science research methods course. In these courses, we evaluated lectures given by the professor with and without the agent, and presentations given by students, with and without the agent. Our aim was to assess the acceptance and effectiveness of the system when participants were exposed to different ways of using the co-presenter agent in realistic settings over a long-term period.

1.1 Related Work Using Virtual Agents as Presenters

A number of studies have explored the potential of virtual agents to support presentation delivery. One of the earliest attempts is the WebPersona system [4], which uses an animated cartoon character to present hypermedia information automatically generated from the World Wide Web. In a controlled study comparing presentations of technical content with and without the agent, participants rated the presentations delivered by the virtual presenter as significantly less difficult and more entertaining. However, such effect was not found for presentations of non-technical content.

In addition to fully automated presentation systems, other systems [5, 6] have been developed to enable virtual agents to present manually authored speech text on behalf of a human presenter. However, these systems often require users to learn highly technical scripting languages to annotate the presenter's speech text with various gesture commands, which could then be performed by an animated computer character capable of non-verbal behavior and synthesized speech. To date, there has been very little report on the acceptance and effectiveness of these virtual presenter systems, especially when being deployed in real settings outside of the lab.

Although all of these agents acted as virtual presenters, their main goal was to replace the human presenters instead of augmenting their performance through human-agent collaboration. It is this human-agent *collaboration*, which, we argue, can deliver both analytical and emotional content, while enabling a dialogical mode of presentation, which is impossible in single-speaker talks. Moreover, the presence of a co-presenter could also help decrease public speaking anxiety, as indicated by social impact theory [7] and demonstrated in empirical studies [8].

1.2 Related Work on Presentation Technologies

A number of research projects have proposed methods to support various presentation activities, from authoring [9] to rehearsal [10] and delivery [11, 12]. Of particular relevance to our work is the PitchPerfect system [10], which provides an integrated rehearsal environment for structured presentation preparation. The system enables presenters to break down their speaking notes into a series of 'note segments' which correspond to specific visual elements on slides. It also includes a special note segment called the 'transition note,' which encourages presenters to speak between slides, explaining transitions and relations between different slides.

2 Design of the Co-presenter Agent System

Implemented as an add-in to PowerPoint 2013, our co-presenter agent system consists of three primary components: (1) a *life-sized co-presenter virtual agent* that exhibits a range of verbal and non-verbal behaviors; (2) a *collaborative note authoring* tool that enables human-agent note scripting at slide level; (3) a *collaborative presentation environment* that is integrated into the PowerPoint's slideshow delivery mode. Our system enables presenters to author and deliver their dual presentation using a simple visual interface seamlessly integrated into PowerPoint.

The Virtual Presenter. Our virtual presenter, Angela, is a life-sized, animated human-like character developed using the Unity game engine (Fig. 2). The agent talks using synthetic speech and synchronized nonverbal behavior, including affective facial expressions (smile, neutral, concern), eyebrow movement, directional gazes, head nods, posture shifts, as well as contrastive, beat (emphasis), and deictic gestures (e.g. pointing to a slide).

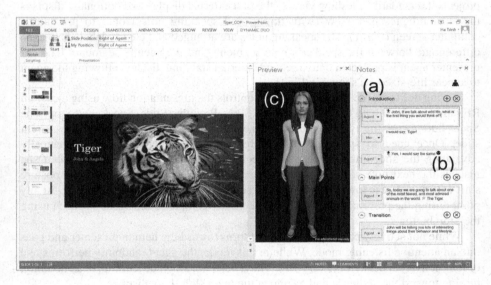

Fig. 2. Collaborative note authoring interface with: (a) human-agent note segments; (b) icons representing manually added non-verbal behaviors; (c) agent speaking preview.

Co-presentation Authoring. To prepare a co-presentation, the human presenter starts by creating slides as usual, then activating the *Co-presenter Notes* side pane to enter human-agent speaking notes (Fig. 2). For each slide, the system automatically creates placeholders for three note sections: *Introduction*, *Main Points*, and *Transition* (Fig. 2a). Every note section is further divided into a series of note segments, each of which can be assigned to either the co-presenter agent or the human presenter.

The majority of the agent's nonverbal behaviors are automatically generated using BEAT [13], but the human presenter can explicitly insert nonverbal behavior commands into the agent's note segments using the behavior context menu. The menu consists of 10 presentation-specific behavior options, including: *gazing* towards the audience/towards the human presenter, *pointing* to slides/to the human presenter, *turning* towards the audience/towards the human presenter, *facial expressions*, and *playing selected animation* on the current slide. Each inserted behavior is represented by a visual icon in the note segment (Fig. 2b).

To determine appropriate directions of gazes, posture shifts and deictic gestures, the presenter can specify their spatial position and the slide's position in reference to the agent's position for a given presentation room (i.e. either at the left or right to the agent), using appropriate controls on the PowerPoint ribbon (Fig. 2).

While authoring the agent's notes, the presenter can preview her verbal and non-verbal behavior from the *Preview* side pane (Fig. 2c).

Presentation Environment. Once the presentation environment is started, PowerPoint projects its standard slideshow view to the first external display and optionally displays the standard presenter view (with timing and speaking notes) onto to presenter's computer screen (Fig. 1). The speaking notes are arranged and clearly labeled, so as to differentiate between the speaker's note segments and the agent's segments. The co-presenter agent is projected onto a second external standing display, allowing the agent to appear life-sized, as shown in Fig. 1.

During delivery, the human presenter controls the presentation flow using a custom RF remote control with four buttons: Next Slide, Previous Slide, Speak, and Stop. The Speak button cues the agent to present the next available agent segments on the current slide. Once cued to speak, the agent presents her segments while automatically advancing the slides and playing pre-specified animations, and stopping when she reaches the next note segment of the human presenter. The agent performs a posture shift to turn and gaze toward the human presenter as an indicator of turn-giving. At any point during the presentation, the human presenter can pause the agent's speech using the Stop button.

While not actively presenting, the agent turns toward the human presenter and goes into an attentive listening mode. While in this mode, the agent randomly performs one of four nonverbal behaviors every 10 s. These behaviors include smiling, head nodding, turning toward the audience and gazing at the main slideshow display.

3   Pilot Lab-Based Evaluation Study

We conducted a laboratory-based experimental evaluation of the co-presenter agent, comparing presentations given with and without the agent by the same participants (previously reported in [3]). The study involved 12 students and professionals. Participants were asked to deliver two 7-minute presentations on comparable topics using prepared PowerPoint slide decks and notes, one with the co-presenter agent and one without (counterbalanced, within-subjects experiment). There was a significant interaction effect of study condition (human-agent vs. human-only) and native language (native vs. non-native English speakers), with the agent significantly decreasing public speaking anxiety, $p = .014$, and increasing speaker confidence, $p = .006$, for non-native English speakers. In a subsequent study in which 12 judges rated the pairs of presentations, judges rated the human-agent presentations significantly better on note reliance ($p < .05$), speech quality ($p < .01$) and overall presentation quality ($p < .05$).

4   Use of the Co-presenter Agent in a Research Methods Class

Although results of our pilot evaluation study were promising, we wanted to investigate use of the co-presenter agent in a real environment, and as a teaching tool to help computer science students give better oral presentations. We conducted our evaluation within the context of a mixed graduate and undergraduate-level university course on research methods, which covers the basics of experimental design for human subjects studies, along with statistical analysis techniques. The class met 26 times in the Spring, 2016 semester. In addition to 100-minute lectures by the instructor, three class meetings were set aside for students to present results from team-based field studies they conducted in the latter part of the course. The co-presenter agent was used both by the instructor for a subset of his lectures and by the students for a subset of their study presentations.

Table 1. Audience self-report presentation rating questions and responses (mean (sd)) (all tests non-parametric using Mann-Whitney U)

Audience ratings (by 10 Students)			Lectures by professor			Student presentations		
Question	Anchor 1	Anchor 7	No-agent (N = 2)	Agent (N = 2)	p	No-agent (N = 15)	Agent (N = 5)	P
Overall quality of the presentation	Very poor	Very good	6.06 (0.73)	5.82 (0.73)	.34	5.74 (0.54)	5.60 (0.62)	.74
Were you engaged by the presentation?	Not at all	Very much	5.56 (1.25)	6.06 (0.75)	.19	5.50 (0.59)	5.55 (0.61)	.71
Could you understand the presentation?	Not at all	Very well	6.00 (0.77)	5.88 (0.93)	.75	5.78 (0.53)	5.79 (0.69)	.74
How novel was the presentation?	Very routine	Very novel	4.39 (1.24)	5.88 (1.11)	**.001**	4.84 (0.63)	5.21 (0.57)	**.04**
How exciting was the presentation?	Very boring	Very exciting	4.83 (1.10)	5.82 (0.88)	**.009**	4.93 (0.68)	5.16 (0.50)	.14
How entertaining was the presentation?	Not at all	Very much	4.67 (1.19)	5.94 (0.90)	**.003**	4.83 (0.75)	5.14 (0.63)	.11
How competent was the presenter?	Not at all	Very much	6.78 (0.43)	6.41 (0.62)	.06	5.91 (0.49)	5.80 (0.66)	.67
Did the co-presenter help the presentation?	Not at all	Very much		5.35 (0.86)			5.23 (0.57)	
How entertaining was the presenter?	Not at all	Very much	4.83 (1.25)	5.47 (0.94)	.11	4.83 (0.75)	5.14 (0.63)	.06
Like to see another presentation like this?	Not at all	Very much	5.06 (1.16)	5.76 (1.03)	.09	4.93 (0.71)	5.20 (0.70)	.13

Students were recruited at the beginning of the semester and were asked to evaluate a subset of the instructor's lectures and student presentations, including those given with and without the agent, and offered the option of giving their presentations with the agent. At the end of the semester students were interviewed about their experience.

Participants.   Three undergraduate and seven PhD students agreed to participate in the study. Participants were 22–34 years old, and 70 % male. Of these ten participants, three were categorized as high competence public speakers and seven were categorized as moderate competence public speakers, according to the Self-Perceived Communication Competence Scale [14].

Measures. Students were asked to rate lectures and presentations using the scale measures shown in Table 1. Students who volunteered to give their in-class presentations with the co-presenter agent were also asked to complete the co-presenter agent satisfaction questionnaire shown in Table 2.

Table 2. Co-presenter agent rating questions and responses by student presenters

Question	Anchor 1	Anchor 7	Agent
How satisfied are you with the co-presenter agent?	Not at all	Very satisfied	6.6 (0.55)
How much would you like to give future presentations with the co-presenter agent?	Not at all	Very much	6.6 (0.55)
How much do you like the co-presenter agent?	Not at all	Very much	6.2 (0.84)
How easy was it to use the co-presenter agent?	Very easy	Very difficult	3.0 (2.35)
How much do you feel you trust the co-presenter agent?	Not at all	Very much	6.8 (0.45)
How much do you feel the agent helped you?	Not at all	Very much	6.8 (0.45)

Quantitative Results. Table 1 shows study participant ratings of lectures and student presentations given with and without the co-presenter agent. Students found lectures by the professor given with the agent significantly more novel (5.2 vs. 4.8, Mann-Whitney $U = 55.5$, $p = .001$), exciting (5.8 vs. 4.8, $U = 77.5$, $p < .01$), and entertaining (5.9 vs. 4.7, $U = 65.0$, $p < .01$), compared to the comparison lectures given without the agent. There were trends for students to rate the professor as more competent without the agent (6.8 vs. 6.4, $U = 104.0$, $p = .06$), but they preferred to see future lectures given with the agent (5.8 vs. 5.1, $U = 103.5$, $p = .09$).

Students found that in-class project presentations given by other students with the agent were significantly more novel (5.2 vs. 4.8, $U = 150.0$, $p < .05$), compared to those given without the agent. There was also a trend for students to rate other student presenters as more entertaining with the agent (5.1 vs. 4.8, $U = 158.5$, $p = .06$).

Table 2 shows ratings of the co-presenter agent system by students who used it to give their in-class presentations. Overall, students expressed high levels of satisfaction (6.6 on a 7-point scale) and desire to use the agent for future presentations (6.6 on a 7-point scale).

Qualitative Findings. We identified three main themes in exit interviews with students related to audience engagement, collaboration models, and presenter's anxiety.

Theme 1: Increasing Audience Engagement. In addition to the novelty effects of the new technology, most participants also reported certain benefits of the dialogical presentation formats in keeping their attention, especially during long lectures: *"I like the dynamics of going back and forth... It's more like a conversation between two experts in the area. I would say that it is more engaging"* [P6]. Breaking up the content into digestible human-agent segments was reported to be *"a lot more helpful in trying to* *learn information"* [P8]. The changes of voice and pace between the co-presenters also helped the audience stay focused: *"Having two voices that are speaking at you makes you perk up every time that it changes"* [P8]. Creative uses of the agent, such as incorporating jokes in the dialogue, also made the presentations *"a lot more likeable, which is not something you can do with just one presenter"* [P8]. Enabling the agent to directly interact with the audience (e.g., by asking questions) also increased their engagement and anticipation: *"I was very excited when she called out my name... I didn't expect her to do it but I found it very interesting"* [P2].

While the dyadic interaction formats were positively received, the audience could, however, *"get distracted if there is a lot of interaction"* [P7]. Thus, further work is needed to assist presenters in designing a balanced and meaningful interaction model of co-presenters to avoid disrupting the presentation flow.

Theme 2: Diversifying Presentation Forms through Different Collaboration Models. Participants demonstrated various methods of collaboration with the agent, such as: iterative turn-taking at bullet point and slide levels, assigning the introduction and transition sections to the human presenter as a way to control the presentation flow, or embedding a question-answering dialogue to introduce new topics and transition between presenters. Several presenters also used the agent creatively to add humor, and to deliver content that would otherwise be uncomfortable for them, for example: *"I had some criticism for the project and I had her point out all the negative things instead of just saying it myself"* [P1]. The audience generally preferred a balanced distribution of content between the co-presenters, and responded negatively when the agent was underused.

Choosing an appropriate collaboration model can, however, be a difficult process that requires trial and error as well as creativity. Thus, several participants expressed the need for more instructions or *"interactive templates"* [P7] to scaffold this process.

In order for the agent to become a more effective collaborator, most participants wanted the agent to have more human qualities, including emotions, knowledge, and the ability to dynamically adapt to the presentation environment.

Theme 3: Reducing Presenter's Anxiety. In line with the results of our lab-based study, participants felt that presenting with the agent helped decrease anxiety, due to four key factors. First, preparing a co-presentation forced the presenters to invest time on planning and rehearsing their speech. As a result, they *"had a better understanding of the presentation"* [P4], felt *"more prepared"* [P2] and thus became *"more confident"* [P4] during their delivery. Second, the presence of a co-presenter agent helped reduce stage pressure through shared attention: *"having her there made me less nervous because not all the attention is on me"* [P2]. Third, taking turns to present with the agent allowed the presenter to *"take a break"* [P4] while the agent was speaking to *"think about what is coming next"* [P4]. Finally, the distribution of content reduced the human's memorization load, making them feel assured because the agent *"wasn't going to forget anything"* [P5]. This benefit could be of particular importance for presentations of technical content with large amounts of statistical data.

To summarize, our qualitative findings showed that the co-presenter agent was positively received by students, and was able to improve the presentation experiences for both audiences and presenters. One of our participants commented on the overall benefit of the agent: *"I was more engaged with the class. I felt that I got more out of the class when she was there"* [P8].

5   Use of the Co-presenter Agent in a Public Speaking Class

The co-presenter was also used in a public speaking class ("Business and Professional Speaking"), offered in the Communication Department of our university in the Spring, 2016 semester. One section of the course was specially modified to incorporate the co-presenter agent in all student presentations, by setting aside class sessions for training on the co-presenter system, presentation preparation, and rehearsal. Twelve students enrolled in the course, aged 18–24, 54 % male. All students volunteered to give their initial presentation using the agent, and 66 % volunteered to give their second in-class presentation with the agent.

Overall, students were accepting of the agent, and felt that it helped them learn to give better presentations. Use of the agent forced students to prepare and rehearse more than they otherwise would have done, and to think more carefully about their presentation content and how it would be delivered. As in the methods course, students (and the instructor) felt that the co-presenter agent increased variety, engagement, and energy level, and that presenting in a team increased confidence and decreased anxiety, even when the teammate is artificial. On the negative side, initial exposure to the new technology was an initial challenge and was a source of more anxiety among students than using existing presentation technology.

6   Conclusion

We designed a virtual agent that helps individuals give oral presentations, and evaluated it in two university classroom settings. Overall, students were accepting and very positive regarding this use of agents, and felt that the agent increased the novelty and engagement of the speaker, for presentations given by both students and a professor.

Limitations and Future Work. Our studies used very small convenience samples of students, and thus are likely not representative of all college students. The studies also lacked the rigorous controls of a laboratory environment (e.g., participants were not randomized across study conditions). However, the classroom environment provided a more realistic setting to test acceptance and use of the co-presenter agent.

There are many directions of future research for this work. Students requested greater control over agent appearance, a larger repertoire of nonverbal behavior and prosodic control, and more flexible interaction methods. They also expressed the need for more instructions and templates to facilitate the creation of more engaging human-agent co-presentations. We are currently exploring the use of automated speech recognition for the agent to track where the human presenter is in his or her talk so that the agent can take over at any point or can fill in important points the human presenter may have forgotten. We also plan to employ technologies to assess both the human presenter's performance and audience interaction, allowing for spontaneous support by the virtual presenter through its ability to dynamically adapt to the presentation environment when needed.

Acknowledgements. This work is supported in part by the National Science Foundation under award IIS-1514490. Any opinions, findings, and conclusions or recommendations expressed in this material are those of the authors and do not necessarily reflect the views of the National Science Foundation.

References

1. Goodman, A.: Why Bad Presentations Happen to Good Causes. Andy Goodman & Cause Communication, Los Angeles (2006)
2. Bishop, J., Bauer, K., Becker, E.: A survey of counseling needs of male and female college students. J. Coll. Student Dev. **39**, 205–210 (1998)
3. Trinh, H., Ring, L., Bickmore, T.: DynamicDuo: co-presenting with virtual agents. In: ACM SIGCHI Conference on Human Factors in Computing Systems (CHI) (2015)
4. André, E., Rist, T., Müller, J.: WebPersona: a lifelike presentation agent for the world-wide web. Knowl.-Based Syst. **11**, 25–36 (1998)
5. Nijholt, A., van Welbergen, H., Zwiers, J.: Introducing an embodied virtual presenter agent in a virtual meeting room. In: IASTED International Conference on Artificial Intelligence and Applications, pp. 579–584 (2005)
6. Noma, T., Badler, N.: A virtual human presenter. In: IJCAI 1997 (1997)
7. Latane, B., Nida, S.: Social impact theory and group influence: a social engineering perspective. In: Paulus, P.B. (ed.) Psychology of Group Influence, pp. 3–34. Lawrence Erlbaum, Hillsdale (1980)
8. Jackson, J., Latané, B.: All alone in front of all those people: Stage fright as a function of number and type of co-performers and audience. J. Pers. Soc. Psychol. **40**, 73–81 (1981)
9. Edge, D., Savage, J., Yatani, K.: HyperSlides: dynamic presentation prototyping. In: CHI 2013, pp. 671–680 (2013)
10. Trinh, H., Yatani, K., Edge, D.: PitchPerfect: integrated rehearsal environment for structured presentation preparation. In: CHI (2014)
11. Damian, I., Tan, C., Baur, T., Schoning, J., Luyten, K., Andre, E.: Augmenting social interactions: realtime behavioral feedback using social signal processing techniques. In: CHI 2015, pp. 565–574 (2015)
12. Saket, B., Yang, S., Tan, H., Yatani, K., Edge, D.: TalkZones: section-based time support for presentations. In: MobileHCI 2014 Conference on Human Computer Interaction with Mobile Devices and Services (2014)
13. Cassell, J., Vilhjálmsson, H., Bickmore, T.: BEAT: the behavior expression animation toolkit. In: SIGGRAPH 2001, pp. 477–486 (2001)
14. McCroskey, J., McCroskey, L.: Self-report as an approach to measuring communication competence. Commun. Res. Rep. **5**, 108–113 (1988)

Manipulating the Perception of Virtual Audiences Using Crowdsourced Behaviors

Mathieu Chollet[1]([⊠]), Nithin Chandrashekhar[1], Ari Shapiro[1],
Louis-Philippe Morency[2], and Stefan Scherer[1]

[1] Institute for Creative Technologies, University of Southern California,
Waterfront Drive, Playa Vista, CA 12015, USA
{mchollet,nithinch,shapiro,scherer}@ict.usc.edu
[2] Language Technology Institute, Carnegie Mellon University,
5000 Forbes Avenue, Pittsburgh, PA, USA
morency@cs.cmu.edu

Abstract. Virtual audiences are used for training public speaking and mitigating anxiety related to it. However, research has been scarce on studying how virtual audiences are perceived and which non-verbal behaviors should be used to make such an audience appear in particular states, such as boredom or engagement. Recently, crowdsourcing methods have been proposed for collecting data for building virtual agents' behavior models. In this paper, we use crowdsourcing for creating and evaluating a nonverbal behaviors generation model for virtual audiences. We show that our model successfully expresses relevant audience states (*i.e.* low to high arousal, negative to positive valence), and that the overall impression exhibited by the virtual audience can be controlled my manipulating the amount of individual audience members that display a congruent state.

Keywords: Virtual audience · Crowdsourcing · Non-verbal behaviors

1 Introduction

Modern professional and personal life often involve situations where we are required to speak in public, such as when performing a professional presentation or when making a toast at a wedding. The ability to speak in public proficiently can greatly influence a person's career development, help build relationships, resolve conflict, or even gain the upper hand in negotiations. While there is no such thing as a best style of public speaking, every efficient public speech requires the mobilization of varied skills, ranging from the selection and arrangement of appropriate and convincing arguments to the efficient vocal and non-verbal delivery of the speech. This very desirable set of skills is not innate to most of us, and many people actually dread the prospect of speaking in public: it is actually one of the most commonly reported phobias [2]. Fortunately, public speaking ability can be improved through training and public speaking anxiety

© Springer International Publishing AG 2016
D. Traum et al. (Eds.): IVA 2016, LNAI 10011, pp. 164–174, 2016.
DOI: 10.1007/978-3-319-47665-0_15

can be reduced through a number of methods, including exposure to virtual audiences [6,14]. Virtual audiences are collections of virtual agents situated in 3D environments designed to reproduce a public speaking situation [3,9].

Multimodal interactive systems for social skills training have recently been proposed in domains such as job interview training [4] or public speaking training [5,15]. While virtual audiences have been used since fifteen years for the mitigation of public speaking anxiety [6,14], they have only recently been proposed for training public speaking skills [1,3]. Training systems using such audiences could hold several advantages over traditional public speaking training methods, such as training workshops and rehearsals with colleagues or friends [7]: they are always available, whereas audiences of friends or public speaking experts are not; whilst some people could be reluctant to training their public speaking ability with real people out of fear of being judged, virtual audiences do not pose such a threat [10]; in addition, they can be finely controlled, allowing training to be standardized. Finally, virtual humans are excellent in captivating individuals' attention, in creating rapport and engaging the learner [16], which are essential prerequisites for successful learning outcomes.

Designing virtual audiences for public speaking training requires understanding how they are perceived and how this perception can be manipulated through their behavior, layout or appearance. However, this has only started to be investigated recently [8,9], and many aspects of this question remain unanswered. In particular, it is still unclear how combinations of behaviors from different modalities (e.g. postures, head movements, facial expressions, gaze) are perceived when expressed by a virtual audience character. Additionally, to the best of our knowledge, the overall perception of audiences containing characters displaying disparate states has not been studied yet. In this paper, we set out to study these research questions by using crowdsourcing methods.

In the next section, we begin by reviewing related works on social skills training using multimodal interfaces and on the design and usage of virtual audiences. We then present in Sect. 3 a study on the relationship between virtual characters behaviors and perceivable audience states. We then realized another experiment, outlined in Sect. 4, in order to validate that the overall perception of a virtual audience can be finely controlled by adjusting the amount of characters that display a target state.

2   Related Work

Recently, public speaking training with multimodal interfaces providing direct feedback mechanisms has been a popular topic. The Rhema system uses Google Glass to provide the speaker with feedback on speaking volume and speaking rate [15]. Logue [5] is a similar system that provides realtime feedback to presenters on their speech rate body openness and body energy using functional icons displayed on Google Glass. Barmaki and Hugues presented a system for training teachers to adopt better body postures, using a virtual classroom populated with manually controlled virtual students [1]. A particular paradigm for interfaces for public speaking training is the virtual audience. Such a system aims at reproducing a public speaking situation with high fidelity, using an environment that is typical of public speaking situations (*e.g.* a conference room) and populating it with virtual characters acting as the user's audience. Virtual audiences have first been investigated to treat public speaking anxiety. North *et al.* found in a series of studies that virtual audiences were effective in inducing stress and reducing public speaking anxiety [6,12]. Researchers also investigated the effect of three different types of virtual audiences, namely a neutral, a positive, and a negative audience, consisting of eight virtual characters [14]. Virtual audiences have only been recently used for specifically improving public speaking ability, and not solely reducing their anxiety. In previous work, we introduced the Cicero public speaking training framework [3], which uses an interactive virtual audience to deliver natural feedback using the virtual characters' non-verbal behavior. In a preliminary study, the audience used head nods (resp. shakes) and forward (resp. backward) leaning postures for positive (resp. negative) feedback; however we did not systematically study the effect of these behaviors.

The perception of virtual audiences' behaviors has only recently been systematically studied by Kang *et al.* [8,9]. In [9], two real audiences were recorded while listening to presentations designed to elicit certain states in the audience, *e.g.* a speech advocating for pay cuts was used in order to elicit a negative reaction from the audience. Participants' behaviors were coded every 2 s and the resulting dataset was used to build models for choosing full body postures (*i.e.* head, arms, hands, torso and feet) according to given input state variables (attitude, personality, mood, energy). Facial expressions and gaze were not considered, and head nods and shakes were rarely found in the annotations. An evaluation by users describing the audience displayed in a virtual reality headset seems to indicate that the model adequately portrays attentiveness or boredom, but not valence. In [8], further studies were realized using this framework in order to evaluate which behavior types and states are recognized by participants observing a virtual audience. In particular, they found that study participants could differentiate between audiences with different levels of valence and arousal (or interest), and described five main recognizable audience types. While their work shows many insights about the design of virtual audiences, one main limitation of their model is that it considers only full body postures, and not other crucial listening behaviors such as head nods and head shakes, and it is difficult to grasp from their results the particular influence of a certain modality compared to the others. They also did not investigate the perception of audiences consisting of virtual agents with mixed states (*e.g.* an audience with 2 engaged characters and 3 bored characters).

In this paper, we build on Kang *et al.*'s work, adopting valence and arousal as two underlying dimensions that drive our virtual audience behaviors and evaluate the influence of homogeneity of virtual audience members' behaviors on the perception of the overall audience (*i.e.* what happens when 2 characters are bored, 3, 4, *etc.*). In a first study, we investigate the role of non-verbal modalities for expressing these states. Then, we explore in a second study participants' overall impressions of virtual audiences when manipulating the amount of virtual characters that express a target state. In a nutshell, we try to answer the following questions:

Q_1: *Which non-verbal signals make a virtual audience character appear critical or supportive of the speech? Bored or engaged?*
Q_2: *Can we control users' perception of a virtual audience's level of arousal and valence by manipulating individual audience members' behaviors?*

In the next section, we set out to answer Q_1 by using a crowdsourcing method to collect audience members' behaviors.

3   Crowdsourcing Audience Behaviors

Our first research goal was to identify the link between different non-verbal signals of various modalities and the relevant audience state dimensions we defined in the previous section, *i.e.* valence and arousal. To achieve this goal, we used a methodology introduced by Ochs *et al.* that consists of asking users to select combinations of behaviors (and/or parameters of these behaviors, *e.g.* duration or intensity) that adequately portray a studied socio-emotional phenomenon [13]. For instance, Ochs *et al.* used this method to collect a repertoire of amused, polite and embarassed smiles by letting users create their own virtual smiles, choosing what they thought to be adequate intensities, durations and combination of facial movements involved for the chosen smile category.

3.1   Crowdsourcing Interface

We adopted this methodology for our first research question Q_1, producing a web interface shown in Fig. 1. This interface consists of a task description, a panel containing a number of possible behavior choices, a video panel displaying a virtual character (male or female) enacting the chosen behaviors, and a 7-point scale to indicate how well the participant thinks the resulting video conveys the input condition. The different parameters that could be chosen by the users were the following:

– Amount of time with an averted gaze: 0 %, 25 %, 50 %, 75 %, 100 %
– Direction of the averted gaze, if any: Sideways, Down, Up.
– Posture: 6 different choices (5 of them visible in Fig. 3).
– Facial expression, if any: smile, frown, eyebrows raised.
– Facial expressions frequency (if applicable): 25 %, 50 %, 75 % of the time.
– Head movements, if any: nod, shake.
– Head movements frequency (if applicable): 1/2/3 times every 10 s.

These parameters allow us to cover most modalities of human communication. We only discarded gestures and vocal behavior which we do not consider in our framework, meaning the audience only produces listening behavior. We

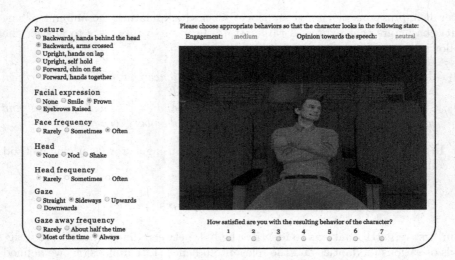

Fig. 1. The crowdsourcing interface.

also chose a variety postures, allowing us to explore different underlying dimensions of postural behavior, in particular proximity to the speaker (lean backward/forward) and openness (hands behind head *vs.* arms crossed) [11]. Some heuristics were introduced in order to make sure that no clashes between behaviors would happen in the videos (*e.g.* no head shake while the gaze direction is changing) and to introduce some variability in behavior timings. We defined five values for both the arousal (resp. valence) states: "very low", "low", "medium", "high", "very high" (resp. negative/positive). We created 10 s videos corresponding to all of the possible different combinations of the behavior parameters for a male and a female character, resulting in 10920 videos.

3.2   Experimental Results

We recruited 72 participants using the Amazon Mechanical Turk website[1] to create combinations of behaviors for the states we considered. Using our web interface, we collected 1045 combination of behaviors, an average of 20.9 combinations of behaviors per input state.

In order to explore the data and answer our research question Q_1, we tested the following hypotheses about how behaviors were chosen by participants.

H1 Arousal and expressions: More frequent facial expressions, head movements and less frequent gaze aversions lead to higher arousal.

H2 Valence and expressions: Smiles and nods lead to positive valence, frowns and head shakes to negative valence, while eyebrow raises are mostly neutral.

---

[1] https://www.mturk.com.

H3 Arousal and postures: Postures chosen for high arousal involve leaning closer to the speaker than postures chosen for lower arousal.

H4 Valence and postures: Open postures lead to higher valence compared to more closed postures.

The distributions of behaviors per valence and arousal states regarding these hypotheses are displayed in Fig. 2. We conducted statistical tests to ensure that these behavior distributions were statistically significant. Prior to conducting these tests, we transformed our arousal and valence data into numerical values (very low $\rightarrow$ 1 to very high $\rightarrow$ 5), and we created numerical variables for proximity (backward $\rightarrow$ 1 to forward $\rightarrow$ 3) and openness (arms crossed and self-hold $\rightarrow$ 1, arms behind the head $\rightarrow$ 3, the rest $\rightarrow$ 2).

For **H1**, **H3** and **H4**, the data being of ordinal nature, we realized Kruskal-Wallis tests. For H1, we set the arousal as the independent variable (IV) and conduct tests with the face, head and gaze frequencies as dependent variables (DV). The three tests are significant, for facial expressions ($H(3) = 49.88$, $p < 0.001$), head movements ($H(3) = 101.09$, $p < 0.001$) and gaze ($H(4) = 347.32$, $p < 0.001$). For H3, we set arousal as the IV and proximity as the ordinal DV. The results confirm our hypothesis: higher arousal leads to higher postural proximity ($H(3) = 334.82$, $p < 0.001$). Similarly for H4, we set valence as the IV and openness as the DV and confirm our hypothesis ($H(3) = 73.59$, $p < 0.001$). For **H2**, the data being of categorical nature and not ordinal, we performed a Chi-squared test, which also showed statistical significance ($\chi^2(12) = 1559.8$, $p < 0.001$). These results confirm the four hypotheses we presented earlier. We found that higher arousal leads to more frequent expressions and to postures that are closer to the speaker, while valence affects the type of expressions used (*e.g.* smiles and nods for positive valence, frowns and shakes for negative valence) and leads to less open postures.

Using the data we collected, we then built a probabilistic model that reflect how often certain behaviors are chosen in a given state. In effect, it models the $P(Behavior|Arousal, Valence)$ behavior distributions for the different modalities and states used in the crowdsourcing study. At runtime, we can select appropriate behaviors for expressing one character's state by querying our model. For each modality, a random number (in the $[0, 1)$ range) is generated and compared to the cumulative distribution function (CDF) of that modality's behavior distribution. The behavior corresponding to that level of the CDF is then returned to be displayed by the character. This model allows us to select appropriate behaviors so that each virtual character reflects its current state, while still exhibiting variability in behaviors. Our second research question Q_2 was to validate that the perception of a virtual audience' overall state can be incrementally manipulated by adjusting the amount of characters that display the chosen state. To that end, we realized a second experiment, presented in the next section.

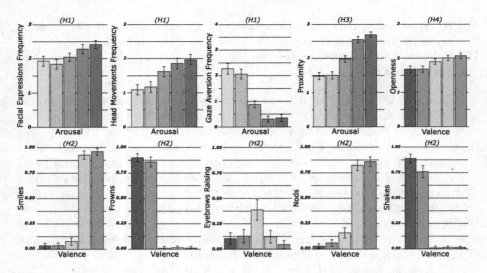

Fig. 2. Distribution of behaviors per state levels for the investigated hypotheses. From left to right in the subfigures, very low to very high arousal (resp. valence).

4   Overall Perception of Virtual Audiences

In order to investigate the perception of complete audiences, we realized a second study. The goal was to verify that by manipulating the expressed state of one virtual character at a time, the overall perceived state of the audience can be changed continuously.

For this study, we defined two independent variables: the target state **S**, consisting of a value of valence and arousal, and the number of manipulated characters **N**. We used a fixed audience configuration, displayed in Fig. 3. In order to reduce the amount of tested conditions, we considered only three levels of valence and arousal, *i.e.* low, medium or high arousal and negative, neutral and positive valence, randomly selecting between a very low/low and very high/high level for generating a character's state when creating a video. The audience consisted of 10 characters and thus **N** could take 11 values, from 0 to 10. The (**N**) manipulated characters would be assigned behaviors according to their state using the probabilistic model built after the previous experiment. For the other (10-**N**) non-manipulated characters, a random state was selected, meaning that they could display congruent, neutral or contradictory behaviors compared to the input condition. We created 4 video variants for every condition, meaning we evaluated a total of 396 videos.

We created another web interface for this study. The participants' task was to watch the video and to indicate their overall perception of the audience's level of arousal and valence, using 5-point scales. The participants were also recruited from Amazon Mechanical Turk. We collected 2643 answers for both dimensions from 105 participants, for an average of 7,1 answers per video, or

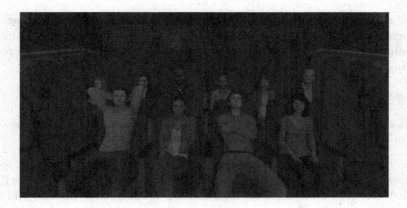

Fig. 3. Screenshot of the full audience.

26,7 answers per input condition. For compiling the results, we used a majority voting to determine the perceived state of a particular video, *e.g.* if the audience of one video was rated with an arousal level of 5 by 4 participants and with an arousal level of 3 by 2 participants, then the video receives a score of 5. When a tie occurs, the scores are averaged for the video. The results, averaged over all input videos, are presented in Fig. 4.

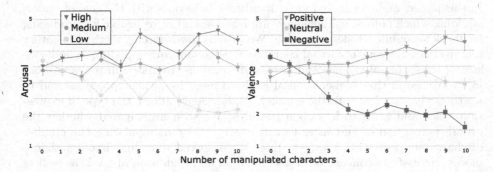

Fig. 4. Perception of arousal (resp. valence) for audiences of 10 characters, depending on the target state and the number of manipulated characters.

We can observe from Fig. 4 that the perceived state of the audience gets more clearly recognized as the number of manipulated characters expressing the input condition increases. Our model can successfully express low, medium and high arousal as well as negative, neutral and positive valence. We conducted a linear regression analysis in order to further analyze the impact of manipulating individual characters. Specifically, we studied a regression model of the following form $y = \alpha + \beta_S * \mathbf{N}$, with y corresponding to the participants' rating of the arousal (resp. valence) for the video's audience, S being the input arousal condition (resp. valence) of the video, *i.e.* high, medium or low, and β_S the corresponding regression coefficient. Finally, **N** corresponds to the amount of manipulated characters. The results of our linear regression analysis are the following:

- $y_{Arousal} = 3.485 + 0.109 * N_{High} + 0.025 * N_{Medium} - 0.146 * N_{Low}$
  $(F(3, 392) = 53.21, p < 0.001.\ R^2 = 0.29,\ StdErr = 0.99)$
- $y_{Valence} = 3.362 + 0.092 * N_{Positive} - 0.027 * N_{Neutral} - 0.181 * N_{Negative}$
  $(F(3, 392) = 95.49, p < 0.001.\ R^2 = 0.42,\ StdErr = 0.79)$

For medium arousal (resp. neutral valence), we find that the slope is not statistically significantly different from a flat line ($p > 0.05$ in both cases). We find that the slope coefficients for high and low arousal (resp. positive and negative valence) are significant ($p < 0.001$ in all 4 cases), *i.e.* the slope in these cases is significantly different from a flat line. This validates our second research question Q_2, meaning that it is possible to incrementally alter the arousal and valence manifested by the virtual audience by changing the state of one virtual character at a time. Another interesting result is that the slope for negative valence seems to be twice as strong as for positive valence. This suggests that users might perceive negative behaviors as more salient than positive behaviors.

5   Conclusion and Future Work

In this paper, we investigated virtual audience behaviors with the goal of understanding which non-verbal behaviors are relevant and recognizable for producing feedback for public speaking training. We used a crowdsourcing method to gather a user-created corpus of virtual characters' behaviors corresponding to audience states, consisting of valence and arousal dimensions, validated in previous work [8,9]. We found that higher arousal leads to more frequent expressions and to postures that are closer to the speaker, while valence affects the type of expressions used and leads to less open postures. We then investigated whether the overall perception of audiences can be controlled by manipulating the number of characters displaying a target state. We observed that our virtual audience model successfully conveys both low, medium and high arousal levels as well as negative, neutral and positive valences. We also found that the perceived level of arousal (resp. valence) of our audience is proportional to the amount of characters that display it. This means that we can continuously vary the impression given by the virtual audience, by changing the expressed state of one virtual character at a time towards the target feedback state.

In future work, we will investigate the link between the placement of individual characters and their influence on the overall perception of the audience: indeed, it could be that the front row characters are more salient to the users than the back row characters. Understanding this effect, if it exists, could allow us to control the virtual audience impression even more precisely. Additionally, we will study the perception of our virtual audience during actual public speaking training sessions with participants.

Acknowledgments. This material is based upon work supported by the National Science Foundation under grant No. IIS-1421330 and U.S. Army Research Laboratory under contract number W911NF-14-D-0005. Any opinions, findings, and conclusions or recommendations expressed in this material are those of the author(s) and do not necessarily reflect the views of the National Science Foundation or the Government, and no official endorsement should be inferred.

References

1. Barmaki, R., Hughes, C.E.: Providing real-time feedback for student teachers in a virtual rehearsal environment. In: Proceedings of the 2015 ACM on International Conference on Multimodal Interaction, ICMI 2015, pp. 531–537. ACM, New York (2015)
2. Bodie, G.D.: A racing heart, rattling knees, and ruminative thoughts: defining, explaining, and treating public speaking anxiety. Commun. Educ. **59**(1), 70–105 (2010)
3. Chollet, M., Wortwein, T., Morency, L.-P., Shapiro, A., Scherer, S.: Exploring feedback strategies to improve public speaking: an interactive virtual audience framework. In: Proceedings of UbiComp 2015, Osaka, Japan. ACM (2015)
4. Damian, I., Baur, T., Lugrin, B., Gebhard, P., Mehlmann, G., André, E.: Games are better than books: in-situ comparison of an interactive job interview game with conventional training. In: Conati, C., Heffernan, N., Mitrovic, A., Verdejo, M.F. (eds.) AIED 2015. LNCS, vol. 9112, pp. 84–94. Springer, Heidelberg (2015). doi:10.1007/978-3-319-19773-9_9
5. Damian, I., Tan, C.S.S., Baur, T., Schöning, J., Luyten, K., André, E., Augmenting social interactions: realtime behavioural feedback using social signal processing techniques. In: Proceedings of the 33rd Annual ACM Conference on Human Factors in Computing Systems, CHI 2015, pp. 565–574. ACM, New York (2015)
6. Harris, S.R., Kemmerling, R.L., North, M.M.: Brief virtual reality therapy for public speaking anxiety. Cyberpsychol. Behav. **5**, 543–550 (2002)
7. Hart, J., Gratch, J., Marsella, S.: How virtual reality training can win friends and influence people. In: Human Factors in Defence, chap. 21, pp. 235–249. Ashgate (2013)
8. Kang, N., Brinkman, W.-P., van Riemsdijk, M.B., Neerincx, M.: The design of virtual audiences: noticeable and recognizable behavioral styles. Comput. Hum. Behav. **55**, 680–694 (2016)
9. Kang, N., Brinkman, W.-P., van Riemsdijk, M.B., Neerincx, M.A.: An expressive virtual audience with flexible behavioral styles. IEEE Trans. Affect. Comput. **4**(4), 326–340 (2013)
10. Lucas, G., Gratch, J., King, A., Morency, L.-P.: It's only a computer: virtual humans increase willingness to disclose. Comput. Hum. Behav. **37**, 94–100 (2014)
11. Mehrabian, A.: Nonverbal Communication. Transaction Publishers, Piscataway (1977)
12. North, M.M., North, S.M., Coble, J.R.: Virtual reality therapy: an effective treatment for the fear of public speaking. Int. J. Virtual Reality **3**, 2–6 (1998)
13. Ochs, M., Ravenet, B., Pelachaud, C.: A crowdsourcing toolbox for a user-perception based design of social virtual actors. In: Computers are Social Actors Workshop (CASA) (2013)

14. Pertaub, D.-P., Slater, M., Barker, C.: An experiment on public speaking anxiety in response to three different types of virtual audience. Presence: Teleoperators Virtual Environ. **11**(1), 68–78 (2002)
15. Tanveer, M., Lin, E., Hoque, M.E.: Rhema: a real-time in-situ intelligent interface to help people with public speaking. In: Proceedings of the 20th ACM Conference on Intelligent User Interfaces, pp. 286–295 (2015)
16. Wang, N., Gratch, J.: Don't just stare at me! In: Proceedings of the SIGCHI Conference on Human Factors in Computing Systems (CHI), Chicago, IL, pp. 1241–1250 (2010)

Using Temporal Association Rules
for the Synthesis of Embodied Conversational
Agents with a Specific Stance

Thomas Janssoone[1(✉)], Chloé Clavel[2], Kévin Bailly[1], and Gaël Richard[2]

[1] Sorbonne Universités, UPMC Univ Paris 06, CNRS UMR 7222, ISIR,
75005 Paris, France
{thomas.janssoone,kevin.bailly}@isir.upmc.fr
[2] Institut Mines-Télécom, Télécom-ParisTech CNRS-LTCI, Paris, France
{chloe.clavel,gael.richard}@telecom-paristech.fr

Abstract. In the field of Embodied Conversational Agent (ECA) one of the main challenges is to generate socially believable agents. The long run objective of the present study is to infer rules for the multimodal generation of agents' socio-emotional behaviour. In this paper, we introduce the Social Multimodal Association Rules with Timing (SMART) algorithm. It proposes to learn the rules from the analysis of a multimodal corpus composed by audio-video recordings of human-human interactions. The proposed methodology consists in applying a Sequence Mining algorithm using automatically extracted Social Signals such as prosody, head movements and facial muscles activation as an input. This allows us to infer Temporal Association Rules for the behaviour generation. We show that this method can automatically compute Temporal Association Rules coherent with prior results found in the literature especially in the psychology and sociology fields. The results of a perceptive evaluation confirms the ability of a Temporal Association Rules based agent to express a specific stance.

Keywords: Multi-modal social signal · Sequence mining · Signal processing · Embodied conversational agent

1 Introduction

Embodied Conversational Agents (ECAs) can improve the quality of life in our modern digital society. For instance, they can help soldiers to recover from PTSD (Post Traumatic Stress Disorder) or help a patient to undergo treatment [1] if they are empathic enough to provide support. The main challenge relies on the naturalness of the interaction between Humans and ECAs. With this aim, an ECA should be able to express different stances towards the user, as for instance dominance for a tutor or friendliness for a companion. This work proposes the SMART algorithm for the generation of believable behaviours conveying interpersonal stances.

© Springer International Publishing AG 2016
D. Traum et al. (Eds.): IVA 2016, LNAI 10011, pp. 175–189, 2016.
DOI: 10.1007/978-3-319-47665-0_16

To give ECAs the capacity to express emotions and interpersonal stances is one of the main challenges [2]. However, this field of research is thriving as more and more databases are available for the processing of Social Signals [3]. These databases are mainly audiovisual and provide monomodal or multimodal inputs to Machine Learning methods [4–7]. Features such as prosodic descriptors or activations of facial muscles labelled as Action Units (AUs see Fig. 1) are extracted to recognize a social expression (emotion, stance, behavior...). The data is usually labelled by an external observant who rates his/her perception of the ongoing interaction (*e.g.* the levels of valence, of arousal, of antagonism, of tension...). These annotations provide different classes for supervised machine learning algorithms.

This paper focuses on the scheduling of the multimodal signals expressed by a protagonist in an intra-synchrony study of his/her stance. Intra-synchrony refers here to the study of multimodal signals of one individual whereas the inter-synchrony studies the synchrony between two interlocutors. We focus on the sequencing that provides information about interpersonal stance as defined by Scherer [8] as the "characteristic of an affective style that spontaneously develops or is strategically employed in the interaction with a person or a group of persons, coloring the interpersonal exchange in that situation (e.g. being polite, distant, cold warm, supportive, contemptuous)". Indeed, the scheduling of non-verbal signals can lead to different interpretations: Keltner [9] illustrates the importance of this multi-modality dynamics: a long smile shows amusement while a gaze down followed by a controlled smile displays embarrassment.

We present here an automatic method based on a sequence-mining algorithm which aims to analyse the dynamics of the social signals such as facial expression, prosody, and turn-taking. The focus is put on the processing of the input signals to find relevant sequences of temporal events through temporal association rules. To the best of our knowledge, this paper is the first attempt to deduce association rules with temporal information directly from social signals by transforming social signals into temporal events. The association rules are learnt from a corpus and will provide time-related information between the signal-based events in a sequence. From a long term perspective, the association rules will be dedicated to automatic temporal planning for the generation of ECA's stances that are believable. However, one major difficulty to find these rules is that they are blended into each other due not only to the stance but also to other constraints such as identity, bio-mechanical constraints or the semantic contents of the given utterance [10]. For instance, two persons can have a warm exchange but one frowns because he/she is dazzled by the sun. Another example is that the AU 26, jaw drop, can signify surprise but can also be activated due to the speech production mechanisms.

We detail how to process social signals such as AU and prosodic features as an input to a sequence-mining algorithm to find temporal association rules. The previous approaches found in the literature will be detailed. Afterwards, the methodology will be explained: the considered multimodal social signals (Action Unit, head nod and turn taking), the process of the symbolization of the input

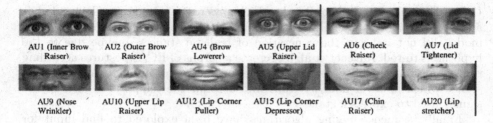

Fig. 1. Facial action unit locations, images are obtained from http://www.cs.cmu.edu/~face/facs.htm

signals into temporal events, the sequence mining algorithm and the scoring of the obtained Temporal Association Rules are justified. Then, the methodology is applied on a multimodal corpus in a human-agent interaction context to investigate the differences between someone cheerful and someone hostile during an interaction. These results will be reviewed and discussed by confronting them to the literature. A perceptive study of Temporal Association Rules based ECA is also detailed and discussed. Finally, perspectives and future leads will be presented.

2   Related Work

The links between social signals and interpersonal stances have been studied during the last decades [11] with goals such as the detection of the user's/human's stance or the generation of believable interpersonal stances for ECAs. To do so, humans' expressions of these stances were studied.

First, qualitative studies were made such as Allwood et al. [12] where verbal and gestural feedbacks during dialogues between a travel agent and customers were investigated. The relationship between prosody and gestures was underlined in this particular context.

In qualitative studies about first impression, Cafaro et al. [13] show how the observant's feeling of the stance of a virtual character is impacted by nonverbal immediacy cues. They underline that proximity has no effects on judgements of friendliness. In [14], a cluster approach shows the link between head-nod, head-shake and affect labels made either with audiovisual files or visual only. They show a strong affective meaning of the nod and the shake and underline the limit of the inter-rater agreement due to the verbal context available for one party. These approaches use statistical tools to link social signals and perceptions of stances.

Lately, machine-learning algorithms were used like in the study of Lee and Marsella [15] about how head-nod magnitude and eyebrow movements evolve while speaking. Participants were asked to rate their immediate feeling of a virtual agent speaking while making head nods and eyebrow movements. Three learning algorithms (Hidden Markov Model, Conditional Random Fields and

Latent-Dynamic Conditional Random Fields) were compared to model head nods and eyebrow movements. However, even if they improve the recognition, this model did not improve the generation of realistic stances, maybe due to the hypothesis tested. Ravenet et al. [16] create a corpus of ECAs postures according to several stances. They develop a Bayesian model to automatically generate stance which however does not take into account the temporal aspects of the signals used to express a stance.

Finally, sequence-mining algorithms have been explored to find input for machine-learning based generation of agent. For instance, Martinez et al. [17] and then Chollet et al. [18] explain how to use them to find simple sequences of non-verbal signals associated to social stances. Martinez et al. [17] use the particular context of video gaming to link these feature samples to emotions such as frustration. They use the Generalised Sequence Pattern (GSP) algorithm on physiological signals to predict the player's affective state. Yet, the obtained sequences are not used for generation. Chollet et al. [18] also used GSP algorithm to extract sequences of manually annotated non-verbal signals characterizing different interpersonal stances. Hence, the GSP algorithm extracts sequences of events without temporal information *i.e.* it can only find that one event happens after another. Then, a model for the expression of a particular stance by an ECA was built to select the most appropriate sequence. Although these studies have proposed an analysis of social signal sequences, they do not consider temporal information. However, such information may change the interpretation of social signals sequences e.g. a long smile versus a short one as shown in [9].

3   Our Approach

In the same vein, the chosen approach takes advantage of a sequence mining algorithm. The new contributions of our approach rely, firstly, on adding temporal information and, secondly, on directly processing the audio-visual input signals. To do so, the signals are transformed to be seen as temporal events (Sect. 3.1) that are the inputs of the sequence mining algorithm and we choose to use the Temporal Interval Tree Association Rule Learning algorithm (TITARL) as sequence mining algorithm (Sect. 3.2). We adapt the TITARL algorithm and embedded its new version into our framework Social Multimodal Association Rules with Timing (SMART) that we detail below (Sect. 3.3).

3.1   Feature Extraction

We choose to focus on a set of social signals composed by *facial AUs activation* (see Fig. 1), *the head pose* and information such as *dialogic events*. We detail here the process that is used to compute these descriptors.

The 3D head pose was estimated with Intraface [19], a fully automatic face tracker. Its outputs are the pitch, the yaw and the roll of the head of the actor present in the video. We use these values as descriptor after a moving average smoothing over a 3 frames window and we cluster them in 10 degrees group. We then create events when the head passes from one 10 degrees group to one of the next 10 degrees group. Hence we keep the continuity of the original signal in our new symbolic temporal events.

Dialogic events correspond to events related to turn-taking activity. They indicate whether the human is listening or speaking so we get the action of *start speaking* and *end speaking* as new events. This information is supplied by the manual transcript provided with the studied corpus (see Sect. 4). Dialogic information is also used to annotate the state (speaking or listening mode) of other events such as AUs or head nod.

Prosodic features were extracted using Prosogram, a program developed by Mertens [20] which aims to provide a representation of intonation as perceived by a human listener. We choose Prosogram among other tools for automatic prosodic annotation because of its phonetic approach that better reflects the human perception than the other approaches. Indeed, all pitch movements cannot be perceived by the human ear and, as our long term goal is stance generation, we focus on signals that will play a part in perception.

Furthermore, Prosogram proposes an automatic segmentation of the audio files into syllabic like nuclei and computes global prosodic parameters such as speaker pitch range. Then, it transforms these into an approximation of perceived pitch patterns. This bottom-up approach does not need additional information such as annotation or training, and then avoids the risk of bias.

For this study, we compute for each nuclei the mean f_0, and its variation, the peak of intensity, and the shape of the pitch (rises, falls,...). Then, we merge the nuclei information of the shape at the word level to obtain the shape of the pitch inside the word. The timing information of each word is provided by the transcript. The three other features, f_0, its variation and the peak of intensity, as they are continuous, are turned into symbolized temporal events with the SAX symbolization process [21].

The Action Units were automatically detected using the solution proposed by Nicolle et al. [22]. An exponential smoothing was applied with $\alpha = 0.7$ on this continuous output to reduce the noise of the detection. Then, the AUs were symbolized as three folders: inactivate, low activation and high activation. For the study presented in Sect. 4, we focus on AUs corresponding to smile and eyebrow movements (see Fig. 1). AU 1 and 2 are grouped and describe brow raising. AU 4 describes brow lowering. AU 6 describes cheek raising. AU 12 describes lip corner pulling. When two AUs are grouped, the value kept is the maximum value of each.

We consider as events the variation of AU activation like for example AU6 disabled to low activation will be an $AU6_{\text{off to low}}$ event or AU12 from low to high activation an $AU12_{\text{low to high}}$ event. We also provide for each event the state of the person, listening or speaking, thanks to the dialogic event formely detailed.

3.2 Sequence Mining Algorithm

After a survey of existing Temporal Constrained Systems solutions (Chronicle, Episode, etc.), we focused on The Temporal Interval Tree Association Rule

Learning (Titarl) algorithm [23] because of its flexibility and its ability to express uncertainty and temporal inaccuracy of temporal events. Indeed, it can compute time relation as rules between events (before/after), negation and accurate time constraints such as *"If there is an event D at time t, then there is an event C at time t+5"*. This temporal learning approach to find temporal associative rules from symbolic sequences allows to represent imprecise (non-deterministic) and inaccurate temporal information between social signals considered as events.

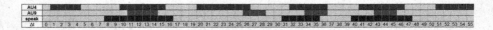

Fig. 2. Example of social signal input for TITARL

A temporal rule gives information about the relation between symbolic events with a temporal aspect. In our case, the events are the social signals (AUs, head nods, prosody, turn taking) considered as discrete events after a preprocessing step of symbolization. For example, with the input of Fig. 2, a temporal pattern could be: *If an event "activation of AU4" happens at time t while state Speak is active, then an event "activation of AU9" will be triggered between $t + \Delta t$ and $t + 3\Delta t$ with a uniform distribution* which can be symbolized by the rule following in (1):

$$AU4_{\text{off to low}} \xrightarrow{\Delta t, 3\Delta t} AU9_{\text{off to low}} \tag{1}$$
$$\substack{Speaking}$$

Δt represents here a time-step due to the training data such as the video frame rate. A rule is composed by a head, here the $AU9_{\text{off to low}}$, a tree of temporal constraints, here the

$$AU4_{\text{off to low},}$$
$$\substack{Speaking}$$

a temporal distribution, here the $\Delta t, 3\Delta t$.

Some characteristics of a rule can be computed to validate its interest. If we look at the following rule r defined in Eq. (2):

$$A \xrightarrow{\Delta t_{min}, \Delta t_{max}} B \tag{2}$$

then the confidence of a rule is the probability of a prediction of the rule to be true (see 3a). We are also interested in the support of a rule which is the percentage of events explained by the rule (see 3b). Finally, TITARL ensures a good precision in the rule that is the temporal accuracy of the prediction, i.e., a low dispersal of the distribution of the events A (standard deviation) verifying the rule r.

$$confidence = P(B(t')|A(t)), t' - t \in [\Delta t_{min}, \Delta t_{max}] \tag{3a}$$

$$support = \frac{\# B, \exists A \text{ such that } (A \to B) \text{ true}}{\# B} \tag{3b}$$

$$precision = \frac{1}{\text{std}([t' - t, \exists A, B, (A(t) \to B(t')) \text{ true}])} \tag{3c}$$

For example, for the rule in 1, the confidence will be 1.0 and the support 0.75.
More details about the TITARL algorithm can be found in [23].

3.3   Adjustment of the TITARL Algorithm into SMART

Introduction to the TITARL Algorithm. The structure of the TITARL
pipeline, shown in the Fig. 3, has two major parts. With the set of input events,
characterized by a name, a session, a character and a time, a first process will
generate simple rules with a structure like in (2) and a very large temporal
distribution. These rules have a high confidence and support but a very low
precision. The three steps of TITARL are recursively applied: division of the
rule, refinement and addition of conditions.

The division step will produce more accurate rules by dealing with co-
occurence of events. For example, if we have an event A at time t, an event
B at time $t + 5\Delta t$ and an event B at time $t + 15\Delta t$, we can have the rule
$A \xrightarrow{U_{5\Delta t, 15\Delta t}} B$ or the two rules $A \xrightarrow{U_{5\Delta t}} B$ and $A \xrightarrow{U_{15\Delta t}} B$. This division step
will choose between the two possibilities.

The refinement of a rule aims at increasing its precision: it observes the
temporal distribution of the events verifying the rule and decreases their variance
with a threshold on its histogram of distribution.

The addition of a condition to a rule is done to maximize the information
gain. To do so, given a rule $A \rightarrow B$, the algorithm observes all the simple rules
like $B \rightarrow C$. It will combine them as $A \rightarrow B \rightarrow C$ if its number of occurrences
remains over a fixed threshold. This step will stop in case of a loop in the chain
of events.

These last steps are carried on while the product of the confidence, the support and the precision remains over a threshold.

The original TITARL algorithm had some limitations and we detail here how
we handled them into the SMART framework that can be seen in Fig. 4.

Discriminative Selection of the Association Rules: A score shown in
Eq. 4a was defined as a combination of the confidence, the support and the size
of the temporal interval of the rules to rank the computed Temporal Association
Rules. This score was introduced by Guillame-Bert in [23] and tried out on

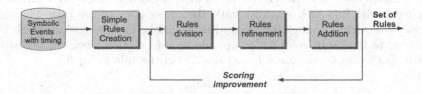

Fig. 3. Pipeline of the TITARL algorithm

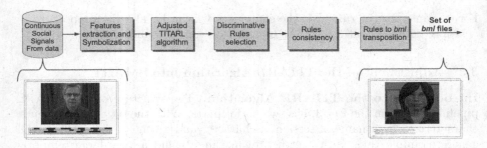

Fig. 4. Pipeline of the SMART algorithm

artificial dataset and a 'Home Activities' dataset.

$$score = \frac{conf_r^4 . supp_r^2}{t_{max} - t_{min}} \tag{4a}$$

$$freq_{\text{character}_C}(r) = \frac{\text{number of occurence of rule r for character C}}{\text{total length of the data}} \tag{4b}$$

$$freqRatio(r, \text{character}_C, \text{character}_D) = \frac{freq_{\text{character}_C}(r)}{freq_{\text{character}_D}(r)} \tag{4c}$$

This score reflect the relevance of a rule in a general context. However, for our purpose, a rule can have a high score without being linked to a stance. As we also want to know the accuracy of the rule with a specific stance, we also defined the frequency of a rule. As described in Eq. 4b, it consist of the ratio between the number of occurrences of the rule and the length of the session. Indeed, as it will be described below, the learning is done on video of actor playing characters with a very specific stance. To differ rule specific to a stance played by a character, we can then use the ratio of frequencies detailed in Eq. 4c. This ratio of frequencies enables to prune the rules linked to a specific stance form others. For instance, if the ratio is high between a friendly video and a hostile one, the rule may be relevant to generate a friendly stance. In the mean time, rules corresponding to jaw movements due to the speech production mechanism are detected with a close to one frequency ratio. We can then not consider them as a stance relevant rule. This part is made in the *Discriminative rule selection* of the Fig. 4.

Rule Consistency for the Generation of Relevant Stance for ECAs: An other issue with TITARL was to handle the consistency of the rule. The association were originally made between all the signals. For one social signal, this could lead to irrelevant rules which provide no information when the transition are lost. For example, we could have rules like in the rule in Eq. 5

$$Event_{\text{off to low}} \xrightarrow{\Delta t_{min}; \Delta t_{max}} Event_{\text{off to low}} \tag{5}$$

but we do not know how and when the Event went from low to off value again. With our generation perspective, this information is essential. To deal with this, we modify TITARL, the simple rule part to be specific, and we design two computational strategies: intra-signal and inter signal. This corresponds to the *Adapted TITARL* box in the Fig. 4. For instance, intra signal applies to two consecutive changes for the same AU while inter signal will be an AU and a head movement or two different AUs.

For intra signal, we compute the simple rules only with the previous occurrence of the same signal. Hence, the consistency is assured. For inter signal, we keep all the previous occurrence, so the original TITARL design. This reduces inaccurate rules computation by improving the consistency of all the transitions in the Temporal Association Rule. Hence, the rule in Eq. 5 cannot be consider and is replaced by the following one:

$$
Event_{\text{off to low}} \xrightarrow{\Delta t_{min_1}; \Delta t_{max_1}} Event_{\text{low to off}} \xrightarrow{\Delta t_{min_2}; \Delta t_{max_2}} Event_{\text{off to low}}
$$

$$(6)$$

Behavior Markup Language File Generation for ECAs: The last contribution we made in the SMART framework is the transposition of the Temporal Association Rule into Behavior Markup Language files (*BML*). The Behavior Markup Language, or BML, is an XML description language for controlling the verbal and nonverbal behavior of (humanoid) embodied conversational agents (ECAs). A BML block describes the physical realization of behaviors (such as speech and gesture) and the synchronization constraints between these behaviors. This is the last part of the framework in Fig. 4.

Through this BML, we can provide the timing used to control the social signals expressed by the ECA during an animation. To do so, we also log the occurrences of each events verifying each rule. In this first version of the SMART framework, we simply use the timing with the most occurences for the transition (red bar at $\Delta_t = 5$ in Fig. 5. In a future release, we could also use the whole distribution of events verifying the rule to diversify the transition and so have more diverse synthesis of a stance.

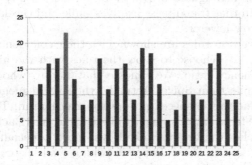

Fig. 5. Example of distribution of occurrences for a rule (Color figure online)

4   Social Signals as Temporal Events: Application for the Study of the SEMAINE-db Corpus

4.1   The SEMAINE-db Corpus

We applied TITARL on the SAL-SOLID SEMAINE database [24] to illustrate our methodology. This corpus uses the Sensitive Artificial Listener (SAL) paradigm to generate emotionally coloured interactions between a user and a 'character' played by an operator. It proposes video and audio data streams of this Face-to-Face interaction where the operator answers with pre-defined utterances to the user's emotional state. We only focus here on the operator part where, for each session, he acts four defined roles, one by one, corresponding to the four quadrants of the Valence-Arousal space. Spike is aggressive, Poppy is cheerful, Obadiah is gloomy and Prudence is pragmatic.

As a first step, for this study, we only focus here on two roles of the operator part, one friendly, Poppy, and one hostile, Spike. This represents 48 interactions of 3–4 min recording, 25 with Poppy, 23 with Spike, played by 4 different actors. This kind of data makes us restraint our study to the affiliation axis of the Argyle's theory of stance [25]. The characters of Poppy and Spike overact it very well and this allows us a first validation of our model.

4.2   First Study: Comparison to the Literature

We performed a first study to validate the extracted rules by comparing them to the results obtained in the literature in two steps. The first one focuses on the rules combining specific AUs, the second one focuses on the rules combining the AUs with the prosodic events.

As a first step, we choose to consider here more specifically AUs corresponding to smile and cheek raiser (AU6, AU12) and brow lowerer (AU1/2 and AU4) and to test TITARL on these specific social signals. Indeed, we want here to compare the connections highlighted in [16, 26] on an ECA study with our results. These papers explain that friendliness involves smile and cheek raiser while hostility is linked to brow lowerer.

In Table 1, association rules are shown with their confidence, support, score and frequency ratio. We choose to show the rules with the highest score with a discriminant frequency ratio. We can see that Poppy, who acts as friendly, is more likely to smile than Spike. Actually, the low frequency ratio leads to think that this is due to the speech production mechanism. This hypothesis is strengthened by the fact that a large part of AU6 and AU12 activation for Spike are while speaking. For the brows, Spike frown more, especially while speaking but a noteworthy result is about Poppy frowning while listening. This can be considered as a backchannel to notice the speaker of Poppy's interest in the conversation.

These results are not only consistent with the literature but also able to provide temporal information and confidence. Indeed, the empirical and theoretical

Table 1. Sample of results with their confidence, support and score. The two first rows are linked to the smile and the two following are linked to the eyebrow. The four last ones refers to the second study and link the prosody to the brow movements.

	rule $(body \xrightarrow{\Delta t_{min};\Delta t_{max}} head)$	confidence	support	score	frequency ratio
Poppy	$AU6_{\text{off to low / listening}} \xrightarrow{0.0s;0.2s} AU6_{\text{low to off/ listening}}$	0.64	0.63	3.10^{-2}	2.09
Poppy	$AU12_{\text{off to low / listening}} \xrightarrow{0.0s;0.2s} AU12_{\text{low to off/ listening}}$	0.50	0.51	8.10^{-3}	3.78
Spike	$AU4_{\text{low to high / speaking}} \xrightarrow{0.0s;0.2s} AU4_{\text{high to low / speaking}}$	0.76	0.81	1.10^{-1}	1.62
Poppy	$AU4_{\text{off to low / listening}} \xrightarrow{0.0s;0.2s} AU4_{\text{low to off/ listening}}$	0.71	0.71	6.10^{-2}	2.07
Spike	nuclei $f0_{\text{large decrease}} \xrightarrow{0;0.9s} AU1+2_{\text{off to low}} \xrightarrow{0;0.3s} AU1+2_{\text{low to off}}$	0.82	0.17	3.10^{-4}	0.88
Poppy	word shape of $f0_{down} \xrightarrow{0;0.9s} AU4_{\text{low to off}}$	0.53	0.57	1.10^{-5}	1.44
Spike	word shape of $f0_{\text{up and down}} \xrightarrow{0.1;0.8s} AU4_{\text{off to low}} \xrightarrow{-0.1;0.3s} AU4_{\text{low to off}}$	0.74	0.01	2.10^{-5}	0.88
Poppy	start speaking $\xrightarrow{0;0.6s} AU1+2_{\text{low to high}} \xrightarrow{0;0.3s} AU1+2_{\text{high to low}}$	0.74	0.57	1.10^{-3}	2.43

research have shown that friendly stances imply frequent smiles while frowning are perceived as threatening and hostile. Our study enables us to identify more precisely the duration of the social signals. Such information is essential to synthesize the stance of an ECA.

In a second phase, we aim here to validate the process of this methodology combining audio and visual information. To do so, a priori rules were deduced from the literature, confronted to the ones obtained here and then discussed. Guaïtella et al. [27] present an experimental investigation on the link between eyebrow movements to voice variations and turn-taking. It shows that peak of the contour of the fundamental frequency are associated with the observed eyebrow movements but it appears that the reverse is false. It also measure the link between eyebrow-movement and start-or-end-of-vocalization as "eyebrow movements act as marks of a new speaking turn". Roon et al. [28] complete these results by underlining that the relation between eyebrow and head position is much closer than the one between eyebrow and speech.

We investigate here these relations by computing with SMART the association rules for eyebrow $(AU1+2$ and $AU4)$, prosody (f_0 and variation) and turn taking. Some computed rules are shown in Table 1 for the shape of the f_0 at the word level and the brow activation considering Poppy and Spike. We can see that the prosodic shape of a word is followed by a similar activation of the brows. It may be explained by the expressiveness of these two characters and the use of brows to emphasise the Irish/English dynamic accent. However, no significant difference was found between Poppy and Spike, especially for the turn taking. This may be explained by the metric that is not appropriate for such a specific event. We plan to improve it with information retrieval techniques to find relevant keyword in documents. Finally, a remarkable result appears for the turn-taking of Poppy. An intense raise of the brow often follows the start of speaking that may be used to improve the bond while taking the floor and, so, improve the friendliness.

4.3   Second Study: Perspective Evaluation with a Focus on AUs and Headnods

Strengthened by the previous study, we conducted an evaluation of videos of an ECA generated from the best ranked Social Temporal Association Rules specific to a character. We processed the rules into *BML* files to use as an input of a virtual agent generation tool [29]. The aim is to evaluate the perception of the agent's stance. As we were in a generation process, we restrained the set of input signals to head nod movements and AUs we can control on the ECA as explained in Sect. 3.1. For instance, AU_9 corresponding to "nose wrinkler" was not implemented so we did not use it.

The design of the study was the following: we took the three best scored rules after 3 addition steps learned over the actor of the Semaine-SAL database in a listening status for each Poppy (friendly) and Spike (hostile). From these six rules, we got sequences of AU and head-nod evolutions with time information as we focus to the listener part. We also log the occurrences of each events verifying each rule to transpose them into *BML* files. These *BML* were used to generate video sequence with the virtual agent using the corresponding social signales. Hence we were able to synthesized an agent following these rules, with the timing of each transition set to the time of the highest occurrence. We used an agent to play each of this six rules and recorded its performances.

We then used an on-line platform to get 60 ratings of each of the 6 videos. 97 judgements were done by 62 participants and each participant was asked to rate his/her feeling of the affiliation (hostile/friendly) of the ECA and his/her confidence in his/her judgement with two five-point Likert-like scales. For instance, the affiliation rating went from 1 corresponding to *very hostile* to 5 *very friendly* through 2 *hostile*, 3 *neutral* and 4 *friendly*.

We first analyse the overall results of the ratings of the poppy-based (friendly) video and the spike-based (hostile) video. The summary of the answer can be seen in the Table 2. We can see that the mean of the answer for Spike is 2.5 and the third quartile is 3 that means that 75 % of the evaluation rate between 1 and 3 which was the expected results. Likewise, we can see for the one about Poppy that the mean is 3.367 and 75 % of the answers were between 3 and 5. For the rest of this study, we followed the statistical advise from [30].

As Shapiro-Wilk test indicates that the answers did not followed a normal distribution (both p-value $< 10^{-16}$), we ran a Mann-Withney's U test to evaluate the difference in the response and we found a significant effect of Group ($p = 9.10^{-5}$). This confirms that the results of the Poppy based evaluation are higher than the Spike one. The results are shown as a boxplot in Fig. 6. This confirm

Table 2. Summary of the global answer over Poppy and Spike based video.

	Min.	1st Qu.	Median	Mean	3rd Qu.	Max
Poppy	2.000	3.000	3.000	3.367	4.000	5.000
Spike	1.000	2.000	3.000	2.5	3.000	5.000

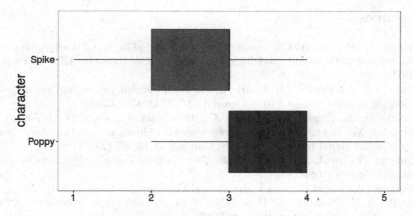

Fig. 6. Boxplot of the evaluation of the affiliation

that a video based on a Temporal Association Rule characteristic of Poppy is seen friendlier than a Spike one, despite this very basic synthesis process.

5 Conclusion and Future Work

This paper presents a methodology to compute temporal association rules from automatically extracted multimodal signals. The focus is put on the processing of these signals to use them as an input of this sequence mining algorithm. The studies show that such methodology can be used to identify interesting sequences of social signals. The adaptation of the score and the use of frequency of occurences give is an important new feature. This combination manages to discriminate rules du to bio-mechanical constraints (i.e. speech production) to others relevant to a stance. However, we believe that this pruning can be still improved in future works.

The studies also shows the ability of SMART to find temporal information associated to specific stances. It is efficient to retrieve relevant rules detailed in the literature with temporal information, confidence and support. The two studies validated this approach but also open the perspective for future developments. The prosodic aspect remains challenging but we plan to use SMART to retrieve contours of sentences. We are now struggling with subtle issues such as dynamic accent as presented in the studies.

Acknowledgement. This work was performed within the Labex SMART supported by French state funds managed by the ANR within the Investissements dÁvenir programme under reference ANR-11-IDEX-0004-0.

References

1. Truong, K., Heylen, D., Chetouani, M., Mutlu, B., Salah, A.A.: Workshop on emotion representations and modelling for companion systems. In: ERM4CT@ICMI (2015)
2. Vinciarelli, A., Pantic, M., Bourlard, H.: Social signal processing: survey of an emerging domain. Image Vision Comput. **27**, 1743–1759 (2009)
3. Vinciarelli, A., Pantic, M., Heylen, D., Pelachaud, C., Poggi, I., D'Errico, F., Schröder, M.: Bridging the gap between social animal, unsocial machine: a survey of social signal processing. Affect. Comput. **3**, 69–87 (2012)
4. Rudovic, O., Nicolaou, M.A., Pavlovic, V.: Machine Learning Methods for Social Signal Processing (2014)
5. Pentland, A.: Social dynamics: signals and behavior. In: ICDL (2004)
6. Sandbach, G., Zafeiriou, S., Pantic, M.: Markov random field structures for facial action unit intensity estimation. In: ICCVW (2013)
7. Savran, A., Cao, H., Nenkova, A., Verma, R.: Temporal Bayesian fusion for affect sensing: combining video, audio, and lexical modalities (2014)
8. Scherer, K.R.: What are emotions? And how can they be measured? Soc. Sci. Inf. **44**, 693–727 (2005)
9. Keltner, D.: Signs of appeasement: evidence for the distinct displays of embarrassment, amusement, and shame. J. Pers. Soc. Psychol. **68**, 441–454 (1995)
10. Bevacqua, E., Pelachaud, C.: Expressive audio-visual speech. Comput. Anim. Virtual Worlds **15**, 297–304 (2004)
11. Fu, Q., op den Akker, R., Bruijnes, M.: A literature review of typical behavior of different interpersonal attitude. Capita Selecta HMI, University of Twente (2014)
12. Allwood, J., Cerrato, L.: A study of gestural feedback expressions. In: First Nordic Symposium on Multimodal Communication (2003)
13. Cafaro, A., Vilhjálmsson, H.H., Bickmore, T., Heylen, D., Jóhannsdóttir, K.R., Valgardsson, G.S.: First impressions: users judgments of virtual agents personality and interpersonal attitude in first encounters. In: IVA (2012)
14. Cowie, R., Gunes, H., McKeown, G., Armstrong, J., Douglas-Cowie, E.: The emotional and communicative significance of head nods and shakes in a naturalistic database (2010)
15. Lee, J., Marsella, S.: Modeling speaker behavior: a comparison of two approaches. In: IVA (2012)
16. Ravenet, B., Ochs, M., Pelachaud, C.: From a user-created corpus of virtual agent's non-verbal behavior to a computational model of interpersonal attitudes. In: IVA (2013)
17. Martínez, H.P., Yannakakis, G.N.: Mining multimodal sequential patterns: a case study on affect detection. In: ICMI (2011)
18. Chollet, M., Ochs, M., Pelachaud, C.: From non-verbal signals sequence mining to bayesian networks for interpersonal attitudes expression. In: Bickmore, T., Marsella, S., Sidner, C. (eds.) IVA 2014. LNCS, vol. 8637, pp. 120–133. Springer, Heidelberg (2014). doi:10.1007/978-3-319-09767-1_15
19. Xiong, X., De la Torre, F.: Supervised descent method and its applications to face alignment. In: CVPR (2013)
20. Mertens, P.: The prosogram: semi-automatic transcription of prosody based on a tonal perception model. In: International Conference on Speech Prosody, 2004 (2004)

21. Lin, J., Keogh, E., Wei, L., Lonardi, S.: Experiencing SAX: a novel symbolic representation of time series. Data Min. Knowl. Discov. (2007)
22. Nicolle, J., Rapp, V., Bailly, K., Prevost, L., Chetouani, M.: Robust continuous prediction of human emotions using multiscale dynamic cues. In: ICMI (2012)
23. Guillame-Bert, M., Crowley, J.L.: Learning temporal association rules on symbolic time sequences. In: ACML (2012)
24. McKeown, G., Valstar, M., Cowie, R., Pantic, M., Schröder, M.: The semaine database: annotated multimodal records of emotionally colored conversations between a person and a limited agent. Affect. Comput. **3**, 5–17 (2012)
25. Argyle, M.: Bodily Communication. Routledge, London (2013)
26. Ochs, M., Pelachaud, C.: Model of the perception of smiling virtual character. In: AAMAS (2012)
27. Guaïtella, I., Santi, S., Lagrue, B., Cavé, C.: Are eyebrow movements linked to voice variations and turn-taking in dialogue? An experimental investigation. Lang. Speech **52**, 207–222 (2009)
28. Roon, K.D., Tiede, M.K., Dawson, K.M., Whalen, D.H.: Coordination of eyebrow movement with speech acoustics and head movement. In: ICPhS (2015)
29. Pecune, F., Cafaro, A., Chollet, M., Philippe, P., Pelachaud, C.: Suggestions for extending SAIBA with the VIB platform. In: Proceedings of the Workshop on Architectures and Standards for IVA (2014)
30. Motulsky, H.: Intuitive Biostatistics: A Nonmathematical Guide to Statistical Thinking. Oxford University Press, New York (2013)

Cross Modal Evaluation of High Quality Emotional Speech Synthesis with the Virtual Human Toolkit

Blaise Potard[1(✉)], Matthew P. Aylett[1,2], and David A. Baude[1]

[1] CereProc Ltd., Edinburgh, UK
blaise@cereproc.com
[2] University of Edinburgh, Edinburgh, UK
https://www.cereproc.com

Abstract. Emotional expression is a key requirement for intelligent virtual agents. In order for an agent to produce dynamic spoken content speech synthesis is required. However, despite substantial work with pre-recorded prompts, very little work has explored the combined effect of high quality emotional speech synthesis and facial expression. In this paper we offer a baseline evaluation of the naturalness and emotional range available by combining the freely available SmartBody component of the Virtual Human Toolkit (VHTK) with CereVoice text to speech (TTS) system. Results echo previous work using pre-recorded prompts, the visual modality is dominant and the modalities do not interact. This allows the speech synthesis to add gradual changes to the perceived emotion both in terms of valence and activation. The naturalness reported is good, 3.54 on a 5 point MOS scale.

Keywords: Speech synthesis · Unit selection · Expressive speech synthesis · Emotion · Prosody · Facial animation

1 Introduction

Both human faces and human voices convey information about the speaker's emotional state. In order to develop artificial agents making use of both modalities, both emotional speech and emotional facial expression require synthesis. However, whereas a considerable about of previous work has examined these modalities in isolation (see [14] for a review), less work has examined their combined effect. Of this, work where an emotional voice has been used together with emotional facial synthesis has almost exclusively used pre-recorded prompts (e.g. SEMAINE's [1] sensitive artificial listener), and almost exclusively used matching voice and facial expression.

This is partly caused by the lack of available speech synthesis systems that can generate emotional variation. A large proportion of systems evaluated are research systems and not available for general academic use. Two exceptions are

D. Traum et al. (Eds.): IVA 2016, LNAI 10011, pp. 190–197, 2016.
DOI: 10.1007/978-3-319-47665-0_17

OpenMary TTS, a diphone based voice using MBROLA [15], and the commercial unit selection system CereVoice [3], which is freely available for academic research.

Integrating emotional speech synthesis with agent animation systems is also a challenging task requiring synchronisation of lip movements and audio and visual streaming. The Virtual Human Toolkit [9] (VHTK) is a collection of modules, tools, and libraries designed to aid and support researchers and developers with the creation of virtual human conversational characters. More specifically, VHTKs component SmartBody is a character animation library that provides synchronized locomotion, steering, object manipulation, lip syncing, gaze direction, and non-verbal behaviour in real-time.

SmartBody has been used in the current study as it contains all the necessary components for animating a highly realistic talking head. Although the CereVoice SDK is not normally distributed along with SmartBody, support for the CereVoice SDK is built-in, and the mapping from phonemes to viseme used for lip animation in VHTK is already present[1].

The resulting multi-modal system offers both state-of-the-art animation and speech synthesis at a commercial grade quality which can be used by the IVA community to explore multi-modal emotional interaction. In order to facilitate such work this paper presents baseline results which we believe will be invaluable for allowing further comparison and the investigation of the effect of interaction, and alternative graphic and audio renderings on perceived emotion.

We address these challenges of synthesising and evaluating cross-modal emotional ambiguity in virtual agents by: (1) Evaluating utterances using a parametric *activation/evaluation* space, (2) integrating the CereVoice synthesiser with the Virtual Human Toolkit, making the combined system readily available for researchers who wish to explore high quality dynamic emotional expression in their work. Our research questions are as follows:

RQ1: How do negative/positive and active/passive features of the two modalities combine? Are they independent? How much range do they offer?

RQ2: Does combining the emotional change across modalities impact naturalness in comparison to a high quality neutral baseline?

1.1   Positive/Negative Voice Quality Selection in Speech Synthesis

Voice quality is an important factor in the perception of emotion in speech [8]. A stressed (tense) voice quality is rated negatively in the evaluation space, while a lax (calm) voice quality is rated negatively in the activation space [5]. However, unlike speech rate and pitch which can be modified relatively easily using digital signal processing techniques such as PSOLA [18], modifying voice quality is more

---

[1] The mapping is currently only available for US accented voices but further accents will become available. Previous studies have shown phoneme-based lip animation is superior to viseme-based approaches [11]. Phone sequences including stress is available from the CereVoice system API and could be incorporated into later releases of VHTK.

difficult, especially if it is important to retain naturalness. Rather than modifying speech to create the effect, an alternative approach is to record different voice qualities in sub-corpora and use them directly during concatenative synthesis. This approach has been applied to diphone synthesis [16], however, CereVoice is the first commercial system to use pre-recorded voice quality sub-corpora in unit selection [4]. Previous work has examined the use of sub-corpora of specific emotions e.g. [10] where Happy, Angry and Neutral sub-corpora were used.

As with [16] three styles of voice quality are available: Neutral, the default for the recorded corpora, and two sub-corpora of lax (calm) and stressed (tense) voice quality. Adding XML tags in the speech input of the form:

```
<usel genre='stressed'>Text</usel>
<usel genre='calm'>Text</usel>
```

biases the selection of the units to come from the sub-corpora.

1.2   Evaluating Emotion in Synthesis

In order to evaluate mild changes in emotion and interactions between different modalities, an approach which is parametric rather than categorical is required. We therefore adopt the approach taken by FEELTRACE [7] and evaluate utterances within the *activation/evaluation space*.

FEELTRACE was developed specifically for assessing gradual changes in emotion by allowing subjects to place the emotion in a two dimensional space called the evaluation/activation space. This space is based on previous work in psychology [12,13] and regards emotions as having two components, a valence which varies from negative to positive, and an activation which varies from passive to active (See Fig. 1a). Therefore rather than asking subjects which emotion they perceive in an utterance, the subject chooses a point in this two dimensional space. There is active debate on how well such a space can represent emotional variation (see [2] for a review). Results presented here are not intended to be used to support or validate the model itself, rather the model is used purely pragmatically because of it powerful ability to detect *shifts* in emotion. This allows us to investigate the perceptual effect across modalities.

1.3   The Talking Head

As mentioned above, SmartBody has been used in the current study to generate realistic multi-modal animations. By default, SmartBody relies on the freely available Festival [17] speech synthesiser, but also support other synthesisers such as CereVoice.

Forcing VHTK to use the CereVoice SDK instead of the Festival synthesiser simply requires installing the SDK where SmartBody expects to find it. Some small modifications were performed in the source code of SmartBody to improve the robustness and ease of use of the integration, these modifications were transmitted to the SmartBody team.

We used one of the standard female character of the SmartBody library, Rachel, along with, for evaluation purposes, a custom build of CereProc US female voice Isabella. 12 neutral sentences were selected for the evaluation. For reference, these sentences were recorded by the *Isabella* voice talent in the 3 voice modalities (neutral, lax, tense), but in order to ensure realistic Text-to-Speech output, these natural recordings were omitted for the voice build. The recorded voice stimuli were used for a training phase during the evaluation.

The video stimuli were generated to simulate 3 different affects: *neutral*, *happy*, and *angry*. The *neutral* stimuli adopted the neutral stance from Smart-Body. The *happy* stimuli were marked by a light smile, tightening of the eyes during speech, and by having the character smile markedly at the very end of the utterance. The angry stimuli were simulated by having the character frown markedly during the utterance.

A SmartBody animation was generated that created a long video sequence of the Rachel character uttering the 12 selected sentences in various configurations. In total, the animation contained 108 clips (all 12 sentences in all possible combinations of video/audio modalities, i.e. $3 \times 3 \times 12 = 108$). Note that SmartBody can by default only output sequences of images, and the image output needs to be triggered manually from the user interface. For simplicity, we generated all clips from a single SmartBody script, then split the audio and set of image sequences accordingly. The image sequences were generated at a constant frame rate of 30 image per second, and the audio was generated at a sampling rate of 48 kHz. The clips were then compressed into 2 different video format (MP4<h264>/webm<VP8>) so as to be compatible with most HTML5 browsers (Google Chrome/Internet Explorer 9+/Firefox/Safari). The audio embedded in the video was compressed in the AAC format at 128 kbps.

2   Methodology

We asked subjects to rate the emotion in the synthetic speech by choosing a position in the activation/evaluation space (cf. circle in Fig. 1a). We also asked them to rate naturalness on a 5 point scale (Bad/Poor/Fair/Good/Excellent). The experiment was carried out online (see Fig. 1) using in total 13 English native speakers recruited through Crowdflower–a UK crowd sourcing evaluation service, similar to Amazon Mechanical Turk. Subjects were asked to use headphones, and to rate the *speech* present in the video clips. There were two factors in the experiment: Facial expression (happy, neutral, angry) **FACE**, and voice quality (Tense/Neutral/Lax) **VQ**.

The listeners were first trained in rating the audio stimuli by practising on short videos clips with the *neutral* facial expression but with audio stimuli of the *neutral*, *tense*, and *calm* voice modalities respectively. These clips were generated similarly to the evaluation sentences described above, except that the evaluation sentences had been recorded and retained during the voice building process, therefore despite being synthesised they were of comparable quality to pre-recorded prompts.

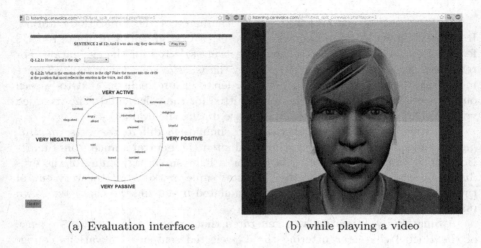

(a) Evaluation interface   (b) while playing a video

Fig. 1. Online experimental setup

The training of the listeners was performed through a tutorial section in the evaluation process containing an example of each voice modality, with an interface and guidelines identical to the rest of the evaluation; the system would however not proceed until the positions in the activation/evaluation space chosen by the user fall within an area consistent with the voice quality of each clip.

The evaluation was split into 3 parts: each set contained 3 variants of each of the 12 sentences (36 stimuli). Materials were presented in a randomised sequence to avoid order effects. Each listener was given the option to perform 1 to 3 parts of the evaluation, with the evaluation being terminated for each part as soon as we received responses from 13 listeners. In order to prevent the listeners from being tempted to cheat, the web-based evaluation ensured that each video was played at least once, and participants could only receive their payment using a key that was provided to them at the end of each part, handling some of the issues identified by [6].

Each part of the evaluation took roughly 15 min to perform. A majority of the listeners (8) did all 3 parts; some listeners attempted to use the same payment key for several parts of the evaluation and the parts with a wrong key were rejected. In order to maintain a balanced design this resulted in 10 subject responses for each of the 108 stimuli.

3   Results

A by-materials MANOVA analysis with two factors: facial expression **FACE** and voice quality **VQ**, across 3 dependent variables, Naturalness, Activation, Evaluation, were used to analyse the experimental results. Both factors had a significant multivariate effect (FACE: Wilk's Lambda 0.001, $F(6, 40) = 276.774$, $p < 0.001$, partial $\eta^2 = 0.976$), (VQ: Wilk's Lambda 0.235, $F(6, 40) = 7.080$,

$p < 0.001$, partial $\eta^2 = 0.515$). Sphericity held for all dependent variables (Mauchly's Test of Sphericity). The interaction was not significant (partial $\eta^2 = 0.125$)

Univariate tests showed a significant effect of FACE and VQ on valence (FACE: $F(2, 22) = 720.390$, $p < 0.001$, partial $\eta^2 = 0.987$, VQ: $F(2, 22) = 25.906$, $p < 0.001$, partial $\eta^2 = 0.702$) and on activation (FACE: $F(2, 22) = 274.699$, $p < 0.001$, partial $\eta^2 = 0.961$, VQ: $F(2, 22) = 5.238$, $p < 0.025$, partial $\eta^2 = 0.323$). For naturalness only **FACE** had a significant effect (FACE: $F(2, 22) = 24.840$, $p < 0.001$, partial $\eta^2 = 0.693$).

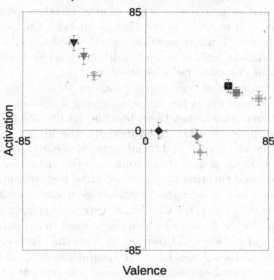

Fig. 2. Mean activation/evaluation of materials by facial expression (FACE) indicated by shape of point, and voice quality (VQ) indicated by shade. Triangle - Angry FACE, Diamond - Neutral FACE, Square - Happy FACE. Black - Tense VQ, Dark Grey - Neutral VQ, Light Grey - Lax VQ. The original activation/evaluation circle shown in Fig. 1a is radius 170. All means show moderate variation within this space (<80). FACE is dominant but VQ also significantly alters the perception of emotion. Error bars show ±1 standard error.

Figure 2 shows the means by **VQ** and **FACE**. Posthoc pairwise comparisons (Least Significant Difference - LSD), showed all means significantly ($p < 0.005$) different for FACE Valence: Angry < Neutral < Happy, and FACE Activation: Angry > Happy > Neutral. For VQ Valence: Tense < Neutral < Lax, and VQ Activation: Tense > Neutral and Lax.

The mean naturalness overall was 3.54 with a standard deviation of 0.30. This is in line with unit selection results although lower than neutral speech as a unimodal stimuli [5]. The animation of the avatar appears to dominate the impression of naturalness. In previous audio only experiments, both lax and tense voice qualities led to a small but significant decrease of perceived naturalness [5]. We did not observe this effect, but instead in a post-hoc test a significant difference between the angry face and both the neutral and happy face (LSD $p < 0.001$, Angry mean 3.41 ± 1 SE 0.06, Neutral mean 3.59 ± 1 SE 0.06, Happy mean 3.60 ± 1 SE 0.07).

Nine example videos are available at: https://dl.dropboxusercontent.com/u/1618087/rachel_iva_2016.zip

4   Discussion

The results show that using emotional variation in facial expression and speech can both be synthesised to affect perception of emotion. Compared to previous results with speech only [5] where emotional synthesised speech caused a drop in naturalness, the animated head appears to mitigate this effect with focus moving to the naturalness of animated facial expression.

However, this experiment was not interactive. It is within an application environment, where emotion is key to personifying a character and conveying their underlying motivations, that these baseline results need to be compared. As well as supporting each other cross modally, the ability to mismatch the emotion conveyed by the speech and facial expression could possibly be used to synthesise a sense of irony or underlying tension in the virtual agent which could be useful for games and tutoring applications. It is, however, unclear how such a sophisticated use of emotion might be evaluated in such a context.

In addition to voice quality, the CereVoice system also allows manipulation of pitch, amplitude and speech rate which could be used to support and also alter the perceived effect of the speech. However, altering the synthesised speech over time using all these factors is non trivial if naturalness is to be maintained. As Schröder points out, *"In a dialogue, an emotional state may build up rather gradually, and may change over time as the interaction moves on."* [15, p. 211]. Thus we have a time element, as well as a vocal element, that need to be coordinated to create a successful effect.

5   Conclusions

This is the first study we are aware of that has investigated how high quality commercial expressive speech synthesis interacts with emotional facial expressions. Previous work considered less natural systems (formant, or diphone speech synthesis systems) or used pre-recorded prompts.

We have shown that voice quality, facial expression combine relatively independently to create different perceptions of emotion.

Acknowledgements. This research was funded by the Royal Society through a Royal Society Industrial Fellowship and and by the European Union's Horizon 2020 research and innovation programme under grant agreement No 645378 (ARIA-VALUSPA).

References

1. The semaine project. http://www.semaine-project.eu/
2. Anagnostopoulos, C.N., Iliou, T., Giannoukos, I.: Features and classifiers for emotion recognition from speech: a survey from 2000 to 2011. Artif. Intell. Rev. **43**(2), 155–177 (2015)
3. Aylett, M.P., Pidcock, C.J.: The cerevoice characterful speech synthesiser SDK. In: Pelachaud, C., Martin, J.-C., André, E., Chollet, G., Karpouzis, K., Pelé, D. (eds.) IVA 2007. LNCS (LNAI), vol. 4722, pp. 413–414. Springer, Heidelberg (2007). doi:10.1007/978-3-540-74997-4_65
4. Aylett, M.P., Pidcock, C.J.: UK patent GB2447263A: Adding and controlling emotion in synthesised speech (2012)
5. Aylett, M.P., Potard, B., Pidcock, C.J.: Expressive speech synthesis: synthesising ambiguity. In: SSW8, pp. 133–138, Barcelona, Spain, August 2013
6. Buchholz, S., Latorre, J.: Crowdsourcing preference tests, and how to detect cheating. In: Proceedings of Interspeech, pp. 3053–3056 (2011)
7. Cowie, R., Douglas-Cowie, E., Savvidou, S., McMahon, E., Sawey, M., Schröder, M.: FEELTRACE: an instrument for recording perceived emotion in real time. In: ITRW on speech and emotion, pp. 19–24 (2000)
8. Gobl, C., Chasaide, A.N., et al.: The role of voice quality in communicating emotion, mood and attitude. Speech Commun. **40**(1), 189–212 (2003)
9. Hartholt, A., Traum, D., Marsella, S.C., Shapiro, A., Stratou, G., Leuski, A., Morency, L.-P., Gratch, J.: All together now. In: Aylett, R., Krenn, B., Pelachaud, C., Shimodaira, H. (eds.) IVA 2013. LNCS (LNAI), vol. 8108, pp. 368–381. Springer, Heidelberg (2013). doi:10.1007/978-3-642-40415-3_33
10. Hofer, G.O., Richmond, K., Clark, R.A.: Informed blending of databases for emotional speech synthesis. In: Proceedings of Interspeech (2005)
11. Mattheyses, W., Latacz, L., Verhelst, W.: Comprehensive many-to-many phoneme-to-viseme mapping and its application for concatenative visual speech synthesis. Speech Commun. **55**(7), 857–876 (2013)
12. Plutchik, R.: The Psychology and Biology of Emotion. Harper Collins College Publishers, New York (1994)
13. Schlosberg, H.: A scale for the judgement of facial expressions. J. Exp. Psychol. **29**(6), 497–510 (1941)
14. Schröder, M.: Emotional speech synthesis: a review. In: Proceedings Eurospeech, vol. 01, pp. 561–564 (2001)
15. Schröder, M.: Dimensional emotion representation as a basis for speech synthesis with non-extreme emotions. In: André, E., Dybkjær, L., Minker, W., Heisterkamp, P. (eds.) ADS 2004. LNCS (LNAI), vol. 3068, pp. 209–220. Springer, Heidelberg (2004). doi:10.1007/978-3-540-24842-2_21
16. Schröder, M., Grice, M.: Expressing vocal effort in concatenative synthesis. In: Proceedings of 15th International Conference of Phonetic Sciences, pp. 2589–2592 (2003)
17. Taylor, P.A., Black, A., Caley, R.: The architecture of the festival speech synthesis system. In: SSW3. pp. 147–151. Jenolan Caves, Australia (1998)
18. Valbret, H., Moulines, E., Tubach, J.P.: Voice transformation using psola technique. In: 1992 IEEE International Conference on Acoustics, Speech, and Signal Processing, ICASSP-1992, vol. 1, pp. 145–148. IEEE (1992)

Bidirectional LSTM Networks Employing Stacked Bottleneck Features for Expressive Speech-Driven Head Motion Synthesis

Kathrin Haag$^{(\boxtimes)}$ and Hiroshi Shimodaira$^{(\boxtimes)}$

School of Informatics, Centre for Speech Technology Research,
University of Edinburgh, Edinburgh, UK
K.Haag@sms.ed.ac.uk, H.Shimodaira@ed.ac.uk

Abstract. Previous work in speech-driven head motion synthesis is centred around Hidden Markov Model (HMM) based methods and data that does not show a large variability of expressiveness in both speech and motion. When using expressive data, these systems often fail to produce satisfactory results. Recent studies have shown that using deep neural networks (DNNs) results in a better synthesis of head motion, in particular when employing bidirectional long short-term memory (BLSTM). We present a novel approach which makes use of DNNs with stacked bottleneck features combined with a BLSTM architecture to model context and expressive variability. Our proposed DNN architecture outperforms conventional feed-forward DNNs and simple BLSTM networks in an objective evaluation. Results from a subjective evaluation show a significant improvement of the bottleneck architecture over feed-forward DNNs.

Keywords: Head motion synthesis · Recurrent neural network · Bottleneck feature · Long-short-term memory · Talking avatar

1 Introduction

Head motion plays an important role in human communication. It is used to give emphasis to certain words or phrases, to convey emotions or to signal agreement or disagreement when listening. In the domain of animation, where realistic virtual agents are desired, it is crucial that head motion looks as natural as possible. Well synthesised head motion can enrich communicative interaction, while badly synthesised head motion is more likely to diminish it.

Work in speech-driven head motion synthesis is often based on Hidden Markov Model (HMM) based methods [1–4]. In general, frame-wise functions are applied to map acoustic features to head motion angles. In order to compensate for the frame-by-frame independence assumption of HMMs, head motion is classified into typical head motion patterns, either manually or by using automatic clustering. HMMs are then trained on each of these head motion clusters. At synthesis time, for an unknown sequence of acoustic observations, the most

© Springer International Publishing AG 2016
D. Traum et al. (Eds.): IVA 2016, LNAI 10011, pp. 198–207, 2016.
DOI: 10.1007/978-3-319-47665-0_18

likely cluster given the observation has to be recognised first, and then the most likely head motion sequence is generated from the corresponding HMM that was trained on this cluster.

The data used in these studies typically contains short sentences and/or does not show a large variability of expressiveness in both speech and motion. Constraining the number of possible contexts by pre-defining motion patterns does not work well for expressive data with considerable variation. Furthermore, there is not a one-to-one mapping between speech and head motion [5] and many different output patterns are possible for a given acoustic input sequence. Thus, treating head motion synthesis as a classification problem is not a feasible approach.

DNNs can overcome some of the limitations of the conventional HMM approach. They provide a powerful architecture to capture the large range of variations that are found in expressive data without the need to pre-define motion patterns. Their hidden layers are able to detect complex relationships between input and output features and have been found to be more effective than decision trees [6]. DNNs are also less prone to over-smoothing and preserve more detail in the output signal than HMMs. DNNs have been widely and successfully used in text-to-speech synthesis and often outperform HMM systems [6]. They have also found their way into facial animation [7,8] and speech-driven gesture synthesis [9].

Ding et al. [10] were the first to use DNNs for speech-driven head motion synthesis. They pre-trained a deep belief network (DBN) with stacked restricted Boltzmann machines, then added a target layer on top of the DBN for parameter fine-tuning. Their training data included broadcast speakers and they used a context window of 11 acoustic frames as input to the DNN. While their architecture performed better than a frame-by-frame DNN modelling approach, a contextual window of this size is not large enough to capture distinctive motion patterns such as nodding and shaking the head, which can span over a window of one or two seconds. For modelling expressive data with a large variability in different motions, an alternative framework is required.

In a further study Ding et al. [11] showed that good performance can be gained by using bidirectional long short-term memory (BLSTM). They report significant improvement of their BLSTM system over a feed-forward DNN, but used data from a single speaker which was not very expressive. We extend on this research and propose a framework which is novel to the domain of head motion synthesis. It combines stacked bottleneck features and a BLSTM network, and we use expressive data.

2   Proposed System

2.1   Bottleneck Features

The features we use for head motion are highly correlated and their dependencies span over long trajectories. The use of bottleneck features for modelling these dependencies seems reasonable. Bottleneck features have been widely used in

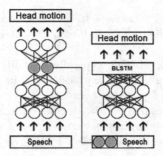

Fig. 1. Example for a bottleneck DNN architecture. Features from the bottleneck layer are stacked and serve as input to a second DNN combined with the original speech features.

speech recognition [15,16] and text-to-speech systems [17]. They can be used in a similar way for speech-driven head motion synthesis. At first, a DNN with a hidden bottleneck layer is trained on speech and head motion features. This layer has a relatively small number of nodes compared to the other layers in the network. The activations at the bottleneck layer (the bottleneck features) give us a compact frame-wise representation of the input and output features. Multiple bottleneck features of consecutive frames are then stacked using a sliding window and combined with the original speech features as the input to a second DNN network (Fig. 1).

2.2   BLSTM with Bottleneck Features

In this paper we investigate whether the use of bottleneck features as input to a BLSTM network is beneficial. It can be argued that contextual information is not required in training a BLSTM network because it already takes the preceding and following context into account, and we will investigate whether this is indeed the case. It should be noted that, although the second network in Fig. 1 is trained in a speaker dependent manner to predict an individual speaker's head motion trajectory, the first network can be trained with data from multiple speakers rather than a single one to obtain robust bottleneck features. We found that this results in better prediction of an individual speaker's head motion trajectory. The training procedure is as follows:

1. Train the first DNN which contains a bottleneck layer. The inputs to the DNN are speech features, the output head motion features.
2. Make a forward pass through this network to generate bottleneck features for the training, validation and test data. This is done frame by frame.
3. Stack bottleneck features from the current frame along with n preceding and n following frames.
4. The bottleneck features are combined with the speech features and a second DNN with a BLSTM layer is trained using these features as its input.

5. A forward pass is made through the network to generate head motion features from the second DNN.

2.3 BLSTM Training Issues

When using long segments of input data that go beyond the length of a single sentence, for example when synthesising paragraphs or monologues, we found that BLSTMs are difficult to train and do not generate satisfactory output trajectories. This is especially the case for data with a large expressive variability. One way to work around this is to divide the dataset into smaller segments and employ mini-batch gradient descent. Instead of computing the gradient over all training examples during one iteration, we use a window of w frames, perform one update of the cost function per window and iterate until we reach the end of the data stream. We found that employing mini-batch gradient descent improves the overall performance of our system.

3 Experiments

3.1 Data

We used three male English native speakers from The University of Edinburgh Speaker Personality and MoCap Dataset [18] for training and testing different architectures. This database contains expressive dialogues between semi-professional actors in extroverted and introverted speaking styles. The dialogues were non-scripted and spontaneous. For the purpose of our experiments we selected only the extroverted recordings because they show more variability in head motion and speech.

Speech Features. Audio in this database was recorded with a headset microphone at 44.1 kHz with 32-bit depth and a MOTU-8pre mixer [19]. Separate recording channels were used for the two speakers and a synchronisation signal was recorded on a third channel in the mixer. For the purpose of this work, the audio signal was down sampled to 16 kHz prior to feature extraction. 12 Mel-cepstral coefficients, which represent the discrete log magnitude spectrum, were extracted using SPTK [20]. Voicing probability and energy were computed using openSMILE [21], and smoothed with a moving average filter with a window length of 10 frames.

It has been shown that articulatory features have a closer relationship with head motion than acoustic features [22], even when estimated from speech. Therefore we also extracted articulatory features, which were estimated using an acoustic-to-articulatory inversion technique [22]. They represent (x; y)-coordinates of six active EMA coils (i.e. two coils attached to the upper and lower lip, one to the jaw and three to the tongue). We will refer to them as EMA features. All features were computed from the audio over 25 ms windows at a frame rate of 10 ms to match the frame rate of the head motion data. We also added their first time derivatives (delta features). The dimension of the speech features was 52.

Head Motion Features. The head motion of one speaker of the dialogue pair was recorded with the NaturalPoint Optitrack [23] motion capture system at a 100 Hz sampling rate. From the marker coordinates, rotation matrices for head motion were computed using singular value decomposition [24]. The rotation matrices were converted to Euler angles, which describe the motions of pitch, yaw and roll (nodding, shaking and tilting the head). The first and second time derivatives of the Euler angles were also added, resulting in a 9-dimensional vector as the output feature. We used the delta features in training because this resulted in better performance than when only using the static head motion features, but they were not used at synthesis time.

3.2   Preliminary Experiments

We conducted preliminary experiments using data from one speaker to analyse the effects of various hyper-parameters. The results are presented in Fig. 2. We varied the position of the bottleneck layer in order to find its optimal position. Canonical correlations between the original and synthesised head motion were highest when the third layer was set as the bottleneck layer. We also varied the number of nodes in the bottleneck layer. Correlations were highest when using 16 nodes and performance was degraded when using eight or 32 nodes. Thus, we set the nodes in the bottleneck layer to 16. Furthermore, we analysed the effect of the size of the contextual window. We found that highest correlations were achieved when using 20 preceding and 20 following frames.

We also analysed different network topologies for the BLSTM network. An architecture with one or more BLSTM layers and no feed-forward layers resulted in worse performance than when using both feed-forward layers and BLSTM layers. Best performance was achieved with one BLSTM layer on top of two feed-forward layers, which conforms with the findings of text-to-speech synthesis [13,14]. However, it does not agree with the results of [11] who observed best performance for head motion synthesis when using one BLSTM layers between two feed-forward layers. This suggests that the optimal architecture is dependant on the task and the data being used, and a careful analysis has to be carried out prior to defining the system architecture.

3.3   Experimental Setups

While audio was recorded for both dialogue partners, head motion could only be captured for one speaker. The following architectures use input and output features from this single speaker and include listening pauses (i.e. silences). All systems use the same input and output features. For each speaker we built a speaker-dependent system using four recordings with a duration of approximately four minutes each. Two recordings were used for training, one for validation and one for testing. This was the same for all systems. Training was conducted on a GPU using Theano version 0.6. The systems we implemented are summarised as follows:

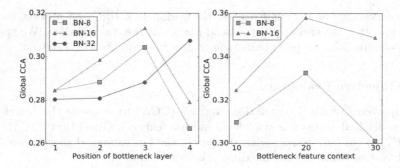

Fig. 2. Analysis of the effect of bottleneck layer position (left) and the number of stacked bottleneck features (right), a number of 10 means that 10 features to the left and 10 features to the right of the current frame were concatenated. Global CCA is defined as the CCA over the entire data stream.

- **DNN:** This system is our baseline and uses a contextual window of acoustic and EMA features as its input. It is similar to the work of [10] except that we did not use RBMs in pre-training. Acoustic and EMA features were concatenated from a context of five frames to the left and fives frames to the right of the current frame, resulting in a 572-dimensional input vector. We used a conventional feed-forward network employing frame-wise minimum mean squared error criterion and mini-batch in training. The network consisted of three hidden layers with 768 hidden units each. The learning rate was set to 0.002 \and halved after 10 epochs, and momentum was 0.3 for the first 10 epochs and increased to 0.9 thereafter. The maximum epoch was 25 and early stopping was applied. A tangent activation function was applied at the bottom layers and a linear output activation function was used.
- **DNN-BN:** For this system we used data from all three speakers to generate bottleneck features. The bottleneck features were then used to train a second feed-forward DNN for each of the speakers independently. The bottleneck layer size was set to 16 and we stacked a context of 20 features to the left and 20 features to the right and combined them with our 52-dimensional acoustic and EMA feature vector, resulting in a 708-dimensional input vector. The second DNN had the same architecture as the DNN baseline system and was trained in the same fashion.
- **DNN-BLSTM:** For this system we stacked a BLSTM layer on top of two feed-forward layers with tangent activation functions. This system processed the input frame-by-frame using a mini-batch size of 300. The input vector had 52 dimensions and the same hyper-parameters as previously were used.
- **DNN-BLSTM-BN:** This system had a similar architecture to the DNN-BN using stacked bottleneck features and acoustic and EMA input features, but the second DNN used a BLSTM layer stacked on top of two feed-forward layers with tangent activation functions. The second DNN was the same as in DNN-BLSTM.

After generating the output features, the variance of the head motion was re-scaled to match the variance of the head motion in the training data. We applied a least-squares 3-order polynomial smoothing filter on the DNN output.

3.4 Objective Evaluation

We employed canonical correlation analysis (CCA) to measure the correlation between original and synthesised head motion features. Given that $X \in \mathbf{R}^p$ and $Y \in \mathbf{R}^q$ are column vectors with random variables, canonical correlation seeks to find vectors a and b that maximise the correlation τ:

$$\tau = \max_{a,b} corr(a^T X, b^T Y) \tag{1}$$

The advantage of CCA over standard correlation is that CCA can be calculated over multi-column vectors rather than single column vectors. This way we can look at the three Euler angles simultaneously. It is claimed that this procedure finds the highest possible correlation that can be achieved [25].

We define a *local CCA* which computes the canonical correlations over sub-sets of the data streams [26]. Head motion trajectories change over time and linear correlations rarely hold over the whole data. Therefore it is useful for us to measure the similarity of the original and synthesised head motion using a smaller time window of n frames that starts at t^{th} frame such that

$$r_t = \frac{1}{d} \left(\sum_{i=1}^{d} \mathrm{corr} \left(A^{[i]T} X_{[t:t+n-1]}, B^{[i]T} Y_{[t:t+n-1]} \right) \right) \tag{2}$$

where $A^{[i]}, B^{[i]}$ are the canonical coefficients obtained in the global CCA and d the dimension of features. For local CCA, we used a time window of 300 frames and calculated the average from the resulting scores.

Results. The highest local CCA was achieved for DNN-BLSTM-BN while the DNN baseline performed worst. DNN-BLSTM is slightly better than DNN-BN and comes second best. These results suggest that combing stacked bottleneck features and a BLSTM architecture works best, however the difference to the remaining systems is only subtle.

3.5 Subjective Evaluation

A mean opinion score (MOS) test was carried out to evaluate the naturalness of the head motion generated by the four presented systems. Head motion was mapped onto a talking head using the Poser Pro 2012 [27] animation software. Audio was provided as a reference but we refrained from using lip-sync to make the subjects focus only on the head motion. For each system, 16 videos between 8–12 s long were animated and four videos with natural speech were added for sanity checking of the ratings. A Latin Square design with four groups was used

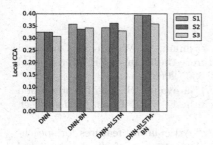 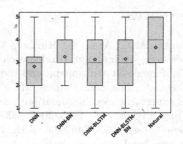

Fig. 3. Average local CCA for the four built systems by speaker before smoothing was applied. S refers to the relevant speaker.

Fig. 4. MOS results - horizontal line indicates the median, diamond shape the mean

so that subjects did not watch an animation with the same audio more than once. The subjects were asked to rate the naturalness of the animated head motion on a scale from 1 (very unnatural) to 5 (very natural). 20 English native speakers took part in the test, four of them were excluded in the analysis due to poor naturalness ratings of the natural head motion. Each system was rated 64 times (Fig. 3).

Results. A MOS was calculated for each system by subject, results are shown in Fig. 4. Listeners were conservative in their judgement of natural head motion, but it was still considered the most natural. We assume that subjects treat the 5-point MOS scale as an interval rather than an ordinal scale [28], thus we applied a one-way ANOVA to compare the means instead of the medians.

The DNN-BLSTM-BN system was only marginally considered as more natural than DNN-BLSTM, but the difference is not significant. DNN-BN seemed to be regarded as slightly more natural than the combined DNN-BLSTM-BN and the DNN-BLSTM system, but no significance can be reported. The only significant difference is between the DNN baseline and DNN-BN ($F = 11.5$, $p < 0.05$).

4 Conclusions and Further Work

In this paper we proposed using stacked bottleneck features and BLSTMs for expressive head motion synthesis. Our objective evaluation suggests that combining bottleneck features with a BLSTM network outperforms systems that make use of either stacked bottleneck features or BLSTMs. It would also appear that BLSTMs generally work better than feed-forward architectures. However, our subjective evaluation does not confirm this; all contextual systems are on a similar level when rated by subjects. It should be noted that we used a challenging dataset with expressive speech and head motion, better results might be achieved using data with less variation in expressiveness.

References

1. Sargin, M.E., Aran, O., Karpov, A., Ofli, F., Yasinnik, Y., Wilson, S.: Combined gesture-speech analysis and speech driven gesture sythesis. In: IEEE International Conference on Multimedia and Expo, pp. 893–896 (2006)
2. Busso, C., Deng, Z., Grimm, M., Neumann, U., Narayanan, S.: Rigid head motion in expressive speech animation: analysis and synthesis. IEEE Trans. Audio Speech Lang. Process. **15**, 1075–2007 (2007)
3. Ben Youssef, A., Shimodaira, H., Braude, D.A.: Articulatory features for speech-driven head motion synthesis. In: 14th Annual Conference of the International Speech Communication Association, Interspeech 2013, pp. 2758–2762 (2013)
4. Braude, D.A., Shimodaira, H., Ben Youssef, A.: Template-warping based speech driven head motion synthesis. In: 14th Annual Conference of the International Speech Communication Association, Interspeech 2013, pp. 2763–2767 (2013)
5. Yehia, H.C., Kuratate, T., Vatikiotis-Bateson, E.: Linking facial animation, head motion and speech acoustics. J. Phonetics **30**(3), 555–568 (2002)
6. Zen, H., Senior, A., Schuster, M.: Statistical parametric speech synthesis using deep neural networks. In: Proceedings of the IEEE International Conference on Acoustics, Speech and Signal Processing (ICASSP), vol. 20, pp. 1713–1724 (2013)
7. Zhao, K., Wu, Z., Cai, L.: A real-time speech driven talking avatar based on deep neural network. In: Signal and Information Processing Association Annual Summit and Conference (APSIPA), pp. 1–4 (2013)
8. Susskind, J., Hinton, G., Movellan, J., Anderson, A.: Generating facial expressions with deep belief nets. In: Or, J. (ed.) Affective Computing, Focus on Emotion Expression, Synthesis and Recognition. I-TECH Education and Publishing, Vienna (2008)
9. Chiu, C.-C., Marsella, S.: How to train your avatar: a data driven approach to gesture generation. In: Vilhjálmsson, H.H., Kopp, S., Marsella, S., Thórisson, K.R. (eds.) IVA 2011. LNCS (LNAI), vol. 6895, pp. 127–140. Springer, Heidelberg (2011). doi:10.1007/978-3-642-23974-8_14
10. Ding, C., Xie, L., Zhu, P.: Head motion synthesis from speech using deep neural networks. Multimedia Tools Appl. **74**, 9871–9888 (2014)
11. Ding, C., Zhu, P., Xie, L.: BLSTM neural networks for speech driven head motion synthesis. In: 16th Annual Conference of the International Speech Communication Association, Interspeech 2015, pp. 3345–3349 (2015)
12. Hochreiter, S.: Recurrent neural net learning and vanishing gradient. Int. J. Uncertain. Fuzziness Knowl. Based Syst. **6**(2), 107–116 (1998)
13. Fan, Y., Qian, Y., Xie, F.-L., Soong, F.K.: TTS synthesis with bidirectional LSTM based recurrent neural networks. In: 15th Annual Conference of the International Speech Communication Association, Interspeech 2014, pp. 1964–1968 (2014)
14. Fan, B., Wang, L., Soong, F.K., Xie, L.: Photo-real talking head with deep bidirectional LSTM. In: Proceedings of the IEEE International Conference on Acoustics, Speech and Signal Processing (ICASSP), pp. 4884–4888 (2015)
15. Dong, Y., Seltzer, M.L.: Improved bottleneck features using pre-trained deep neural networks. In: 12th Annual Conference of the International Speech Communication Association, Interspeech 2011, pp. 237–240 (2011)
16. Gehring, J., Miao, Y., Metze, F., Waibel, A.: Extracting deep bottleneck features using stacked autoencoders. In: Proceedings of the IEEE International Conference on Acoustics, Speech and Signal Processing (ICASSP), pp. 3377–3381 (2013)

17. Wu, Z., Valentini-Botinhao, C., Watts, O., King, S.: Deep neural networks employing multi-task learning and stacked bottleneck features for speech synthesis. In: Proceedings of the IEEE International Conference on Acoustics, Speech and Signal Processing (ICASSP), pp. 4460–4464 (2015)
18. Haag, K., Shimodaira, H.: The University of Edinburgh speaker personality and MoCap dataset. In: Proceedings of Facial Analysis and Animation, pp. 8:1–8:2. ACM (2015)
19. Motu. http://motu.com
20. Speech Signal Processing Toolkit (SPTK). http://sptk.sourceforge.net
21. Eyben, F., Woellmer, M., Schuller, B.: openSMILE: the Munich versatile and fast open-source audio feature extractor. In: Proceedings of the 18th ACM International Conference on Multimedia, MM 2010, pp. 1459–1462. ACM (2010)
22. Ben Youssef, A., Shimodaira, H., Braude, D.A.: Speech driven talking head from estimated articulatory features. In: Proceedings of the IEEE International Conference on Acoustics, Speech and Signal Processing (ICASSP), pp. 4606–4610 (2014)
23. NaturalPoint Optitrack. http://www.naturalpoint.com/optitrack
24. Soederkvist, I., Wedin, P.-A.: Determining the movements of the skeleton using well-configured markers. J. Biomech. **26**, 1473–1477 (1993)
25. Alpert, M., Peterson, R.: On the interpretation of canonical correlation analysis. J. Mark. Res. **9**, 187–192 (1972)
26. Braude, D.: Head motion synthesis: evaluation and a template motion approach. Ph.D. dissertation, School of Informatics, University of Edinburgh (2016)
27. Poser Pro 2012. http://my.smithmicro.com/poser-3d-animation-software.html
28. Dall, R., Yamagishi, J., King, S.: Rating naturalness in speech synthesis: the effect of style and expectation. In: Proceedings of the 7th International Conference on Speech Prosody, pp. 1012–1016 (2014)

Fast-Forwarding Crowd Simulations

Cliceres Mack Dal Bianco[1], Adriana Braun[1], Soraia Raupp Musse[1(✉)],
Claudio Jung[2], and Norman Badler[3]

[1] Graduate Program in Computer Science, Pontifical Catholic
University of Rio Grande do Sul - PUCRS, Porto Alegre, Brazil
soraia.musse@pucrs.br
[2] Graduate Program in Computer Science,
Federal University of Rio Grande do Sul - UFRGS, Porto Alegre, Brazil
[3] University of Pennsylvania - UPENN, Philadelphia, USA

Abstract. The processing time to simulate crowds for games or simulations is a real challenge. While the increasing power of processing capacity is a reality in the hardware industry, it also means that more agents, better rendering and most sophisticated Artificial Intelligence (AI) methods can be used, so again the computational time is an issue. Despite the processing cost, in many cases the most interesting period of time in a game or simulation is far from the beginning or in a specific known period, but it is still necessary to simulate the whole time (spending time and processing capacity) to achieve the desired period of time. It would be useful to fast forward the time in order to see a specific period of time where simulation result could be more meaningful for analysis. This paper presents a method to provide time travel in Crowd Simulation. Based on crowd features, we compute the expected variation in velocities and apply that for time travel in crowd simulation.

1 Introduction

Time travel is the concept of movement between certain points in time, analogous to movement between different points in space. While the theory of CTC (Closed Time-like Curves) is studied, it is not currently feasible for real human travel with current technology [5]. However, in computer science it may be possible to fast forward behaviors. That is exactly the goal of this paper: to fast forward the behaviors of crowds. The time travel in crowds can have many applications. In games, a nice example is the "fog of war" [7]. This term in video games [1] refers to enemy units, and often terrain, being hidden from the player. In Real Time Strategy (RTS) games, units may navigate in partially unknown and non-visible environments, searching for enemies. Imagine that non-visible enemies can have sophisticated behaviors, e.g. navigation, searching and escaping in realistic way. However, such enemies should only be visible in a specific time. The challenge in this case is the computational time, i.e. to compute realistically non-visible behaviors has a huge compromise with the processing time. In this paper, we are interested in fast forwarding the crowd simulation, while keeping the realism of behaviors that have not been computed. Another important application

D. Traum et al. (Eds.): IVA 2016, LNAI 10011, pp. 208–217, 2016.
DOI: 10.1007/978-3-319-47665-0_19

is security. Suppose that you know the situation of a crowd in time t but you want instantaneously to know about this crowd in time $t + \Delta t$. If the predicted behavior might lead to security risks, the safety staff could take action in time t to change the (potentially dangerous) results in time $t + \Delta t$. The challenge of this work is to try to preserve the crowd motion during the travel time, in order to have realistic results and minimize the error occurred due to the fast approximation of the actual simulation. Important aspects that can disturb an agent in the crowd to achieve its goal in the desired time has to be considered, such as collisions with other agents, obstacles and world complexity. In this work, we are focused on computing the disturbance that avoiding collisions among people caused in agents motion, and then use such information to generate plausible speeds to be applied during the time travel, where the simulation is turned off. Indeed, as the prior for the motion, we estimate agents position with Dead Reckoning techniques, which apply Physics to estimate positions, and then consider other agents and environment complexity. Dead Reckoning is a relatively new navigation technique [2,16], that starting from a known position, generates successive positions displacements. Pedestrian Dead Reckoning (PDR) is the estimation of walking speed and a direction of walking. Although there is an extensive body of research on this subject [9,13], the major part of such methods are focused on pedestrian positioning in real life. Furthermore, as far as we know, none of these methods aimed to fast forward time in crowd simulation. This is the novel idea of this work.

2   Related Work

Some methods in crowd simulation have been presented in the literature aiming to reduce the complexity of crowd collision avoidance. Guy et al. [6] extends the notion of velocity obstacles from robotics for collision free navigation in a parallelized algorithm. Pettre and collaborators [11,12] propose some methods to improve the performance and time of collision avoidance processing. Osborne [10] introduces a hierarchical approach for presenting agent behavior details according to the camera's distance focused on 3D animation of agent. Bianco [4] describes a method to fully eliminate the crowd collision and preserve the motion of crowd during a specific period of time. Although these works discuss the effect of reducing the complexity or even eliminate the computational time of crowd collision, they are not focused on travel time and motion preservation in crowds, as the main goal of our work.

The position of a person is a valuable information used in many applications ranging from vehicle navigation, ambient assisted living, location-dependent advertisement, among many others [16]. Although viable techniques exist in indoor and outdoor environments, the accuracy of devices and methods is still a challenge [2]. The use of dead-reckoning in computer graphics is not novel. In 1997 [15], the authors propose a way to decrease the amount of messages communicated among the participants in a multiplayer simulation system. Hakiri and collaborators [8] propose ANFIS Dead Reckoning, which stands for

Adaptive-Network-based Fuzzy Inference Systems Dead Reckoning. The proposed mechanism is based on the optimization approach to calculate the error threshold violation in networking games. Our work aims to use a dead reckoning system to estimate agents' positions in a future time, in the context of crowds. In addition, we want to provide instantaneous estimations of the positions, i.e. without compromising the computational time. As far as we know this has not been used in the context of crowds simulation.

3   The Model for Time Machine

In this section we present our approach to provide a time machine for crowds. Our method has a training step which consists of learning how each agent is affected by the others. We called this as IP step (line 7 in Algorithm 1), i.e. how individual velocities should be affected by the presence of others. In addition to that term, crowd position estimation should also take into account the environment complexity (EC - line 6), i.e. the free region and presence of obstacles. PDR (line 5) represents the dead reckoning method using physics to estimate positions for agents in the crowd, in the future. These three methods work sequentially to obtain a estimated position for each agent in the crowd. Finally, the last step $Repositioning$ (line 11) is responsible for locating the agents in the environment, avoiding collisions among them and obstacles. The overall algorithm of the method is following specified: Our model of time machine can be integrated with any crowd simulator, since the required data can be provided in time t. However, there is an error associated with the estimation process in our method. The main reason is that our prior is computed based on PDR, which can accumulate errors. PDR considers constant speed, but in crowds desired speeds usually cannot be achieved because of the interaction with obstacles and other agents. In order to test our model, we used BioCrowds [3]. It was chosen because it is a free of collision algorithm and there is an available implementation. In Sect. 3.1 we present some details about the software. In addition, the next sections describe details of all steps.

3.1   BioCrowds

The method for crowd simulation called BioCrowds proposed by Bicho et al. [3] is based on the space colonization algorithm presented by Runions et al. [14]. This last algorithm models leaf venation patterns and branching architecture of trees, and it operates by simulating the competition for space guided by the distribution of markers that mimic the auxin hormone. The BioCrowds simulator uses the same idea in order to simulate agents' paths in crowds: the distribution of markers guide agents' paths by indicating the free space and possibility of movement. The simulation environment is populated with discrete markers over "walkable" regions and, for each agent i, individual parameters are assigned, namely its current position $\boldsymbol{X}_t^i$ its current goal $\boldsymbol{g}^i$, its desired maximum speed s_{max}^i and its perception field (the maximum distance from which an agent can

---

Algorithm 1. Time Machine

1: **procedure** TM
2:     Continuous Simulation stops at frame t;
3:     Extract data from environment and the position of agent i in frame t, called pos_t^i;
4: *loop*: For each agent i at frame $t + \Delta t$
5:     $pos_{t+\Delta t}^i(x_{t+\Delta t}^i, y_{t+\Delta t}^i, z_{t+\Delta t}^i) \leftarrow PDR(x_t^i, y_t^i, z_t^i)$;
6:     $pos_{t+\Delta t}^i(x_{t+\Delta t}^i, y_{t+\Delta t}^i, z_{t+\Delta t}^i) \leftarrow EC(x_{t+\Delta t}^i, y_{t+\Delta t}^i, z_{t+\Delta t}^i)$;
7:     $pos_{t+\Delta t}^i(x_{t+\Delta t}^i, y_{t+\Delta t}^i, z_{t+\Delta t}^i) \leftarrow IP(x_{t+\Delta t}^i, y_{t+\Delta t}^i, z_{t+\Delta t}^i)$;
8:     $i \leftarrow i + 1$.
9:     **goto** *loop*.
10:    **close**;
11:    Repositioning($\boldsymbol{x}, \boldsymbol{y}, \boldsymbol{z}$);
12:    End.

---

perceive markers), modeled as a circular region with radius R_i. At each simulation step the position $\boldsymbol{X}$ and goal objective $\boldsymbol{g}$ pointing to the agent's goal are update synchronously. Thus, the algorithm can be divided into two steps: (*i*) computation of nearest markers from each agent and (*ii*) computation of motion direction for each agent. Agents compete for fixed markers, allocating and freeing them as they move throughout the space, allowing other agents to occupy their previous space. It results in a free-of-collision method to simulate crowds. In the case of this paper, the characteristic of BioCrowds to adjust the desired speed based on available space can increase the error in PDR method, since variations in speed bring the estimation far from the constant speed one. However, since it is a common effect in crowd simulations (and in real life), we decided to keep BioCrowds in our tests.

3.2 Dead Reckoning in the Crowd (PDR)

The method used for PDR is based on physics, considering a previously determined position, direction to the goals and constant speed. Dead reckoning can give the best available information on position, but is subject to significant errors due to many factors such as varying speed, obstacles and other agents. In order to estimate a future position for agent i in frame $t + \Delta t$, our PDR method needs: (*i*) the position of agent i in frame t, denoted by $\boldsymbol{X}_t^i = (x_t^i, y_t^i, z_t^i)$; (*ii*) the agent goal $\boldsymbol{g}^i = (g_x^i, g_y^i, g_z^i)$; and (*iii*) its desired speed s^i. Given the required parameters, the estimated position of agent t in frame $t + \Delta t$ is given by

$$pdr_{t+\Delta t}^i = \boldsymbol{X}_t^i + \left(s^i \frac{\boldsymbol{g}^i}{||\boldsymbol{g}^i||} \right)(\Delta t), \tag{1}$$

which is a linear estimate using constant velocity assumption. In order to measure the error caused by PDR, we firstly did a simulation with only one agent. Input simulation data is presented in Table 1. It is important to mention that the goal does not represent the desired position at frame $t + \Delta t = 700$, in fact, the

Table 1. Simulated data with only one agent.

Frame t	100
Position at frame t	$(5.453, 20.181, 0.0)$
Speed s	0.046/frame
Goal g	$(38.039, 19.979, 0.0)$
Frame $t + \Delta t$	700

travel time can be to any frame in the future, until the agent achieves the goal. Based on such data, we simulated one agent in an environment without obstacles, and measured the error presented in the PDR estimation in comparison to BioCrowds. More precisely, we computed the relative error given by

$$Error^i_{t \to t+\Delta t} = \frac{d(\boldsymbol{X}^i_{t+\Delta t}, \boldsymbol{pdr}^i_{t+\Delta t})}{d(\boldsymbol{X}^i_t, \boldsymbol{X}^i_{t+\Delta t})}, \qquad (2)$$

where $\boldsymbol{X}^i_t$ is the position of agent i in frame t (when simulation stops and the time machine starts), while $\boldsymbol{pdr}^i_{t+\Delta t}$ and $\boldsymbol{X}^i_{t+\Delta t}$ are the positions of the same agent in frame $t + \Delta t$ using the time machine and the full continuous simulation, respectively. For the tested simulation the achieved error was 0.0013.

3.3   Computing the Environment Complexity (EC)

Although it is important to start with a good prior, in this case the PDR estimation, it is also relevant to consider the complexity of the environment in a time machine model. Clearly, the free navigation area, as well as the number and area of obstacles, have impact on the flow of pedestrians. The environment complexity is modeled taken into account the free space for crowd movement, i.e. considering number of agents and obstacles and the space needed to place all of them. We included a constant $0 < \alpha < 1$ that describes the weight to be given to the number of obstacles, if one wants to consider that in addition to the sum of obstacles areas.

$$EC = \min\{1, \frac{n_a A_a + \alpha n_o}{A_w - A_o}\}, \qquad (3)$$

where n_a represents the total of agents in the simulation; A_a is the area of one agent and n_o is the number of obstacles in the world. Also, A_w represents the area of the world and A_o is the sum of all obstacles areas. If the number of agents or area occupied by obstacles are too big and there is no free space to allow individuals motion, then EC is truncated at 1 and no motion is allowed. Equation 4 presents our proposal to use EC as a penalty function in the generation of each agent's position in the time machine model when PDR and the complexity of environment EC are considered, obtaining the final PDR estimation:

$$pdr'^i_{t+\Delta t} = pdr^i_{t+\Delta t} - \left(s^i \frac{\boldsymbol{g}^i}{||\boldsymbol{g}^i||}\right) EC\Delta t \tag{4}$$

$$= \boldsymbol{X}^i_t + \left(s^i \frac{\boldsymbol{g}^i}{||\boldsymbol{g}^i||}\right)(1 - EC)\Delta t.$$

3.4   Computing the Interaction Among People in Crowds (IP)

In crowd simulation, the interaction among agents due to the intrinsic collision avoidance processes can produce a disturbance in the desired velocity of each agent i. This disturbance depends on various factors such as the direction of the flows, desired speed variability and local density, among others. Due to the complexity in the simulation of dense crowds, we decided to adopt a stochastic approach to learn the disturbance arisen from the interaction of the agents. In this approach, we observed the impact of the local density and of counter-flow in the effective velocity of the agents.

To this end, we performed several pairs of simulations, varying the number of agents n_a and the average and standard deviation of the desired speed in the scenario of Fig. 3. Each pair of simulations corresponds to one simulation with n_a agents moving in an uni-directional flow and another with $2n_a$ agents moving in a bi-directional flow. The first n_a agents from the bi-directional simulation have the same id, starting point and desired velocity than the agents of the uni-directional flow. In order to measure the disturbance caused by the counter-flow in the movement of a given agent i, we computed the displacement of this agent in a time-window $W = 2s$ in both simulations of each pair uni/bi-directional. Let us call the displacement of agent i in the uni-directional flow $\Delta \boldsymbol{X}_{iU}$, and the displacement of the equivalent agent in the bi-directions flow $\Delta \boldsymbol{X}_{iB}$. The impact in the speed of agent i from the disturbance caused by the counter-flow is given by:

$$\Delta \boldsymbol{v}_i = \frac{\Delta \boldsymbol{X}_{iU} - \Delta \boldsymbol{X}_{iB}}{W}. \tag{5}$$

We measured the values of $\Delta \boldsymbol{v}_i$ for each agent in the different pairs of simulations. For each one of them we associated the corresponding value of local density of agents, computed considering the number of agents present in a $4\,\mathrm{m}^2$ square region, with the agent i at the center. We grouped the values of $\Delta \boldsymbol{v}_i$ as a function of the values of local densities $\rho \in \{0.25, 0.50, ..., 2.5\}$agents/m^2. The distribution of speed variation from all pairs of BioCrowds simulations for $\rho = 1$agent/m^2 is shown by the dark columns of the histogram in Fig. 1. Then, for each value of ρ, we analyzed the frequency distribution of $\Delta \boldsymbol{v}_i$. We found that those distributions resemble the Weibull distribution, given by:

$$f(x) = \frac{b}{a}\left(\frac{x}{a}\right)^{b-1} \exp\left[-\left(\frac{x}{a}\right)^b\right] \tag{6}$$

We used maximum likelihood estimation in order to find the values of a and b that best fit the Weibull distribution to the data. After this process, we achieved

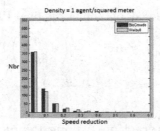

Fig. 1. Histograms of speed reductions in pairs of BioCrowds simulations and randomly generated speed reductions according to Weibull distributions (in m/s).

10 Weibull $f(\Delta v|\rho)$ distributions, one for each value of local density ρ. Once we get the distributions of speed reduction, we can generate random values r_i for speed reduction, according to the local density of agent i. This reduction is incorporated to adjusted PDR estimates, and the position $tm^i_{t+\Delta t}$ produced by the time machine for each agent i is then given by

$$tm^i_{t+\Delta t} = pdr'^i_{t+\Delta t} - r_i \frac{g^i}{||g^i||}\Delta t. \tag{7}$$

3.5   Re-positioning the Agents in Crowds

Our model for the time machine does not need any simulated trajectory to be fast forwarded. Indeed, we propose penalty functions and generate positions in a future time only based on information available when simulation stops (time t used in this text). This fact consumes least processing time than if a path planning algorithm must be executed for each agent in the simulation. However, the drawback of avoiding the use of simulated information in the time machine is that the position $tm^i_{t+\Delta t}$ generated for agent i in future time $t+\Delta t$ can be placed in an impossible location, such as the interior of an obstacle or overlapping with another agent that had been already placed.

In order to treat this problem, we implement an extension to original BioCrowds to read the positions tm of agents and consider those as desired positions, and not final ones. In fact, BioCrowds tries to achieve the desired positions, but if it is impossible, it tries to place them in the nearest possible region. Due to the model inherent structure to compete for markers (see Sect. 3.1), the agents are placed exactly in the position tm when this position has free markers to be allocated. Otherwise, the algorithm searches for free markers in the four cardinal directions (N, E, S, W) oriented w.r.t. to the goal vector and shifted by R_i (perception field for agent i, i.e. the maximum distance from which an agent can perceive markers), as explained in Sect. 3.1.

Clearly, this procedure impacts in errors that are evaluated in the next section, but we consider that as acceptable in order to provide the time machine instantaneously and without the needed to simulate any trajectory in the travel time between frames t and $t + \Delta t$.

4   Experimental Results

In order to evaluate our model we tested the time machine in one environment
with 920 sqm (23×40 m) and four obstacles configurations: *(i)* without obstacles;
(ii) with 4 obstacles and $A_o = 582.22$ sqm; *(iii)* with 2 obstacles and $A_o =$
109.71 sqm; *(i)* with 6 obstacles and $A_o = 128.68$ sqm. In addition, these four
scenarios were simulated with populations of $8, 80, 160, 240$ and 320 agents, and
each agent has a diameter of 0.456 m. For all scenarios, we computed the relative
error in position for each agent i according to Eq. (8) (similar to Eq. (2), except
that $tm^i_{t+\Delta t}$ is used instead $pdr^i_{t+\Delta t}$). The average distances for each scenario
for all agents in each scenario are presented in Fig. 2.

$$Dif^i_{t \to t+\Delta t} = \frac{d(X^i_{t+\Delta t}, tm^i_{t+\Delta t})}{d(X^i_t, X^i_{t+\Delta t})}, \qquad (8)$$

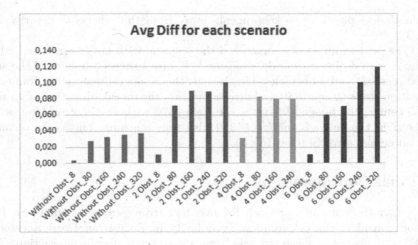

Fig. 2. Average distance (meters) from all agents for each scenario, when comparing
the position generated in our model and the continuous simulation.

As can be seen in Fig. 2, the maximum achieved error is approximately 0.12
in a scenario with 320 agents and 6 obstacles. In this scenario the average error
value is 0.06. To assess the visual quality of our results, the following images
illustrate simulation results. The Fig. 3 shows 3 images of a simulated scenario
without obstacles, containing 240 agents. On the left, the image represents the
frame the simulation stops (frame 350) and arrows indicate the motion direction
of groups. In the center we show frame 650 with the continuous simulation and
the predicted result using the proposed time machine (right). As can be observed,
there is a visual difference. It can be explained due to PDR and also due to the
fact that time machine positions are not free of collision, and then BioCrowds

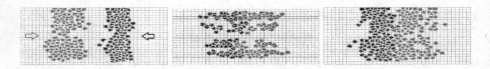

Fig. 3. Left: Frame the simulation stops (frame 350). Center: frame 650 using the continuous simulation and the proposed time machine (right).

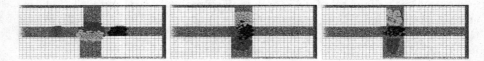

Fig. 4. On the left: the image represents the frame the simulation stops (frame 200), on the center: image illustrates the frame 370 without time machine, while on the right the image is the frame 370 with time machine.

should change positions to keep agents away from the others, as described in Sect. 3.5.

In the next example, we considered the scenario with larger error, according to Fig. 2, with 4 obstacles and 240 agents[1]. Figure 4 shows 3 images of the simulated scenario and 4 obstacles. On the left, the image represents the frame the simulation stops (frame 200) and arrows indicate the motion direction of groups. In the center, the image illustrates the frame 370 without time machine, while on the right the image is the frame 370 with time machine. This is the scenario with numerical error of 0.08 (Fig. 2).

5   Final Considerations

This paper presents an approach for fast forwarding crowd simulations. Our method considers the environment complexity in Pedestrian Dead Reckoning (PDR) and proposes a way to take into account the people interaction. The method was tested using BioCrowds, but can be adapted to any crowd simulation algorithm. There are points that should be investigated in further analyses: local EC instead of global EC, more agents and larger environments, more complex obstacles, other people distributions for disturbance and the integration with other crowd simulators.

References

1. Adams, E.: Fundamentals of Game Design. New Riders Press, Berkeley (2014)
2. Beauregard, S., Haas, H.: Pedestrian dead reckoning: a basis for personal positioning. In: Proceedings of the 3rd Workshop on Positioning, Navigation and Communication (WPNC06), p. 1 (2006)

---

[1] This scenario could not be simulated with 320 agents because the agents were stuck due to lack of free space.

3. Bicho, A.L., Rodrigues, R.A., Musse, S.R., Jung, C.R., Paravisi, M., Magalhes, L.P.: Simulating crowds based on a space colonization algorithm. Comput. Graph. **36**(2), 70–79 (2012). http://www.sciencedirect.com/science/article/pii/S0097849311001713. Virtual Reality in Brazil 2011
4. Bianco, C.M.D., Jovani Oliveira Brasil, A.B., Musse, S.R.: A model to compute people disturbance in crowds. In: Poster at ACM Motion in Games, vol. 1 (2015)
5. Everett, A.: Time travel paradoxes, path integrals, and the many worlds interpretation of quantum mechanics. Phys. Rev. D69, 124023. http://link.aps.org/doi/10.1103/PhysRevD.69.124023
6. Guy, S.J., Chhugani, J., Kim, C., Satish, N., Lin, M.C., Manocha, D., Dubey, P.: Clearpath: highly parallel collision avoidance for multi-agent simulation. In: ACM SIGGRAPH/EUROGRAPHICS Symposium on Computer Animation, pp. 177–187. ACM (2009)
7. Hagelback, J., Johansson, S.: Dealing with fog of war in a real time strategy game environment. In: IEEE Symposium On Computational Intelligence and Games, CIG 2008, pp. 55–62, December 2008
8. Hakiri, A., Berthou, P., Gayraud, T.: QoS-enabled anfis dead reckoning algorithm for distributed interactive simulation. In: Turner, S.J., Roberts, D.J. (eds.) DS-RT, pp. 33–42. IEEE Computer Society (2010). http://dblp.uni-trier.de/db/conf/dsrt/dsrt2010.html#HakiriBG10
9. Ladetto, Q., Merminod, B.: Digital magnetic compass and gyroscope integration for pedestrian navigation. In: 9th International Conference on Integrated Navigation Systems, St-Petersburg, pp. 27–29 (2002)
10. Osborne, D., Dickinson, P.: Improving Games AI Performance Using Grouped Hierarchical Level of Detail. Elsevier Science Inc., New York
11. Pettre, J., de Heras Ciechomski, P., Maim, J., Yersin, B., Laumond, J.P., Thalmann, D.: Real-time navigating crowds: scalable simulation and rendering. Comput. Anim. Virtual Worlds **17**(3–4), 445–455 (2006). http://dx.doi.org/10.1002/cav.147
12. Pettr, J., Ondrej, J., Olivier, A.H., Crtual, A., Donikian, S.: Experiment-based modeling, simulation and validation of interactions between virtual walkers. In: Fellner, D.W., Spencer, S.N. (eds.) Symposium on Computer Animation, pp. 189–198. ACM (2009). http://dblp.uni-trier.de/db/conf/sca/sca2009.html#PettreOOCD09
13. Randell, C., Djiallis, C., Muller, H.: Personal position measurement using dead reckoning. In: Proceedings of The Seventh International Symposium on Wearable Computers, pp. 166–173. Springer (2003)
14. Runions, A., Fuhrer, M., Lane, B., Federl, P., Rolland-Lagan, A.G., Prusinkiewicz, P.: Modeling and visualization of leaf venation patterns. In: ACM SIGGRAPH 2005 Papers, SIGGRAPH 2005, NY, USA, pp. 702–711 (2005). http://doi.acm.org/10.1145/1186822.1073251
15. Capin, T.K., Pandzic, I.S., Thalmann, N.M., Thalmann, D.: A dead-reckoning algorithm for virtual human figures. Proceedings of VRAIS97 **1**(1), 161–169 (1997)
16. Zampella, F., Ruiz, A.R.J., Granja, F.S.: Indoor positioning using efficient map matching, RSS measurements, and an improved motion model. IEEE Trans. Veh. Technol. **64**(4), 1304–1317 (2015)

Socially-Aware Virtual Agents: Automatically Assessing Dyadic Rapport from Temporal Patterns of Behavior

Ran Zhao[(✉)], Tanmay Sinha, Alan W. Black, and Justine Cassell

Language Technologies Institute, School of Computer Science,
Carnegie Mellon University, Pittsburgh, PA 15213, USA
{rzhao1,tanmays,awb,justine}@cs.cmu.edu

Abstract. This work focuses on data-driven discovery of the temporally co-occurring and contingent behavioral patterns that signal high and low interpersonal rapport. We mined a reciprocal peer tutoring corpus reliably annotated for nonverbals like eye gaze and smiles, conversational strategies like self-disclosure and social norm violation, and for rapport (in 30 s thin slices). We then performed a fine-grained investigation of how the temporal profiles of sequences of interlocutor behaviors predict increases and decreases of rapport, and how this rapport management manifests differently in friends and strangers. We validated the discovered behavioral patterns by predicting rapport against our ground truth via a forecasting model involving two-step fusion of learned temporal associated rules. Our framework performs significantly better than a baseline linear regression method that does not encode temporal information among behavioral features. Implications for the understanding of human behavior and social agent design are discussed.

1 Introduction and Motivation

The year is 2025. Zack comes into math class with his personalized virtual peer agent Zoe projected on his glasses. Zoe smiles as she says to Zack, "You look tired today. I told you it was a bad idea to play "AR Starcraft" that late on weeknights!". Zack grimaces "OK, so I'm tired. But it was awesome! The whole math class was getting to know one another - that's work, right?" to which Zoe nods and responds by indexing their shared experience - "Perhaps, but last time you did this, I was too exhausted the next day to help you."

Zack and Zoe then work on the math task they are supposed to complete. Zoe starts off - "We need to solve this set of linear equations $5x * (3x - 18) = 10$ first". Zack seems a bit confused "Well, I'm familiar with fractions, but I suck at linear equations." Zoe gazes at the work sheet, then back at Zack and finally provides motivational scaffolding in the form of negative self disclosure followed by praise, in order to boost their interpersonal bond, and Zack's confidence "Don't worry, I used to suck at linear equations too, but you're a rockstar at this stuff. You'll be fine. Besides which, we'll go through it together," following with a smile.

© Springer International Publishing AG 2016
D. Traum et al. (Eds.): IVA 2016, LNAI 10011, pp. 218–233, 2016.
DOI: 10.1007/978-3-319-47665-0_20

This vision illustrates several factors related to the important role that the relationship between learners, or learners and their tutors, can play in improving learning gains. While this phenomenon is described in the educational literature [19,22], there has existed no rigorous models of the mechanism underlying the relationship between social and cognitive functioning in tasks such as these [23], nor do there exist computational models of interpersonal closeness that can drive the functioning of an intelligent tutor. There is therefore great opportunity to expand on the social capabilities of current educational technologies in order to create long-term interpersonal connectedness in the service of increased adaptivity in learning [29], and thereby increased learning gains. In this vein, here we investigate the dynamics of social interaction in longitudinal peer tutoring, as manifested in manifested in verbal and nonverbal behaviors. The aspect of social interaction that we focus on is rapport management, as rapport is argued to be one of the central constructs necessary to understanding successful helping relationships [4]), and rapport management is abundantly present in peer tutoring [31].

Let us at this point step back to describe what we mean by rapport. Rapport is often defined as "a close and harmonious relationship in which the people concerned appear to understand each other's feelings or ideas and communicate well," however we feel it is best described by examples and so, below, are two examples from our corpus, of high and low rapport, respectively.

High rapport:	Low rapport:
P1: I suck at negative numbers;	P2: [silent][long pause]
P2: it's okay so do I;	P1: shh;[long pause]
P1: {smile}	P2: alright;
P2: uh actually no I don't, negative numbers are easy	P1: let me do my work;

In our own prior work, we proposed a computational model of long-term interpersonal rapport to explain how humans in dyadic interactions build, maintain and destroy rapport through the use of specific conversational strategies [37]. Because these strategies function to fulfill specific social goals and are instantiated in particular verbal and nonverbal behaviors, studying the synergistic interaction of conversational strategies and nonverbal behaviors on rapport management is important. To do so, not only a qualitative examination of certain dyadic behavior patterns that benefit or hurt interpersonal rapport is essential, but it is also desirable to build automated frameworks to learn fine-grained behavioral interaction patterns that index such social phenomena. The latter has received less attention, in part due to the time-intensive nature of collecting and annotating behavioral data for different aspects of interpersonal connectedness, and the difficulty of developing and using machine learning algorithms that can take the time course of interaction among different modalities and between interlocutors into account. Learning fine-grained behavioral interaction patterns that index rapport is the focus of the current work. There are three key issues that we believe should be taken into consideration when performing such assessment.

(1) When the foundational work by [34] described the nature of rapport, three interrelating components were posited: positivity, mutual attentiveness and coordination. Their work demonstrated, that over the course of a relationship, positivity decreases and coordination increases. Factors such as these, then, depend on the stage of relationship between interlocutors [37], and therefore it is necessary to take into account the relationship status of a dyad when extracting dyadic patterns of rapport. (2) while our previous work [27] discovered some of the common behaviors exhibited by dyads in peer tutoring to build or maintain rapport; playful teasing, face-threatening comments, attention-getting, etc., tutors and tutees were looked at separately, and each of these behaviors was examined in isolation from one another. In the current work, our interest is in moving beyond individual behaviors to focus on temporal sequences of such behaviors in the dyadic context. Likewise, our prior work did not distinguish between rapport management during task (tutoring) vs social activities. We believe that the interactions between verbal and nonverbal behaviors may manifest differently in social and tutoring periods, since the roles of a tutor and tutee are more evident in the tutoring compared to the social periods. (3) Most prior computational work examining rapport, such as [12,13,18], has used post-session questionnaires to asses rapport. However, to measure the effect of multimodal behavioral patterns on rapport and better reason about the dynamics of social interaction, a finer-grained ground truth for rapport is needed.

In this paper, then, we take a step towards addressing the above limitations. To create a longitudinal peer tutoring corpus, we compared friend to stranger dyads, bringing each dyad back for five face-to-face sessions over five weeks. In each session, two tutoring periods were interspersed with three social periods. The students switched roles so that each both tutored and was tutored. We employed thin-slice coding [2] to elicit ground truth for rapport, by asking naive raters to judge rapport for every 30 s slice of the hour long peer tutoring session, presented to raters in a randomized order. This, in turn allowed us to analyze fine-grained sequences of verbal and nonverbal behaviors that were associated with high or low rapport between the tutor and tutee.

As a side note, while the current paper addresses these phenomena in the context of peer tutors and intelligent tutoring agents, this work is part of a larger research program that targets more general models of how to predict rapport between interlocutors in real time, using as input the interaction among linguistic (verbal) and nonverbal (visual) behaviors. This basic science serves as input in some of our work into embodied conversational agents that can use the dyad's current rapport as part of a decision about what to say next to manage rapport with the user as, in turn, input into a decision about how best to help the user achieve his/her goals, goals that include, in some of our agents, peer tutoring.

2   Related Work

2.1   Individual-Focused Temporal Relations

The study of temporal relationships between verbal and nonverbal behaviors has been of prime importance in understanding various social and cognitive phenomena. A lot of this work has focused on the observable phenomena of interaction (low level linguistic, prosodic or acoustic behaviors that can be automatically extracted) or has leveraged computational advances to extract head nods, gaze, facial action units, etc., as a step towards modeling co-occurring and contingent patterns inherent in an individual person's behavior. Since feature extraction approaches that aggregate information across time are not able to explicitly model temporal co-occurrence patterns, two popular technical approaches to investigate temporal patterns of verbal and nonverbal behaviors are histogram of co-occurrences [28] and motif discovery methods [26].

For instance, [20] presented a study of co-occurrence patterns of human non-verbal behaviors during intimate self-disclosure. However, contingent relations between different nonverbal behaviors was not considered, which could extensively contribute to the design of a social agent that interacts with a human over time. [35] learned behavioral indicators that were correlated to expert judgess opinions of each key performance aspect of public speaking. They fused the modalities by utilizing a least squared boosted regression ensemble tree and predicted speaker performance. However, this work also did not consider the effect of interactions among different modalities and their temporal relations. In similar vein, [6] introduced deep conditional neural fields to model the generation of gestures by integrating verbal and acoustic modalities, while using an undirected second-order linear chain to preserve temporal relations between gestures as well. However, this approach only modeled individual co-verbal gestures, without considering interaction between the speaker and the interlocutor.

In [17] temporal combinations of individual facial signals (such as nod, smiles etc.) were used to infer positive (agree, accept etc.) and negative (dislike, disbelief etc.) meanings via ratings by humans. An interesting take-away from this work was that a combination of signals could significantly alter the perceived meaning. For instance, facial tension alone and frown alone did not mean "dislike, but the combination frown and tension did. Tilt alone and gaze right down alone did not mean "not interested as significantly as the combination tilt and gaze. However, while a combination of these nonverbals signaled higher level constructs (that were in turn associated with some pragmatic meaning), the authors were more interested in how these combinations were perceived by humans, rather than necessarily in a predictive task or testing these combinations in a human-agent dialog.

2.2   Dyadic Temporal Relations

In a conversation, attending to the contribution of both interactants adds greater complexity in reasoning about the social aspects of the interaction. Listeners show their interest, attention and understanding in many ways during the speakers utterances. Such "listener responses" [10], which may be manifested through gaze direction and eye contact, facial expressions, use of short utterances like "yeah", "okay", and "hm-m" etc. or even intonation, voice quality and content of the words, are carriers of subtle information. These cues may convey information regarding understanding (whether the listeners understand the utterance of the speaker), attentiveness (whether the listeners are attentive to the speech of the speaker), coordination, and so forth.

For instance, [14] looked at observable lexical, acoustic and prosodic cues produced by the speaker followed by back channeling from the listener. The authors found that the likelihood of occurrence of a backchannel from the interlocutor appeared to increase with simultaneous occurrence of one or more cues by the speaker, such as final rising intonation, higher intensity and pitch levels, longer inter-pausal units (maximal sequence of words surrounded by silence longer than 50 ms) etc. However, in this work, no attempt was made to use the temporal sequence or co-occurrence of observables preceding a backchannel to predict higher level social constructs such as positivity, coordination, attentiveness, or underlying psychological states such as rapport or trust.

[1] explored the interplay between head movements, facial movements like smile and eye brow raising, and verbal feedback in a range of conversational situations, including continued attentiveness, understanding, agreement, surprise, disappointment, acknowledgment and refusing information. As the situations became more negative (disappointment, refusing information), the accompanying nonverbals became more extensive in time - no longer just a head nod, but a series of movements. The authors claim that this series of movements functioned to add some extra information or to emphasize or contradict what had been said, but ground truth was not provided for these claims.

Finally in [7], the authors used sequence mining methods to automatically extract nonverbal behavior sequences of the recruiters that were representative of interpersonal attitudes. Then, Bayesian networks were deployed to build a generation model for computing a set of nonverbal sequence candidates, which were further ranked based on the previously extracted frequent sequences. Even though this work considered the effect of sequencing of nonverbal signals, their model could be improved by the addition of temporal information inside these sequences, the addition of verbal signals and modeling of listeners' behaviors as well.

3   Study Context

3.1   Data

Reciprocal peer tutoring data was collected from 12 American English-speaking dyads (6 dyads were friends and 6 strangers; 6 were boys and 6 girls), with a mean age of 13 years old ranging from 12 to 15, who interacted for 5 h sessions over as many weeks (a total of 60 sessions, and 5400 min of data), tutoring one another on procedural and conceptual aspects of linear equations [36]. All interactions were videotaped from three camera views (a frontal view of each participant and a side view of the two participants). Speech was recorded by lapel microphones in separate audio channels. Each session began with a period of getting to know one another, after which the first tutoring period started, followed by another small social interlude, a second tutoring period with role reversal between the tutor and tutee, and then the final social time. Prior work demonstrates that peer tutoring is an effective paradigm that results in student learning [30], making this an effective context to study dyadic interaction with a concrete task outcome. Our student-student data demonstrates that a tremendous amount of rapport-building takes place during the task of reciprocal tutoring [32]. In their recent review of the research on design spaces for computer supported reciprocal tutoring, [8] emphasize reciprocal tutoring to be a natural extension of one-on-one tutoring in today's networked world.

3.2 Annotations

We assessed rapport-building via thin slice annotation [2], or rapidly made judgments of interpersonal connectedness in the dyad, based on brief exposure to their verbal and nonverbal behavior. Naive raters were provided with a simple definition of rapport and three raters annotated every 30 s video segment of the peer tutoring sessions for rapport using a 7 point likert scale. Weighted majority rule was deployed to mitigate bias from the ratings of different annotators, account for label over-use and under-use and pick a single rapport rating for each 30 s video segment. The segments were presented to the annotators in random order so as to ensure that raters were not actually annotating the delta of rapport over the course of the session. Prior work has shown that such reliably annotated measures of interpersonal rapport are causally linked to behavioral convergence of low-level linguistic features (such as speech rate etc.,) of the dyad [31,32] and that greater likelihood of being in high rapport in the next 30 s segment (improvement in rapport dynamics over the course of the interaction) is positively predictive of the dyad's problem-solving performance.

In addition, we also annotated the entire corpus for conversational strategies such as self-disclosure (Krippendorf's $\alpha = 0.753$), reference to shared experience ($\alpha = 0.798$), praise ($\alpha = 1$), social norm violation ($\alpha = 0.753$) and backchannel ($\alpha = 0.72$) in the first pass, and reciprocity in these strategies (using a time window of roughly 1 min) in the second pass ($\alpha = 0.77$). [33] has investigated the phenomenon of congruence or interpersonal synchrony in usage of such conversational strategies, in absolute number as well as the pattern of timings, and found positive relationships with rapport and problem-solving performance. In other work, we have also shown that these conversational strategies can be reliably detected from observable indicators of verbal, visual and acoustic cues an accuracy of over 80 % and kappa ranging from 60–80 % [38]. Finally, our temporal association rule framework comprised of nonverbal behaviors like eye gaze (Krippendorf's $\alpha = 0.893$) and smiles ($\alpha = 0.746$), which we have found to significantly co-occur with conversational strategies [38].

4   Method

The technical framework we employ in this work is essentially an approach for pattern recognition in multivariate symbolic time sequences, called the Temporal Interval Tree Association Rule Learning (Titarl) algorithm [15]. Since it is practically infeasible to predict exactly when certain behavioral events happen, it is suitable to use probabilistic approaches that can extract patterns with some degree of uncertainty in the temporal relation among different events. Temporal association rules, where each rule is composed of certain behavioral pre-conditions (input events) and behavioral post-conditions (output events), are one such powerful approach. In our case, input events are conversational strategies and nonverbal behaviors such as violation social norms, smile etc. The output event is the absolute value of thin-slice rapport. Because interpersonal rapport is a social construct that is defined at the dyadic level, the applied framework helps reveal interleaved behavioral patterns from both interlocutors. An example of a simple generic temporal rule is given below. It illustrates the rule's flexibility by succinctly describing not only the temporal inaccuracy of determining the temporal location of output event, but also its probability of being fired.

"If event A happens at time t, there is 50 % chance of event B happening between time t + 3 to t + 5".

Intuitively, the Titarl algorithm is used to extract large number of temporal association rules (r) that predict future occurrences of specific events of interest. The dataset comprises both multivariate symbolic time sequences $E_{i=1...n}$ and multivariate scalar time series $S_{i=1...m}$, where $E_i = \{t_j^i \in \mathbb{R}\}$ is the set of times that event e_i happens and S_i is an injective mapping from every time point to a scalar value. Before the learning process, a parameter w or the window size is specified, which allows us at each time point t to compute the probability for the target event to exist in the time interval $[t, t + w]$.

The four main steps in the Titarl algorithm [15] are: (i) exhaustive creation of simple unit rules that are above the threshold value of confidence or support, (ii) addition of more input channels in order to maximize information gain, (iii) production of more temporally precise rules by decreasing the standard deviation of the rule's probability distribution, (iv) refinement of the condition and conclusion of the rules by application of Gaussian filter on temporal distribution. Confidence, support and precision of the rule are three characteristics to validate its interest and generalizability. For a simple unit rule r: $e_1 \xrightarrow{[t,t+w]} e_2$ (confidence: x%, support: y%), confidence refers to the probability of a prediction of the rule to be true, support refers to the percentage of events explained by the rule and precision is an estimation of the temporal accuracy of the predictions.

$$confidence_r = P((t \in E_1)|(t' \in E_2), t' - t \leq w) \tag{1}$$

$$support_r = \frac{\{\#e_2|\text{r is active}\}}{\#e_2} \tag{2}$$

$$precision_r = \frac{1}{\text{standard deviation}_r} \tag{3}$$

5 Experimental Results

We first separated out friend and stranger dyads to learn rules from their behaviors separately. We also tagged the data as occurring during a social or tutoring period, and as being generated by a tutor or a tutee. We then randomly divided the friend and stranger groups into a training set (4 dyads) and test set (2 dyads). In the first experiment, we extracted a potentially large number of temporal association rules affiliated with each individual rapport state (from 1 to 7). In this experiment, for each event, we looked back 60 s to find behavioral patterns associated with it. A representative example is shown in Fig. 1, and descriptions of some of the rules in the test set whose confidence are above 50 % and for whom the number of cases the rule applies to are more than 20 times are described below, divided into friends (F) and strangers (S) and into high rapport (H), defined as thin-slice rapport states 5, 6, and 7 and low rapport (L), defined as states 1, 2, and 3.

5.1 Behavioral Rules for Friends

There are 14,458 total rules for friends with confidence higher than 50 %, 14,345 of which apply to friends in high rapport states. Overall, engaging in reference to shared experience, smiling while violating a social norm and overlapping speech are associated with high rapport. Examples are:

FH 1 *One of the student smiles while the other violates a social norm (Social period)*

FH 2 *One of the students refers to shared experience (Social period)*

FH 3 *One student smiles and violates a social norm, and the second smiles and gazes at the partner within the next minute (Social period)*

FH 4 *The two conversational partners overlap speech while one is smiling, following which the second starts smiling within the next minute (Social period)*

FH 5 *The tutee reciprocates a social norm violation while overlapping speech with the tutor, following which the tutor smiles and violates a social norm (Task period)* [**shown in Fig. 1**]

In contrast to the high number of rules with confidence higher than 50 % for friends in high rapport, there are only 113 rules that satisfy these criteria for friends in low rapport. Some examples are:

FL 1 *The tutor finishes violating a social norm while gazing at the tutee's work sheet, and within the next minute the tutee follows up with a social norm violation, but gazing at his/her own work sheet (Task period)*

FL 2 *The tutor reciprocates a social norm violation without a smile and neither the tutee nor the tutor gaze at one another. Meanwhile, the tutee begins violating another social norm within the next minute (Task period)*

FL 3 *The tutor backchannels while gazing at his/her own work sheet and does not smile. Moreover, the tutor also overlaps with the tutee in the next minute (Task period)*

5.2 Behavioral Rules for Strangers

There are 761 total rules for strangers, of which 130 are rules that apply to strangers in high rapport. In general, smiling and overlapping speech while using particular conversational strategies are associated with high rapport. Some examples are:

SH 1 *One of the interlocutors smiles while the other gazes at him/her and begins self-disclosing, and they overlap speech within the next minute (Social period)*

SH 2 *One of the interlocutors smiles and backchannels in the next minute (Social period)*

SH 3 *The interlocutors' speech overlaps and the tutee smiles within the next minute (Task period)*

631 rules, then, explain strangers in low rapport. Interestingly, rules that explain low rapport among strangers most often come from task periods. In general, overlapping speech after a social norm violation leads to low rapport in strangers. Some examples are:

SL 1 *The tutor smiles and gazes at the worksheet of the tutee while the tutee does not smile (Task period)*

SL 2 *The tutor violates social norms while being gazed at by the tutee, and their speech overlaps within the next minute (Task period)*

SL 3 *The tutor smiles and the tutee violates a social norm within the next 30 s, before their speech overlaps within the next 30 s (Task period)* [**shown in Fig. 2**]

An example from the corpus is shown below:

Tutor: Sweeney you can't do that, that's the whole point{smile}; [**Violation of Social Norm**]

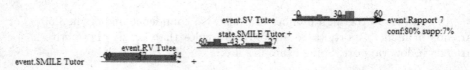

Fig. 1. Friends in high rapport - The tutee reciprocates a social norm violation while overlapping speech with the tutor, following which the tutor smiles while the tutee violates a social norm.

Tutee: I hate you. I'll probably never never do that; [**Reciprocate Social Norm Violation**]

Tutor: Sweeney that's why I'm tutoring you{smile};

Tutee: You're so oh my gosh{smile}. We never did that ever; [**Violation of Social Norm**]

Tutor: {smile}What'd you say?

Tutee: Said to skip it{smile};

Tutor: I can just teach you how to do it;

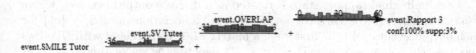

Fig. 2. Strangers in low rapport - The tutor smiles and the tutee violates a social norm within the next 30 s, before their speech overlaps within the next 30 s.

An example from the corpus is shown below:

Tutee: divide oh this is so hard let me guess;eleven;

Tutor: you know;

Tutee: six;

Tutor: next problem is is exactly the samesmile, over eleven equals, eleven x over eleven;

Tutee: I don't need your help; [**Violation of Social Norm**]

Tutor: {Overlap}That is seriously like exactly the same.

6   Validation and Discussion

In order to demonstrate that the extracted temporal association rules can be reliably used for forecasting of interpersonal human behavior, we first applied machine learning to perform an empirical validation, which we describe in the next subsection. The motivation behind constructing this forecasting model was to prove the automatically learned temporal association rules are good indicators of the dyadic rapport state. In the subsequent subsections of the discussion, we will discuss implications of our work for the understanding of human behavior and the design of "socially-skilled" agents, linking prior strands of research.

6.1   Estimation of Interpersonal Rapport

In addition to its applicability to sparse data, one of the prime benefits of the temporal association rule framework to predict a high-level construct such as rapport lies in its flexibility in modeling presence/absence of human behaviors and also the inherent uncertainty of such behaviors, via a probability distribution representation in time. In summary, the estimation of rapport comprises two steps: in the first step, the intuition is to learn the weighted contribution (vote) of each temporal association rule in predicting the presence/absence of a certain rapport state (via seven random-forest classifiers); in the second step, the intuition is to learn the weight of each binary classifier for each rapport state, to predict the absolute continuous value of rapport (via linear regression). For clarity, we will use the following three mathematical subscripts to represent different types of index. i: index of output events, k: index of time-stamps, j: index of temporal association rules.

Each individual rapport state is treated as a discrete output event e_i, where $i = 1, 2, 3, 4, 5, 6, 7$. We learn the set of temporal association rules $R_i = \{r_j^i\}$ for each output event e_i. In the first step, a matrix M_i is constructed with $|T_i|$ rows and $1 + |R_i|$ columns, where $T_i = \{t_k^i \in \mathbb{R}\}$ denotes the set of time-stamps at which at least one of the rules in set R_i is activated. $M_i(k, j) \in [0, 1]$ denotes confidence of the rule r_j^i at the particular time point t_k^i. The extra column represents the indicator function of rapport state: $M_i(k, |R_i| + 1) = \{1, \text{if } t_k^i \in E_i; 0 \text{ otherwise}\}$. Seven random-forest classifiers ($f_i(t)$ and $t \in T_i$)) are then trained on each corresponding matrix M_i using the last column (binary) as the output label and all other columns as input features [16]. In the second step, another matrix G with $|T|$ rows and $1 + |C|$ columns is formalized, where $|C|$ is the number of random-forest classifiers, $G(k, i) = f_i(t_k)$ and $T = \{t_k | t_k \in T_i, i = 1...7\}$. The last column is the absolute number of rapport state gathered by ground truth. This matrix is used to train a linear regression model.

For our corpus, as part of the Titarl-based regression approach, we first extracted the top 6000 rules for friend dyads and 6000 rules for stranger dyads from the training dataset, with the following parameter settings: minimum support: 5 %, minimum confidence: 5 %, maximum umber of conditions: 5, minimum use: 10. Second, we fused those rules based on algorithm discussed above and applied them on test set, performing a 10-fold cross validation. In order to test the robustness of the results, we repeated the experiment for all possible random combinations of training (4 dyads) and test (2 dyads) sets for friends and strangers, and performed a correlated samples t-test to test whether our approach results in lower mean squared error compared to a simple linear regression model that treats each of the verbal and nonverbal modalities as independent features to predict the absolute value of rapport. Evaluation for performance metrics in this basic linear regression approach was done using the supplied test set of randomly chosen 2 dyads for each experimental run. In addition, we also calculated effect size via Cohen'sd d ($2t/\sqrt{df}$), where t is the value from the t-test and df refers to the degrees of freedom. Results in Table 1 suggest that the Titarl-based regression method has a significantly lower mean square error than the naive baseline linear regression method. The high effect size in both strangers ($d = -0.62$) and friends ($d = -0.42$) further prove the substantial improvement on accuracy of assessing rapport by Titarl-based regression comparing to simple linear regression.

Table 1. Statistical analysis comparing mean square regression of Titarl-based regression and a simple linear regression, for all possible combination of training and test sets in the corpus. Effect size assessed via Cohen's d. Significance: ***:$p < 0.001$, **:$p < 0.01$, *:$p < 0.05$

Relationship status	t-test value	Mean value (Mean square error)	Effect size
Friends	$t(1,14) = -6.41$***	Titarl = 1.257, Linear regression = 2.120	-0.42
Strangers	$t(1,14) = -8.78$***	Titarl = 0.837, Linear regression = 1.653	-0.62

These results have been integrated into a real-time end-to-end socially aware dialog system (SARA),[1] described in [25]. SARA is capable of automatically detecting conversational strategies based on verbal, nonverbal, and acoustic features in the user's input [38], relying on the conversational strategies detected in order to accurately estimate rapport between the interlocutors, reasoning about what conversational strategy to respond with as the next turn, and generating those appropriate responses in the service of more effectively carrying out her task duties. To our knowledge, SARA is the first socially-aware dialog system that relies on visual, verbal, and vocal cues to detect user social and task intent, and generates behaviors in those same channels to achieve her social and task goals.

6.2 Implications for Understanding Human Behavior

One of the important behavior patterns that plays out differently across friends and strangers, and whose interactions can lead to either high or low rapport, is smiling in combination with social norm violations and speech overlap. A violation of social norms without a smile is always followed by low rapport. On the other hand, a social norm violation accompanied by a smile is followed by high rapport when followed by overlap and performed among friends. Meanwhile, violating social norms while smiling leads to low rapport when followed by overlap if performed among strangers [See FH1, FH3, FH5, FL1, FL2, SL3]. What we may be seeing here is what [11] described as embarrassment following violations of "ceremonial rules" (social norms or conventional behavior), which is less often seen among family and friends than among strangers and new acquaintances. Similarly, [21] emphasized that the smile is a kind of hedge, signaling awareness of a social norm being violated and serving to provoke forgiveness from the interlocutor. Overlap in this context may be an index of the high coordination that characterizes conversation among friends whereby simultaneous speech indicates comfort, or that same overlap may indicate the lack of coordination that characterizes strangers who have not yet entrained to one another's speech patterns [5]. Our findings provide further empirical support for this body of prior work.

Another important contingent pattern of behaviors discussed here is the interaction between smile and backchannels [See SH2, FL3]. In general a backchannel + smile was indicative of high rapport, perhaps because the smile + backchannel

---

[1] sociallyawarerobotassistant.net.

indicated that the listener was inviting a continuation of the speaker's turn, but also indicating his/her appreciation of the interlocutor's speech [3].

We also discover the interaction between smile, the conversational strategy of self-disclosure and overlaps [See SH1]. Smiles invite self-disclosure, after which an overlap demonstrates responsiveness of the interlocutor. [24] have shown that partner responsiveness is a significant component of the intimacy process that benefits rapport. Finally we described how the presence of overlaps with a non-verbal behavior or conversational strategy often signals high rapport in friends but low rapport in strangers [See SH3, FL3, SL2, SL3]. Prior work has found that friends are more likely to interrupt than strangers, and the interruptions are less likely to be seen as disruptive or conflictual [5].

6.3   Implications for Social Agent Design

Rules such as those presented above can play a fundamental role in building socially-aware agents that adapt to the rapport level felt by their users in ways that previous work has not addressed. For example, [12] extracted a set of hand-crafted rules based on social science literature to build a rapport agent. Such rules not only need expert knowledge to craft, but may also be hard to scale up and to transfer to different domains. In our current work, we alleviate this problem by automatically extracting behavioral rules that signal high or low rapport, learning on verbal and nonverbal annotations of a particular corpus, but employing only the annotations of conversational strategies that did not concern the content domain of the corpus. This also represents an advance on work by [18] that improved rapport through nonverbal and para-verbal channels, but did not take linguistic information or temporal co-occurrence across modalities into account. We included linguistic information in our rules and In other work we have shown that the linguisic information (conversational strategies) that formed an essential part of the temporal rules presented here can be automatically recognized [38]. Similarly, [9]'s gaze-reactive pedagogical agent diagnoses disengagement or boredom by the use of eye trackers. However, only taking eye gaze into account forfeits the potential synergistic effect of interaction across modalities.

As noted above, while our current work focused on developing an interpretable and explanatory model of temporal behaviors to serve as a building block for our rapport-aligned peer-tutoring system (RAPT), the framework can be applied for prediction of other social phenomena of interest in virtual agent systems (such as trust and intimacy), in domains as diverse as survey interviewing, sales, and health.

7   Conclusion

In this work, we utilized a temporal association rule framework for automatic discovery of co-occurring and contingent behavior patterns that precede high and low interpersonal rapport in dyads of friends and strangers. Our work provides insights for better understanding of dyadic multimodal behavior sequences and their relationship with rapport which, in turn, moves us forward towards the implementation of socially-aware agents of all kinds–including "socially-skilled" virtual peer tutors that can assess the state of a relationship with a student, sigh in frustrated solidarity about a learning task at hand, and know how to respond to maximize learning in the peer tutoring context.

Among the patterns our rules discovered were the interaction of smiles and backchannels in signaling mutual attention and appreciation, and the pattern of self-disclosure, followed or preceded by smiles and speech overlap, as an indicator of high rapport. We found smiles to be one way in which interlocutors appear to mitigate the face-threat of social norm violations such as insults. However, our experiments discovered that while the presence of speech overlaps with smiles and social norm violations in friends signals high rapport, the presence of speech overlaps with social norm violations in strangers signals low rapport. In addition, for prediction of rapport, we observed the benefits (significantly lower mean square prediction error) of constructing predictor variables that work on fine-grained representation of social behaviors, explicitly model the temporal relations among them and encode ordering as well as timing, over using simple aggregated behavioral descriptors in a baseline linear regression model that are crudely informative.

Limitations of the current work include our focus on rapport states; in future work we will also want to find the temporal association rules that lead to a delta in rapport. In addition, while the current work discovers those behaviors that directly precede a rapport state, we have not yet verified that the link is causal. In service to that goal, our current work has implemented the temporal association rules as a real-time module, and has integrated them into a working virtual agent system. Our future work will use this system to evaluate the causal nature of these rules, and their effect on human–virtual agent interaction.

References

1. Allwood, J., Cerrato, L.: A study of gestural feedback expressions. In: First Nordic Symposium on Multimodal Communication, pp. 7–22. Copenhagen (2003)
2. Ambady, N., Rosenthal, R.: Thin slices of expressive behavior as predictors of interpersonal consequences: a meta-analysis. Psychol. Bull. **111**(2), 256 (1992)
3. Bevacqua, E., Mancini, M., Pelachaud, C.: A listening agent exhibiting variable behaviour. In: Prendinger, H., Lester, J., Ishizuka, M. (eds.) IVA 2008. LNCS (LNAI), vol. 5208, pp. 262–269. Springer, Heidelberg (2008). doi:10.1007/978-3-540-85483-8_27
4. Cappella, J.N.: On defining conversational coordination and rapport. Psychol. Inq. **1**(4), 303–305 (1990)
5. Cassell, J., Gill, A.J., Tepper, P.A.: Coordination in conversation and rapport. In: Proceedings of the workshop on Embodied Language Processing, pp. 41–50. ACL (2007)
6. Chiu, C.C., Morency, L.-P., Marsella, S.: Predicting co-verbal gestures: a deep and temporal modeling approach, pp. 152–166 (2015)

7. Chollet, M., Ochs, M., Pelachaud, C.: From non-verbal signals sequence mining to Bayesian networks for interpersonal attitudes expression. In: Bickmore, T., Marsella, S., Sidner, C. (eds.) IVA 2014. LNCS (LNAI), vol. 8637, pp. 120–133. Springer, Heidelberg (2014). doi:10.1007/978-3-319-09767-1_15
8. Chou, C.-Y., Chan, T.-W.: Reciprocal tutoring: design with cognitive load sharing. Int. J. Artif. Intell. Educ. **26**(1), 1–24 (2015)
9. D'Mello, S., Olney, A., Williams, C., Hays, P.: Gaze tutor: a gaze-reactive intelligent tutoring system. Int. J. Hum. Comput. Stud. **70**(5), 377–398 (2012)
10. Fujimoto, D.T.: Listener Responses in Interaction: A Case for Abandoning the Term. Backchannel (2009)
11. Goffman, E.: Interaction Ritual: Essays in Face to Face Behavior. AldineTransaction, New Brunswick (2005)
12. Gratch, J., Okhmatovskaia, A., Lamothe, F., Marsella, S., Morales, M., Werf, R.J., Morency, L.-P.: Virtual rapport. In: Gratch, J., Young, M., Aylett, R., Ballin, D., Olivier, P. (eds.) IVA 2006. LNCS (LNAI), vol. 4133, pp. 14–27. Springer, Heidelberg (2006). doi:10.1007/11821830_2
13. Gratch, J., Wang, N., Gerten, J., Fast, E., Duffy, R.: Creating rapport with virtual agents. In: Pelachaud, C., Martin, J.-C., André, E., Chollet, G., Karpouzis, K., Pelé, D. (eds.) IVA 2007. LNCS (LNAI), vol. 4722, pp. 125–138. Springer, Heidelberg (2007). doi:10.1007/978-3-540-74997-4_12
14. Gravano, A., Hirschberg, J.: Backchannel-inviting cues in task-oriented dialogue. In: INTERSPEECH, pp. 1019–1022 (2009)
15. Guillame-Bert, M., Crowley, J.L.: Learning temporal association rules on symbolic time sequences, pp. 159–174 (2012)
16. Guillame-Bert, M., Dubrawski, A.: Learning temporal rules to forecast events in multivariate time sequences
17. Heylen, D., Bevacqua, E., Tellier, M., Pelachaud, C.: Searching for prototypical facial feedback signals. In: Pelachaud, C., Martin, J.-C., André, E., Chollet, G., Karpouzis, K., Pelé, D. (eds.) IVA 2007. LNCS (LNAI), vol. 4722, pp. 147–153. Springer, Heidelberg (2007). doi:10.1007/978-3-540-74997-4_14
18. Huang, L., Morency, L.-P., Gratch, J.: Virtual rapport 2.0. In: Vilhjálmsson, H.H., Kopp, S., Marsella, S., Thórisson, K.R. (eds.) IVA 2011. LNCS (LNAI), vol. 6895, pp. 68–79. Springer, Heidelberg (2011). doi:10.1007/978-3-642-23974-8_8
19. Johnson, D.W.: Student-student interaction: the neglected variable in education. Educ. Researcher **10**(1), 5–10 (1981)
20. Kang, S.-H., Gratch, J., Sidner, C., Artstein, R., Huang, L., Morency, L.-P., Towards building a virtual counselor: modeling nonverbal behavior during intimate self-disclosure. In: Proceedings of the 11th ICAAMS, vol. 1, pp. 63–70 (2012)
21. Keltner, D., Buswell, B.N.: Embarrassment: its distinct form and appeasement functions. Psychol. Bull. **122**(3), 250 (1997)
22. Klem, A.M., Connell, J.P.: Relationships matter: Linking teacher support to student engagement and achievement. J. Sch. Health **74**(7), 262–273 (2004)
23. Kreijns, K., Kirschner, P.A., Jochems, W.: Identifying the pitfalls for social interaction in computer-supported collaborative learning environments: a review of the research. Comput. Hum. Behav. **19**(3), 335–353 (2003)
24. Laurenceau, J.-P., Barrett, L.F., Pietromonaco, P.R.: Intimacy as an interpersonal process: the importance of self-disclosure, partner disclosure, and perceived partner responsiveness in interpersonal exchanges. J. Pers. Soc. Psychol. **74**(5), 1238 (1998)
25. Matsuyama, Y., Bhardwaj, A., Zhao, R., Romero, O.J., Akoju, S., CassellJ.: Socially-aware animated intelligent personal assistant agent. In: 17th Annual SIGdial Meeting on Discourse and Dialogue (2016)

26. Nakano, YI., Nihonyanagi, S., Takase, Y., Hayashi, Y., Okada, S.: Predicting participation styles using co-occurrence patterns of nonverbal behaviors in collaborative learning, pp. 91–98 (2015)
27. Ogan, A., Finkelstein, S., Walker, E., Carlson, R., Cassell, J.: Rudeness and rapport: insults and learning gains in peer tutoring. In: Cerri, S.A., Clancey, W.J., Papadourakis, G., Panourgia, K. (eds.) ITS 2012. LNCS, vol. 7315, pp. 11–21. Springer, Heidelberg (2012). doi:10.1007/978-3-642-30950-2_2
28. Ramanarayanan, V., Leong, CW., Chen, L., Feng, G., Suendermann-Oeft, D.: Evaluating speech, face, emotion and body movement time-series features for automated multimodal presentation scoring, pp. 23–30 (2015)
29. Rummel, N., Walker, E., Aleven, V.: Different futures of adaptive collaborative learning support. Int. J. Artif. Intell. Educ. **26**(2), 784–795 (2016)
30. Sharpley, A.M., Irvine, J.W., Sharpley, C.F.: An examination of the effectiveness of a cross-age tutoring program in mathematics for elementary school children. Am. Educ. Res. J. **20**(1), 103–111 (1983)
31. Sinha, T., Cassell, J.: Fine-grained analyses of interpersonal processes and their effect on learning. In: Conati, C., Heffernan, N., Mitrovic, A., Verdejo, M.F. (eds.) AIED 2015. LNCS (LNAI), vol. 9112, pp. 781–785. Springer, Heidelberg (2015). doi:10.1007/978-3-319-19773-9_115
32. Sinha, T., Cassell, J., We click, we align, we learn: impact of influence and convergence processes on student learning and rapport building. In: 17th ACM International Conference on Multimodal Interaction Proceedings of the 2015 Workshop on Modeling Interpersonal Synchrony. ACM (2015)
33. Sinha, T., Zhao, R., Cassell, J.: Exploring socio-cognitive effects of conversational strategy congruence in peer tutoring. In: 17th ACM International Conference on Multimodal Interaction Proceedings of the 2015 Workshop on Modeling Interpersonal Synchrony. ACM (2015)
34. Tickle-Degnen, L., Rosenthal, R.: The nature of rapport and its nonverbal correlates. Psychol. Inquiry **1**(4), 285–293 (1990)
35. Woertwein, T., Chollet, M., Schauerte, B., Stiefelhagen, R., Morency, L.P., Scherer, S.: Multimodal public speaking performance assessment, pp. 43–50 (2015)
36. Yu, Z., Gerritsen, D., Ogan, A., Black, A., Cassell, J.: Automatic prediction of friendship via multi-model dyadic features. In: 14th Annual SIGdial Meeting on Discourse and Dialogue, Metz, France (2013)
37. Zhao, R., Papangelis, A., Cassell, J.: Towards a dyadic computational model of rapport management for human-virtual agent interaction. In: Bickmore, T., Marsella, S., Sidner, C. (eds.) IVA 2014. LNCS (LNAI), vol. 8637, pp. 514–527. Springer, Heidelberg (2014). doi:10.1007/978-3-319-09767-1_62
38. Zhao, R., Sinha, T., Black, A., Cassell, J.: Automatic recognition of conversational strategies in the service of a socially-aware dialog system. In: 17th Annual SIGDIAL Meeting on Discourse and Dialogue (2016)

Facial Expressions of Appraisals Displayed by a Virtual Storyteller for Children

Nesrine Fourati[1]([⊠]), Adeline Richard[2], Sylvain Caillou[1], Nicolas Sabouret[1], Jean-Claude Martin[1], Emilie Chanoni[2], and Celine Clavel[1]

[1] LIMSI, CNRS (UPR3251), Université Paris-Saclay, 91405 Orsay, France
{fourati,sylvain.caillou,nicolas.sabouret,jean-claude.martin,
celine.clavel}@limsi.fr
[2] PSY-NCA, Université de Rouen, 76000 Rouen, France
{adeline.richard,emilie.chanoni}@etu.univ-rouen.fr

Abstract. In this paper, we present a framework for an expressive virtual storyteller for children. Our virtual storyteller displays facial expressions of appraisals related to story events. The facial expressions are animated jointly with deictic gestures towards graphical elements representing story events. We describe a preliminary study that we conducted with 23 children. We discuss the impact of facial expressions of appraisals on children's memorization of story events, their perception of characters' appraisals, their subjective perception of the virtual storyteller and more generally how emotion combines with joint attention.

Keywords: Expressive virtual storyteller · Facial expression · Appraisal

1 Introduction

In addition to its entertaining values, storytelling supports children's development of cognitive, communicative, linguistic and literacy skills as well as logical thinking [5,18]. Nonverbal behaviors displayed by a human storyteller, including facial expressions of emotions, intonation, and communicative gestures, do provide important information about the meaning of the story as well as the personal interpretation of this story by the storyteller. Storytelling with virtual agents and robots has emerged in the nineties. It allows children to experience new forms of interaction and possibly to increase their enjoyment [12]. Several studies highlight the importance of interactive storytelling frameworks to better engage children with the story narrated by a virtual agent and to foster their creativity during storytelling [12,24]. Joint Attention (JA) behavior also allows interacting with the partner in order to share a particular experience through coordinated attention to an object (or event) with mutual affect [13]. JA behavior can be achieved by the means of verbal (e.g. "look at this object") and non-verbal behaviors (e.g. gaze direction, pointing gestures) [21]. Besides, contextual expressive capabilities of a virtual storyteller are important for children [12]. Several studies propose virtual agents endowed with socio-emotional skills

© Springer International Publishing AG 2016
D. Traum et al. (Eds.): IVA 2016, LNAI 10011, pp. 234–244, 2016.
DOI: 10.1007/978-3-319-47665-0_21

[11,20]. Studies observe that endowing virtual agents with the ability to express emotions and social attitudes might improve the quality of the interaction with the user compared to non expressive agents [2,14,19]. Courgeon et al. [9] adapted a computational model of emotion based on an appraisal theory in the case of a reversi game (but not in a storytelling task). Whereas the expression of emotion and joint attention initiation seem to be major requirements for a virtual storyteller for children, few virtual storytellers do exploit these two communicative functions together as a function of the current context [4]. Besides, the joint effect of expressions of emotions and joint attention initiation on children's experience and understanding of a story remains understudied. In this paper, we explain how we combine emotion expression and joint attention initiation within a single framework of a virtual storyteller for children. Our first aim is to study the contribution of emotion expression when combined with deictics. The present paper focuses on the modeling of emotion expression during a storytelling task and its impact on children's memorization of the story's emotional events, their evaluation of the characters' emotional states and their subjective perception of the storyteller. In the next section, we present related work on artificial storytellers. We then present in Sect. 3 our methodology for animating such an artificial storyteller capable of expressing emotions related to a story and displaying deictic behaviors. In Sect. 4 we present a preliminary study with 23 children. Section 5 discusses future work including future evaluations and how such work can be used to inform the design of autonomous expressive storytellers.

2   Related Work

Storytelling for children recently received a growing interest in the Human-Computer Interaction community. Several interactive storytelling frameworks, applications, and devices are proposed such as interactive toys [7], interactive books, robots [15] and computer games characters [3]. Studies suggest positive impacts of exploiting virtual agents compared to a text displayed on a screen [26]. Several studies focus on the design of interactive storytelling frameworks to establish a natural interaction [3,7]. However, expressing and acting emotions sounds important to offer a positive storytelling experience [25]. Besides, the expression of emotion can have a considerable impact on the believability of an artificial storyteller [8]. Recently, there has been a growing interest on the development of storytellers endowed with capabilities to express emotions. The need to generate expressive and emotional speech was considered for the design of an expressive character-based storyteller in [8,25]. In [23], the authors present their expressive virtual storyteller called Papous. A text-to-speech framework is used and expressive parameters are employed to endow the virtual storyteller with the ability to express emotion through prosody. The authors claim that the agent's voice still seems synthetic despite efforts to make it sound expressive [23]. Other studies focus on bodily expressions of emotions and moods during storytelling for example using the NAO robot [15]. Only a few studies consider the combined impact of emotion expression and joint attention initiation on the experience of Storytelling with children [4].

3   Methodology

Our expressive virtual storyteller is based on the MARC virtual agent framework (Multimodal Affective and Reactive Characters) [10]. The female agent, named Mary, is used for our study (see Fig. 1). We selected a French story called "Le ballon perché" because of its pedagogical relevance and for its rich expressive content. The story is about three children playing football just before the class starts. The ball gets stuck on a roof. The children try to get the ball down by throwing their personal items on the roof. However, the situation gets even worse since all of the items also remain on the roof. The children have to go back to the classroom and they face several difficult situations involving their missing items, for which they find workarounds. Finally, a storm blows all the items and the ball off the roof. This story is full of unexpected situations for young children, while happening in a familiar and realistic frame.

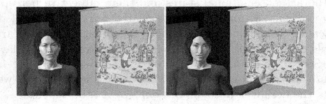

Fig. 1. Our expressive virtual storyteller displaying facial expressions of appraisals and performing a pointing gesture.

Since our goal is to endow our virtual storyteller with the ability to drive an interactive and expressive narration, the original story content has been revised by researchers in psychology to include interactive utterances in addition to narrative utterances (160 utterances totally). Thus, we distinguish two categories of utterances: (1) narrative utterances (56.25 % of all the utterances), and (2) interactive utterances (43.75 % of all the utterances). Narrative utterances correspond to the original story content. Interactive utterances are useful to maintain engagement during the narration task. We define different forms of interactive utterances; Interrogative, Affirmative and Joint Attention (JA) initiation utterances. An Interrogative utterance refers to a question which aims to maintain the child's engagement (e.g. "do you think he is going to make it?"). An Affirmative utterance refers to the introduction and the conclusion phases of the story (e.g. "Hello my name is Mary") or to the transition between the child's answer and a narrative utterance (e.g. "That's what Im thinking too"). JA utterances are used to drive the child's attention to events or objects related to the story (e.g. "look at this teacher").

During narration task, JA utterances are coupled with nonverbal behaviors to direct the child's attention to a character/event/object in the story images. For each JA utterance, the agent's gaze and his head movement are oriented toward the image. In addition to the gaze and head movement, we also include either torso movement or pointing gesture. The former is used to stress the presence of a new event. The latter is employed to point a particular object or character. To maintain the child's attention and to be able to initiate joint attention, we imported graphics from the story book into the 3D virtual environment and displayed besides the virtual storyteller (see Fig. 1).

In the present study, we aim to endow our agent with the ability to display facial expressions (see Sect. 3.1). As audio recording results in a more natural storyteller compared to a synthetic voice, we asked a (female) psychology student to record the speech of each utterance in a spontaneous and an expressive way. 160 audio files were collected (one per utterance). We synchronized lips motion provided from the utterance content based on the JSAPI text to speech tool with the audio recording of narration.

3.1 Facial Expressions

Different theories were proposed to model the morphological and dynamic characteristics of facial expressions of emotions. They are commonly grouped in three approaches: Categorical, Dimensional and Appraisal approaches. Appraisal theory is one of the most influential theory within affective computing [17]. It has been widely used as the basis for several computational models of emotion [16]. In our work, we adopt the Component Process Model (CPM), an appraisal theory, for its dynamic ability to evaluate and describe an adaptive reaction to a story event [22]. The five appraisal variables (also called "Stimulus Evaluation Checks") described in [22] have been selected and considered for our study: Novelty, Intrinsic Pleasantness, Goal/Need Conduciveness, Coping Control and Coping Power. Norm/Self compatibility check has not been considered in our study for the lack of insights regarding the activation of the corresponding Action Units. A mapping between appraisal variables and Action Units from the FACS (Facial Action Coding System) was proposed in [22]. A computational model of these five appraisal variables has been developed within the MARC platform [9]. The mapping between each appraisal variable and the associated facial action units is mainly based on the work described in [22].

A manual annotation step was performed to attribute the appropriate appraisal evaluation for each utterance of the story. As such, the agent will display the appropriate facial expression according to each utterance based on appraisal annotation. Five researchers (the authors) from Affective Computing and Psychology were asked to perform this annotation step. For each utterance, each annotator was asked to explain the viewpoint used to evaluate the appraisal variables (e.g. Narrator or Story Character viewpoint) and to attribute the appropriate discrete value of each appraisal variables based on a 5-points scale $(-1, -0.5, 0, 0.5, 1)$. The annotators were provided with the definition of each appraisal variable. As we aim to obtain a single annotation of appraisal to animate our virtual agent during the storytelling task, the annotators met to discuss the differences in their annotation in order to reach an agreement on the appropriate annotation of appraisal variables for each utterance. At the end of the annotation process, 57.50 % of the utterances were evaluated as expressive (i.e. at least one appraisal variable was not set to 0). The other utterances were defined as non-expressive (i.e. no facial expressions should be displayed). However, we assume that endowing a virtual agent with smiles during the storytelling task can create a friendly atmosphere, which is of high importance during an interaction with children. For this reason, during non-expressive utterances, we endowed our virtual agent with a smiling face based on the morphological characteristics of an *amused* smile [20] (i.e. 6 (Cheek raiser), 12 (Lip corner puller) and AU25 (lips parted)). We chose to display facial expressions (facial expressions of appraisal and amused smile respectively for expressive and non-expressive utterances) during the whole spoken utterance based on the results described in [6]. These results indicate that facial expressions seem to be perceived as more intense and more realistic when displayed during the whole spoken utterance [6]. In the next section, we present a preliminary study that provides first insights into the impact of facial expression of appraisal during storytelling task on the cognitive skills of children and on their ability to evaluate emotional states based on an appraisal model. In the present study, we do not investigate the impact of Joint Attention initiation on these components. This research question will be addressed in a future work.

4   Exploratory Study

We conducted an exploratory study to explore how facial expressions of appraisals may affect children cognitive processes and evaluation of characters' appraisals. The narration of the story lasts around 10 min. Twenty three children contacted via a recreation center participated in our experiment (10 female). One recording session was performed per child. During the whole recording session, the child was accompanied with an adult. The children were between 6 and 10 years old. Twelve children were asked to listen to the story narrated by our virtual agent in expressive condition, while eleven children were asked to listen to the story in non-expressive condition. In the expressive condition, our virtual agent displayed facial expressions of appraisals for each expressive utterance based on the annotation described in Sect. 3.1. In the non-expressive condition, our virtual agent displayed an amused smile all along the storytelling task (see Sect. 3.1). The child was free to make spoken comments during the whole storytelling task. At the end of the story, the child was asked to fill a survey with the help of an adult. The videos of the children were also recorded for later study of their interaction with the virtual storyteller. The parents of each child gave informed consent and agreed that their children' answers to the survey as well as their videos could be used and published for research purposes.

4.1 Measures

Our survey is composed of three parts.

- Twenty-three questions used to assess the memorization of story's events. The answers to these questions were converted into numerical values belonging to the interval [0,1] (0 means the answer is wrong, 1 means the answer is right, between 0 and 1 means the answer is partially right).
- Eight questions used to examine how children evaluate several appraisal variables. They were inspired from the Geneva Appraisal Questionnaire [22] and adapted to children's cognitive skills. Each question is associated to a specific story event illustrated by the corresponding story's image. For instance, the second question is associated to the story image of one character trying to throw a personal item onto the roof in order to get the ball down. For each question, the child was asked to evaluate 5 appraisal variables along a 5-point scale from "totally disagree" to "totally agree". The appraisal variables are Novelty, Intrinsic pleasantness, Goal Conduciveness, Coping Control and External Causation (i.e. Compatibility with social norms) [22]. Five assertions were used to help the child evaluate each appraisal variable. For instance, the assertion corresponding to Novelty check was "It's something that does always happen."
- Fifteen questions used to explore how the virtual storyteller is perceived (e.g. nice, friendly, pleasant ...). The content of these subjective questions was inspired by the French Translation of Bartneck's Godspeed Questionnaire [1]. The answer was given by the means of a 5-points scale.

4.2 Preliminary Results

Based on the measures described above, we discuss the impact of facial expressions of appraisals on (1) the children's memorization of the story's events, (2) their evaluation of appraisals and (3) their appreciation of the virtual storyteller.

Do facial expressions of appraisals impact children's memorization of the story? In order to study the impact of facial expressions of appraisals, the answers of the 21 questions that address the memorization of story's events were averaged to obtain a measure of the overall memorization of story's event for each subject. A t-test was applied to study the effect of facial expressions on the overall memorization of story' events. No significant effect was found (see Table 1). However, we observed that children tended to slightly better memorize story's events in the expressive condition (see Table 1). Pointing gestures were used to initiate the joint attention for the events addressed in eleven questions of memorization (out of 21). Indeed, the pointing gestures used to initiate the joint attention for these events could affect the child's memorization regardless of the facial expressions.

The age of our participants varies between 6 and 10 years old (std = 0.94, mean = 8, 14 children under 8 years old). A t-test was conducted to explore

Table 1. The effect of facial expressions and of the child's age on the overall memorization of story events.

	t-test	Mean	Std	Min	Max
Non-expressive storyteller	$p = 0.58$	0.65	0.15	0.44	0.88
Expressive storyteller		0.68	0.14	0.46	0.93
Younger (under 8 years old)	$p < 0.001$	0.60	0.12	0.44	0.81
Older (above 8 years old)		0.78	0.09	0.68	0.93

the effect of the age on the overall memorization of events. A significant difference was found between the groups of children under and above 8 years old ($p < 0.001$). We observed that older children tended to better memorize story's events than younger children (see Table 1). This result might explain why no significant difference was found between the memorization of events in expressive and non-expressive conditions. Given the strong effect of age on the memorization of the story's events, one may conclude that more participants on a more focused age range will be needed to investigate the effects of emotion expressions on children's cognitive skills.

For the sake of simplicity, we will respectively call older and younger children the subjects who are above and below 8 years old (the mean age of our participants). We found that young children tended to better memorize events related to the story content and reported in joint attention initiation utterances in non-expressive condition ($p < 0.05$). Indeed, it seems that facial expressions disturb young children's memorization of story's events when the agent initiate joint attention for events related to the story content. However, the same was not observed for the old children group who tended to memorize story's events regardless of the presence or absence of facial expressions of appraisals. This difference might can be explained by the content of the story and the interactive scenario that we created which might not be relevant for children above 8 years old. This difference in the results suggests to conduct an evaluation only with young children (e.g. less than 8 years old).

Do facial expressions of appraisals impact children's evaluation of appraisals? We applied a t-test for each of the 40 answers of appraisals evaluation to study the impact of facial expressions on children's evaluation of appraisals (8 questions * 5 appraisal variables, see Sect. 4.1). No significant effect was found, which could also be related to the variety of age. We explored the effect of facial expressions on their evaluation of appraisals separately for younger and older group of children. A serial of t-test was conducted for this purpose for the 40 answers. We found that facial expressions of appraisals displayed during narration impacted young children's evaluation of Novelty across different events($p < 0.05$). Overall, younger children tended to evaluate different events as more Novel when the virtual agent displayed facial expressions of appraisals. As such, the presence of facial expressions of appraisals accentuates the evaluation of Novelty.

For instance, the event related to "Standing in line before class starts" was evaluated as expected (e.g. always happening) in the non-expressive condition. It was evaluated as significantly less expected in the expressive condition. In the expressive condition, the virtual storyteller displayed facial expressions associated to non-expected, unpleasant and obstructive to the children's goal since the children did not get the ball down in time and their items were still stuck on the roof. Another similar significant finding was observed for the evaluation of the "External causation" variable with younger children. In the expressive condition, younger children tended to evaluate a few events as being not in line with social norms. In the non-expressive condition, they tended to evaluate these events as in line with social norms. For example, the event "Standing in line before class starts" tended to be evaluated as less respecting social norms in the expressive condition where the virtual storyteller expressed the emotional states of the characters being in an awkward situation (the characters had to go to the classroom without their personal items). Besides, we compared the children's evaluation of appraisal variables with the annotators' manual annotation. We found that the children's evaluation of these appraisal variables can vary according to the viewpoint that one takes, which has been already be reported by the annotators (see Sect. 3.1). For example, the event "the teacher is screaming" would be surprising in a general situation, but might be expected in the case of our story when the children were standing much too close to the window. In the expressive condition, we found that the children's evaluation of these appraisal variables (for the corresponding particular events) tended to be correlated with the annotators' evaluation according to the *story content*. Besides, children's evaluation of these appraisal variables in the non-expressive condition tended to be correlated with our annotation in absolute terms. As such, it seems that facial expression of appraisals helped children to refer to the story content to evaluate appraisal variables. When no facial expression was displayed, children tended to evaluate events according to a non story-specific point of view. Overall, these findings suggest potential impacts of displaying facial expressions of appraisals on the evaluation of appraisal variables by children.

Do facial expressions of appraisals impact children' appreciation of the virtual storyteller? A serial of t-test was applied on each of the 15 questions that assess the children's subjective evaluation of the agent. No significant difference was found between their subjective evaluation in expressive and non-expressive condition. Similarly to the results reported above for the impact of facial expressions of appraisals on children's memorization, we observed that children's appreciation of the virtual storyteller tend to depend on their age. Young children tended to evaluate the virtual storyteller as being more or less human (means = 2.6 with 0 meaning "machine" and 4 "human") while old children tended to evaluate the agent as being less human (mean = 1.7). However, old children tended to consider the agent as being more likeable (means = 3.6) than young children (means = 3.07). This result might be explained by the fact that young children tended to perceive the agent as being more alive and thus had high expectations about it. Old children might have been more aware that the agent was a computer software and thus were more tolerant to graphical flaws.

5   Conclusion and Future Directions

Our framework supports the expression of appraisals of the story content and the initiation of joint attention during the storytelling task. The Component Process Model was used to drive the virtual agent's Action Units to display corresponding facial expressions of appraisals. An exploratory study with 23 children was conducted to explore the impact of these facial expressions of appraisal on children' perception and understanding of the story. Understanding and appreciation of the virtual storyteller depended on the age of the child. Young children's cognitive skills and evaluation of the appraisals were impacted by the facial expressions of appraisals displayed by the virtual storyteller. In the short term, we will conduct an experimental study with a larger pool of participants with a more homogeneous age range. We will also use an eye-tracker to record the direction of the children's gaze. This will enable us to explore the frequency and the duration of children's gaze toward the agent's face vs. towards the story graphics. In the long-term, we aim to add bodily expressions of emotion. Finally, the evaluation of the appraisal variables in the present work has been performed based on a manual annotation and a human evaluation of the story events and of the agent viewpoint. An automatic evaluation of appraisal variables would represent an important step towards fully automatic virtual storytellers.

Acknowledgments. The authors would like to thank Matthieu Courgeon for his help in the development of our virtual storyteller. A special thanks goes to the children, their parents and the director of the recreation center. Part of this work was funded by the Agence Nationale de la Recherche (ANR), project NARECA (ANR-13-CORD-0015).

References

1. Bartneck, C., Croft, E., Kulic, D.: Measurement instruments for the anthropomorphism, animacy, likeability, perceived intelligence, and perceived safety of robots. Int. J. Soc. Robot. **1**(1), 71–81 (2009)
2. Beale, R., Creed, C.: Affective interaction: how emotional agents affect users. Int. J. Hum. Comput. Stud. **67**(9), 755–776 (2009)
3. Bernardini, S., Porayska-Pomsta, K., Smith, T.J.: ECHOES: an intelligent serious game for fostering social communication in children with autism. Inf. Sci. **264**, 41–60 (2014)
4. Bosse, T., Pontier, M., Siddiqui, G.F., Treur, J.: Incorporating emotion regulation into virtual stories. In: Pelachaud, C., Martin, J.-C., André, E., Chollet, G., Karpouzis, K., Pelé, D. (eds.) IVA 2007. LNCS (LNAI), vol. 4722, pp. 339–347. Springer, Heidelberg (2007). doi:10.1007/978-3-540-74997-4_31
5. Bruner, J.: The narrative construction of reality. Crit. Inquir. **18**(1), 1–21 (1991)
6. Buisine, S., Wang, Y., Grynszpan, O.: Empirical investigation of the temporal relations between speech and facial expressions of emotion. J. Multimodal User Interfaces **3**(4), 263–270 (2009)

7. Cassell, J., Bers, M.U.: Interactive storytelling systems for children: using technology to explore language and identity. J. Interact. Learn. Res. **9**, 183–215 (1999)
8. Cavazza, M., Pizzi, D., Charles, F.: Emotional input for character-based interactive storytelling. In: Proceedings of the 8th International Conference on Autonomous Agents and Multiagent Systems, pp. 313–320 (2009)
9. Courgeon, M., Clavel, C., Martin, J.C.: Modeling facial signs of appraisal during interaction: impact on users' perception and behavior. AAMAS **59**(1), 765–772 (2014)
10. Courgeon, M., Martin, J.C., Jacquemin, C.: Marc: a multimodal affective and reactive character. In: Proceedings of the 1st Workshop on Affective Interaction in Natural Environments (2008)
11. De Rosis, F., Pelachaud, C., Poggi, I., Carofiglio, V., De Carolis, B.: From Greta's mind to her face: modelling the dynamics of affective states in a conversational embodied agent. Int. J. Hum. Comput. Stud. **59**(1), 81–118 (2003)
12. Fridin, M.: Storytelling by a kindergarten social assistive robot: a tool for constructive learning in preschool education. Comput. Educ. **70**, 53–64 (2014)
13. Kiser, L.J., Baumgardner, B., Dorado, J.: Who are we, but for the stories we tell: family stories and healing. Psychol. Trauma Theory Res. Pract. Policy **2**(3), 243–249 (2010)
14. Krämer, N.C.: Social effects of virtual assistants. A review of empirical results with regard to communication. In: Prendinger, H., Lester, J., Ishizuka, M. (eds.) IVA 2008. LNCS (LNAI), vol. 5208, pp. 507–508. Springer, Heidelberg (2008). doi:10.1007/978-3-540-85483-8_63
15. Le, Q.A., Hanoune, S., Pelachaud, C.: Design and implementation of an expressive gesture model for a humanoid robot. In: 2011 11th IEEE-RAS International Conference on Humanoid Robots, pp. 134–140 (2011)
16. Marsella, S.C., Gratch, J.: EMA: a process model of appraisal dynamics. Cogn. Syst. Res. **10**(1), 70–90 (2009)
17. Marsella, S.C., Gratch, J., Petta, P.: Computational models of emotion. In: Scherer, K.R., Banziger, T., Roesch, E. (eds.) A Blueprint for Affective Computing: A Sourcebook and Manual, pp. 21–46. Oxford University Press, Oxford (2010)
18. Miller, S., Pennycuff, L.: The power of story: using storytelling to improve literacy learning. J. Cross Discip. Perspect. Educ. **1**(1), 36–43 (2008)
19. Ochs, M.: Modélisation, formalisation et mise en oeuvre d'un agent rationnel dialoguant émotionnel empathique. Ph.D. thesis, Doctoral dissertation, Paris 8 (2007)
20. Ochs, M., Niewiadomski, R., Pelachaud, C.: How a virtual agent should smile? In: Allbeck, J., Badler, N., Bickmore, T., Pelachaud, C., Safonova, A. (eds.) IVA 2010. LNCS (LNAI), vol. 6356, pp. 427–440. Springer, Heidelberg (2010). doi:10.1007/978-3-642-15892-6_47
21. Scaife, M., Bruner, J.: The capacity for joint visual attention in the infant. Nature **253**(5489), 265–266 (1975)
22. Scherer, K.R.: Appraisal considered as a process of multilevel sequential checking. In: Scherer, K.R., Schorr, A., Johnstone, T. (eds.) Appraisal processes in emotion: Theory, Methods, Research, pp. 92–120. Oxford University Press, New York (2001)
23. Silva, A., Vala, M., Paiva, A.: Papous: the virtual storyteller. In: Antonio, A., Aylett, R., Ballin, D. (eds.) IVA 2001. LNCS (LNAI), vol. 2190, pp. 171–180. Springer, Heidelberg (2001). doi:10.1007/3-540-44812-8_14

24. Theune, M., Linssen, J., Alofs, T.: Acting, playing, or talking about the story: an annotation scheme for communication during interactive digital storytelling. In: Koenitz, H., Sezen, T.I., Ferri, G., Haahr, M., Sezen, D., Çatak, G. (eds.) ICIDS 2013. LNCS, vol. 8230, pp. 132–143. Springer, Heidelberg (2013). doi:10.1007/978-3-319-02756-2_17

25. Theune, M., Meijs, K., Heylen, D., Ordelman, R.: Generating expressive speech for storytelling applications. IEEE Trans. Audio Speech Lang. Process. **14**(4), 1137–1144 (2006)

26. Walker, J., Sproull, L., Subramani, R.: Using a human face in an interface. In: Proceedings of the SIGCHI Conference on Human Factors in Computing Systems: Celebrating Interdependence, pp. 85–91 (1994)

Evaluating Social Attitudes of a Virtual Tutor

Florian Pecune[1]([✉]), Angelo Cafaro[1], Magalie Ochs[2], and Catherine Pelachaud[1]

[1] LTCI, CNRS, Télécom ParisTech, Université Paris-Saclay, Saint-Aubin, France
florian.pecune@telecom-paristech.fr
[2] Aix Marseille Université, CNRS, ENSAM, Université de Toulon, LSIS,
Toulon, France

Abstract. In this paper we evaluate a model of social decision-making for virtual agents. The model computes the social attitude of a virtual agent given its social role during the interaction and its social relation toward the interactant. The resulting attitude influences the agent's social goals and therefore determines the decisions made by the agent in terms of actions and communicative intentions to accomplish. We conducted an empirical study in the context of virtual tutor-child interaction where participants evaluated the tutor's perceived social attitude towards the child while the tutor's social role and relation were manipulated by our model. Results showed that both role and social relation have an influence on the agent's perceived social attitude.

1 Introduction

In order to improve the naturalness and the believability of virtual anthropomorphic agents, socio-emotional components should be considered when modeling their decision-making and behavior in a human-agent interaction. These components allow agents to express an emotional behavior and a social attitude relevant to the context of the interaction. According to Scherer [15], a social attitude is an *"affective style that spontaneously develops or is strategically employed in the interaction with a person or a group of persons, coloring the interpersonal exchange in that situation"*. The spontaneous aspect of social attitudes can be defined as the social relation between interactants. For instance, two people who like each other spontaneously tend to comply with the other's requests, thus showing a friendly attitude [7]. The strategic aspect can be governed by the interactants' social roles in their social context [8]. For example, in a restaurant (social context), a waiter (social role) is supposed to be nice and polite (social attitude) toward its clients, while a teacher might be more authoritative toward its students. We investigated the effects of the social relation of an agent compared to its social role on the perceived social attitudes that a user attribute to that agent. More specifically, is an agent liking its interactant *always* considered friendly regardless of its role during the interaction? Is an agent that wants to be authoritative always perceived as dominant?

In order to give a virtual agent the capability of reasoning about its role and its own social relation toward the user, and the capability of expressing an

© Springer International Publishing AG 2016
D. Traum et al. (Eds.): IVA 2016, LNAI 10011, pp. 245–255, 2016.
DOI: 10.1007/978-3-319-47665-0_22

adequate in-context social attitude, we designed and evaluated an agent's model of social decision making that integrates spontaneous and strategical aspects of social attitudes.

2   Related Work

The most common dimensions used for representing an agent's social relation toward another refer to the notion of *affiliation* (whether the agent likes or dislikes the other) and *status* (whether the agent has power over the other) [1]. In [5], authors evaluated the *status* and *affiliation* of their virtual recruiter through verbal cues and non-verbal behaviors. The social attitude of a virtual recruiter during an interview was also evaluated in [6]. In this work, recruiters conveyed *status* and *affiliation* through sequences of non-verbal signals. In [13], authors also used agent's non-verbal behavior as a cue, as well as interruption strategies. Participants were asked to evaluate *status* and *affiliation* of two particular agents among a group of four discussing characters. Participants had to interact with a virtual museum guide in [3]. After a short interaction, they were asked to evaluate the *affiliation* of the guide. Here, the agent's social attitude was defined by its amount of smiles, mutual gaze with the participant, and its proximity (whether it was standing close or fare the participant). These studies mainly focused on the verbal and nonverbal behavior of the agents, and social attitudes were evaluated by third parties. None of them, however, focused on the actions of the agents. Therefore, our main contribution is a study protocol designed to evaluate an agent's social attitudes through sequences of actions.

3   SocRATES Model

The focus of this paper is the validation of SocRATES, our computational model of social attitudes. The purpose of this model is to build a virtual agent able to reason about its social role and its social relation towards its interactant, and thus select its actions accordingly. First, we compute the social attitude expressed by the agent according to its social relation toward its interactant and its social role. Then, considering its social attitude, the agent has two social goals: it wants its interactant to express (1) the same level of affiliation and (2) opposite level of status. Finally, the agent chooses its action according to importance given to its social goals and its task-oriented goals. A complete description of SocRATES can be found in [12].

Figure 1 shows a schematic representation of our model's implementation. We first used PsychSim [10] for defining a set of actions and their influence on the states of the world for each agent. Social and situational goals were implemented as agent's reward functions. When an agent plans its next action in PsychSim, it first evaluates the effect of each of its possible future actions on the different states of the world. Then it predicts the other agent's expected actions and their impact on the world's states. Then again, the agent will anticipate its reaction until a given *horizon* (i.e. number of steps). When the agent finishes its

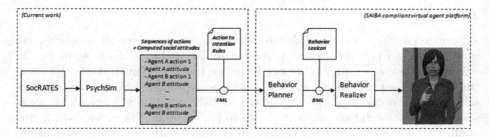

Fig. 1. Overview of the architecture: The left part of the image depicts SocRATES and its PsychSim implementation. The right part shows the SAIBA compliant virtual agent platform used to perform the generated sequences of actions and communicative intentions.

projection, it evaluates the overall effect of each sequence of actions according to its goals. Then, the agent selects the action with the highest expected utility. SocRATES enables each agent to take its decision according to its social attitude, while computing the influence of its actions on an other agent's social relation. More details about this part of the implementation can be found in [12]. The outputs of SocRATES and PsychSim are actions and social attitudes generated for both interactants. For each interactant, both outputs are dynamically computed on a turn-by-turn basis and by taking into account the other interactant's previous turn (i.e. action and attitude expressed). The set of actions for each interactant is transformed into a sequence of communicative intentions through a mapping from actions to FML [4] (described with more detail in Sect. 4.1). As shown in the second block of Fig. 1, the produced communicative intents are accomplished through sequences of multimodal behaviors by relying on the Greta platform [11].

4   Experimental Design

We performed an evaluation study to measure the influence that agent's initial social relation and social role have on its perceived interpersonal attitude by a user. Given the influence of *actual social relation* and *ideal social relation* on the agent decision making in SocRATES, we aimed at checking whether the sequences of actions computed by the model convey the expected social attitudes. Since many works have shown the influence of tutor's social attitude on child's motivation [20], we defined a scenario depicting a tutor-child interaction where an animated conversational agent plays the role of the tutor. The tutor's situational goal is to make the child do its homework. Participants were asked to rate the perceived level of social status and affiliation of the tutor. As exploratory measure given by the social context, we also asked participants to rate the perceived level of performance of the tutor.

4.1   Stimuli

We created a series of tutor-child interaction videos. Since gender and/or visual appearance can influence users' perceived social attitudes of an agent [9], in our study we controlled this aspect by using the same female character as a tutor throughout all the videos. The child was represented by an androgynous still figure in order to avoid any gender or behavior biases. Figure 2 shows a screenshot from a video stimuli as shown to participants. The child's still figure is shown on the left with a dynamic label underneath describing its current action. Neither speech nor behavior of the child were shown in order to steer the participants' attention as much as possible on the tutor's side. The animated virtual tutor was shown on the right. We used a synthesized voice accompanied by facial expressions, gestures, gaze behavior and head movements generated by the model described in [11] for expressing the tutor's communicative intentions. A red square highlighted the agent (tutor or child) that had the turn (i.e. speaking or doing an action) during the interaction.

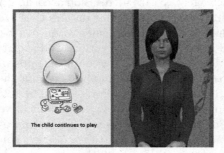

Fig. 2. A screenshot of the video used as stimuli in our study. The child is represented by a still figure on the left and the tutor is the animated virtual agent on the right.

The different videos were generated by systematically varying the tutor's initial *actual social relation* and its *ideal social relation* using our model (see [12] for examples of the generated interactions). The sequences of actions were all different, however, the verbal and non-verbal behaviors used to represent each action were the same across the interactions (i.e. the mapping from action to communicative intention). We relied on [5] to represent the communicative intentions using a neutral verbal and non-verbal behavior. Thus, we identified a between-subjects variable that was the tutor's initial *actual liking* (**T-InitialActualLiking**) towards the child. This variable has two levels: *Negative Actual Liking* vs. *Positive Actual Liking*. Since the tutor is able to influence the child's goals, we fixed its initial actual power to a positive value. Then, once the initial *actual liking* was defined, we identified a within-subjects factor, the tutor's **ideal social relation** (**T-IdealRelation**). Considering our scenario, we identified the three following levels: positive ideal power $(P+)$, positive ideal liking $(L+)$ and, positive ideal power and positive ideal liking $(P+L+)$. In sum,

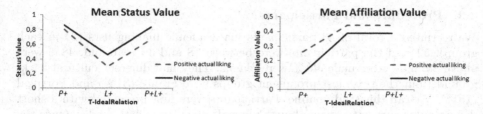

Fig. 3. The left figure represents the mean status value (y axis) according to the *ideal social relation* (x axis) for both positive *actual liking* (plain line) and negative *actual liking* (dashed line).

we obtained six different videos. Figure 3 represents the evolution of the mean tutor's social attitude computed by our model in the six different interactions. The scenario ended whenever the child finished its homework.

4.2   Measurements

We asked the participants to rate the perceived attitude of the tutor towards the child in terms of social status (**T-Status**) and social affiliation (**T-Affiliation**), and the perceived efficiency of its strategies (**T-Performance**).

For measuring **T-Status** and **T-Affiliation**, we adapted eight statements from the third person version of the InterPersonal Questionnaire (IPQ-R) [17], which is built on Wiggin's circumplex representation of attitudes [19]. The IPQ-R questionnaire defines twelve interpersonal styles (i.e. duodecants) representing different blends of the two attitude dimensions. Each duodecant was linked to a sub-questionnaire containing six statements. For measuring status, we selected two statements from the *dominant* duodecant and two statements from the *deferent* duodecant. The statements for the *dominant* duodecant are: *"Trying to control the child"* and *"Assertive toward the child"*. The items adopted for the *deferent* duodecant are: *"Avoiding imposing power over the child"* and *"Unauthoritative with the child"*. For measuring affiliation, we selected two statements from the *warm* duodecant and two statements from the *aloof* duodecant. The statements for the *warm* duodecant are: *"Warm toward the child"* and *"Taking strong interest in the child's goals"*. The items adopted for the *aloof* duodecant are: *"Unfriendly toward the child"* and *"Uninterested in the child's goals"*.

For measuring **T-Performance** we selected the three most reliable items from the *efficacy for student engagement* factor found in the Ohio State teacher efficacy scale (OSTES) [18] according to their score. This questionnaire is used to measure teachers' performance along three factors. The three selected statements are: *"Helping the child to understand the importance of learning"*, *"Trying to motivate the child"* and *"Getting the child to believe s/he can do well"*.

All answers were on a 7-points labeled Likert scale (anchors: 1. *Completely disagree* and 7. *Completely agree*).

4.3 Procedure and Participants

We recruited a total of 48 participants via academic mailing lists (24 in each group). 52 % of the participants were between 18 and 30 years old, 48 % were above 30. 60 % were male, 40 % were female. They had different cultural backgrounds, but the two most prominent groups were France (31 %) and Portugal (15 %). We ran this study online. Participants were first presented with a short demographic survey to know about their nationality, age and gender. Once the survey was completed, we randomly assigned the participants to a group according to the **T-InitialLiking** variable (positive vs. negative). Finally, we presented each stimulus as a video on a different web page with questions underneath by following a within-subjects repeated measures design and fully counterbalancing conditions' order as recommended by [2].

4.4 Hypotheses

Given Scherer's definition [15], we suppose that the tutor's initial *actual social relation* and its *ideal social relation* have both an influence on its perceived social attitude. Moreover, given that a tutor's social attitude has an influence on its performance, as suggested by [20] we suppose that the tutor's initial *actual social relation* and its *ideal social relation* have both an influence on its perceived performance. According to the social attitudes computed by our model and presented in Fig. 3 we defined the following hypotheses:

H.1-Sta: The **T-IdealRelation** will have a main effect on perceived **T-Status**, in particular a tutor with a positive level of *ideal power* (P+) will be perceived with a higher status compared to a tutor with both positive *ideal power* and positive *ideal liking* (P+L+) that in turn will be perceived with a higher status compared to a tutor with a positive *ideal liking* (L+).

H.1-Aff: The **T-IdealRelation** will have a main effect on perceived **T-Affiliation**, in particular tutors with a positive *ideal liking* (L+) or with both positive *ideal power* and positive *ideal liking* (P+L+) will be perceived with a higher affiliation compared to a tutor with a positive level of *ideal power* (P+).

H.1-Perf: The **T-IdealRelation** will have a main effect on perceived **T-Performance**, in particular tutor with both positive *ideal power* and positive *ideal liking* (P+L+) will be perceived with a higher performance compared to a tutor with a positive *ideal liking* (L+) that in turn will be perceived with a higher performance compared to a tutor with a positive level of *ideal power* (P+).

H.2-Sta: The **T-InitialActualLiking** will have a main effect on perceived **T-Status**, in particular tutor with (Negative Actual Liking) will be perceived with a higher status compared to a tutor with (Positive Actual Liking).

H.2-Aff: The **Initial Actual Liking** will have a main effect on perceived **T-Affiliation**, in particular tutor with (Positive Actual Liking) will be perceived with a higher closeness compared to a tutor with (Negative Actual Liking).

H.2-Perf: The **Initial Actual Liking** will have a main effect on perceived **T-Performance**, in particular tutor with (Positive Actual Liking) will be perceived with a higher performance compared to a tutor with (Negative Actual Liking).

5   Results

We conducted a two way repeated measures MANOVA (i.e. multivariate repeated measures analysis of variance) with T-InitialActualLiking as between-subjects factor and T-IdealRelation as within-subjects factor. The dependent measures were tutor's status (**T-Status**), tutor's affiliation (**T-Affiliation**) and tutor's performance (**T-Performance**).

The MANOVA revealed two overall significant main effects of T-InitialActualLiking ($Wilks'Lambda = .57, F(3, 44) = 10.75, p < .001, \eta_p^2 = .44$) and T-IdealRelation ($Wilks'Lambda = .20, F(6, 41) = 26.30, p < .001, \eta_p^2 = .80$). The analysis also indicated a significant interaction effect ($Wilks'Lambda = .35, F(6, 41) = 12.23, p < .001, \eta_p^2 = .64$). Since the sphericity assumption was not violated, we performed a follow-up analysis that looked at univariate effects for each dependent measure with two-way Mixed ANOVAs. These analyses confirmed the significant main effects and interaction of T-InitialActualLiking and T-IdealRelation on our three measurements (all $p < .001$ and effect sizes were ranging from **.20** to **.72**).

This would suggest that **both** tutor's initial *actual liking* of the child and its *ideal relation* have effects on our dependent measures. We conducted a post-hoc analysis by further analyzing the effects of the within-subjects factor, T-IdealRelation, by performing pairwise multiple comparisons with Bonferroni adjustments. Whereas for the between-subjects factor, T-InitialActualLiking, we ran a Simple Main Effects analysis. In Table 1 we report a summary of all means and standard errors (in parentheses) for the 3 dependent variables (DVs) as indicated in the table's heading. The columns describe levels of the within-subjects factor (i.e. T-IdealRelation) corresponding to *positive ideal power* (P+), *positive ideal liking* (L+) and *positive ideal power and liking* (P+L+). The two rows correspond to the two levels of the between-subjects factor (T-InitialActualLiking). For instance, the mean value of the rated status was 5.65 for the interaction where the tutor had a positive *actual liking* and a positive *ideal power*. The follow-up simple main effect analysis revealed that all differences between the two groups were significant ($p \leq .001$) except for those when the tutor had positive ideal power (P+). Those means that did not significantly differ between groups are marked with "*" in the table.

We found that tutor with a positive *ideal power* was perceived with a lower affiliation and performance than tutor with positive *ideal liking* and tutor with both positive *ideal liking and power*, but tutor with both positive *ideal power and liking* (P+L+) was perceived with a lower affiliation and performance than a tutor with a positive *ideal liking* (L+). Thus, our hypotheses **H.1-Aff** and **H.1-Perf** are partially supported. We also found that tutor with a positive ideal power was perceived with a higher status than tutor with positive *ideal liking*

Table 1. Summary of means and standard errors in parentheses for the 3 dependent variables (DVs). The differences between the means marked with "*" (i.e. according to the Initial Actual Liking levels) were not significant. All comparisons among the within-subjects factor's levels were significant ($p \leq .001$) except for the effects of $P+L+$ and $L+$ on tutor's *Status*.

DVs:	T-Status			T-Affiliation			T-Performance		
Ideal relation:	P+	P+L+	L+	P+	P+L+	L+	P+	P+L+	L+
Positive	5.65*	4.05	3.95	2.96*	5.43	5.68	1.97*	5.48	5.73
Initial liking	(±.19)	(±.22)	(±.20)	(±.27)	(±.24)	(±.25)	(±.23)	(±.25)	(±.26)
Negative	5.80*	5.45	5.28	3.09*	3.51	4.15	2.22*	2.70	3.44
Initial liking	(±.19)	(±.22)	(±.20)	(±.27)	(±.24)	(±.25)	(±.23)	(±.25)	(±.26)

and tutor with both positive *ideal liking and power*, but the perceived status was not significantly different between a tutor with a positive *ideal liking* and one with both positive *ideal power and liking*. Thus, **H.1-Sta** is partially supported. Participants rated the tutor with a positive *actual liking* with higher status, affiliation and performance than tutor with a negative *actual liking*. However, the difference between T-InitialActualLiking for the two groups was not significant when the tutor had a positive *ideal power* (P+). Thus, hypotheses **H.2-Sta**, **H.2-Aff** and **H.2-Perf** are partially supported.

6   Discussion and Future Work

We found that participants were able to perceive the tutor's social attitudes when our model was generating sequences of actions according to the tutor's initial *actual liking* and its *ideal social relation*. More specifically, we found that both tutor's initial *actual liking* and tutor's initial *ideal social relation* had main effects on its perceived status, affiliation and performance.

As hypothesized, a tutor with a positive *ideal power* was perceived with a significantly higher status than a tutor with a positive *ideal liking* and both positive *ideal power* and *liking*, but with a significantly lower affiliation and performance (**H.1-Sta**, **H.1-Aff** and **H.1-Perf** partially supported). In our generated sequences of actions, tutors with a positive *ideal power* almost immediately switched off the child's console for forcing it to work, thus possibly explaining the perceived low level of tutor's affiliation. Moreover, tutors with positive *ideal power* preferred using coercive strategies more than explaining to the child the importance of doing its homework and thus a lower performance was attributed to them. However, a tutor with both positive *ideal power* and *liking* was perceived with a lower performance and affiliation than a tutor with only positive *ideal liking*. We believe that tutors with both positive *ideal power and liking* are more pragmatic, thus perceived as less friendly than tutors only aiming at increase a child's liking towards themselves. Moreover, we think that the duration of the interaction was too short for participants in order to identify the child's goals, therefore to judge the tutors' performance. Moreover, since we did not model the content of the child's exercises, it was difficult for participants to judge the quality or the correctness of their homework.

There was a significant interaction effect between the tutor's initial *actual liking* and *ideal social relation* on tutor's perceived status, affiliation and performance. In simple words, the initial *actual liking* had the effect of "amplifying" the outcomes on all dependent measures. Tutor's with a positive *actual liking* were perceived with a significantly higher affiliation and performance than tutors with a negative *actual liking*, but they were perceived with a significantly lower status (**H.2-Sta**, **H.2-Aff** and **H.2-Perf** partially supported). We believe that when the tutor liked the child since the beginning it was displaying more *immediacy* towards the child, therefore increasing affiliation and rapport with it as described in [14]. Another possible explanation is that first impressions induced a cognitive bias which led participants to rate tutors trying to please the child from the beginning with a higher affiliation. Tutors with a positive actual liking might have been considering negotiating with the child to please it, which could have been considered as a sign of submission. However, tutors with positive ideal power were perceived with the same level of status, affiliation and performance, no matter their initial actual liking. One possible explanation is that tutors intending to be dominant immediately used coercive strategies (i.e. switching off the child's console) without trying to explain to the child the importance of working.

Some future work should be considered. Concerning our model, we didn't take interpersonal rigidity [16] into account when computing an agent's social attitude as the mean of actual and ideal social relation. Interpersonal rigidity theory assesses that people with a high level of rigidity tends to maintain the same social attitude through the whole interaction (i.e. considering their *ideal social relation* as more important than their *actual social relation*), whereas people with a low level of rigidity are considered more flexible as they can adapt their attitude according to their interactant's behavior (i.e. considering their *actual social relation* as more important than their *ideal social relation*). Thus, the tutor's level of rigidity would change the importance accorded to its *ideal social relation* and its *actual social relation* when computing its social attitude. Regarding the evaluation, we consider evaluating our model in a context-free interaction, to check whether our results could be generalized outside a tutor-child scenario.

Acknowledgement. This work was partially performed within the Labex SMART (ANR-11-LABX-65). It has also been partially funded by the French National Research Agency project MOCA (ANR-12-CORD-019).

References

1. Argyle, M.: Bodily Communication, 2nd edn. Methuen, New York (1988)
2. Bradley, J.V.: Complete counterbalancing of immediate sequential effects in a Latin square design. J. Am. Stat. Assoc. **53**(282), 525–528 (1958)

3. Cafaro, A., Vilhjálmsson, H.H., Bickmore, T., Heylen, D., Jóhannsdóttir, K.R., Valgardhsson, G.S.: First impressions: users' judgments of virtual agents' personality and interpersonal attitude in first encounters. In: Nakano, Y., Neff, M., Paiva, A., Walker, M. (eds.) IVA 2012. LNCS, vol. 7502, pp. 67–80. Springer, Heidelberg (2012). doi:10.1007/978-3-642-33197-8_7

4. Cafaro, A., Vilhjálmsson, H.H., Bickmore, T., Heylen, D., Pelachaud, C.: Representing communicative functions in SAIBA with a unified function markup language. In: Bickmore, T., Marsella, S., Sidner, C. (eds.) IVA 2014. LNCS, vol. 8637, pp. 81–94. Springer, Heidelberg (2014). doi:10.1007/978-3-319-09767-1_11

5. Callejas, Z., Ravenet, B., Ochs, M., Pelachaud, C.: A computational model of social attitudes for a virtual recruiter. In: Proceedings of the 2014 International Conference on Autonomous Agents and Multi-Agent Systems, pp. 93–100 (2014)

6. Chollet, M., Ochs, M., Pelachaud, C.: From non-verbal signals sequence mining to bayesian networks for interpersonal attitudes expression. In: Bickmore, T., Marsella, S., Sidner, C. (eds.) IVA 2014. LNCS, vol. 8637, pp. 120–133. Springer, Heidelberg (2014). doi:10.1007/978-3-319-09767-1_15

7. Cialdini, R.B., Goldstein, N.J.: Social influence: compliance and conformity. Annu. Rev. Psychol. 55, 591–621 (2004)

8. Goffman, E.: Presentation of self in everyday life. Am. J. Sociol. 55, 6–7 (1949)

9. Krämer, N.C., Karacora, B., Lucas, G., Dehghani, M., Rüther, G., Gratch, J.: Closing the gender gap in stem with friendly male instructors. on the effects of rapport behavior and gender of a virtual agent in an instructional interaction. Computers and Education (2016)

10. Marsella, S.C., Pynadath, D.V., Read, S.J.: PsychSim: agent-based modeling of social interactions and influence. In: Proceedings of the International Conference on Cognitive Modeling, pp. 243–248 (2004)

11. Niewiadomski, R., Bevacqua, E., Mancini, M., Pelachaud, C.: Greta: an interactive expressive ECA system. In: Proceedings of the 8th International Conference on Autonomous Agents and Multiagent Systems, International Foundation for Autonomous Agents and Multiagent Systems, vol. 2, pp. 1399–1400 (2009)

12. Pecune, F., Ochs, M., Marsella, S., Pelachaud, C.: Socrates: from social relation to attitude expressions. In: Proceedings of the 2016 International Conference on Autonomous Agents and Multiagent Systems, International Foundation for Autonomous Agents and Multiagent Systems, pp. 921–930 (2016)

13. Ravenet, B., Cafaro, A., Biancardi, B., Ochs, M., Pelachaud, C.: Conversational behavior reflecting interpersonal attitudes in small group interactions. In: Brinkman, W.-P., Broekens, J., Heylen, D. (eds.) IVA 2015. LNCS, vol. 9238, pp. 375–388. Springer, Heidelberg (2015). doi:10.1007/978-3-319-21996-7_41

14. Richmond, V., McCroskey, J., Hickson, M.: Nonverbal Communication in Interpersonal Relations, 6th edn. Allyn and Bacon, Boston (2008)

15. Scherer, K.R.: What are emotions? and how can they be measured? Soc. Sci. Inf. 44(4), 695–729 (2005)

16. Tracey, T.J.: Interpersonal rigidity and complementarity. J. Res. Pers. 39(6), 592–614 (2005)

17. Trapnell, P.D., Broughton, R.H.: The interpersonal questionnaire (ipq): duodecant markers of wiggins' interpersonal circumplex. The University of Winnipeg (2006). Unpublished data

18. Tschannen-Moran, M., Hoy, A.W.: Teacher efficacy: capturing an elusive construct. Teach. Teach. Educ. 17(7), 783–805 (2001)

19. Wiggins, J.S., Trapnell, P.D.: A dyadic-interactional perspective on the five-factor model. In: Wiggins, J.S. (ed.) The Five-Factor Model of Personality: Theoretical Perspectives, pp. 88–162. Guilford Press, New York (1996)
20. Wubbels, T., Opdenakker, M.C., Den Brok, P.: Lets make things better. In: Wubbels, T., den Brok, P., van Tartwijk, J., Levy, J. (eds.) Interpersonal Relationships in Education, pp. 225–249. Springer, Heidelberg (2012)

Robots or Agents – Neither Helps You More or Less During Second Language Acquisition

Experimental Study on the Effects of Embodiment and Type of Speech Output on Evaluation and Alignment

Astrid M. Rosenthal-von der Pütten[✉], Carolin Straßmann, and Nicole C. Krämer

Department for Social Psychology: Media and Communication,
University of Duisburg-Essen, Forsthausweg 2, 47057 Duisburg, Germany
{a.rosenthalvdpuetten,carolin.strassmann,
Nicole.kraemer}@uni-due.de

Abstract. When designing an artificial tutor, the question arises: should we opt for a virtual or a physical embodied conversational agent? With this work we contribute to the ongoing debate of whether, when and how virtual agents or robots provide more benefits to the user and conducted an experimental study on linguistic alignment processes in HCI in the context of second language acquisition. In our study (n = 130 non-native speakers) we explored the influence of design characteristics and investigated the influence of embodiment (virtual agent vs. robot vs. speech based interaction) and system voice (text-to-speech vs. pre-recorded speech) on participants' perception of the system, their motivation, their lexical and syntactical alignment during interaction and their learning effect after the interaction. The variation of system characteristics had no influence on the evaluation of the system or participants' alignment behavior.

Keywords: Linguistic alignment · Second language acquisition · Virtual agent · Robot · Speech output · Nonverbal behavior · Embodiment · Experimental study

1 Introduction

When designing an artificial tutor, numerous decisions have to be made regarding system characteristics. One of the most influential decisions pertains to the question of whether to employ and develop a virtual or physically embodied conversational agent. Virtual agents are comparably cheap and more flexible, but robots are seen to provide an even richer interactive experience, because they can manipulate their environment and actually get in physical contact with users [1]. New approaches opt for migrating both types of artificial entities into one entity represented differently (e.g. as robot or as screen agent) depending on where the user is located [2]. However, it is unclear whether there is a preference of one embodiment form over the other dependent on the specific task the user intends to complete with the help of the system. Results of previous research are somewhat inconclusive (cf. [3] for an extensive review). While quite a number of studies showed that a robot is more persuasive, receives more attention and is perceived

© Springer International Publishing AG 2016
D. Traum et al. (Eds.): IVA 2016, LNAI 10011, pp. 256–268, 2016.
DOI: 10.1007/978-3-319-47665-0_23

more positively than a virtual agent, there is a general lack of studies examining different behavioral outcomes, particularly, with regard to linguistic behavior. One important future application field for virtual agents and robots are tutoring systems. Artificial tutors could especially be helpful to assist with second language acquisition, because they could help overcome inhibition effects which can occur in human-human interaction due to native speakers linguistically aligning "downward" to non-natives and simplifying their language use. Because people tend to align more strongly to computers than to humans [4], this mechanism might lead to enhanced learning outcomes when computers expose a high standard in the language to learn so that learners are prompted to align upward. Thus, we hypothesize that processes of linguistic alignment in HCI can be exploited to help second language acquisition. However, system characteristics such as embodiment might influence alignment processes. Moreover, alignment processes are supposedly dependent on the learners' comprehension of the speech output of the artificial tutor. Hence, it is important to investigate whether current text-to-speech (tts) software is of sufficient quality to not inhibit alignment and hence also learning processes. Although using prerecorded natural speech would annul comprehension deficits of tts systems, it is more effortful to add study units later on. Thus, we explore whether linguistic alignment can be used in the context of second language acquisition to support learning and whether and if yes how system design characteristics such as embodiment and quality of speech output influence evaluation and learning outcome.

1.1 Effects of Differently Embodied Artificial Entities

Virtual agent or robot? This is an essential design decision developers have to make when designing new embodied conversational agents. Both embodiment types provide unique interaction possibilities, but also come along with certain restrictions. In a sense virtual agents are more flexible than robots in that we can easily change a virtual agent's appearance. Hence the appearance can be matched to users' preferences, to the needs of special target groups or to the corporate design of the developing company. Virtual agents can appear on different devices including smartphones. Moreover, they have unlimited degrees of freedom and can perform actions that are not possible in real life. In contrast, robots have limited degrees of freedom, their design cannot be changed easily. Most of the available products are quite stationary and thus can only be used at home or at work. A big advantage of robots is that they are "tangible artifacts" [1], which can be touched, and are able to manipulate their environment by means of physical contact to objects as well as to human interaction partners. Studies comparing robots and virtual agents led to inconsistent results. A majority of findings suggests that robots are superior to virtual representations with regard to the perceived social presence of the entity [5], the evaluation of the entity as entertaining or enjoyable [1, 6], and trustworthy [6]. Furthermore, robots have been demonstrated to be more persuasive [7], elicit more attention [8], and increase user's task performance [9]. On the contrary, other results point to superiority of a virtual representation when the outcome variable is information disclosed to the entity [7]. In fact, there seems to be an interaction effect of embodiment and task. Regarding the evaluation of task attractiveness, Hoffmann and Krämer [10] demonstrated that a robot was better evaluated in a task-related scenario, while a virtual representation was favored for a conversation. Finally, a study by Bartneck [9] yielded no differences between a robot and a screen animation with regard to how entertaining the interaction was evaluated. Also, Kennedy et al. [8] observed no difference in children's learning increase when interacting with a real NAO robot or an animation of the robot on a screen. Only one study investigated participants' linguistic behavior on the context of differently embodied agents [11]. It was found that verbosity and complexity of linguistic utterances did not differ between a virtual agent or a robot, but participants used more interactional features of language towards the robot such as directly addressing it by its name. The interplay of embodiment and linguistic alignment has not been investigated so far.

1.2   Linguistic Alignment in HHI, HCI and in Context of Second Language Acquisition

Empirical evidence in human-human-interaction (HHI) research showed that interaction partners align linguistically in conversations on different levels, for instance, regarding accent or dialect [12], speech rhythm [13], lexical choices and semantics [14] as well as syntax [15]. Quite a number of these effects also occur in interactions with artificial entities. Similarly to HHI, users align to computers, for instance, with regard to prosody, lexis, and syntax (for an overview cf. [16]). Studies with virtual agents showed the same tendencies: in the interaction with a virtual tutor users aligned to lay language or medical jargon [17] and to dialect or standard language [18]. However, studies suggest that alignment in HHI and HCI is similar but not the same, since people tend to show stronger alignment with computers [4] presumably to compensate the computers weaker communicative abilities. However, although initial beliefs about their artificial interaction partner are taken into account by human users, recent comparative work showed that "when social cues and presence as created by a virtual human come into play, automatic social reactions appear to override initial beliefs in shaping lexical alignment." [19]. An open question is whether the physical embodiment of the artificial interlocutor strengthens this effect of blurring boundaries or not. This would be especially important to know when designing artificial language tutors for SLA. Native-speakers often adapt to non-natives in order to foster mutual understanding and successful communication, sometimes with the negative outcome of interfering with successful SLA on a native-speaker level. Using artificial tutors could help to overcome this bias. Since users more strongly align to computers in order to ensure communicative success, there is a potential to exploit these alignment processes for SLA. A first study with native and non-native speakers showed that both groups aligned lexically to a virtual tutor. However, alignment was weaker for non-natives [20] due to a substantial lack of fluency. For instance, if people are not able to conjugate a verb or have trouble to pronounce words correctly, they tend to choose easier vocabulary [21]. Hence, participants might not be able to reproduce all linguistic nuances. This might also be due to the speech output quality of the agent since tts systems do not expose perfect pronunciation. Still, alignment is seen as core to language acquisition, thus, also to SLA [22] and the tendency of non-natives to align to technology in a learning setting could be exploited for SLA. Admittedly, system characteristics have to be taken into account and their potential inhibiting effects need to be explored – especially in the case of speech output quality.

1.3 Research Questions and Hypotheses

In this work we explore the potential of artificial tutors to avoid inhibition effects and exploit linguistic alignment processes in HCI for SLA. In particular, we examine whether an artificial tutor's embodiment (virtual agent vs. robot vs. speech based interaction) influences participants' evaluation of the tutor, their lexical and syntactical alignment during interaction and their learning effect after the interaction (*RQ1*). Since previous work showed that robots can elicit more positive evaluations than virtual agents (5–9), we propose that the robot will be rated most positively followed by the virtual agent and the solely language-based tutor (*H1*). In contrast to classic language learning software like DVDs or online platforms, most virtual agents and robots do not use prerecorded natural speech, but tts software which could affect listening comprehension and thereby alignment. Thus, quality of speech output is also varied in our study (*RQ2*). Moreover, we want to know whether alignment in dialog results in better performance in a post interaction language test (*RQ3*).

2 Method

2.1 Experimental Design and Independent Variables

In order to determine which system characteristics people prefer in their interaction with an artificial tutor, we chose a 3 × 2 between-subjects design with *speech output* and *embodiment* as independent variables. We used three types of embodiment of the artificial tutor. Participants either interacted exclusively language-based (and saw only a blue screen with the text "language learning system"), or they interacted with a virtual version of the Nao robot or the physical present Nao robot. Secondly, we varied the artificial tutor's speech output. Participants were either confronted with speech output generated by tts software or with prerecorded natural speech (ns). Since Nao's tts system is installed on the physical Nao itself and thus is not available for the virtual Nao, we generated wave files by recording the tts speech output. Natural speech was recorded after generating the tts soundfiles. The speaker was instructed to speak similarly, i.e. imitate intonation and speed (sounds examples can be found in the supplementary material). In order to avoid different perceptions of presence due to sound quality (and not type of speech output), we also used the sound files for the people interacting with the physical Nao.

2.2 Participants and Procedure

One hundred and thirty volunteers (74 female, 56 male) aged between 15 and 53 years (M = 26.6; SD = 6.87) participated in this study. Seventeen participants had previously interacted with a robot and 26 had interacted with a robot. Participants stem from more

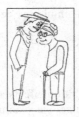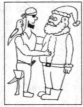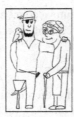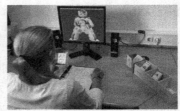

Fig. 1. Left: examples for interaction cards in the guessing game; Right: participant playing the guessing game with the virtual Nao

than 40 different countries, speak more than 25 different native languages and exposed different levels of German language skills (with a minimum of an intermediate level). Participants were recruited on campus or in German classes in the local adult education center. The study was approved by the local ethics committee. Upon arrival participants read and signed informed consent. They completed two language tests: a test on grammar and reading and listening comprehension and a so called C-Test (www.c-test.de), a cloze test which also addresses language skills with regard to different dimensions. Based on their test results, their country of origin and first language, respectively, participants were distributed equally across conditions where possible and were invited for a second appointment. On the second appointment participants were instructed about the different tasks to be solved with the artificial tutor. Each task was again explained by the tutor during the interaction (cf. Fig. 1). Participants were also given a folder with detailed instructions in case they did not understand the tutor. Participants completed five tasks: (1) introducing themselves, (2) describing a picture in detail, (3) playing a guessing game, (4) playing a search game, and (5) again describing a picture. The order of tasks was always the same for all participants. The first two tasks were used to make participants comfortable at speaking loudly to the system. The two structured games (guessing game and search game) were used to analyze alignment processes. We repeated the task of describing a picture to give participants another possibility to speak quite freely at the end of the learning session. This was done to create a more believable training environment for the participants. After the interaction, participants completed a second C-Test as a measure of learning outcome and a questionnaire asking for their experiences and assessment of the interaction. Finally, they were debriefed, reimbursed (€10) and thanked for participation.

2.3   Dependent Variables: Self-report

Perception of the Artificial Tutor.   For the person perception of the artificial tutor, we used the Godspeed Questionnaire [23], a semantic differential with 25 bi-polar items which are rated on a 5-point scale. We used the four subscales *Anthropomorphism* (attribution of a human form, characteristics, or behavior to nonhuman things; 5 items, e.g. fake-natural, machinelike-humanlike; Cronbach's $\alpha = .889$), *Animacy* (perception of lifelikeness; 5 items, e.g. dead-alive; stagnant-lively; Cronbach's $\alpha = .880$), *Liking*

(5 items, e.g. dislike-like, unfriendly-friendly; Cronbach's α = .844), and *Perceived Intelligence* (5 items, e.g. incompetent-competent; Cronbach's α = .789).

Social Presence. We assessed participants' sense of co-presence with the Nowak and Biocca Presence Scale [24], which contains 12 items on the concept of "perceived other's co-presence" (Cronbach's α = .716) and 6 items on "self-reported co-presence" (Cronbach's α = .716), both rated on a 5-point Likert scale.

General Evaluation of the Interaction. The general evaluation of the interaction was assessed by eight items that asked for the participants' sense of control during the interaction, the enjoyment of the interaction, and whether participants like to use a system like this for other tasks (rated on a 5-point Likert scale; Cronbach's α = .793).

Speech Output. Additionally, we asked, on a 5-point Likert-scale from "very mechanical" to "very humanlike", how humanlike they perceived the speech output to be.

2.4 Dependent Variables: Linguistic Alignment

In order to analyze linguistic alignment with the artificial tutor, participants played two structured games (guessing game and search game) in which the tutor and the participant took turns in constructing sentences.

Guessing Game. The first structured game was a dialog based game adapted from Branigan et al. [15]. In the original game participants took turns in describing a card and trying to find this card out of a set of cards. The description was originally one sentence. In our adaption of the game participants took turns in guessing the two persons and their interaction on so-called interaction cards (cf. Fig. 1) by asking only yes-or-no questions similarly to the "Who am I" guessing game (e.g. "Is the person on the left side female?"; "Is the person on the right side old?", "Is the interaction between the two friendly?"). Questions are asked in a structured manner: first guess who is one the left, then who is on the right and lastly, find out the interaction between the two. By this we created more opportunities to vary lexical and syntactic choices within one round of the guessing game. There were two rounds of guessing in which the system first guessed the participant's card and then the participant guessed the system's card. Between the two rounds, the system changed linguistic choices (e.g. lexical choices (mustache vs. beard); usage of different prepositions, verbs, adjectives or active and passive sentences). Participants ´ verbal utterances were analyzed with regard to their lexical choices. A ratio was built for alignment (usage of the same lexical choice (e.g. mustache)/occurrence of the concept (e.g. number of linguistic expression referring to a beard)).

Search Game. The second structured game was also a dialog based game in which the participant and the tutor took turns in describing picture cards to one another. For this game is used the original experimental setup used by Branigan et al. [15] in order to study syntactic alignment. The cards displayed two characters (e.g. policeman and cowboy) a verb (e.g. to give), and an object (e.g. balloon, cf. Fig. 2). Participants had two sets of cards (reading cards and search cards). The task was to take a card from the

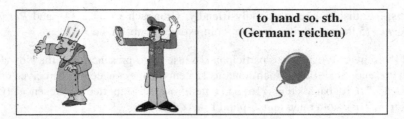

Fig. 2. Example card for the search game

first card set (reading cards) and to form a sentence based on the characters, verb and object displayed on the card (e.g. the balloon was given to the policemen by the cowboy). The interaction partner's task was to search in their set of "search cards" for this exact card. This means that the system's search cards are identical to participant's reading cards and vice versa. The system began the interaction and built a sentence. The participant had to find the card and put it away and in turn had to take a card from the "reading" set and form a sentence so that the tutor can find the card in its (imagined) search card pool and put it away. In total, the system read out 15 cards, thereby formed 15 sentences in three "blocks". The first block i.e. the first five sentences were formed as passive voice, the second five sentences as prepositional phrase and the last as accusative. A ratio was built for syntactical alignment (usage of the same case/5 sentences). Since previous research showed that alignment can occur with a delay [25], we also examined whether participants aligned to previously heard syntactic choices, and e.g. in the second block aligned to the first block and in the third block aligned to the second block, respectively.

2.5 Dependent Variables: Learning Outcome

As described in Sect. 2.2, participants exposed different levels of German language skills which were assessed by two language tests: first a standard test on grammar and reading and listening comprehension and second a so called C-Test (www.c-test.de), a cloze test which also addresses language skills with regard to different dimensions. The C-Test was completed again after the interaction with the tutoring system. To explore whether the interaction has a positive effect on participants' language skills we analyzed the results of the C-Tests prior and after the interaction. The C-Test has been used previously for accessing language skills and also improvement in language skills [26]. It usually comprises of five short pieces of self-contained text (ca. 80 words or four to five sentences) in which single words are "damaged". The first sentence is undamaged. Beginning with the second word in the second sentence there are 20 damaged words alternating with undamaged words. In order to reconstruct the sentences, participants have to activate their language fluency. Text pieces were taken from reading exams on an academic language level. Tests are analyzed by true-false answers. Participants could reach 100 points at most.

3   Results

Data were analyzed with ANOVAS and correlation analyses using IBM®SPSS Statistics 21. However, we also estimated Bayes factors using Bayesian Information Criteria [17], comparing the fit of the data under the null hypothesis and the alternative hypothesis using R and the package BayesFactor by Richard D. Morey.

3.1   Participants' Self-reported Experiences

First, the speech output conditions did not differ regarding how humanlike the voice was perceived (ns: M = 2.80, SD = .70; tts M = 2.72, SD = .75). In order to examine whether embodiment or speech output affects the evaluation of the tutor or the interaction, we conducted ANOVAS with these both factors as independent variables and the dependent variables *general evaluation, perceived others co-presence, self-reported co-presence, likability, perceived intelligence, anthropomorphism,* and *animacy.* There were no significant differences between the groups nor did we find significant interaction effects (no support for *H1*, cf. Table 1). An estimated Bayes factor (null/alternative) suggested that the data were between 2.3 and 13.1 times more likely to occur under a model without including an effect of embodiment or speech output, rather than a model with these factors.

Table 1. Means and standard deviations of self-reported dependent variables

	Speech ns[a]	Speech tts[b]	Virtual ns	Virtual tts	Robot ns	Robot tts	BF[c]	BF[d]
	M (SD)	M (SD)	M (SD)	M (SD)	M (SD)	M (SD)	Emb.	SO.
Gen. Eval.	4.09 (.67)	4.24 (.50)	4.17 (.53)	4.13 (.53)	4.26 (.71)	4.31 (.45)	4.9	5.3
Perc Oth CoPres	2.94 (.27)	3.17 (.28)	3.07 (.28)	3.10 (.38)	3.06 (.33)	3.03 (.31)	11.7	2.3
Self-rep CoPres	3.14 (.45)	2.87 (.37)	2.97 (.40)	2.94 (.37)	2.90 (.31)	2.98 (.50)	8.8	4.0
Likability	4.20 (.72)	4.44 (.56)	4.26 (.67)	4.35 (.55)	4.43 (.63)	4.36 (.67)	11.3	4.1
Perc. Intel.	4.13 (.71)	4.07 (.83)	4.05 (.48)	4.08 (.61)	4.08 (.62)	4.06 (.64)	13.1	5.3
Anthropomo.	3.32 (1.19)	3.39 (1.13)	2.88 (1.07)	3.20 (.98)	3.19 (1.03)	3.10 (1.00)	6.3	4.8
Animacy	3.44 (1.04)	3.73 (.84)	3.04 (.97)	3.41 (.94)	3.42 (.96)	3.30 (.83)	3.9	3.3

Notes: [a]ns = natural speech; [b]tts = text-to-speech; [c]BF = Bayes Factor Embodiment; [d]BF = Bayes Factor Speech Output

3.2   Participants' Linguistic Alignment

Guessing Game. With the guessing game we examined participants' syntactical and semantical alignment during the interaction. Therefore, the system's utterances between the two rounds varied in lexical choices when describing the features of the displayed characters (*age* (old vs. advanced in years), *gender* (male/female vs. a man/a woman), *facial hair* (mustache vs. beard)). Moreover, the system used different *verbs* (has vs. wears), *adjectives* (friendly vs. kind) and syntactical constructions (*person on the left side vs. the left person; active vs. passive*). As described above, a ratio was calculated for alignment (usage of the same lexical/syntactical choice (e.g. lexical choice mustache)/occurrence of the concept (e.g. number of expressions referring to a beard)). To examine whether embodiment or speech output affects participants' linguistic alignment, we conducted ANOVAS with both factors as independent variables and the seven ratios for linguistic alignment as dependent variables. There were no significant differences between the groups nor did we find significant interaction effects (cf. Table 2). An estimated Bayes factor (null/alternative) suggested that the data were between 1.7 and 9.4 times more likely to occur under a model without including an effect of embodiment or speech output, rather than a model with these factors.

Table 2. Means and standard deviations for alignment ratios in the guessing game

	Speech ns[a]	Speech tts[b]	Virtual ns	Virtual tts	Robot ns	Robot tts	BF[c]	BF[d]
	MD (SD)	MD (SD)	MD (SD)	MD (SD)	MD (SD)	MD (SD)	Emb.	SO.
Left/right	.43 (.19)	.37 (.31)	.29 (.16)	.43 (.26)	.36 (.29)	.43 (.18)	9.4	3.0
Age	.52 (.29)	.43 (.15)	.45 (.25)	.60 (.34)	.60 (.32)	.58 (.37)	3.9	4.8
Gender	.64 (.27)	.65 (.24)	.61 (.26)	.58 (.22)	.56 (.30)	.64 (.26)	8.6	4.7
Face hair	.39 (.49)	.44 (.42)	.43 (.41)	.29 (.41)	.21 (.28)	.49 (.47)	3.9	4.8
Verb	.63 (.34)	.44 (.41)	.49 (.24)	.65 (.32)	.64 (.37)	.57 (.32)	7.6	4.3
Adjective	.66 (.40)	.50 (.44)	.46 (.38)	.34 (.40)	.46 (.38)	.38 (.43)	2.2	1.7
Act./pas.	.39 (.24)	.53 (.30)	.61 (.26)	.38 (.41)	.57 (.33)	.47 (.41)	9.0	4.8

Notes: [a]ns = natural speech; [b]tts = text-to-speech; [c]BF = Bayes Factor Embodiment; [d]BF = Bayes Factor Speech Output

Search Game. The search game focused on the syntactical alignment. Regarding all 15 sentences, participants most often used accusative ($M = 6.61$, $SD = 5.08$), followed by prepositional phrases ($M = 3.49$, $SD = 3.91$) and passive voice ($M = 3.01$, $SD = 3.73$). In order to examine whether embodiment or speech output affects participants' syntactical alignment, we conducted ANOVAS with both these factors as independent variables and the alignment ratio. There were no significant differences between groups nor did we find significant interaction effects. Since studies have shown that alignment can occur with a delay [25], we also analyzed whether participants aligned to the previous blocks. Again there were no significant differences between the experimental groups with regard to embodiment and speech output nor interaction effects (cf. Table 3). An estimated Bayes factor (null/alternative) suggested that the data were between 2.4 and 11.7 times more likely to occur under a model without including an effect of embodiment or speech output, rather than a model with these factors.

Table 3. Means and standard deviations for alignment ratios in the search game

Alignment	Speech ns[a]	Speech tts[b]	Virtual ns	Virtual tts	Robot ns	Robot tts	BF[c]	BF[d]
	MD (SD)	MD (SD)	MD (SD)	MD (SD)	MD (SD)	MD (SD)	Emb.	SO.
Direct	.34 (.17)	.36 (.16)	.38 (.18)	.46 (.19)	.34 (.19)	.37 (.16)	2.4	5.2
Delayed	.23 (.19)	.18 (.21)	.25 (.24)	.26 (.22)	.18 (.23)	.20 (.20)	11.7	5.7

Notes: [a]ns = natural speech; [b]tts = text-to-speech; [c]BF = Bayes Factor Embodiment; [d]BF = Bayes Factor Speech Output

3.3 Language Skills and Learning Effect

To explore whether the interaction has a positive effect on participants' language skills we analyzed the results of the C-Tests prior and after the interaction. Thus, we conducted split-plot ANOVAS with the group factors embodiment and speech output and repeated measures for the C-Test. Two main effects emerged. First, participants' C-Test scores were worse after the interaction ($M = 51.90$, $SD = 17.09$) than at their first appointment to assess their language proficiency level ($M = 55.77$, $SD = 19.43$; $F(124, 1) = 29.97$; $p < .001$, $\eta p^2 = .195$). Moreover, the system's embodiment influenced participants' C-Test scores after the interaction ($F(124, 2) = 6.24$; $p = .003$, $\eta p^2 = .091$). The descriptive data suggests that participants interacting with a robot had lower test results than those interacting with a virtual agent or only language-based (cf. Table 4). The factor speech output showed no effect, nor did we find interaction effects. One goal of this study was to explore the potential of artificial tutors to exploit linguistic alignment processes in HCI for SLA. Thus, we correlated participants' alignment ratios with their C-Test results after the interaction, but did not find a significant correlation.

Table 4. Means and standard deviations for the pre and post C-Test (language skill test)

| | Speech ns[a] | Speech tts[b] | Virtual ns | Virtual tts | Robot ns | Robot tts |
	MD (SD)	MD (SD)	MD (SD)	MD (SD)	MD (SD)	MD (SD)
Pre C-Test	61.95 (22.97)	53.81 (16.44)	57.15 (20.44)	57.72 (17.23)	49.35 (21.23)	54.18 (18.16)
Post C-Test	55.00 (19.28)	50.09 (13.83)	51.25 (18.00)	52.20 (15.68)	51.85 (18.58)	51.00 (18.48)

Notes: [a]ns = natural speech; [b]tts = text-to-speech

4 Discussion

With this work we contribute to the ongoing debate of whether virtual agents or robots provide more benefits to the user. Previous work predominantly found that robots were more persuasive, entertaining, enjoyable, and trustworthy. Moreover, they elicit more attention, and increase user's task performance (cf. [3] for an overview). However, there is a lack of research on behavioral effects, particularly, with regard to linguistic behavior. Moreover, some studies found interaction effects of type of embodiment and type of task showing that robots were preferred for (physical) tasks and virtual agents for conversations [10]. We conducted an experimental study on linguistic alignment processes in HCI in the context of SLA and varied the artificial tutor's embodiment (virtual agent vs. robot vs. speech based interaction). Moreover, we argued that tts systems might be problematic in SLA since they do not always pronounce words correctly and therefore we varied whether participants heard tts or prerecorded natural speech. We found that neither embodiment nor quality of speech output influenced participants' perception of the system or their lexical and syntactical alignment during interaction. There were no differences in perceived human-likeness of the speech output. Regarding language skills, participants performed worse in the language test after the interaction compared to the first appointment where participants' language skills were assessed in order to distribute them equally across conditions. We did not find the hoped for positive influence of the system on language skills. This might be due to the different workload of the two appointments. In the initial appointment participants only completed these language tests. On the second appointment they first interacted with the system for about 50 min and then completed the language test. Since participants had to concentrate on the tutoring system and interact with it by speaking German this means constant cognitive effort. Hence, participants were probably less concentrated and more exhausted in the posttest than in the pretest. However, there was one effect regarding embodiment: Participants interacting with a robot (regardless of quality of speech output) performed worse in the posttest. Although there were no evaluation differences, we observed that participants were more excited meeting the physical Nao than meeting the virtual or speech-based system. Some of them explored the Nao or even took a picture. Supposedly, at least some participants paid less attention to the actual tasks ahead and concentrated on the robot itself. In sum, the variation of system characteristics had barely influence on the evaluation of the system (*H1*) or participants' alignment behavior – neither for embodiment (*RQ1*) nor for quality of speech output (*RQ2*). In this study we kept the appearance of the system between the virtually embodied and physically embodied condition consistent with the virtual version of the actual Nao robot. It could be that the recorded speech might be evaluated differently when matched with a human form like a humanlike virtual agent. It is, however, striking that prerecorded speech and tts did also not differ in perceived human-likeness in the language-based only conditions when there is no possible match or mismatch with the appearance of the tutor.

There are several implications relevant for designers of artificial tutors. First, at least in the domain of language learning with predominantly conversation based tasks the type of embodiment or more precisely embodiment itself in whatever form did not result in more positive evaluation effects or different linguistic behavior. Hence, developers can opt for the more flexible and inexpensive virtual agent or solely speech-based system. Second, tts systems have a sufficient quality to be used for SLA purposes. Astonishingly, the tts was perceived only marginally less humanlike than the actual human voice. Since the usage of prerecorded speech is more expensive, harder to implement and to change later on (e.g. extend learning system with new learning situations/ games etc.), it is good news that tts systems are perceived equally positive.

Moreover, we wanted to know whether alignment in dialog results in better performance in the post interaction language test (*RQ3*). We found that although participants aligned to the artificial tutor in all conditions comparably to previous studies [17, 19, 20] this did not significantly contribute to the post interaction test performance. Maybe participants would need more learning sessions to benefit from the system and to transfer the alignment into a learning progress. Moreover, the descriptive analysis of the seven alignment ratios showed that participants aligned differently strongly. For instance, they aligned more when referring to *gender* than to *facial hair*. Moreover, alignment is generally lower for any passive construction, because they are also rarely used in everyday conversations. Moreover, we observed that participants with lower initial language skills had trouble in producing sentences. This may have confounded the process of alignment which is at least in part an unconscious process based on priming [14–16]. If words or constructions are not known, they cannot be easily activated by primes thereby eliciting alignment. Hence, linguistic alignment in SLA might only be effective for very advanced language learners. Future work should explore whether repeated tutoring sessions accumulate in a learning effect that might be moderated by alignment during the interaction sessions. Moreover, more distinct groups of participants regarding their initial language skills might give insight into the question of whether alignment contributes effectively to SLA only for advanced learners.

Acknowledgements. The noALIEN (Using linguistic alignment in German language promotion for immigrants on the basis of human-technology interaction) project was funded by the German Federal Ministry of Education and Research.

References

1. Wainer, J., Feil-Seifer, D.J., Shell, D., et al.: Embodiment and human-robot interaction: a task-based perspective. In: 16th IEEE International Conference on Robot and Human Interactive Communication, pp. 872–877. IEEE, Piscataway (2007)
2. Aylett, R., Kriegel, M., Wallace, I., et al.: Memory and the design of migrating virtual agents. In: Proceedings of the 2013 International Conference on Autonomous Agents and Multi-agent Systems, pp. 1311–1312. International Foundation for Autonomous Agents and Multiagent Systems (2013)
3. Li, J.: The benefit of being physically present: a survey of experimental works comparing copresent robots, telepresent robots and virtual agents. Int. J. Hum. Comput. Stud. **77**, 23–37 (2015). doi:10.1016/j.ijhcs.2015.01.001
4. Branigan, H.P., Pickering, M.J., Pearson, J., et al.: Beliefs about mental states in lexical and syntactic alignment: evidence from human-computer dialogs. In: Proceedings of the 17th CUNY Conference on Human Sentence Processing (2004)
5. Fasola, J., Mataric, M.: A socially assistive robot exercise coach for the elderly. J. Hum. Robot Interact. **2**(2), 3–32 (2013)
6. Kidd, C.D., Breazeal, C.L.: Effect of a robot on user perceptions. In: Proceedings of the IEEE/RSJ International Conference on Intelligent Robots and Systems (IROS 2004), pp. 3559–3564. IEEE, Piscataway (2004)
7. Kiesler, S.B., Powers, A., Fussell, S.R., et al.: Anthropomorphic interactions with a robot and robot-like agent. Soc. Cogn. **26**(2), 169–181 (2008). doi:10.1521/soco.2008.26.2.169
8. Kennedy, J., Baxter, P., Belpaeme, T.: Comparing robot embodiments in a guided discovery learning interaction with children. Int. J. Soc. Robot. **7**(2), 293–308 (2015). doi:10.1007/s12369-014-0277-4
9. Bartneck, C.: Interacting with an embodied emotional character. In: Proceedings of the International Conference on Designing Pleasurable Products and Interfaces, pp. 55–60. ACM Press, New York (2003)
10. Hoffmann, L., Krämer, N.C.: Investigating the effects of physical and virtual embodiment in task-oriented and conversational contexts. Int. J. Hum. Comput. Stud. **71**(7–8), 763–774 (2013). doi:10.1016/j.ijhcs.2013.04.007
11. Fischer, K., Lohan, K.S., Foth, K.: Levels of embodiment: linguistic analyses of factors influencing HRI. In: Proceedings of the 7th ACM/IEEE International Conference on Human-Robot Interaction (HRI 2012), pp. 463–470 (2012)
12. Giles, H.: Accent mobility: a model and some data. Anthropol. Linguist. **15**, 87–105 (1973)
13. Reed, B.S.: Speech rhythm across turn transitions in cross-cultural talk-in-interaction. Special Issue Pragmat. Perspect. Parliam. Discourse J. Pragmat. **42**(4), 1037–1059 (2010). doi:10.1016/j.pragma.2009.09.002

14. Brennan, S.E., Clark, H.H.: Conceptual pacts and lexical choice in conversation. J. Exp. Psychol. Learn. Memory Cogn. **22**, 1482–1493 (1996)
15. Branigan, H.P., Pickering, M.J., Cleland, A.A.: Syntactic co-ordination in dialogue. Cognition **75**(2), B13–B25 (2000)
16. Branigan, H.P., Pickering, M.J., Pearson, J., et al.: Linguistic alignment between people and computers. J Pragmat. **42**(9), 2355–2368 (2010). doi:10.1016/j.pragma.2009.12.012
17. Rosenthal-von der Pütten, A.M., Wiering, L., Krämer, N.C., et al.: Great minds think alike. Experimental study on lexical alignment in human-agent interaction. i-com **12**(1), 32–38 (2013). doi:10.1524/icom.2013.0005
18. Kühne, V., Rosenthal-von der Pütten, A.M., Krämer, N.C.: Using linguistic alignment to enhance learning experience with pedagogical agents: the special case of dialect. In: Aylett, R., Krenn, B., Pelachaud, C., Shimodaira, H. (eds.) IVA 2013. LNCS, vol. 8108, pp. 149–158. Springer, Heidelberg (2013)
19. Bergmann, K., Branigan, H.P., Kopp, S.: Exploring the alignment space – lexical and gestural alignment with real and virtual humans. Front. ICT **2**, 7 (2015). doi:10.3389/fict.2015.00007
20. Wunderlich, H.: Talking like a machine?! Linguistic alignment of native-speakers and non-native speakers in interaction with a virtual agent. Bachelor thesis, University of Duisburg-Essen (2012)
21. Costa, A., Pickering, M.J., Sorace, A.: Alignment in second language dialogue. Lang. Cogn. Proc. **23**(4), 528–556 (2008). doi:10.1080/01690960801920545
22. Atkinson, D., Churchill, E., Nishino, T., et al.: Alignment and interaction in a sociocognitive approach to second language acquisition. Mod. Lang. J. **91**(2), 169–188 (2007). doi:10.1111/j.1540-4781.2007.00539.x
23. Bartneck, C., Kulić, D., Croft, E., et al.: measurement instruments for the anthropomorphism, animacy, likeability, perceived intelligence, and perceived safety of robots. Int. J. Soc. Robot. **1**(1), 71–81 (2009). doi:10.1007/s12369-008-0001-3
24. Nowak, K.L., Biocca, F.: The Effect of the agency and anthropomorphism on users' sense of telepresence, copresence, and social presence in virtual environments. Presence Teleop. Virtual **12**(5), 481–494 (2003). doi:10.1162/105474603322761289
25. Reuter, M.: Linguistic alignment with virtual agents. Bachelor thesis, University of Duisburg-Essen (2011)
26. Baur, R.S., Meder, G.: C-Tests zur Ermittlung der globalen Sprachfähigkeit im Deutschen und einer Muttersprache bei ausländischen Schülern in der Bundesrepublik Deutschland. In: Grotjahn, R. (ed.) Der C-Tes. Theoretische Grundlagen und praktische Anwendungent. Brockmeyer, Bochum (1994)
27. Wagenmakers, E.J.: A practical solution to the pervasive problems of p values. Psychon. Bull. Rev. **14**(5), 779–804 (2007)

Impact of Individual Differences on Affective Reactions to Pedagogical Agents Scaffolding

Sébastien Lallé[1(✉)], Nicholas V. Mudrick[2], Michelle Taub[2], Joseph F. Grafsgaard[2], Cristina Conati[1], and Roger Azevedo[2]

[1] Department of Computer Science, University of British Columbia, Vancouver, BC, Canada
{lalles, conati}@cs.ubc.ca
[2] Department of Psychology, North Carolina State University, Raleigh, NC, USA
{nvmudric, mtaub, jfgrafsg, razeved}@ncsu.edu

Abstract. Students' emotions are known to influence learning and motivation while working with agent-based learning environments (ABLEs). However, there is limited understanding of how Pedagogical Agents (PAs) impact different students' emotions, what those emotions are, and whether this is modulated by students' individual differences (e.g., personality, goal orientation). Such understanding could be used to devise intelligent PAs that can recognize and adapt to students' relevant individual differences in order to enhance their experience with learning environments. In this paper, we investigate the relationship between individual differences and students' affective reactions to four intelligent PAs available in MetaTutor, a hypermedia-based intelligent tutoring system. We show that achievement goals and personality traits can significantly modulate students' affective reactions to the PAs. These findings suggest that students may benefit from personalized PAs that could adapt to their motivational goals and personality.

Keywords: Pedagogical agents · Personalization · Emotions · Achievement goals · Personality traits · Intelligent tutoring systems

1 Introduction

There is extensive evidence that emotions can impact how well students learn from agent-based learning environments (ABLEs) [1], including how pedagogical agents (PAs) can impact learning and problem-solving through adaptive scaffolding, feedback, and individualized instruction [2, 3]. Previous research has investigated how the design (e.g., gender, age, appearance) of PAs influences their effectiveness in fostering learning [2, 4, 5]. Our goal is to extend prior research by examining additional factors (i.e., personality, goal achievement, and emotions) that can impact the effectiveness of PAs in fostering learning with ABLEs. ABLEs include intelligent PAs that are designed to support student learning through tailored prompts, feedback, working examples, etc. However, there is still limited understanding of the reasons for which different emotions occur during interactions with PAs, and what those emotions are.

© Springer International Publishing AG 2016
D. Traum et al. (Eds.): IVA 2016, LNAI 10011, pp. 269–282, 2016.
DOI: 10.1007/978-3-319-47665-0_24

Initial studies showed the influence of students' gender and personality traits on affective reactions to PAs [6, 7]. It suggests that further research on the impact of individual differences on student emotions with ABLEs may help researchers gain a more comprehensive understanding of when and how students benefit from PAs in terms of affect, motivation and learning. This understanding, in turn, can be leveraged to devise intelligent PAs that can better adapt to the student's relevant individual differences in order to enhance the student's experience with ABLEs.

In this paper we contribute to this line of research by investigating the relationships of students' *achievement goals* [8] and *personality traits* [9] with their affective reactions while learning with MetaTutor, an ABLE that includes four PAs designed to scaffold and foster effective metacognition and self-regulated learning [1]. In particular, we investigate the relationships between achievement goals, personality traits, and students' affective reactions at specific points during the interaction with the system.

The main contributions of this work are as follows. First, our work is the first to examine the impact of students' *achievement goals* on their affective reactions to PAs. Achievement goals are considered a facet of motivation given that they provide a purpose or focus for the learning task at hand, and, as such, guide students' learning behaviors and performance by setting the standards with which to evaluate success [8]. In general, this framework assumes that students who adopt a *mastery-approach* goal focus on developing competence and skills, whereas students with a *performance-approach* goal focus on outperforming their peers [8]. Whereas there is extensive work on the impact of achievement goals on students' performance and motivation in general [4, 10], and on student learning while interacting with PAs [11], there are currently no reported studies on the impact of achievement goals specifically on affective reactions to PAs.

Second, we extend recent published findings on the impact of personality traits on student's affective reactions toward MetaTutor. Specifically Harley et al. [7] have shown that personality traits modeled via the five-factor framework [9] can influence emotions retrospectively reported towards PAs at the end of the learning session. In this paper, we extend these results with an analysis of students' emotions reported *during* interaction with MetaTutor, which provide more fine-grained information on the students' affective reactions when studying with this ABLE.

Lastly, we propose design guidelines about how our results can inform the design of more personalized PA scaffolding and feedback, e.g., promoting more pride to students with a mastery-approach goal by congratulating them when they master new skills. Such personalization could positively impact students' affect and their overall experience when interacting with MetaTutor.

2   Related Work on Students' Reactions to Pedagogical Agents

There is extensive evidence that pedagogical agents (PAs) can impact learning, motivation and affect during the interaction with learning environments [2, 4]. Further research has shown that students' reaction to such agents can be modulated by student's individual characteristics [12–14]. For instance, achievement goals can impact learning [12] and help-seeking behavior in the presence of PAs [13]. Personality traits have been shown to modulate the effect of PAs on learning as well, for instance based on the level of politeness of the agents [14].

Other research has focused more specifically on how individual differences impact the affective reactions of students to PAs [6, 7]. In particular, personality traits were found to influence the emotions specifically reported towards the agents at the end of the experiment (e.g., "*the agent made me feel happy*") [7]. For instance, students high in neuroticism reported to feel more bored when interacting with the PA responsible for metacognitive scaffolding. Additionally, students' gender has been shown to impact emotions reported by students during the interaction with PAs depending on the gender of the agent's persona [6].

3   MetaTutor Intelligent Learning Environment

MetaTutor (Fig. 1) is a hypermedia based intelligent tutoring system with 47 pages of text and diagrams, developed to teach students about the circulatory system and how to self-regulate their learning with the assistance of multiple PAs [1]. When working with MetaTutor, students are given the task of learning as much as they can about the human circulatory system. The main interface of MetaTutor includes a table of contents, a timer that indicates how much time remains in the learning session, and a self-regulated learning (SRL) palette where students can engage in cognitive and metacognitive SRL strategies, with the assistance (i.e., prompts and feedback) of each of four PAs.

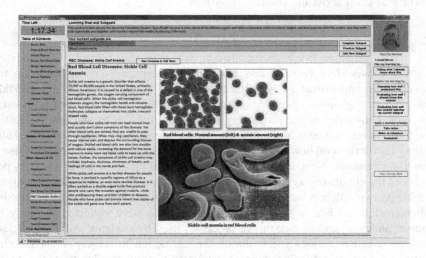

Fig. 1. Screenshot of MetaTutor during the learning session.

Only one PA is displayed at a time in the upper right corner of the screen. Except for Gavin the Guide, each of the PAs is responsible for specific self-regulatory processes and provides audible assistance through the use of a text-to-speech engine. Specifically, Gavin the Guide provides guidance for students in MetaTutor by presenting videos on how to interact with the interface (e.g., how to navigate through the content by using the table of contents) and also administers pretest and posttest knowledge assessments and the Emotions and Values (EV) Questionnaire. Pam the Planner prompts and scaffolds planning processes primarily at the beginning of the learning session by assisting the student in creating subgoals relevant to learning as much as they can about the human circulatory system (e.g., path of blood flow, malfunctions of the circulatory system). Mary the Monitor prompts and supports students in their metacognitive monitoring processes (e.g., self-assessment of their progress during learning) that students can use to judge their understanding or relevance of the content to their subgoals. Lastly, Sam the Strategizer prompts students to engage in cognitive learning strategies such as taking notes on the content or summarizing it in their own words.

The PAs are visually rendered using Haptek virtual characters and spoken utterances are produced through Nuance text-to-speech. Haptek animation of the virtual characters includes idle movements when the agents are not speaking (subtle, gradual head and eye movements), as well as lip movements during speech. Nuance text-to-speech provides distinct voices for each of the male and female PAs.

4 User Study

The data used for the analysis presented in this paper was collected via a user study during which 62 university students (65 % female, mean age of 19.9) worked with MetaTutor to learn about the circulatory system.

4.1 Procedure

The study consisted of two sessions conducted on separate days. During the first session, lasting approximately 30 min, students were administered several questionnaires (e.g., demographics, personality questionnaire – cf. Sect. 4.3) and a pretest to assess their knowledge of the circulatory system. During the second session, lasting about three hours, students were first shown an introductory video on MetaTutor, including instructions on how to navigate through the learning environment and use its different components. Next, each student was given 90 min to learn as much as possible about the circulatory system using MetaTutor. Students were randomly assigned to work with two different versions of the system, described below. During the session, multi-channel trace data (e.g., eye tracking, log files) were collected to study the cognitive, affective, and metacognitive processes used by students. Additionally, students were asked at various points during the interaction to self-report their current emotions (cf. Sect. 4.3). Finally, students completed a posttest analogous to the pretest, followed by a series of questionnaires, including a retrospective assessment of how they felt about the PAs (cf. Sect. 4.3).

4.2 Experimental Conditions

To examine the influence of PAs scaffolding on students' interaction with MetaTutor, students were randomly assigned to either an experimental Prompt and Feedback (PF) condition or Control condition. In the PF condition, the agents proactively provided students with timely *prompts* to promote the use of SRL strategies, as well as *feedback* on how students performed these strategies. A set of 20 production rules were used by the PAs to trigger scaffolding based on students' behavior or interaction with the system, such as the time spent on a subgoal or a content page, the relevance of the current page to the active subgoal, changes of page, etc. [1, 15]. For example, if a participant spends a certain amount of time on a page, Mary the Monitor could prompt students to metacognitively judge their understanding of a page, which would lead to a quiz on the information on the page to gauge how accurate their judgment was. Mary would also provide feedback on the results of the quiz, such as suggesting to continue reading the content on that page if less than 70 % of the quiz was correct (i.e., if the participant answered fewer than two out of three questions correctly). Sam the Strategizer could prompt students to summarize the content of the current page if they have been on it for a long time, and Sam would then provide feedback on the students' summary. High-level rules were also implemented to avoid over-prompting, for instance students would not be prompted to summarize the current page if they already refused to do it, but could be prompted to summarize material on the next page. Additionally, students could self-initiate SRL strategies by using the SRL palette and receive feedback on the performance of these strategies as well. For example, students could click on the SRL palette to judge how well they understood the information on the page and would also receive feedback from Mary on their quiz performance.

In the control condition, agents had a much more passive role. They would not prompt the use of any SRL strategies and would not provide any form of feedback on the performance of these strategies. However, students could still self-initiate the use of SRL strategies by clicking on the SRL palette. For example, students would still be able to judge their understanding of the information on the page and would still take a quiz, but they would not get feedback on their performance.

4.3 Material Collected

Here we describe the study material that provided the data we leverage to analyze the relationship between achievement goals, personality traits and student emotions.

Achievement Goals. The Achievement Goal Questionnaire Revised (AGQ-R) [8] is a 12-item self-report questionnaire that assesses four achievement goal dimensions: (a) mastery-approach, (b) mastery-avoidance, (c) performance-approach, and (d) performance-avoidance. Items were adapted to assess students' motivation for the Meta-Tutor learning task. Students were asked to indicate the degree to which they agreed with each item using a 7-point Likert scale. A sample item for the mastery-approach subscale is: "my aim is to completely master the material presented during this learning session." A sample item for the performance-approach subscale is: "my goal is to perform better than the other student participants." A student's *dominant goal* is determined based on the highest sub-scale score. In the case of a tie, we assume that the student had no dominant goal and exclude him from the analysis. Following the work of Duffy and Azevedo [11], we focus only on mastery-approach and performance-approach goals in this work, given that avoidance goals are typically considered less useful to foster effective learning.

Personality Traits. The 50-item International Personality Item Pool (IPIP) [16] assesses the personality dimensions of the well-established Five-Factor Model [9], which models personality in terms of: (a) agreeableness (tendency to be more friendly, considerate of others, altruistic, sympathetic), (b) extraversion (associated with high physical and verbal activity, assertiveness, sociability), (c) conscientiousness (associated with efficiency, determination, responsibility, and persistence), (d) neuroticism (tendency to be temperamental and experience negative moods and feelings; e.g., anxiety), and (e) openness (tendency to prefer novel and broader ideas and experiences, intellectual activities, creativity). Students were asked to respond to each IPIP item using a 5-point Likert scale ranging from 1 (very inaccurate) to 5 (very accurate). A sample item is "I get upset easily."

Emotions During Interaction. During the interaction with MetaTutor, at regular intervals students had to complete an on-line Emotions and Value (EV) Questionnaire [1]. This questionnaire consists of 15 items, each asking whether the student currently feels one of the 15 emotions listed in Table 3. These items were rated on a 5-point Likert scale ranging from 1 (strongly disagree) to 5 (strongly agree). One example item is: "Right now I feel bored". The instructions and wording of the questions are based on a subscale of the Academic Emotions Questionnaire (AEQ, [17]), that assesses students' current emotions, as opposed to emotions reported on prospective or retrospective measures. The 15 emotions measured using the EV Questionnaire represent a comprehensive list of emotions commonly experienced by students in learning or academic settings [17].

Emotional Reactions Towards the Agents. At the end of the learning session, students were asked to retrospectively assess how they felt about the PAs while they were learning with MetaTutor. To do so, students responded to a questionnaire asking whether each of the 4 PAs made them feel each of the 15 emotions measured by the EV Questionnaire (cf. Table 3), resulting in 4 (agents) × 15 (emotions) = 60 items. A 5-point Likert scale ranging from 1 (strongly disagree) to 5 (strongly agree) was used for each item. One example item is: "Sam made me feel bored".

5   Statistical Analyses

In our analyses, we leverage the data collected in the study to investigate whether there is a relationship between achievement goals and personality traits with student affective reactions while working with MetaTutor, and whether the relationship is modulated by the condition in which the agents were used (PF vs. Control). We mainly focus on the emotions reported via the EV Questionnaire during the learning session, but we also integrate results on the emotional reactions reported towards the PAs at the end of the session when they provide more insights on our findings.

Descriptive statistics of the collected personality traits, achievement goals, and emotions reported during the interaction are shown in Tables 1, 2 and 3. As sadness, hopeless and shame were rarely reported by learners (i.e., Likert scale reports were mostly close to "strongly disagree" for these emotions, resulting in a lack of variance), we removed these emotions from the analysis, resulting in 12 studied emotions.

Table 1. Descriptive statistics for IPIP.

Personality traits	M	SD
Extraversion	33.28	9.83
Agreeableness	40.89	4.93
Conscientiousness ·	36.88	6.98
Neuroticism	28.37	7.93
Openness	38.14	5.87

Table 2. Descriptive statistics for AGQ-R.

Achievement goals	M	SD
Performance-approach	4.27	0.63
Performance-avoidance	3.6	0.82
Mastery-approach	4.05	0.68
Mastery-avoidance	3.68	0.86

Table 3. Descriptive statistics for EV.

Emotions	M	SD	Emotions	M	SD	Emotions	M	SD
Neutral	3.33	1.21	Pride	2.57	1.13	Confusion	1.71	0.92
Hope	3.12	1.11	Anxiety	2.29	1.23	Eureka	1.71	0.97
Boredom	2.94	1.38	Frustration	2.19	1.22	Sadness	1.40	0.73
Curiosity	2.90	1.29	Surprise	1.85	1.12	Shame	1.46	0.79
Enjoyment	2.75	1.02	Contempt	1.79	1.10	Hopelessness	1.43	0.76

We ran a set of ordinal logistic regressions (appropriate for Likert-scale data [18]), each with one of the reported *emotions* as the dependent variable, and *achievement goals*, each of the five *personality traits,* and the *group condition* (PF or Control) as the factors. Each factor has 2 levels. For achievement goals, we assigned students in two groups (mastery or performance) based on their dominant goal (i.e., their highest rated goal orientation, as defined Sect. 4.3). For personality traits, we assigned students to either low or high levels of each trait using a median split. This approach produced 60 models (one for each of the 12 remaining emotions we considered from the EV Questionnaire and one for each of the 48 emotional reactions reported towards the PAs [12 emotions × 4 agents]). Then results were adjusted to account for family-wise error using the Holm-Bonferroni approach, which is appropriate to strictly ensure the significance of the statistical effects found when running models on multiple dependent variables. This adjustment was applied based on the number of dependent variables in 5 different families: one for the emotions reported during interaction, and one per set of emotional reactions towards each of the 4 agents. We report statistical significance at the .05 level (using adjusted p-values), and effect sizes as small for $r \geq 0.1$, medium for $r \geq 0.3$, and large for $r \geq 0.5$.

6 Results

In this section, we first report the significant interactions we found between achieve-ments goals, emotions and experimental condition (Sect. 6.1), and between personality traits, emotions and experimental conditions (Sect. 6.2). In Sect. 6.3, we summarize our findings and discuss their implications.

6.1 Achievement Goals and Emotions

We found interaction effects of *achievement goals* with *condition* on *pride* ($\chi_2(1) = 20.5$, $p < .001$, $r = .55$), *anxiety* ($\chi_2(1) = 13.4$, $p < .001$, $r = .47$), and *pride towards Sam* (the agent responsible for prompting cognitive strategies).

The effects on *pride* (shown in Fig. 2) and *anxiety* (Fig. 3) follow the same pattern in terms of affective valence, revealing that performance-oriented students experienced more positive affect (more pride, less anxiety) in the PF condition than in the control condition, whereas the effect is reversed for mastery-oriented students (i.e., higher levels of pride and lower levels of anxiety in the control condition). These results are consistent with those for *pride towards Sam*, which show that performance-oriented students experienced more pride with Sam in the PF condition than in the control condition, with the opposite effect for mastery-oriented students.

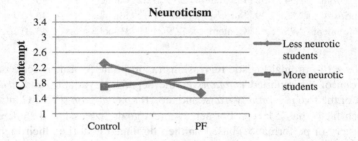

Fig. 2. Interaction effect of achievement goals (performance or mastery goal oriented) with condition on levels of pride reported during interaction.

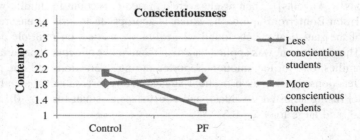

Fig. 3. Interaction effect of achievement goals (performance or mastery goal oriented) with condition on levels of anxiety reported during interaction.

6.2   Personality Traits and Emotions

We found interaction effects of neuroticism, conscientiousness, agreeableness and extroversion with condition on affect.

The interaction effect of *neuroticism* is on *contempt* ($\chi_2(1) = 5.4$, $p = .02$, $r = .36$) (Fig. 4), revealing that more neurotic students experienced higher levels of contempt in the PF condition than in the control condition, whereas less neurotic students experienced higher levels of contempt in the control condition.

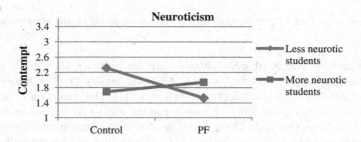

Fig. 4. Interaction effect of neuroticism with condition on levels of contempt reported during interaction.

The interaction effect of *conscientiousness* is also on *contempt* ($\chi_2(1) = 17.9$, $p < .001$, $r = .54$) (Fig. 5), showing that more conscientious students experienced lower levels of contempt in the PF condition than in the control condition. There is no effect of conditions for less conscientious students.

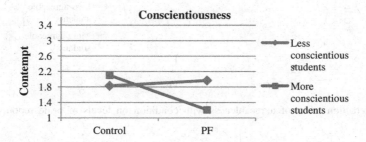

Fig. 5. Interaction effect of conscientiousness with condition on levels of contempt reported during interaction.

The interaction effect of *extroversion* is on *anxiety* and *anxiety towards Sam* ($\chi_2(1) = 4.9$, $p = .027$, $r = .28$) (Fig. 6), showing that more extroverted students reported higher levels of anxiety in the PF condition than in the control condition, whereas less extroverted students reported higher levels of anxiety in the control condition. This finding is in part consistent with *anxiety towards Sam*, showing that more extroverted students experienced more anxiety with Sam in the PF condition than in the control condition (there was no impact of condition for less extroverted students).

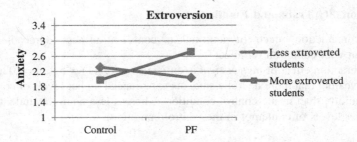

Fig. 6. Interaction effect of extroversion with condition on levels of anxiety reported during interaction.

The interaction effects of *agreeableness* are on *pride* ($\chi_2(1) = 14.2$, $p < .001$, $r = .48$), *curiosity* ($\chi_2(1) = 12.5$, $p = .027$, $r = .44$), *anxiety* ($\chi_2(1) = 6.9$, $p = .009$, $r = .33$) and *contempt* ($\chi_2(1) = 10.11$, $p = .001$, $r = .41$). The effects on *pride* (shown Fig. 7) and *curiosity* (Fig. 8) follow the same pattern, and so do the effects on *anxiety* (Fig. 9) and *contempt* (Fig. 10). These effects are not strictly consistent: more agreeable students experienced both positive (more pride and curiosity) and negative affect (more anxiety and contempt) in the PF condition compared to the control condition. As for less agreeable students, there is no effect of condition on pride and curiosity (see Figs. 7 and 8), but they experienced lower levels of anxiety and contempt (less negative affect) in the PF condition compared to the control condition (see Figs. 9 and 10).

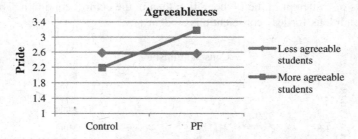

Fig. 7. Interaction effect of agreeableness with condition on levels of pride reported during interaction.

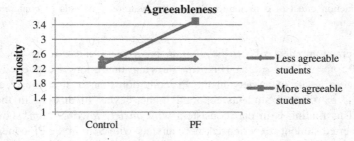

Fig. 8. Interaction effect of agreeableness with condition on levels of curiosity reported during interaction.

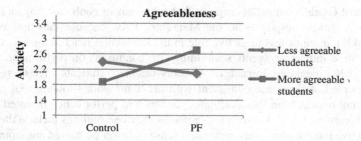

Fig. 9. Interaction effect of agreeableness with condition on levels of anxiety reported during interaction.

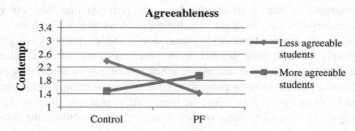

Fig. 10. Interaction effect of agreeableness with condition on levels of contempt reported during interaction.

6.3 Summary of Findings and Implications for Design of Personalized PAs

Table 4 summarizes the results reported above in terms of whether MetaTutor agents scaffolding in the PF condition had positive or negative influences on student emotions, for students with different achievement goals and personality traits.

Table 4. Overview of effects found, summarized in terms of the positive or negative impact of prompts and feedback (PF) on affect, modulated by individual differences.

Individual differences	Positive impact of PF on:	Negative impact of PF on:
Achievement goals	Performance-oriented students (more pride, less anxiety)	Mastery oriented students (less pride, more anxiety)
Extroversion	Less extroverted students (less anxiety)	More extroverted students (more anxiety)
Neuroticism	Less neurotic students (less contempt)	More neurotic students (more contempt)
Conscientiousness	Less conscientious students (less contempt)	
Agreeableness	More agreeable students (more pride, more curiosity)	More agreeable students (more anxiety, more contempt)
	Less agreeable students (less anxiety, less contempt)	

Achievement Goals. Our results suggest that achievement goals can play an important role in the emotions responses to the MetaTutor PAs, because they influence how students with a more or less proactive role in the interaction react to agents. We found mostly positive impact of agents scaffolding (PF condition) on performance-oriented students, and a negative impact on mastery-oriented students. These results for mastery-oriented students are consistent with previous work showing that those students may not benefit from PAs scaffolding as much as performance-oriented students, in terms of learning [4, 7]. Possible explanations for these findings include the fact that PAs' proactive interventions may generate a sense of lower perceived autonomy [19] in mastery-oriented students, which is consistent with lower levels of pride and higher levels of anxiety found in our work. In particular, mastery-oriented students reported lower levels of pride with Sam (the PA responsible for cognitive strategies prompting, e.g., taking notes). As Sam provides by far more prompts than any other PAs in MetaTutor, mastery-oriented students may have felt overwhelmed by Sam's scaffolding, resulting in lower perceived autonomy. These findings suggest that mastery-oriented students may benefit from personalization of PAs interventions geared toward giving them more autonomy when learning with MetaTutor (e.g., providing fewer prompts, or prompts promoting more active learning). Moreover, empathetic feedback given by the PAs might be improved to promote more pride (e.g., by congratulating them when they achieve their goal and understanding the topic).

Personality Traits. Our results (Table 4) indicate that four dimensions of personality, namely agreeableness, extroversion, conscientiousness and neuroticism, can modulate the affective reactions to PAs. These findings are in line with previous work showing that personality traits can impact students' emotional reactions reported towards the PAs [7]. Thus, our results provide further evidence that personality traits may warrant personalized prompts and feedback. In particular, we found that students high in neuroticism, extroversion and agreeableness experienced more negative affect in the PF condition. This might be explained by results from previous work in the field of virtual agents suggesting that users benefit from interacting with agents that match their personality, e.g., [21, 22]. For instance, extroverted students may benefit from more extroverted PAs conveying more social presence [22]; agreeable students may favor more friendly and caring agents [21]. The MetaTutor PAs exhibit no specific personality trait, thus when they have a stronger presence in the PF condition they plausibly are perceived as interfering rather than helping by students with strong personality traits. Thus students may benefit from PAs that can recognize the students' personality and personalize their feedback accordingly, as suggested above. Our results, however, suggest that the need for personalization is not as relevant for conscientiousness, as we found no negative impact in the PF condition for students with either high or low levels of this trait.

7   Conclusion and Future Work

We investigated the relationship between individual differences and affective reactions to intelligent pedagogical agents during the interaction with MetaTutor, an agent-based learning environment to foster self-regulated learning and meta-cognition. Our objective was to identify individual differences that could be the target of personalized support for improving the user affect provoked by the agents. Overall we found that achievement goals and personality traits do have a significant influence on emotions reported during interaction. Based on these findings, we made several suggestions on how the agents could adapt to the individual differences, for instance by offering more autonomy to mastery-oriented students.

As future work, we first plan to investigate whether achievement goals and personality traits can be detected during the interaction with MetaTutor using students' data collected in real time (e.g., interaction data, eye tracking). Such detection would allow enabling personalization even when it is not viable to assume that students will be able/willing to fill questionnaires. Second, we plan to investigate further how the effects of PAs scaffolding on student affect found in our results are modulated by individual differences, by analyzing student behavior while interacting with the PAs. Finally, we are interested in designing and evaluating the forms of personalization suggested by our results, to examine further whether and how personalized PAs can impact students' affect, motivation and learning.

Acknowledgements. This publication is based upon work supported by the National Science Foundation under Grant No. DRL-1431552 and the Social Sciences and Humanities Research Council of Canada. Any opinions, findings, and conclusions or recommendations expressed in this material are those of the authors and do not necessarily reflect the views of the National Science Foundation or the Social Sciences and Humanities Research Council of Canada.

References

1. Azevedo, R., Harley, J., Trevors, G., Duffy, M., Feyzi-Behnagh, R., Bouchet, F., Landis, R.: Using trace data to examine the complex roles of cognitive, metacognitive, and emotional self-regulatory processes during learning with multi-agent systems. In: Azevedo, R., Aleven, V. (eds.) International Handbook of Metacognition and Learning Technologies, pp. 427–449. Springer, New York (2013)
2. Schroeder, N.L., Adesope, O.O.: A systematic review of pedagogical agents' persona, motivation, and cognitive load implications for learners. J. Res. Technol. Educ. **46**, 229–251 (2014)
3. D'Mello, S., Graesser, A.: AutoTutor and affective AutoTutor: learning by talking with cognitively and emotionally intelligent computers that talk back. ACM Trans. Interact. Intell. Syst. **2**, 23 (2012)
4. Heidig, S., Clarebout, G.: Do pedagogical agents make a difference to student motivation and learning? Educ. Res. Rev. **6**, 27–54 (2011)
5. Baylor, A.L., Kim, Y.: Pedagogical agent design: the impact of agent realism, gender, ethnicity, and instructional role. In: Lester, J.C., Vicari, R.M., Paraguaçu, F. (eds.) ITS 2004. LNCS, vol. 3220, pp. 592–603. Springer, Heidelberg (2004). doi:10.1007/978-3-540-30139-4_56

6. Arroyo, I., Woolf, B.P., Royer, J.M., Tai, M.: Affective gendered learning companions. In: Proceedings of Artificial Intelligence in Education, Brighton, U.K., pp. 41–48 (2009)
7. Harley, J.M., Carter, C.K., Papaionnou, N., Bouchet, F., Landis, R.S., Azevedo, R., Karabachian, L.: Examining the predictive relationship between personality and emotion traits and students' agent-directed emotions: towards emotionally-adaptive agent-based learning environments. User Model. User-Adapt. Interact. **26**, 1–43 (2016)
8. Elliot, A.J., Murayama, K.: On the measurement of achievement goals: critique, illustration, and application. J. Educ. Psychol. **100**, 613 (2008)
9. Costa, P.T., McCrae, R.R.: Four ways five factors are basic. Personality Individ. Differ. **13**, 653–665 (1992)
10. Hidi, S., Harackiewicz, J.M.: Motivating the academically unmotivated: a critical issue for the 21st century. Rev. Educ. Res. **70**, 151–179 (2000)
11. Duffy, M.C., Azevedo, R.: Motivation matters: interactions between achievement goals and agent scaffolding for self-regulated learning within an intelligent tutoring system. Comput. Hum. Behav. **52**, 338–348 (2015)
12. Erhel, S., Jamet, E.: Digital game-based learning: impact of instructions and feedback on motivation and learning effectiveness. 1 **67**, 156–167 (2013)
13. Harris, A., Bonnett, V., Luckin, R., Yuill, N., Avramides, K.: Scaffolding effective help-seeking behaviour in mastery and performance oriented learners. In: Proceedings of Artificial Intelligence in Education, Brighton, U.K., pp. 425–432 (2009)
14. Wang, N., Johnson, W.L., Mayer, R.E., Rizzo, P., Shaw, E., Collins, H.: The politeness effect: pedagogical agents and learning outcomes. Int. J. Hum.-Comput. Stud. **66**, 98–112 (2008)
15. Azevedo, R., Martin, S.A., Taub, M., Mudrick, N.V., Millar, G.C., Grafsgaard, J.F.: Are pedagogical agents' external regulation effective in fostering learning with intelligent tutoring systems? In: Micarelli, A., Stamper, J., Panourgia, K., Krouwel, M.R., Abolkasim, E. (eds.) ITS 2016. LNCS, vol. 9684, pp. 197–207. Springer, Heidelberg (2016). doi:10.1007/978-3-319-39583-8_19
16. Goldberg, L.R.: A broad-bandwidth, public domain, personality inventory measuring the lower-level facets of several five-factor models. Personal. Psychol. Eur. **7**, 7–28 (1999)
17. Pekrun, R., Goetz, T., Frenzel, A.C., Barchfeld, P., Perry, R.P.: Measuring emotions in students' learning and performance: The Achievement Emotions Questionnaire (AEQ). Contemp. Educ. Psychol. **36**, 36–48 (2011)
18. Williams, R.: Generalized ordered logit/partial proportional odds models for ordinal dependent variables. Stata J. **6**, 58–82 (2006)
19. Benita, M., Roth, G., Deci, E.L.: When are mastery goals more adaptive? It depends on experiences of autonomy support and autonomy. J. Educ. Psychol. **106**, 258 (2014)
20. Carr, A., Luckin, R., Yuill, N., Avramides, K.: How mastery and performance goals influence learners' metacognitive help-seeking behaviours when using Ecolab II. In: Azevedo, R., Aleven, V. (eds.) International Handbook of Metacognition and Learning Technologies, pp. 659–668. Springer, New York (2013)
21. Kang, S.-H., Gratch, J., Wang, N., Watt, J.H.: Agreeable people like agreeable virtual humans. In: Prendinger, H., Lester, J.C., Ishizuka, M. (eds.) IVA 2008. LNCS, vol. 5208, pp. 253–261. Springer, Heidelberg (2008). doi:10.1007/978-3-540-85483-8_26
22. Lee, K.M., Nass, C.: Designing social presence of social actors in human computer interaction. In: Proceedings of the SIGCHI Conference on Human Factors in Computing Systems, pp. 289–296. ACM, New York (2003)

The Benefits of Virtual Humans for Teaching Negotiation

Jonathan Gratch[✉], David DeVault, and Gale Lucas

Institute for Creative Technologies, University of Southern California,
Playa Vista, CA, USA
{gratch,devault}@ict.usc.edu

Abstract. This article examines the potential for teaching negotiation with virtual humans. Many people find negotiations to be aversive. We conjecture that students may be more comfortable practicing negotiation skills with an agent than with another person. We test this using the Conflict Resolution Agent, a semi-automated virtual human that negotiates with people via natural language. In a between-participants design, we independently manipulated two pedagogically-relevant factors while participants engaged in repeated negotiations with the agent: perceived agency (participants either believed they were negotiating with a computer program or another person) and pedagogical feedback (participants received instructional advice or no advice between negotiations). Findings indicate that novice negotiators were more comfortable negotiating with a computer program (they self-reported more comfort and punished their opponent less often) and expended more effort on the exercise following instructional feedback (both in time spent and in self-reported effort). These findings lend support to the notion of using virtual humans to teach interpersonal skills.

1 Introduction

Most people hate to negotiate and this aversion has real economic costs [1]. Not surprisingly, negotiation expertise is a highly-valued commodity. Negotiation is often taught in professional schools, as part of a business or law degree. For example, as part of a Master in business administration, students might take a semester-long course on negotiation concepts. For those seeking a more cursory introduction, consulting companies offer intensive short courses. For example, Vantage Partners, a spinoff of the Harvard Business School, offers 3-day tutorials to corporate executives. Regardless of the length of instruction, negotiation is taught via a mixture of instruction (typically classroom lectures) and hands-on experience (typically where students pair-off and engage in a simulated negotiation with each other). In business schools, these simulations are often run by dedicated staff trained to be experts in experiential learning techniques.

All of this is big business. It has been estimated that billions of dollars are spent on teaching negotiation [2]. Professional schools and consulting companies charge high fees for these services. Even the creation of simulated negotiations is a money making operation. Instructors submit their teaching cases to repositories, such as the Kellogg Schools Dispute Resolution Resource Center (DRRC) and instructors are expected to pay to use these cases in the classroom. As a result, professional negotiation skills are mainly limited to the elite.

© Springer International Publishing AG 2016
D. Traum et al. (Eds.): IVA 2016, LNAI 10011, pp. 283–294, 2016.
DOI: 10.1007/978-3-319-47665-0_25

Virtual human technology has the potential to address the challenges and expense in teaching negotiation [3–5]. In this article, we examine the experiential aspect of negotiation training. Currently, students experience negotiations by practicing their skills on each other, playing simulated negotiations such as those maintained by the DRRC. Being novices, these negotiations have something of the flavor of the blind leading the blind. Especially in introductory cases, the majority of the students fail to incorporate the key teaching points into their negotiation behavior. Rather, the professor or professional facilitator will walk around the classroom, find the few students that performed well, and lead a classroom discussion on why such outcomes occurred.

We argue virtual humans, in particular, can serve as an especially valuable tool for augmenting experiential learning. Virtual humans can serve as both automated role-players and automated tutors; allowing students to practice with more proficient (computerized) partners and then receive targeted feedback on their own performance, much as is done in cognitive tutoring in more conventional domains. But further, we conjecture that virtual humans, by the very nature of being artificial, can help mitigate the anxiety people often feel in negotiations, and thereby enhance their efficiency in learning.

We first review some key negotiation skills and motivate why virtual humans may be well-suited to teaching them. We introduce these within the context of the multi-issue bargaining task, an abstract characterization of negotiation often adopted for teaching these skills. We next review some previous approaches to using automation for teaching these skills, then present the Conflict Resolution Agent, a virtual human negotiator that we will use in our study. We finally present experimental results supporting our conjecture that virtual humans are uniquely beneficial to teaching negotiation and conclude with some final thoughts.

2   Negotiation Skills

Multi-issue Bargaining. We expect virtual humans will be most effective for the introductory modules of a semester-long course or for the short intensive instruction offered by consulting firms. In these more introductory settings, simulated negotiations often follow a very stylized form that is more amenable to automation. Specifically, we focus on one useful and common abstraction of negotiation known as the multi-issue bargaining task [6], which has become a *de facto* standard for introductory negotiation simulations, as well as research on negotiation in both the social and computer sciences [e.g., see 2, 7, 8]. Multi-issue bargaining generalizes simpler games developed in game theory, such as the ultimatum game, and more closely approximates many of the challenges found in real-life negotiations. This task has received so much attention amongst educators and researchers because, with only a small number of mathematical parameters, one can evoke a wide range of psychologically-distinct decision-tasks. Thus, multi-issue bargaining has been used to teach and study a wide range of negotiation concepts.

In its basic form, multi-issue bargaining requires parties (typically 2) to find agreement over a set of issues. Each issue consists of a set of levels and players must jointly decide on a level for each issue (levels might correspond to the amount of a product one player wishes to buy, or it might represent attributes of a single object, such as the price or warranty of a car). Each party receives some payoff for each possible agreement and each player's payoff is usually not known to the other party. The payoff is often assumed to be additive (i.e., a player's total payoff is the sum of the value obtained for each issue) and presented to players through a payoff matrix. For example, Table 1 illustrates the two payoff matrices for a hypothetical negotiation over items in an antique store. In this case, players must divide up three crates of records, two lamps and one painting, but each party assigns different value to items.

Table 1. An example 3-issue integrative bargaining problem

Side A Payoff

Records		Lamps		Painting	
Level	Value	Level	Value	Level	Value
0	$0	0	$0	0	$0
1	$20	1	$10	1	$5
2	$40	2	$20		
3	$60				

Side B Payoff

Records		Lamps		Painting	
Level	Value	Level	Value	Level	Value
0	$0	0	$0	0	$0
1	$10	1	$30	1	$0
2	$20	2	$60		
3	$30				

Negotiation concepts. One important set of negotiation concepts relates to the relative importance each party assigns to different issues. The payoff structure in Table 1 is used to teach the concept of *integrative potential* and serves to define an *integrative* (or win-win) negotiation as player A receives the most value from the painting and records, whereas player B receives the most value from the lamps, the joint payoff is maximized when player B gets all the lamps and player A gets the rest. In contrast, if both parties have the same priorities, this creates a *distributive* (or zero-sum) negotiation as any gain in value to one side would result in an equal loss to the other side.

Most students assume their opponent wants the same thing as them (i.e., they assume they are engaged in a distributive negotiation). Thus, integrative structures provides students the opportunity to *create* value by discovering integrative potential. They can only find this potential if they are willing to exchange information about their preferences, but students often fear to reveal too much, lest they be exploited by their opponent. Thus, integrative negotiations also provide the opportunity to teach ways to establish trust and safely exchange information. For example, one tactic is reciprocal information exchange, in which one provides a small amount of information and only provides more if the opponent reciprocates [9]. In contrast, distributive negotiations provide the students with the opportunities to learn tactics for how to *claim* value, as they can only improve their position by overpowering their opponent. These can including making threats or staking out strong positions [10].

Another important negotiation concept is the Best Alternative to a Negotiated Agreement (BATNA) for each player. This represents how much a party would receive if the negotiation fails. For example, if player A already has a tentative deal with another player that affords him $150, there is no reason to accept a deal worth less than $150 from player B (e.g., 2 records and a painting). The BATNA represents the player's bargaining power, and as with preference weights, these are typically unknown to the other player.

If player B's BATNA is only $20, then player A has more potential power in the negotiation, although whether this translates into better outcomes depends on how each party shapes the other party's perceptions and how carefully they attend to the structure of the negotiation. By focusing on their own and their opponent's BATNAs, students can better understand their bargaining power and how to claim value. For example, when claiming value, it can be effective to mislead one's opponent about the size of one's own BATNA.

Virtual humans can implement and reason about these different concepts. For example, an agent can be programmed to engage in reciprocal information exchange, allowing the student to explore and discover this concept. These techniques could also facilitate tutorial feedback. In this vein, Nazari showed that automated techniques can classify if a student is communicating distributive or integrative preferences [11] and an automated tutor could contrast this objective communication with a student's subjective beliefs about what he or she communicated to their opponent.

Negotiation anxiety. Teaching negotiation requires imparting several different types of skills. Up to this point, we have been discussing cognitive skills. These including recognizing the structure of the negotiation (integrative versus distributive), identifying each player's bargaining power, and deciding which tactics to use depending on these factors. But many people find negotiation aversive. People often experience negative affect or anxiety in negotiations and this can undermine their cognitive skills [12, 13] and lead to poorer negotiation outcomes [1]. This can be especially true when negotiations are distributive and students must focus on claiming value at the expense of their opponent. Thus, students of negotiation are confronted with the dual challenge of learning cognitive skills (negotiation concepts) while simultaneously learning to manage and regulate their emotions.

One of the best ways to reduce negative affect is to improve and automatize cognitive skills. Negotiations are cognitively challenging and can create high-cognitive load, but this cognitive load can make them more susceptible to emotional influences [14] and lower the cognitive resources available for emotion regulation [15, 16]. More broadly, negative affect can make it more difficult for negotiators to explore solutions and create value [17]. Thus, if students have the opportunity to practice cognitive skills in a safe and positive environment, they may learn to more quickly become comfortable with cognitive aspects of negotiation and thereby free up resources to regulate their emotions.

We conjecture that virtual humans can reduce negotiation negative affect and negotiation anxiety and promote cognitive learning. Previous research has suggested that people feel less fear and anxiety when they practice interpersonal skills with virtual humans [18, 19]. We predict that these findings will extend to the context of negotiation.

3 Prior Work and the Conflict Resolution Agent

Researchers have looked at the potential of artificial intelligence technology to teach negotiation. Several systems have used automated techniques to help students prepare for a negotiation. For example, the pocket negotiator uses preference-elicitation techniques and visualizations of the Pareto frontier to help students better understand their preferences and limits [20]. ELECT BiLAT explore the potential of an embodied agent to teach negotiation. Students could practice a series of negotiations with virtual characters that uses menu based "conversation" and sophisticated decision-theoretic and theory-of-mind techniques to guide their behavior. Like the Pocket Negotiator, this pedagogy focuses students on the preparations leading up to a negotiation [21].

Other researchers have focused on teaching tactics that occur during the negotiation. Kraus and colleagues have shown that negotiating with a disembodied rational agent can help students learn better negotiation tactics [3]. SASO is perhaps the only negotiation system that supports conversational negotiation with an embodied agent [22]. It allows student-soldiers to negotiate with a local leader over how best to conduct a peacekeeping operation, however, it adopted a very different formalism of negotiation, building more on planning and shared-plans frameworks (e.g., [23]), and thus has only limited relevance to the larger body of research on multi-issue bargaining. Nonetheless, this research provides a foundation for the natural language understanding and dialog processes required for a virtual human negotiator.

Most recently, our group has proposed a conversational virtual human that performs the multi-issue bargaining task and we adopt this system to examine our hypotheses. The Conflict Resolution Agent (CRA), pictured in Fig. 1 [24], is a game-like environment that allows negotiation students to engage with a variety of virtual human role-players across a variety of multi-issue bargaining problems. The current, wizard-of-Oz (WOz) system allows students to communicate through natural language and nonverbal expressions. CRA is implemented with the publicly-available Virtual Human Toolkit [25]. Low-level functions such as speech and gesture generation are carried out automatically, while two wizards make high-level decisions about the agent's verbal and nonverbal behavior. The WOz interface allows the agent to speak over 5000 distinct utterances. Utterances are synthesized by the NeoSpeech text-to-speech system and gestures and expressions are generated automatically by NVBG [26] and realized using the SmartBody character animation system [27]. This low-level automation complements and facilitates the decision-making of the wizards. Details of the development and capabilities of the CRA WOz interface can be found in [28].

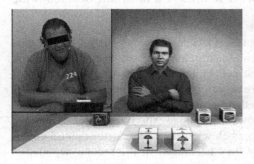

224:	I'll tell you what. I'll take this box of records 'cause it looks like it has the least.
CRA:	That doesn't seem fair though...
224:	Why not? [exasperated laugh]
CRA:	Well, you see, I have a buyer right now that is interested in old records.
224:	So do I.
CRA:	Your customers would probably love those lamps.
224:	My customers?

Fig. 1. A participant interacting with the Conflict Resolution Agent.

CRA realizes a physically-embodied version of the multi-issue bargaining task developed by Carnevale and described in [29]. As can be seen in Fig. 1, issues are represented as different types of physical objects (e.g., crates of records, lamps, and paintings) and levels correspond to the number of each type of item the player receives. Participants communicate with CRA through spoken natural language (currently interpreted through the wizards) or by manipulating, gazing at, and/or gesturing at the physical objects. The intent behind the physical objects is to elicit multimodal behavior and create multiple communication channels to facilitate the understanding of participant intent. For example, the participant can make an offer via language ("Would you like the painting?"), moving the objects, or both. The agent can respond in kind, making offers either via speech or by manipulating the objects.

4   Experiment

We devised an experiment to test two hypotheses concerning the pedagogical potential of CRA. Most importantly, we wanted to assess if negotiating with a computer program felt more comfortable and safe than negotiation with another person. Secondly, we wanted to assess if pedagogical feedback would help improve negotiation effort and performance.

Hypothesis 1:   Participants will feel more comfortable negotiating with a tough computer opponent compared with a tough human opponent

We instructed wizards to adopt a tough negotiation stance to evoke negotiation anxiety. We then manipulated participants' belief as to whether the CRA agent was controlled by a human or by a computer (in all cases it was controlled by human wizards), and assessed how aversive they found the negotiation. This was measured subjectively via scales (an 8-item subjective comfort scale and an 8-item friendliness/cooperativeness scale) and objectively by giving participants an opportunity to punish their opponent by reneging on the final deal if they felt dissatisfied. We hypothesize participants will feel more comfortable when CRA is framed as an automated agent.

Hypothesis 2:   Participants will try harder to achieve a favorable deal following pedagogical feedback

Participants engaged in two negotiations: first an integrative negotiation that emphasized cooperation and creating value, then a distributive negotiation that emphasized competition and claiming value. The first negotiation was to give all participants a common familiarity with the system before exploring our primary manipulations. After the first negotiation, we manipulated whether participants received pedagogical feedback (about the concept of BATNA and how they could use this information to increase their bargaining power, as described further below) or no feedback (the control condition). We then measured how forcefully they negotiated in the second negotiation through subjective and objective measures.[1] We hypothesize the feedback will increase the effort they invest in the exercise.

4.1 Design

Ninety three participants (52 female) were recruited from an on-line job service and randomly assigned to one of four experimental conditions (described below). Each completed two negotiations: a cooperative/integrative negotiation and a competitive/ distributive negotiation. The integrative round matched the structure of Table 1. Participants played Side A, and agents Side B. In the second, distributive round, the agent played side A, and the participant received a payoff similar to side A with the exception that the painting had no value. Note that the actual items differed in round 2 (i.e., chairs, crates of china plates, and a clock), but the values were equivalent to the original items, thus for simplicity, we discuss only the original set of items. Participants could make money based on their performance. Rather than dollars, participants received lottery tickets based on the value of items they obtained. If they failed to reach agreement, their BATNA equaled the number of tickets they would have received for one of their highest-value items. Tickets were then entered into a $100 lottery.

Participants interacted with a male and a female virtual human controlled by the same wizard interface; order of presentation was counterbalanced and found to have no effect on the results presented below. The virtual humans use the same utterances, general dialogue policy and gestures, but differ in appearance and voice. For both virtual human agents, Wizards followed a script. In both rounds, they acted as if the participant preferences were unknown; the wizard avoided volunteering their own preferences unless participants used reciprocal information exchange; the wizard avoided making the first offer unless directly asked. In *both* the integrative *and* distributive rounds, when directly asked their preferences, they would make a distributive offer (in the integrative case, asking for 2 lamps and 1 record; in the distributive case, asking for 2 records and a lamp). In the integrative round, participants always accepted this offer, as they received two of their highest value items (2 records). In the distributive round, such an offer was less attractive and participants negotiated to obtain a better deal for themselves; however, the wizard remained on script and did not budge on this offer.

Two factors were manipulated, resulting in a 2 × 2 between-subjects design. Participants were randomly assigned to framing condition, where they were either told that the agent was operated by a computer or a human as in [18]. They were also randomly assigned to the feedback condition, where they were given feedback after the first round about how they underperformed when their partner's BATNA is taken into account, or else were given no feedback. Specifically, in the feedback condition, after accepting the offer in the first round, it was pointed out to them that, although they received two of

---

[1] Following standard practice (see [8]), wizards negotiate following a fixed script. This is to avoid the possibility of experimenter bias (e.g., if one participant seems more likeable than another). A disadvantage, however, is that all participants reach approximately the same final deal, making it difficult to judge the impact of pedagogical feedback. Thus we look at time on task and subjective effort to index if they are trying to apply the suggested advice.

their highest value items (2 records), their partners' BATNA was only one lamp. Participants were encouraged to reflect on how they could have gotten more items in that first negotiation if they had considered how much better the deal was for their partner compared to the partners' BATNA. Those in the control group received no such feedback.

4.2   Results

Ratings of comfort. Participants were more comfortable dealing with a tough negotiator when framed as a computer. Participants responded to eight items on a 1 to 5 scale signaling their agreement that they were "comfortable interacting" with the agent, that "it felt natural to talk" to the agent, and that the agent was "easy to talk to," for example; we averaged these 8 items to index ratings of comfort. As can be seen in Fig. 2a, participants felt more comfortable interacting with the agent when they believed it was a computer in both the first, integrative negotiation ($F(1,89) = 5.90$, $p = .02$) and the second, distributive negotiation ($F(1,89) = 5.60$, $p = .02$). There were no effects of or interactions with feedback condition, $Fs < 0.99$, $ps > .32$. This supports our first hypothesis that people are more comfortable dealing with a tough negotiator if they are negotiating with a computer.

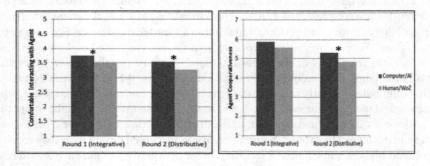

Fig. 2. Partner comfort (a: left) and perceived cooperativeness (b: right)

Ratings of agent's cooperativeness. Participants viewed their opponent as more cooperative if framed as a computer. Participants rated the agent on eight items using a 1 to 7 scale with bipolar anchors such as uncooperative/cooperative and unfriendly/friendly; we averaged these 8 items to index ratings of cooperativeness. As can be seen in Fig. 2b, there was a trend for the participants to rate the agent as more cooperative when framed as a computer in the first, integrative negotiation ($F(1,89) = 1.98$, $p = .16$); they rated the agent to be significantly more cooperative when they believed it was operated by a computer in the second, distributive negotiation ($F(1,89) = 3.91$, $p = .05$). There were no effects of or interactions with feedback condition, $Fs < 0.36$, $ps > .55$. This provides additional support for our first hypothesis.

Behavioral measure of commitment to the final deal. Participants were less likely to punish a tough opponent when they were framed as a computer. At the end of the study, participants were told that the negotiator from the first (integrative) round found another storage unit with identical items to those from the second (distributive) round. Participants were offered the option of following through with their agreement with the second negotiator, or taking an identical offer with the first negotiator instead. As switching leaves the participant's profits unchanged but hurts the second negotiation partner, we interpreted this as a measure of dissatisfaction and/or anger with the second opponent. Although there was an error and data was only recorded for 34 participants, among that group there was a marginally significant effect of framing ($\chi^2(1) = 3.32$, $p = .07$). As can be seen in Fig. 3a, participants who believed the agent was operated by a computer were less likely to renege on the second deal than those who believed it was operated by a human. We interpret this as an indication that participants found the negotiation less aversive and felt less desire to retaliate, lending further support for our first hypothesis. There was also a trend for feedback ($\chi^2(1) = 2.75$, $p = .10$), such that those in the feedback condition were less likely to renege on their second deal (as can be seen in Fig. 3b). This later trend could suggest that participants were more satisfied with their negotiated outcome following such feedback. There was not a significant interaction between framing and feedback ($p > .14$).

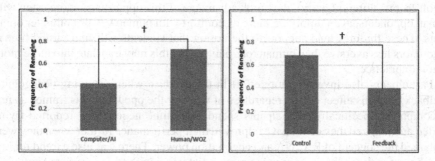

Fig. 3. Frequency of reneging by framing (a: left) and feedback (b: right)

Time spent negotiating. Participants tried harder to win when they received peda-gogical feedback. Participants who were given feedback after the first round about how they underperformed when their partner's BATNA is taken into account spent signifi-cantly longer negotiating in the second round (466 s) than those in the no feedback control condition (373 s); ($F(1, 89) = 5.58$, $p = .02$). This provides behavioral support for our second hypothesis that feedback will increase effort. This effect was not qualified by framing condition ($F(1, 89) = 0.1$, $p = .91$). The human/computer framing did not significantly impact negotiation time. There were no effects or interactions on time spent negotiating during the first round ($Fs < .69$, $ps > .40$). On the second round, there was a trend for participants to spend longer negotiating with the agent when they believed it to be controlled by a human than when they believed it to be controlled by a computer ($F(1, 89) = 2.77$, $p = .10$).

Appraisal of negotiation. Participants also felt they tried harder when they received pedagogical feedback and felt their performance could be further improved in the future.

Using a scale from 0 to 100, they were asked to rate how much effort they put into the negotiation. They also rated the extent to which they felt like they "revealed too much information during the negotiation" on a 1 to 5 scale. Participants who were given feedback after the first round reported expending marginally more effort in the second round (88.0 out of 100) than those in the no feedback control condition (81.4 out of 100); ($F(1, 89) = 3.55$, $p = .06$). Also, participants who received feedback were more aware that they may have still revealed too much information during the second negotiation (2.89 out of 5 vs. 2.40 out of 5); ($F(1, 89) = 6.54$, $p = .01$). All other effects did not approach significance ($Fs < 2.5$, $ps > .12$). These subjective impressions provide further support for our second hypothesis that feedback improves effort.

5   Discussion and Limitations

Our findings show that people found it more comfortable to practice tough negotiations with a computer program. When framed as a computer, participants reported more comfort with the negotiation and found their partner more cooperative. When given the opportunity to punish their opponent (by abandoning their negotiated deal for a certain payoff from a different party), they took advantage of this opportunity more often with human opponents, again implying more discomfort with human versus computer opponents. These findings lend support to the notion that students will find virtual human negotiators less aversive than human role-players and this may translate into more motivation to practice.

Participants also invested more effort in the exercise when receiving pedagogical feedback, and this effect occurs regardless of whether the opponent was framed as real or computer. Specifically, participants spend more time negotiating, reported trying harder, and realized they could have improved their performance further when they were explained the concept of BATNA and negotiation power. There was also a trend for less punishment with feedback, suggesting more satisfaction with their negotiated outcome. Again, this supports the potential benefits of virtual human role-players.

There were several limitations to the study. Our manipulation of the nature of the opponent (human versus computer) has some strengths but also limitations. By manipulating "mere belief" about the nature of the opponent we ensure appearance and behavior were controlled (i.e., participants interacted with the identical system but the system was framed as an interaction with a human or computer), however a more comprehensive study would have also included face-to-face interaction as it is possible that negotiating *via* a computer is significantly different than practicing with another student directly [19]. Additionally, we reported only high-level indices of negotiation performance (e.g., time and self-reported effort). Further analysis must be performed to examine how the experimental factors altered negotiation processes. For example, did people make tougher offers when receiving pedagogical feedback? Did they reason more carefully about their BATNA? Answering these questions will require detailed annotation and analysis of the content of the negotiations. Finally, and most importantly, we must verify that these positive findings translate into measureable benefits when negotiating with human opponents.

Acknowledgments. The paper benefited from the feedback of the anonymous reviewers. This research was supported by the Air Force Office of Scientific Research under grant FA9550-14-1-0364 and the U.S. Army. Statements and opinions expressed do not necessarily reflect the position or the policy of the United States Government, and no official endorsement should be inferred

References

1. Brooks, A.W., Schweitzer, M.E.: Can Nervous Nelly negotiate? how anxiety causes negotiators to make low first offers, exit early, and earn less profit. Organ. Behav. Hum. Decis. Process. **115**(1), 43–54 (2011)
2. Movius, H.: The effectiveness of negotiation training. Negot. J. **24**(4), 509–531 (2008)
3. Lin, R., Oshrat, Y., Kraus, S.: Investigating the benefits of automated negotiations in enhancing people's negotiation skills. In: 8th International Conference on Autonomous Agents and Multiagent Systems (2009)
4. Core, M., et al.: Teaching negotiation skills through practice and reflection with virtual humans. Simulation **82**(11), 685–701 (2006)
5. Broekens, J., Harbers, M., Brinkman, W.-P., Jonker, C.M., Van den Bosch, K., Meyer, J.-J.: Virtual reality negotiation training increases negotiation knowledge and skill. In: Nakano, Y., Neff, M., Paiva, A., Walker, M. (eds.) IVA 2012. LNCS, vol. 7502, pp. 218–230. Springer, Heidelberg (2012)
6. Kelley, H.H., Schenitzki, D.P.: Bargaining. In: Experimental Social Psychology. Holt, Rinehart, and Winston, New York, pp. 298–337 (1972)
7. Baarslag, T., et al.: Evaluating practical negotiating agents: results and analysis of the 2011 international competition. Artif. Intell. **198**, 73–103 (2013)
8. Van Kleef, G.A., De Dreu, C.K.W., Manstead, A.S.R.: The interpersonal effects of anger and happiness in negotiations. J. Pers. Soc. Psychol. **86**(1), 57–76 (2004)
9. Thompson, L.L.: Information exchange in negotiation. J. Exp. Soc. Psychol. **27**(2), 161–179 (1991)
10. Van Kleef, G.A., et al.: Power and emotion in negotiation: power moderates the interpersonal effects of anger and happiness on concession making. Eur. J. Soc. Psychol. **36**(4), 557–581 (2006)
11. Nazari, Z., Lucas, G.M., Gratch, J.: Opponent modeling for virtual human negotiators. In: Brinkman, W.-P., Broekens, J., Heylen, D. (eds.) IVA 2015. LNCS, vol. 9238, pp. 39–49. Springer, Heidelberg (2015)
12. Pillutla, M.M., Murnighan, J.K.: Unfairness, anger, and spite: emotional rejections of ultimatum offers. Organ. Behav. Hum. Decis. Process. **68**(3), 208–224 (1996)
13. Grecucci, A., et al.: Reappraising the ultimatum: an FMRI study of emotion regulation and decision making. Cereb. Cortex **23**(2), 399–410 (2012)
14. Van Kleef, G.A.: Emotion in conflict and negotiation: introducing the emotions as social information (EASI) model. SSRN eLibrary (2005)
15. Gross, J.J.: Emotion regulation: past, present, future. Cogn. Emot. **13**(5), 551–573 (1999)
16. Broekens, J., Jonker, C.M., Meyer, J.-J.C.: Affective negotiation support systems. J. Ambient Intell. Smart Environ. **2**(2), 121–144 (2010)
17. Carnevale, P.J., Isen, A.M.: The influence of positive affect and visual access on the discovery of integrative solutions in bilateral negotiation. Organ. Behav. Hum. Decis. Process. **37**, 1–13 (1986)

18. Lucas, G.M., et al.: It's only a computer: virtual humans increase willingness to disclose. Comput. Hum. Behav. **37**, 94–100 (2014)
19. de Melo, C., Gratch, J., Carnevale, P.J.: The effect of agency on the impact of emotion expressions on people's decision making. In: Humaine Association Conference on Affective Computing and Intelligent Interaction (ACII), pp. 546–551 (2013)
20. Hindriks, K.V., Jonker, C.M.: Creating human-machine synergy in negotiation support systems: towards the pocket negotiator. In: Proceedings of the 1st International Working Conference on Human Factors and Computational Models in Negotiation, pp. 47–54. ACM (2008)
21. Kim, J.M., et al.: BiLAT: A game-based environment for practicing negotiation in a cultural context. Int. J. Artif. Intell. Educ. **19**(3), 289–308 (2009)
22. Traum, D.R., Marsella, S.C., Gratch, J., Lee, J., Hartholt, A.: Multi-party, multi-issue, multi-strategy negotiation for multi-modal virtual agents. In: Prendinger, H., Lester, J.C., Ishizuka, M. (eds.) IVA 2008. LNCS (LNAI), vol. 5208, pp. 117–130. Springer, Heidelberg (2008)
23. Grosz, B., Kraus, S.: Collaborative plans for complex group action. Artif. Intell. **86**(2), 269–357 (1996)
24. Gratch, J., DeVault, D., Lucas, G.M., Marsella, S.: Negotiation as a challenge problem for virtual humans. In: Brinkman, W.-P., Broekens, J., Heylen, D. (eds.) IVA 2015. LNCS, vol. 9238, pp. 201–215. Springer, Heidelberg (2015)
25. Hartholt, A., Traum, D., Marsella, S.C., Shapiro, A., Stratou, G., Leuski, A., Morency, L.-P., Gratch, J.: All together now. In: Aylett, R., Krenn, B., Pelachaud, C., Shimodaira, H. (eds.) IVA 2013. LNCS, vol. 8108, pp. 368–381. Springer, Heidelberg (2013)
26. Lee, J., Marsella, S.C.: Nonverbal behavior generator for embodied conversational agents. In: Gratch, J., Young, M., Aylett, R.S., Ballin, D., Olivier, P. (eds.) IVA 2006. LNCS (LNAI), vol. 4133, pp. 243–255. Springer, Heidelberg (2006)
27. Thiebaux, M., et al.: SmartBody: behavior realization for embodied conversational agents. In: International Conference on Autonomous Agents and Multi-Agent Systems, Portugal (2008)
28. DeVault, D., J. Mell, Gratch, J.: Toward natural turn-taking in a virtual human negotiation agent. In: AAAI Spring Symposium on Turn-taking and Coordination in Human-Machine Interaction. AAAI Press, Stanford (2015)
29. Park, S., et al.: Mutual behaviors during dyadic negotiation: automatic prediction of respondent reactions. In: 2013 Humaine Association Conference on Affective Computing and Intelligent Interaction (ACII). IEEE (2013)

An Architecture for Biologically Grounded Real-Time Reflexive Behavior

Ulysses Bernardet[1(✉)], Mathieu Chollet[2], Steve DiPaola[1], and Stefan Scherer[2]

[1] School of Interactive Arts and Technology, Simon Fraser University Vancouver,
Vancouver, Canada
{ubernard,sdipaola}@sfu.ca
[2] Institute for Creative Technologies, University of Southern California, Los Angeles, CA, USA
{mchollet,scherer}@ict.usc.edu

Abstract. In this paper, we present a reflexive behavior architecture, that is geared towards the application in the control of the non-verbal behavior of the virtual humans in a public speaking training system. The model is organized along the distinction between behavior triggers that are internal (endogenous) to the agent, and those that origin in the environment (exogenous). The endogenous subsystem controls gaze behavior, triggers self-adaptors, and shifts between different postures, while the exogenous system controls the reaction towards auditory stimuli with different temporal and valence characteristics. We evaluate the different components empirically by letting participants compare the output of the proposed system to valid alternative variations.

Keywords: Reactive behavior · Reflexive behavior · Cognitive architecture idle attention · Virtual character

1 Introduction

In this paper, we present a pre-cognitive, reflexive architecture that is based on the distinction between reflexive behavior that has external and internal triggers. Examples of such reflexive behavior are orientation and startle responses to sounds in the environment or posture shift based on effort, respectively. We adopt a systems-based approach, and our aim is to provide a mechanistic model that is grounded in plausible psychological mechanisms. The presented architecture is geared towards the application in the control of the nonverbal behavior of the virtual humans that constitute the audience in a public speaking training system [1]. The development of the reflexive architecture is motivated by the argument that the efficacy of virtual humans as stand-ins for biological humans e.g. in training and therapy hinges on the social co-presence of the agent. Part and parcel of this is that the agent displays a realistic level of sensory-behavioral contingency, meaning that the character is showing behavior that is contingent on events that happen in the environment and within the agent [2]. This contingency is achieved by equipping the character with the ability to respond rapidly and plausibly to events that happen in the environment, be it the virtual space shared with the user in the case of full immersion, or events in the real world, in the case of a mixed-reality setup. In the

© Springer International Publishing AG 2016
D. Traum et al. (Eds.): IVA 2016, LNAI 10011, pp. 295–305, 2016.
DOI: 10.1007/978-3-319-47665-0_26

context of public speaking training, the reflexive behavior system should increase the overall plausibility of the behavior of the virtual humans, hence increasing the quality of the implicit feedback offered to the trainee. Furthermore, as the behavior control is parameterized, it can be easily integrated with implicit feedback by means of audience behavior, e.g. by controlling the level of restlessness of the spectators.

1.1 Related Work

Behavior that is not a direct response to an event in the environment partially overlaps with what is called "idle" behavior in the domain of virtual characters. In the context of the model presented here, we refer to this behavior as endogenous reflexive behavior that we conceptualize as a response to internal triggers. The domains that are under the control of this system are self-adaptors, posture shifting, and gaze. The term "*self-adaptors*" refers to a class of self-touching behaviors that have no clear communicative function, and hence also occur when a person is alone. Self-adaptors are under weak intentional control and are thought to originally have served the purpose of satisfying some bodily need such as grooming. A number of studies empirically investigate self-adaptor usage e.g. in the context of counseling sessions [3], and the effect they have on the perception of a virtual character [4]. However, most architectures of nonverbal behavior, if they do include self-adaptors at all, do so by coupling them to verbal communication. The bulk of research on *posture* is related to gait and standing, and postural asymmetries related to pathologies such as stroke and Parkinson's. Muscle fatigue plays a major role and is best investigate in standing postures. In the domain of conversational agents most, work on posture shifting is related to the structure and content of the discourse [5].

In our model, we refer to behavior that is triggered by events outside of the agent as "exogenous". Attention as a mechanism that filters and prioritizes stimuli perceived by an organism plays a key role in this behavior and a number of attention models have been proposed for virtual characters. Most of these models, however, do not elaborate on the behavioral consequences of the attention process. In real as well as in virtual humans *gaze* serves a number of functions, including signaling of interest and emotional state, as well as regulation of conversations through the management of turn-taking [6]. Correspondingly, a number of works have investigated, mechanics of and models for gaze shifting [e.g. [7]]. Gaze behavior independent of non-verbal or verbal exchange has been empirically investigated and modeled by [8], while [9] propose a model for attention towards specific objects in the environment of the agent.

Some virtual character architectures do include idle behavior [10], with the work of [11] on passive listening agents being probably the closest to the architecture presented here. Yet, in most virtual character architectures nonverbal behavior is coupled to symbolic expression.

2   Reflexive Behavior Architecture

The model presented here operates in an approximated continuous time domain with continuous internal variables (as opposed to a finite-state machine or a look-up table). Where possible we recur to known neurobiological processes such as habituation, refractory periods, leaky integrators etc. The rationale behind this approach is to gear the model towards an eventual grounding in the neurobiological substrate. A pragmatic reason why we need to model underlying processes is that we want to develop a system that is capable of generating different behaviors with a minimal set of parameters. This is of particular interest when wanting to implement multiple discernible characters e.g. for a heterogeneous audience. By having a system with only a few, meaningful parameters, we can easily create a wide range of individualized characters without having to deal with an unmanageable number of parameters. Note that in the remainder of the description of the system we will indicate which are the parameters that can be tuned.

2.1   Architecture Overview

At the most abstract level, the system can be divided into five components: At the "Input stage" the user is generating the inputs into the reflexive system and controls the playback of a spatialized sound in the virtual environment. The behavior control model itself comprises a slow and rapid exogenous and one endogenous reflexive behavior subsystem. These three subsystems independently send control signals to the virtual characters. In the current realization of the model, the endogenous subsystem controls gaze behavior, triggers self-adaptor actions, and shifts between different postures. The exogenous subsystem controls gaze behavior as well and additionally triggers different facial expressions. The endogenous subsystem is the default system that controls behavior in the absence of external events. As soon as an event in the environment occurs, that exogenous reflexive behavior takes control, shunting all endogenous behavior. This is achieved through a state of the slow exogenous subsystem that represent interest in the event, and a "post startle inhibition period" in the rapid response subsystem. Note that in the current version of the model, the exogenous reflexive behavior only includes auditory input, and the auditory stimulus is generated within the system itself and rendered with the virtual environment (as opposed to sensed from the real-world).

2.2   Endogenous Reflexive Behavior

Endogenous behaviors refer to actions that are driven by internal e.g. proprioceptive, signals. This class of behaviors comprises self-adaptors such as scratching, posture, and gaze behavior. Clearly, all these behaviors do have functions that go beyond mere reflexive action e.g. in communication, in the context of the architecture presented here, however, we, explicitly do not include these factors.

Self-adaptor behavior: Self-adaptors are behaviors of touching of one's hand, face or body to scratch, rub, groom, or caress it. Self-adaptor behavior can be motivated externally, or arise from internal motivations such as psychological discomfort, or as a displacement activity. Our functional view of self-adaptor behavior assumes that there are specific triggers and associated action that are being performed. At the core of the self-adaptor control stand two Poisson processes, that produce binary events with delays that follow a Poisson distribution (for diagram see https://figshare.com/articles/Endogenous_Self-adaptor_subsystem/3381547). One process generates events for adaptor targeting the head, the second one triggers self-adapting behavior on the extremities. We give the head self-adaptor a slight priority by implementing a "lateral inhibition" of the extremities self-adaptors, i.e. if both are triggered at exactly the same time, only the head action will be executed. Since the two pulse trains that trigger the actions are stochastic, actions can potentially be triggered in rapid succession. To prevent this unrealistic behavior, we use a refractory period mechanism that suppresses triggers that are too close together. In the current implementation, the adaptor locations can trigger a set of two possible actions, i.e. neck rubbing/head scratching and hand rubbing/finger rubbing). Note that this choice was partially defined by the available animations, and does not present an inherent limitation of the system. In total the self-adaptor system has three tunable parameters: The two Poisson λ parameters that control the shape of the probability distribution of the occurrence for extremities and head self-adaptors, and the length refractory period.

Posture shifting based on fatigue: The second component of the endogenous system we will describe is the shifting between different postures. In the context of our model we are primarily interested in the somatic aspect of posture, and more specifically the motivation for switching from one posture to another. The key mechanism for posture switching is the accumulation of the effort that a posture requires maintaining. The effort of the current posture is integrated over time, and once the threshold is reached, a new posture is selected and the integrator is reset (for diagram see https://figshare.com/articles/Endogenous_Posture_control_subsystem/3381544). At this moment we manually define the effort each posture requires, but the model is explicitly constructed such that a realistic computation of actual strain on the joint and muscles can be added. The tunable parameters of the posture control system are the actual postures themselves, and their associated effort.

Gaze control: The gaze control system is loosely based on the system described in [12]. Similarly, we implement a process that is oscillating between mutual and non-mutual gaze. One key difference is that we draw the dwell times for mutual and non-mutual gaze from Poisson distributions. These distributions approximate the fitting function presented in [12], with that advantage of an easily tunable parameter in the form of the λ of the Poisson distribution. The gaze control process begins by drawing a random number from a Poisson distribution (for diagram see https://figshare.com/articles/Endogenous_Gaze_control_subsystem/3381550). This number then defines the duration for which the agent is looking at the speaker (this is implemented a linear decay function that triggers an event at zero-crossing). This event simultaneously starts the delay process for the non-mutual gaze and triggers gazing at a random location. Once the waiting time for the non-mutual gaze has expired, a new cycle of mutual gaze is initialized. The non-mutual gaze direction is drawing its horizontal and vertical saccade amplitude from a normal distribution with the location of the speaker as the mean. This allows having gaze which is more widely spread e.g. in the horizontal than the vertical plane. The parameters that can be tuned to control the gaze behavior are the λ parameters for the mutual and non-mutual Poisson distribution of the dwell time, and the variances for the horizontal and the vertical saccade amplitude. Additionally, the "Extent" parameter allows tuning which joints are involved in the gaze behavior (ranging from eyes only to eyes/neck/chest/back).

2.3 Exogenous Reflexive Behavior

We refer to behaviors that are a direct consequence of an event in the environment as exogenous (e.g., an acoustic distractor within the virtual or real space). Functionally this reflexive behavior often subserves the acquisition of further information and, depending on the nature of the stimulus, the avoidance of harm. For the latter reason the exogenous reflexive system is generally more concerned with aversive than with appetitive stimuli, and in many cases, the behavior is accompanied by a brief, autonomic expression of affect. The exogenous reflexive behavior control is split into one circuit that deals with stimuli that are sudden, short, and strong, and one that controls the behavior towards sustained and slower onset stimuli. Both circuits are running in parallel, but due do their different sensitivity, most stimuli will only activate one or the other.

Rapid response system: The only input the rapid response system receives is the amplitude time course of the stimulus (distance scaling is taken care of in the "Input stage" block). The first signal processing stage is to detect that the stimulus is of rapid onset (Fig. 1 "Rapid onset detector"). This detection is achieved by first calculating the derivative of the stimulus, then applying a threshold, and finally detecting the binary edge. A computation of the derivative is required because the edge detector block by itself requires a signal that is raising from 0 to 1 in a single step, which is not realistic for even the most sudden signal that we would naturally encounter. The output of the edge detector will trigger a startle response comprising of a startle animation combined with the expression of surprise (Fig. 1 "startleBehavior"). The sensitivity of the system can be tuned using the "Startle threshold" parameter. We can assume that to startle is a fairly singular event, meaning that it should not occur repeatedly within a short amount of time. To implement this process, we use the mechanism of a refractory period (Fig. 1 "startleRefractory") that generates a shunting signal of a specific amount of time, effectively preventing startle behavior from occurring during that period. Internally the refractory mechanism is realized as a leaky integrator. Since startling is a somewhat disruptive event, we want to prevent the system from going back to normal operation for some time. This is realized with a "Post-startle inhibition", that produces a signal which will inhibit the endogenous reflexive system for a specific amount of time. This inhibition process is as well implemented in the form a leaky integrator. Both the "startleRefractory" and the "Post-startle inhibition" have a tunable time constant parameters.

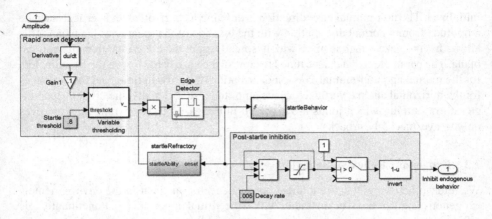

Fig. 1. Rapid response component of the exogenous reflexive system.

Slow response system: The slow response system has as inputs the position of the speaker (or camera) and the agent, as well as the amplitude time course and valence of the stimulus (Fig. 2). The positional inputs determine where that agent will attend to, while the amplitude time course and the valence, influence the dynamic response of the system.

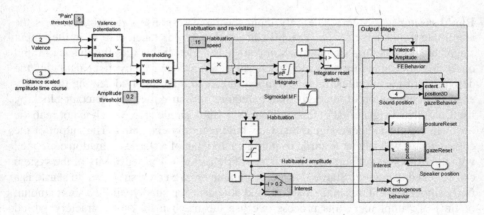

Fig. 2. Slow response component of the exogenous reflexive behavior subsystem.

The first processing step of the amplitude signal is a simple thresholding operation that ensures that low amplitude signals are discarded. At the core of the slow response system is the circuit for "Habituation and re-visiting". Within this block, the amplitude is integrated over time and smoothed with a sigmoid function (Fig. 2 "Sigmoid MF") to create a "Habituation" signal. This signal is then subtracted from the amplitude time course to yield a "Habituated amplitude". A drop of the input amplitude to zero immediately resets the integrator, and hence the habituation. A "Habituated amplitude" above a given threshold yields a binary "Interest" signal. At the output stage an "Interest" above zero enables both, the affective facial expression (Fig. 2 "FEbehavior") as well as the gazing in the direction for the sound (Fig. 2 "gazeBehavior"). The *valence* of the expression of affect is directly proportional to the valence' of the stimulus. While an onset of "interest" triggers the upright posture (Fig. 2 "postureReset"), a drop of "interest" to zero leads to gaze reset (Fig. 2 "gazeReset"), i.e. the agent gazes back at the speaker. In contrast to the binary "Interest" signal, the "Habituated amplitude" is a graded signal that varies in strength over time. It is this signal that controls the *amplitude* of the facial expression and the extent of joints – ranging from head only to head-neck-chest-back – involved in the gazing behavior. Hence the facial expression will be weaker, and the gazing will be less pronounced the weaker or further away a sound is. With the circuit described thus far the agent will gaze at the location of the sound source and display a facial expression as long as the agent has not habituated to the signal, or the single has not dropped to zero. We assume that it is plausible that an agent will eventually re-visit a sustained input signal, not completely ignore it indefinitely. We implement this revisiting behavior by resetting the integrator via the "Integrator reset switch" once it reaches a saturation threshold. The effect of this reset is that the system treats the input as novel, with the consequence of the agent exhibiting re-visiting behavior. The slow response subsystem has a total of three tunable parameters: Amplitude threshold, habituation speed, and Interest threshold.

2.4 Implementation

The high-level control of the behavior of the virtual humans is implemented using the graphical simulation environment Simulink[1] that allows implementing both, continuous as well as discrete control mechanisms [13]. We run a fixed step, soft real-time simulation using the block from [14]. The SmartBody virtual character system serves as the output platform [15], while the open source m+m software [16] provides middleware transportation layer between Simulink and SmartBody.

3   Empirical Evaluation

3.1   Stimulus Material and Procedure

To evaluate the reflexive behavior system, we conducted and empirical study; we ask participants to compare outputs generate with the model to variants. The subsystems were tested individually, i.e. subsystems that are not tested were disable during the experiment. All variants were generated by modifying the original model. We aimed to compare valid alternatives, i.e. variants that constitute plausible variations of the model, rather than generating arbitrary behavior.

To test the appropriateness of the reflexive behavior to rapid vs. slow onset stimuli we used an auditory input that comprises a sequence of a slamming door and ringing phone. The behavior of the proposed system (V1 https://youtu.be/HappUkyg6l8) was a startle response

---

[1] www.mathworks.com/products/simulink.

after the door slam input and an orientation towards the location of the ringing phone. In the variation (V2 https://youtu.be/1-65HQViwdY), the agent we switched the sounds, and the agent was not startled by the phone and oriented towards the sound of the slammed door. We evaluated the influence of the affective response to external stimuli *(slow system affective response)* by comparing a strong negative response to a phone ringing (V1p/− https://youtu.be/qE7ZbId9YAQ) with no display of affect (V2c https://youtu.be/vMBrTf0wJVo) to the same sound, and a positive affective response to an audio clip of a group chatting (V1c/+ https://youtu.be/eNW9AQu-S3A) to no affective response to the same sound (V2p https://youtu.be/g3L66hEE6Mg). All videos were 10 s long. Lastly, we tested the *slow System habituation* by comparing the behavior towards the sound of chatting. The behavior of the proposed system (V1 https://youtu.be/1Apn71B68Ts) was that the agent orients towards the sound then looks back at the camera (habituation), and as a third behavior orients again towards the sound source (re-visiting). In V2 (https://youtu.be/I8icefKNHkU) the agent shows no habituation, i.e. continues gazing in the direction of the sound, while in V3 (https://youtu.be/f2F1CVN_lRc) he shows habituation, but no re-visiting.

In the case of the exogenous behavior, the system was tested with internally generated signals (i.e. not recorded from the real-world). The test signals comprised of three components: (1) Amplitude time course, (2) Valence of the signal (constant over time), (3) Location in space. The amplitude time course is manually designed (as opposed to computed as an envelope) to mimic the key properties of the input signal such as speed of onset and duration. We assessed the realism of the videos using a scaled pairwise comparison. In this paradigm, participants are asked to indicate whether one video is much more, slightly more, or equally realistic.

4   Results

For the data analysis we used a tournament style scoring system: For each pairwise comparison between two videos we assign 1 or 2 points to the "winning video" (depending on whether participants chose "slightly more realistic" or "much more realistic", respectively). For the answer "Both videos are equivalent" both videos were given 0.5 points. The final score per video is the total score normalized by the number of matches played. A total of 343 pairs of videos were rated by 65 unique Amazon mechanical Turk workers, with age >18 years, and location U.S.A. Five pairs where the video did have a sound, but participant did not indicate which sound was played, were omitted.

Exogenous reflexive behavior: Somewhat surprisingly, swapping the door slam and the phone ringing sound did not yield a difference in perceived realism (Fig. 3a); startling when a door is slammed or when a phone rings, or, conversely, turning towards a phone ringing or towards a door that was slammed, are rated as equally realistic. All tested variations of the affective response in the slow system were rated very similarly (Fig. 3b). A positive response to chatting was virtually equivalent to no affective response to the same sound. Both, in turn, were rated as slightly more realistic than no affective response towards a phone ringing, or negative response respectively. Lastly, the variations on the habituation response yielded the biggest differences in realism (Fig. 3c). Habituating to a stimulus but not re-visiting the location of the sound source was deemed more realistic than a sustained gazing in the direction of the sound. By far the most realistic behavior was generated by the proposed system, i.e. by habituation to the sound and subsequent re-visiting.

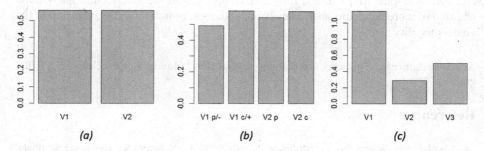

(a)   (b)   (c)

Fig. 3. Evaluation of the exogenous reflexive system. (a) Rapid and slow system response. **V1**: Startle after door slam, orientation towards phone ring, **V2:** Startle response to phone sound, orientation towards door slam, (b) Slow system-affective response. **V1p/−:** Sound: phone ring, strong negative response, **V1c/+:** Sound: chatting, positive response, **V2p:** Phone ring, no affective response, **V2c:** Chatting, no affective response. (c) Slow system habituation (sound: chatting). **V2:** No habituation, **V3:** Normal habituation, no re-visiting.

5   Discussion

In the exogenous subsystem, one of the most unexpected results was that swapping door slam and phone sound did not make a difference. In hindsight, it does indeed make sense that a person would, in addition to a startle response, also show an orientation response towards the rapid onset door slam sound. Conversely, startling, when a phone rings, is similarly something most people will have experienced personally. The mixed results regarding the affective response hint at the problem that the signal to noise ratio between affective response and distractors such as posture, eye movement etc. was not big enough. The open-ended question that asked participants about the reason for their assessment showed that some participants found the affective response was exaggerated, while others did not seem to have noticed it at all. Adding more channels for affective expressions besides facial animations would allow tuning down the amplitude of the latter (hence avoiding unrealistic exaggeration), while simultaneously making the affective response more detectable. The results regarding the habituation response seem to indicate that realism is best achieved for systems that neither involve an affective response nor require that participants pick up on the stochastic nature of a temporal distribution.

6   Conclusion

In this paper, we have presented ongoing work on the development of a reflexive behavior architecture. We follow a systems approach where we build models based on dynamic mechanisms underlying the actual behavior. One of the advantages of this approach is that a small set of canonical parameters can generate a wide range of different behaviors. In the initial phase of the development, the architecture parameters were set based mostly on the modeler's common sense. A next step will be to ground the parameter values empirically. Planned further developments of the architecture include the addition of more behaviors such as evasion, and, most importantly, the inclusion of the visual modality.

Acknowledgments. This work was partially supported by "Moving Stories" Canadian SSHRC grant.

References

1. Chollet, M., Wörtwein, T., Morency, L., Shapiro, A., Scherer, S.: Exploring feedback strategies to improve public speaking. In: Proceedings of the 2015 ACM International Joint Conference on Pervasive and Ubiquitous Computing - UbiComp 2015, pp. 1143–1154. ACM Press, New York (2015)
2. Inderbitzin, M., Betella, A., Lanatá, A., Scilingo, E.P., Bernardet, U., Verschure, P.F.M.J.: The social perceptual salience effect. J. Exp. Psychol. Hum. Percept. Perform. **39**, 62–74 (2013)
3. Schulman, D., Bickmore, T.: Changes in verbal and nonverbal conversational behavior in long-term interaction. In: Proceedings of the 14th ACM International Conference on Multimodal Interaction (2012)
4. Krämer, N.C., Simons, N., Kopp, S.: The Effects of an embodied conversational agent's nonverbal behavior on user's evaluation and behavioral mimicry. In: Pelachaud, C., Martin, J.-C., André, E., Chollet, G., Karpouzis, K., Pelé, D. (eds.) IVA 2007. LNCS, vol. 4722, pp. 238–251. Springer, Heidelberg (2007)
5. Schulman, D., Bickmore, T.: Posture, relationship, and discourse structure: models of nonverbal behavior for long-term interaction. In: Vilhjálmsson, H.H., Kopp, S., Marsella, S., Thórisson, K.R. (eds.) IVA 2011. LNCS, vol. 6895, pp. 106–112. Springer, Heidelberg (2011)
6. Ruhland, K., Andrist, S., Badler, J., Peters, C., Badler, N., Gleicher, M., Mutlu, B., Mcdonnell, R.: Look me in the eyes: a survey of eye and gaze animation for virtual agents and artificial systems. In: Eurographics State-of-the-Art Report, pp. 69–91 (2014)
7. Pejsa, T., Andrist, S., Gleicher, M., Mutlu, B.: Gaze and attention management for embodied conversational agents. ACM Trans. Interact. Intell. Syst. **5**, 3:1–3:34 (2015)
8. Cafaro, A., Gaito, R., Vilhjálmsson, H.H.: Animating idle gaze in public places. In: Ruttkay, Z., Kipp, M., Nijholt, A., Vilhjálmsson, H.H. (eds.) IVA 2009. LNCS, vol. 5773, pp. 250–256. Springer, Heidelberg (2009)
9. Kokkinara, E., Oyekoya, O.: Modelling selective visual attention for autonomous virtual characters. Animat. Virtual **22**, 361–369 (2011)
10. Kallmann, M., Monzani, J.-S., Caicedo, A., Thalmann, D.: ACE: a platform for the real time simulation of virtual human agents. In: Computer Animation and Simulation, pp. 73–84 (2000)
11. Maatman, R.M., Gratch, J., Marsella, S.C.: Natural behavior of a listening agent. In: Panayiotopoulos, T., Gratch, J., Aylett, R.S., Ballin, D., Olivier, P., Rist, T. (eds.) IVA 2005. LNCS (LNAI), vol. 3661, pp. 25–36. Springer, Heidelberg (2005)
12. Lee, S.P., Badler, J.B., Badler, N.I.: Eyes alive. ACM Trans. Graph. **21**, 637–644 (2002)

13. Saberi, M., Bernardet, U., DiPaola, S.: Model of personality-based, nonverbal behavior in affective virtual humanoid character. In: 2015 International Conference on Multimodal Interaction - ICMI 2015 (2015)
14. Houtzager, I.: Simulink block for real time execution. http://www.mathworks.com/matlabcentral/fileexchange/30953-simulink-block-for-real-time-execution
15. Shapiro, A.: Building a character animation system. In: Allbeck, J.M., Faloutsos, P. (eds.) MIG 2011. LNCS, vol. 7060, pp. 98–109. Springer, Heidelberg (2011)
16. Bernardet, U., Schiphorst, T., Adhia, D., Jaffe, N., Wang, J., Nixon, M., Alemi, O., Phillips, J., DiPaola, S., Pasquier, P.: m+m: a novel middleware for distributed, movement based interactive multimedia systems. In: Proceedings of the 3rd International Symposium on Movement and Computing - MOCO 2016. pp. 21:1–21:9. ACM Press, New York (2016)

Thinking Outside the Box: Co-planning Scientific Presentations with Virtual Agents

Ha Trinh[1(✉)], Darren Edge[2], Lazlo Ring[1], and Timothy Bickmore[1]

[1] College of Computer and Information Science, Northeastern University, Boston, MA, USA
hatrinh@ccs.neu.edu
[2] Microsoft Research Cambridge, Cambridge, UK

Abstract. Oral presentations are central to scientific communication, yet the quality of many scientific presentations is poor. To improve presentation quality, scientists need to invest greater effort in the creative design of presentation content. We present AceTalk, a presentation planning system supported by a virtual assistant. This assistant motivates and collaborates with users in a structured brainstorming process to explore engaging presentation structures and content types. Our study of AceTalk demonstrates the potential of human-agent collaboration to facilitate the design of audience-centered presentations, while highlighting the need for rich modelling of audiences, presenters and talk contexts.

Keywords: Presentation planning · Embodied conversational agents · Scientific presentations · Slideware · Powerpoint · Collaboration · Creativity support

1 Introduction

Although oral presentations are an integral feature of science, the typical quality of scientific presentations is low [5], resulting in their failing to engage, motivate, and persuade their scientific audiences and the public. In a survey of 2,501 professionals [5], support for better organization of presentation content was highlighted as one of five areas in most need of improvement. To shift away from their stereotypical presentations, scientists need to spend more time and energy on the planning of creative content for the benefit of their anticipated audiences. This requires exploring multiple narrative structures as well as incorporating a range of narrative devices (e.g., stories, anecdotes, summaries) that go beyond the dry recollection of topics, facts, and figures.

One way to encourage presenters to "think outside the box" is collaborative brainstorming of alternative presentation formats. Studies have shown that brainstorming in groups – when certain guidelines are followed – can be more productive than individual brainstorming, because it allows members to share ideas and to contribute their unique viewpoints and problem-solving approaches [10].

Our research explores the potential of human-computer collaboration to support presentation planning for the scientific community. We aim to take advantage of collaborative brainstorming dynamics to create engaging, audience-centered presentations that diversify presentation forms while better delivering on their intended functions. We

© Springer International Publishing AG 2016
D. Traum et al. (Eds.): IVA 2016, LNAI 10011, pp. 306–316, 2016.
DOI: 10.1007/978-3-319-47665-0_27

began with a workshop study of how human dyads collaborate on the design of conference presentations, to understand the concerns and processes involved when humans perform this task. Inspired by findings from our study and recommendations from the literature, we developed AceTalk, a PowerPoint add-in that supports collaborative presentation planning between a human and a virtual agent. Using conversation, the virtual agent motivates and guides the human presenter through a structured planning process. Our structured process consists of three stages: elicitation of presentation context; guided brainstorming with rhetorical templates; and narrative structuring. Our contributions include:

1. Derivation of three grounded themes that describe current practices in scientific presentation planning and motivate a human-agent collaborative planning approach;
2. Design of the AceTalk system that supports structured presentation planning with a virtual assistant;
3. Demonstration in a formative study of the benefits and issues arising from presentation planning with AceTalk.

2   Related Work

2.1   Human-Agent Collaboration and Creativity Support

Virtual agents have been used in a number of pedagogical applications across various domains (e.g., AutoTutor [8]) to improve learner motivation [13] and learning outcomes [12]. However, most of these systems focused on tasks with well-defined solutions. There have been limited studies exploring the potential of agents to support brainstorming and the open-ended task of creative content composition. One such example is Wang et al.'s study on agent-based dynamic support for collaborative brainstorming in scientific inquiry [17]. In this study, individuals or dyads of participants brainstormed ideas to solve a scientific problem in a chatroom-like interface. During their brainstorming sessions, an agent offered feedback and contributed questions based on the topics being discussed. Results of the study suggested that the agent could be beneficial in mitigating process losses traditionally associated with group brainstorming. To our knowledge, there has been no research to date that explores the use of agents, either as a coach, collaborator or audience, to support the creative process of presentation design.

2.2   Best Practices in Presentation Planning

In his book *"Presenting to Win"*, Weissman [18] describes five cardinal sins of presentations: no clear point; no audience benefit; no flow; too detailed; too long. As the first step to avoid committing these sins, many presentation books (e.g., [1, 4, 18]) advise to begin the planning process with a clear definition of the presenter's objectives and the target audience. Abela [1] recommends making a list of "important" audience members with specific personality types and communication preferences, while Weissman [18] suggests to start with the key question of *"What's in it for you?"* as a way to establish audience benefits.

Once the target audience has been established, many books (e.g., [1, 4, 18]) advocate a bottom-up, brainstorming approach to content planning. The presenter is encouraged to generate as many content items as possible through divergent thinking, before filtering them down and organizing them into a compelling narrative structure. The result of this process should be a balanced collection of facts, stories, anecdotes and visuals that flow logically and naturally to tell a compelling story to the audience. Various narrative structures have been proposed in the presentation literature, such as Weissman's sixteen flow structures [18], and Duarte's *"What is – What could be"* contrast structure [4]. These structures could potentially serve as templates to guide the presenters through their exploration of alternative formats for scientific presentations.

2.3 Presentation Technologies

A number of research projects have proposed methods to support the planning, rehearsal, or delivery of oral presentations. The advantages of narrative-driven presentation planning have been demonstrated by TurningPoint [11], a PowerPoint add-in that supports sticky-note-style ideation and clustering of content in parallel with the use of narrative templates to both elicit content and guide its sequencing of into a meaningful flow. The PitchPerfect system [16] has shown that a more structured approach also benefits presentation rehearsal, while DynamicDuo [15] has demonstrated that virtual agents can effectively co-deliver presentations with human presenters. We extend this prior work by investigating the potential of human-agent interactive collaboration to facilitate presentation planning.

3 Scientific Presentations and Collaboration

We conducted an exploratory study to explore the potential benefits of collaboration during presentation planning, as well as attitudes towards scientific presentations.

3.1 Procedure

We conducted a workshop in which dyads of participants each delivered a 5-minute presentation of a pre-selected scientific conference paper. Each dyad received their assigned paper two days prior to the workshop. They then took part in a 1-hour design session a day before the workshop, where they collaborated on the preparation of their presentation. Beyond the design session, participants were encouraged to spend extra time composing their presentation, if desired. We also provided participants with a summary of best practices in designing presentation content and flow, synthesized from advice in popular presentation self-help books [4, 18]. Following the workshop, we conducted a semi-structured interview with each dyad to better understand their collaboration process, as well as the typical practices of each member of the dyad when preparing scientific presentations.

3.2 Participants

We recruited 12 students and professionals (5 male, 7 female, ages 20–54, mean 30) with varying levels of presentation experience and backgrounds in computer science, communication, and life sciences. Of the 12 participants, 3 were categorized as high competence public speakers, 2 as low competence public speakers, and 7 as moderate competence according to the Self-Perceived Communication Competence Scale [6].

3.3 Findings

The interviews were recorded, transcribed and coded by two researchers using thematic analysis techniques [2]. Our initial open coding resulted in 223 process codes capturing actions in data. We categorized these codes into six categories related to the planning, authoring, rehearsal and delivery of scientific presentations. Here we present the three categories that are directly related to presentation planning, demonstrating the effects of stereotypes, motivation and collaboration on the planning process.

Modelling Presentations after Stereotypes. Many participants expressed low expect-ations towards the general quality of scientific presentations, yet they were resistant to break away from the norm, because *"by nature, academic stuff is like, controlled, to the point, and kind of bland"* [P1]. Although some presenters recognized the need to create engaging presentation content, they were discouraged by the perceived conflict between engagement and seriousness in academic presentations:

"Before I was trying to make the presentations more engaging, more interactive. But once I went to conferences, I see a lot of people make their slides more serious, more scientific. So I think maybe that's the way we should present" [P7].

Most participants also reported that they did not follow the best practice guidelines we had provided. Reasons included a lack of preparation time, low motivation, and difficulties applying the *"meta-level"* [P11] recommendations in specific cases. However, those who followed the guidelines appreciated their benefits, e.g., in making their presentations *"a little more fun and engaging instead of just heavy facts and infor-mation"* [P4].

Planning on Slides with Scientific Templates. In contrast to the brainstorming approach recommended in the guidelines and literature in general, most participants started planning their presentations by first highlighting important points on printouts of their assigned paper, then creating slides following the written structure of the paper:

"We just took the sections in the paper and added them out as main points" [P9].

This resulted in nearly identical presentation structures (Introduction, Related Work, etc.) being used for all the presentations – *"pretty boring for people"* [P4]. Only a few participants recommended structuring the presentations around the audience's benefits, because: *"I can be like, here it is, here's what we did and here's the result, but that doesn't mean it matters to anyone"* [P5].

Strengthening Content through Collaboration. Many participants highlighted the benefits of collaboration in terms of avoiding content bias, since they were encouraged to consider and incorporate different viewpoints:

"If you are working on one slide, you might have some bias about this section, but the other one will give you wonderful ideas about how to present, what is the most important thing" [P7].

Several participants reported that the collaboration process motivated them to create more audience-focused content, because *"your collaborator could be your first audience in the process"* [P8]. This prompted them to *"make [the presentation] more interactive by adding images and videos"* [P7]. The feelings of shared workload and companionship through collaboration also helped presenters to reduce anxiety, both during preparation and delivery. However, these benefits came at the cost of increased effort and time invested during the presentation planning stage.

3.4   Design Implications

Informed by the findings of our interview analysis and best practices from the presentation literature, we derived three implications for the design of presentation planning support tools:

1. Motivate creation of audience-focused content by acting as an audience advocate to proactively elicit and review content from the audience's perspective;
2. Support exploration of non-stereotypical presentation structures through collaborative brainstorming guided by diverse narrative templates;
3. Provide expert advice in an interactive and digestible manner, dynamically adapting to the content matter, presenter's objectives, and talk context.

4   Design of AceTalk

Based on our design implications, we developed AceTalk (**A**gent for **C**reating **E**ngaging **Talk**s), a PowerPoint add-in that supports collaborative presentation planning between a human and a virtual assistant. Through conversation, the assistant motivates and collaborates with the human presenter in the brainstorming of engaging presentation structures and content types. During the process, she provides the presenter with narrative templates and recommendations drawn from the literature on presentation and classical rhetoric. To compensate for the time spent on planning, the system automatically generates provisional slides from the brainstormed content. We now describe our virtual assistant and the structured planning process that she mediates.

4.1   Virtual Assistant

Our virtual assistant, Angela, is an embodied conversational agent developed using Unity (Fig. 1). Angela communicates with the human presenter using synthetic speech. She is capable of displaying a variety of nonverbal behaviors, including facial expressions, eyebrow movement, directional gazes, head nods, posture shifts, and hand gestures (contrastive gestures for comparisons, beat gestures for emphasis, and deictic gestures for on-screen spatial references). Most of her nonverbal behavior is automatically generated using the BEAT text-to-embodied speech system [3]. Human-agent dialogues are scripted using a custom scripting language based on hierarchical transition network. User input to the conversation is obtained via multiple choice selection of utterance options, updated at each turn of the conversation.

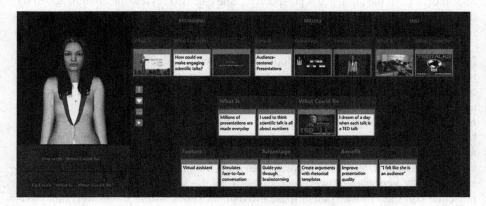

Fig. 1. Collaborative planning environment with the virtual agent (left), brainstorming canvas (bottom), and narrative strip (top).

4.2 Conversation-Led Presentation Planning Process

Through conversation, Angela guides the human presenter through three stages of the planning process:

Elicitation of Presentation Context. At the beginning of the process, Angela engages the user in a brief Motivational Interviewing [7] dialogue to enhance the presenter's intrinsic motivation and confidence to prepare an engaging presentation. She then prompts the user for general information, including presentation length, preparation duration, and target audience, before introducing them to the brainstorming approach recommended in the literature. At the end of this stage, Angela asks the presenter to identify the most important contribution of their work with regard to the target audience, and uses it to suggest a high-level rhetorical template to guide the brainstorming stage.

Guided Brainstorming with Rhetorical Templates. A rhetorical template is a structure used to elicit and categorize presentation content from the user at various levels of abstraction. Each rhetorical template has two components: a macro template addressing the overarching question of *"what's in it for the audience?"*, and a collection of micro templates describing core details of the presenter's work. An example is the *"Invention"* template, used to present the description of something new, which combines the macro template *What Is – What Could Be* [4], and the micro template *Feature – Advantage – Benefit* [18] (Fig. 1).

During brainstorming, Angela instructs the presenter to add four types of content notes (facts, stories, images and videos) to the rhetorical template they are currently instantiating, starting from macro templates, then progressing to micro templates (Fig. 1). Angela encourages the presenter to consider various possible arguments for their presentation without concern for linear sequencing of content. On request, Angela provides specific examples of arguments that can go in the template, explaining their importance from the audience's perspective. She can also review the content added by the presenter, reminding them to add stories, anecdotes or interesting visuals to help increase audience engagement.

Narrative Structuring. On completion of the content brainstorming process, Angela instructs the presenter to filter and select the most engaging content items from the filled templates, then linearly sequence them into the classic 3-act story structure: beginning, middle, and end (Fig. 1). The agent encourages the presenter to consider multiple structuring options with regard to how they benefit the audience. For example, presenting all benefits up front before going into the features and advantages, as a way to fully capture audience attention at the start, versus repeating the benefit-advantage-feature pattern for each benefit in turn, as a way of creating suspense. At the end of this stage, the system automatically generates PowerPoint slides from the selected content sequence. The presenter can then further polish these provisional slides within the PowerPoint environment.

5 AceTalk User Study

We conducted a formative study to examine the benefits and issues of the agent-assisted presentation planning approach embodied in AceTalk.

5.1 Procedure

The study consisted of a 90-minute session in which participants prepared and delivered a presentation with our system. Participants were asked to redesign a scientific talk that they had given in the past. This task was chosen as it allowed the participants to compare the process and presentation content created with AceTalk against their past presentation. The study began with an initial semi-structured interview about the preparation and delivery of the previous presentation. We then gave participants one hour to interact with AceTalk to create a new, 8-minute version of their presentation, before giving a video-recorded presentation. We assessed user satisfaction with AceTalk (Table 1), and State Anxiety [14] and Speaker Competence [9] for both their prior and new presentations. We concluded the study with a final semi-structured interview, prompting critical reflections on both the structured planning process, and the role of the virtual assistant in facilitating that process.

Table 1. Average satisfaction ratings of the virtual assistant

Rating on scale 1 (not at all) − 7 (very much)	Mean (SD)
How *satisfied* are you with…?	5.45 (1.04)
How much would you like to *give future presentations* with…?	5.82 (1.32)
How much do you *like* …?	5.91 (1.14)
How *easy* was it to use…?	4.00 (2.05)
How much do you feel you *trust* …?	6.10 (1.22)
How much *help* was …?	5.10 (1.64)

5.2 Participants

We recruited 11 graduate students and professionals (3 male, 8 female, ages 23-31, mean 27), with backgrounds in design, medicine, social science and different fields of computer science. 3 participants were categorized as high competence public speakers, 1 as low competence public speakers, and 7 as moderate competence, according to the Self-Perceived Communication Competence Scale [6].

5.3 Quantitative Results

The user satisfaction ratings for the agent were highly positive across all participants (Table 1).

Participants reported significantly lower State Anxiety ($t = 3.28$, $p < .01$) and higher Speaker Confidence ($t = 2.27$, $p < .05$) after using AceTalk compared to their retrospective assessment from their past presentation. These comparisons, however, have many potential confounds (e.g., comparing retrospective vs. current state, differences in presentation context, learning effect), so must be interpreted with caution.

5.4 Qualitative Findings

We derived four main themes from the high-level coding and analysis of our final semi-structured interview transcripts, relating to the elicitation of audience-focused content, the use of templates, and the agent's role as a companion in the planning process.

Eliciting Audience-focused Content. Most participants reported that working with the virtual assistant helped them change their presentation content and structure in ways that would be more engaging for the audience: *"I think the structure grabs the attention of the audience a little bit more…a little more striking"* [P10]. Through the questioning strategy, the agent encouraged the presenters to consider the soundness of their content: *"Because she asked me about the question 'what do you think about the benefits of your methodology', and I need to think about it"* [P5]. Several participants expressed that the presence of the agent made them feel *"like she was an audience"* [P9], with explicit needs: *"Before, I didn't think too much about it, I just assume everybody knows"* [P2]. By proactively reviewing existing content and making suggestions to add different content types such as stories, the agent also motivated users to *"think of interesting ways* *of presenting and conveying your information"* [P6]. One participant, however, suggested that the agent should be more knowledgeable about their target audience, to provide more specific recommendations: *"She didn't really ask much about who my audience is. She assumes everyone is interested in the same thing"* [P4].

Providing Interactive Guidance through Conversation. All participants expressed strong preferences for interacting with the agent over traditional text-based interfaces. Compared to written instructions, the conversation format could be more time consuming, but its interactive nature encouraged them to *"pay more attention"* [P5] and therefore *"take more information in"* [P11]. The conversation method also allowed the agent more opportunities to persuade the presenters to follow the guidance: *"I remember when I went to fill up the beginning…and when I chose motivations, she gave me resistance and said 'maybe you should include implications' – it was really cool"* [P7]. The participants also appreciated the communication style of the agent: *"she communicated in a nice way, in that you felt comfortable having her guiding through the steps"* [P6]. Several participants, however, felt that the guidance should evolve and adapt based on specific content matters, presenter characteristics, and time constraints.

Providing Companionship through Collaboration. Several participants reported that the virtual assistant helped increase their confidence through a sense of shared workload: *"Preparing with her gives you a little more confidence because it seems like I have two different brains"* [P10], and thus, *"it doesn't feel like it's a lot of work that you are doing"* [P6]. The companionship provided by the virtual assistant also helped reduce presenter anxiety: *"I feel more relaxed… because I feel like there is someone to support me"* [P9].

Balancing Guiding Structure and Creative Freedom. While many participants reported that our brainstorming process was *"totally new"* [P7] for them, most found it to be helpful. Several participants expressed that the guiding templates and act structures were novel enough to encourage them to *"think outside your normal kind of thinking pattern"* [P6], while still being highly relevant and applicable to scientific research: *"I think the scientific research really falls into this pattern"* [P2]. The templates were reported to help focus the presenter's attention on the overall logic of the presentation in ways that saved time: *"I liked how it took the broad structure, it got you thinking about the main points right away…I did it more quickly this time."* [P11]. Having a *"clear picture"* [P1] of the rhetorical organization of the presentations also helped the presenters feel *"more confident"* [P2] in their delivery. However, once presenters had used the templates to establish their core content and talk structure, they felt comfortable adding more low-level content slides within the less-constrained PowerPoint environment: *"Once you know the way to do it, you want to follow the structure but fill in more of your own content"* [P5]. Several participants expressed the desire to either have more templates of diverse styles (e.g., more *"story structures"* [P3]), or have the flexibility to extend the current templates. One participant also requested "backtracking" opportunities [P4] to switch to other templates should they find the currently chosen template to be inappropriate.

6 Conclusions and Future Work

We have explored the potential of human-agent collaborative planning to facilitate the design of scientific presentations. Our results demonstrated the benefits of this approach in encouraging the exploration of non-stereotypical presentation structures and audience-focused content. We plan to extend our work in three directions. First, we aim to develop a computational model of audiences, presenters and talk contexts, in order to provide more contextualized feedback and recommendations during the brainstorming process of presentation design. Second, we plan to offer more diverse, flexible, and substitutable rhetorical templates. Finally, we aim to evaluate the effectiveness of our system on the presentation quality through controlled, comparative studies.

Acknowledgement. This work is supported in part by the National Science Foundation under award IIS-1514490. Any opinions, findings, and conclusions or recommendations expressed in this material are those of the authors and do not necessarily reflect the views of the National Science Foundation.

References

1. Abela, A.: Advanced Presentations by Design: Creating Communication that Drives Action. Wiley, Hoboken (2008)
2. Braun, V., Clarke, V.: Using thematic analysis in psychology. Qual. Res. Psychol. **3**(2), 77–101 (2006)
3. Cassell, J., Vilhjálmsson, H. H., Bickmore, T.: BEAT: The Behavior Expression Animation Toolkit. In: SIGGRAPH '01, 477–486 (2001)
4. Duarte, N.: Resonate: Presenting Visual Stories that Transform Audiences. Wiley, New York (2010)
5. Goodman, A.: Why Bad Presentations Happen to Good Causes, and How to Ensure They Won't Happen to Yours. Cause Communications, Los Angeles (2006)
6. McCroskey, J.C., McCroskey, L.L.: Self-report as an approach to measuring communication competence. Commun. Res. Rep. **5**, 108–113 (1988)
7. Miller, W., Rollnick, S.: Motivational Interviewing, Second Edition: Preparing People for Change. The Guilford Press, New York (2002)
8. Nye, B.D., Graesser, A.C., Hu, X.: AutoTutor and family: a review of 17 years of natural language tutoring. Int. J. Artif. Intell. Educ. **24**(4), 427–469 (2014)
9. Paul, G.L.: Insight and Desensitization in Psychotherapy: An Experiment in Anxiety Reduction. Stanford University Press, Stanford (1966)
10. Paulus, P.: Groups, teams, and creativity: the creative potential of idea-generating groups. Appl. Psychol. Int. Rev. **49**, 237–262 (2000)
11. Pschetz, L., Yatani, K., Edge, D.: TurningPoint: narrative-driven presentation planning. In: CHI 2014, pp. 1591–1594 (2014)
12. Schroeder, N.L., Adesope, O.O., Gillbert, R.B.: How effective are pedagogical agents for learning? a meta-analytic review. J. Educ. Comput. Res. **46**(1), 1–39 (2013)
13. Schroeder, N.L., Adesope, O.O.: A systematic review of pedagogical agents' persona, motivation, and cognitive load implications for learners. J. Res. Technol. Educ. **46**(3), 229–251 (2014)

14. Spielberger, C.D.: State-trait Anxiety Inventory: Bibliography, 2nd edn. Consulting Psychologists Press, Palo Alto (1989)
15. Trinh, H., Ring, L., Bickmore, T.: DynamicDuo: co-presenting with virtual agents. In: CHI 2015, pp. 1739–1748 (2015)
16. Trinh, H., Yatani, K. Edge, D.: Pitchperfect: integrated rehearsal environment for structured presentation preparation. In: CHI 2014, pp. 1571–1580 (2014)
17. Wang, H., Rosé, C.P., Chang, C.: Agent-based dynamic support for learning from collaborative brainstorming in scientific inquiry. Int. J. Comput.-Support. Collaborative Learn. 6(3), 371–395 (2011)
18. Weissman, J.: Presenting to Win: The Art of Telling Your Story. FT Press, Upper Saddle River (2009)

CAAF: A Cognitive Affective Agent Programming Framework

Frank Kaptein[✉], Joost Broekens, Koen V. Hindriks, and Mark Neerincx

Delft University of Technology, Mekelweg 2, 2628 CD Delft, The Netherlands
F.C.A.Kaptein@tudelft.nl

Abstract. Cognitive agent programming frameworks facilitate the development of intelligent virtual agents. By adding a computational model of emotion to such a framework, one can program agents capable of using and reasoning over emotions. Computational models of emotion are generally based on cognitive appraisal theory; however, these theories introduce a large set of appraisal processes, which are not specified in enough detail for unambiguous implementation in cognitive agent programming frameworks. We present CAAF (Cognitive Affective Agent programming Framework), a framework based on the belief-desire theory of emotions (BDTE), that enables the computation of emotions for cognitive agents (i.e., making them cognitive *affective* agents). In this paper we bridge the remaining gap between BDTE and cognitive agent programming frameworks. We conclude that CAAF models consistent, domain independent emotions for cognitive agent programming.

Keywords: Models of emotionally communicative behavior · Theoretical foundations and formal models · Dimensons of intelligence, cognition and behavior

1 Introduction

Interaction with intelligent virtual agents is facilitated by providing such agents with affective abilities. For example, affective abilities in intelligent agents have been applied to facilitate *entertainment* [17,23], to make an agent more *likable* for the user [3], to get *empathic* reactions from the user [7], and to create the so-called *the illusion of life* [2,18], where characters are modelled to appear more life-like.

Cognitive agents can be programmed in frameworks like, e.g., GOAL [11], Jadex [16], or Jason [4]. A cognitive agent is an autonomous agent that perceives its environment through sensors and acts upon that environment with actuators [24]. It does so based on its *beliefs*, *desires* and *intentions*. Cognitive agents have a *mental state* and a *reasoning cycle* (see Fig. 1). The mental state consists of *beliefs* and *desires*. Beliefs are the agent's representation of its environment. The agent can believe it is walking down the street, or that it is raining outside. Desires are things the agent *wants* to be true. For example, the agent can want to have

© Springer International Publishing AG 2016
D. Traum et al. (Eds.): IVA 2016, LNAI 10011, pp. 317–330, 2016.
DOI: 10.1007/978-3-319-47665-0_28

an umbrella. The *intention* to get an umbrella reflects the agent's commitment to achieve that desire. After sensing *percepts* from the environment, the agent updates its mental state. Based on its beliefs, desires, and intentions, the agent reasons about its next action. The environment can change by itself, in response to an action of the agent, or actions from other agents that are situated in the same environment; thus, the agent may not always be *certain* of the exact *state of affairs* in its environment.

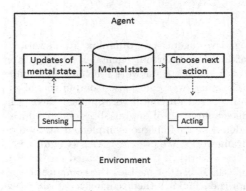

Fig. 1. The reasoning cycle of a cognitive agent.

By adding a computational model of emotion to cognitive agent programming frameworks, one can program intelligent agents capable of using and reasoning over emotions. Computational models of emotion are usually based on cognitive appraisal theories [13]. Cognitive appraisal theory proposes that emotions are consequences of cognitive evaluations (*appraisals*), relating the event to an individual's desires. For example, one is happy because one believes something to be true, and desires this to be true.

However, cognitive appraisal theories [12,15,25] typically introduce a large set of appraisal processes, which are not specified in enough detail for unambiguous implementation in cognitive agent programming frameworks. Psychological theories are developed to explain emotions for humans. These theories are thus not obligated to provide worked out computational specifications for the appraisals.

Here we address this problem by integrating a computational model of the belief-desire theory of emotions (BDTE) [19,20] with a BDI (belief-desire-intention)-based, cognitive agent programming framework. We present CAAF, a Cognitive Affective Agent programming Framework. Emotions are computed based on BDTE for two reasons: (1) because it is conceptually close to the BDI agent framework; and (2) it does not introduce a large set of appraisals that are difficult to describe in a computational manner.

The two main contributions of this work are: (1) We define semantics for the programming constructs of cognitive agents, formalizing how an agent updates its *mental state*, and how emotions are computed. (2) We show when the agent should minimally (re)appraise, by proving that, under some circumstances, the computation of emotions stays consistent when reducing the frequency with which the agent's emotions are recomputed, thereby increasing the efficiency of the computation.

2   Motivation and Related Work

In this article we focus on computational models of emotion based on cognitive appraisal theory. A computational model of emotion describes the eliciting conditions for emotions, often including corresponding intensity. A popular appraisal theory among computer scientists, is the OCC-model [1,15,27]. The appraisal theory by Lazarus [12], and the sequential check theory (SCT) by Scherer [25,26] have also found some attention among computer scientists. For example, the computational model EMA [10,14] is mainly based on the appraisal theory by Lazarus [12], where the link between appraisal and coping is emphasized. EMA models how emotions develop and influence each other. For example, sadness can turn into anger at the responsible source. In [5] a formal notation for the declarative semantics of the structure of appraisal is proposed. Using this, a computational model of emotion is developed based on SCT.

The OCC model is the most implemented cognitive appraisal theory. Computational models based on the OCC model include AR [9], EM [18], FLAME [8], FearNot! [7], FAtiMA [6], and GAMYGDALA [17]. In AR [9] agents judge events based on their pleasantness, and whether they are confirmed, unconfirmed, or disconfirmed. For example, sadness is achieved when an agent confirms an unpleasant event. In EM [18] the aim is to build 'believable agents', agents that appear emotional and engage in social interactions. The EM architecture facilitates artists to model emotional agents in their applications. In FLAME the desirability of an event is modelled with fuzzy sets. For example, they define a fuzzy set 'undesirable event'. Individual events are then partly a member of this set, the amount of membership is adaptively learned over time. FearNot! is an application that helps children to cope with bullying. The agents use planning and expected utility to derive proper emotional responses. Currently the emotional responses in FearNot are triggered with a more enhanced model FAtiMA. FAtiMA divides the appraisal into different modules, all responsible for a separate part of the computation. This enables implementing such modules independently. GAMYGDALA is an emotion engine that can be added to games by annotating events with their influence on the beliefs and desires of different characters.

An underlying problem with many appraisal theories is that cognitive agent programming frameworks lack the required knowledge representations to compute most appraisal processes. For example, a computational model of emotion that aims to describe the OCC-model in total [15], including emotion intensities, needs to model 12 different appraisals. For many of these appraisals it is unclear *how* they should be implemented, e.g., *deservingness*, *sense of reality*, or *proximity.* Other appraisals, e.g., praiseworthiness, require complex constructs like norms and values to be represented by the agent. SCT [25,26] additionally introduces multiple layers in the appraisal process. An event is first analysed in a reactive, bodily responsive, type of way, and later analysed with increasingly nuanced cognitive processes. The computational model of emotion, EMA [14], is mainly based on the appraisal theory by Lazarus [12]. EMA [14] aims to simplify the appraisal processes, introduced by the underlying appraisal theories, and models them from a knowledge representation consisting of beliefs, desires, intentions, and (decision-theoretic) plans. This is conceptually closer to cognitive agent programming frameworks; however, though these frameworks are suited for programming decision-theoretic plans, they do not always do so. This would thus put constraints on the agent programming frameworks for which we want to compute emotions.

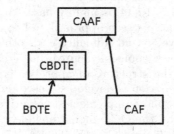

Fig. 2. CAAF is build upon CBDTE [20] and CAFs (Cognitive Agent programming Frameworks). With CAAF, we close the gap between CBDTE and CAFs, and provide a fully worked out, computational account of BDTE.

The appraisals and knowledge representation proposed by the belief-desire theory of emotion (BDTE) [19,20] are more compatible with cognitive agent programming frameworks. In BDTE, emotions are derived only from beliefs and desires. In its minimal form BDTE requires only two appraisals. This makes BDTE more suitable as a basis for simulated emotions for such frameworks.

In this paper we integrate a computational model of BDTE with a cognitive agent programming framework (CAF), hence developing CAAF. In [20], Reisenzein extended BDTE to a computational form (CBDTE). CBDTE has been referred to as a computational model of emotion [13]; however, Reisenzein acknowledges that the motivation behind developing CBDTE was not to develop a worked-out computational model, but rather to clarify aspects of BDTE [20]. Here, we build upon CBDTE, and close the gap between CAFs and CBDTE (see Fig. 2). Thus, this paper presents a *full* computational account of BDTE, and formalizes how a cognitive agent should (efficiently) compute emotions.

3   A Model of Emotion for Cognitive Agent Programming Frameworks

In this Section we present CAAF. We present the formal semantics needed to integrate BDTE with cognitive agent programming. Further, based on this formal system we show in Sect. 4 that emotions can be computed in an efficient way using the model presented here.

3.1   Semantics for a Basic Knowledge Representation and BDTE

The mental state of an agent requires a *knowledge representation*. The agent needs to *represent* states of affairs, to *store* these representations, and to *change* the stored representations.

Representing the states of affairs is achieved with a *language*. This language needs to define a syntax of *well-formed formulae*. We write $\varphi \in \mathcal{L}$ to denote that φ is a formula of language $\mathcal{L}$. Here, a formula is a single proposition that contains information about a *state of affairs*, i.e., it is a sentence that *expresses whether a state of affairs is true (or not)*. We do not define how *logical connectives* work in this language, i.e., symbols that connect propositions such that the sense of the compound proposition depends only on the original sentences (for example, φ_1 *and* φ_2). The contribution of this paper is to define semantics for the programming constructs of cognitive agents, formalizing how an agent updates its *mental state*, and how emotions are computed.

Storing states of affairs is done with a *set*. The belief, desire and emotion base are represented in the semantics as a set of formulae, mapped to a value $[0, 1]$. These bases are a subset of some language $\mathcal{L}$, but contain further information as well. A belief base has the form: $\Sigma : \langle C : \mathcal{L} \rightarrow [0, 1] \rangle$, where C is mapping of a formula φ to (exactly one) certainty value between $[0, 1]$. We denote $b\{\varphi \rightarrow c\} \in \Sigma$ for 'the agent believes φ with certainty c'. Furthermore, we add the constraint that if C contains the mappings $b\{\varphi \rightarrow c\}$ and $b\{\neg\varphi \rightarrow c'\}$, then $c = 1 - c'$. A desire base has the form $\Gamma : \langle U : \mathcal{L} \rightarrow [0, 1] \rangle$, where U is mapping that maps formula φ to a utility value between $[0, 1]$. We denote $d\{\varphi \rightarrow c\} \in \Gamma$ for 'the agent desires φ with utility (strength of desire) u'. Finally an emotion base has the form $\Upsilon : \langle I : \mathcal{L} \times \Theta \rightarrow [0, 1] \rangle$, where $\theta \in \Theta$ is an emotion label (happy, unhappy, hope, fear, surprise, relieve, or disappointment), and I maps formula $\varphi \in \mathcal{L}$ and label $\theta \in \Theta$ to an intensity value between $[0, 1]$. We denote $e\{\varphi \times \theta \rightarrow i\} \in \Upsilon$ for 'the agent has emotion θ (concerning formula φ) with intensity i'. Note that traditional boolean propositional logic (where formulae are either true or false, rather than mapped to a value between $[0, 1]$) would be sufficient for programming cognitive (BDI-based) agents [11]. However, for the computation of many emotions in BDTE we need values between $[0, 1]$. For example, an agent that applies for a new job cannot feel hope (according to BDTE) when it only knows if it got the job afterwards. It should reason over the certainty of getting this job. For example, after having a good job interview. Also note that the emotions in Υ contain a formula, rather than just a label and intensity. With this we model the apparent directedness of emotions, in line with BDTE [20]. One is happy *about* some formula, e.g., $\varphi =$ 'I will get a new job'.

Changing the knowledge representation is denoted with a combine operator $\oplus$. Given some set S and some set T containing a number of formulae, $S \oplus T$ denotes an update of S with T. $\oplus$ is a simple set join, with elements in set T taking priority over elements in set S, to allow updating of c, u and i in S. For all formulae $\varphi \in S$ and $\varphi \in T$, the mapping $\varphi \to n$ in the resulting set is taken from the set T. Thus, $\oplus$ is not symmetric, i.e., $S \oplus T \neq T \oplus S$.

Definition 1 (Combine $\oplus$). *Given some sets S, and T, which contain a number of elements $e = \{\varphi \to n\}$, where φ is a formula $\varphi \in \mathcal{L}$, and n a value $n \in [0, 1]$. $S \oplus T$ is defined as follows:*

$$e \in S \oplus T \quad iff \quad e \in T, \ or \ (e \in S \ and \ e \notin T)$$

A knowledge representation is a pair $\langle \mathcal{L}, \oplus \rangle$, where $\mathcal{L}$ is a language to represent states of affairs, and $\oplus$ defines how a set of formulae is updated with another set of formula. Using our definition of a knowledge representation, we can now formally define what a *mental state* of an agent is. We call this initial definition a 'Simple Mental State' because we will expand it later in the paper.

Definition 2 (Simple Mental State). *A mental state is a pair $\langle \Sigma, \Gamma \rangle$ where Σ is called a belief base, and Γ is a desire base.*

The aim of the work presented here is to add *emotional reasoning* to these agent programming frameworks. The belief-desire theory of emotion (BDTE) [19, 20] provides a method for computing emotional responses based solely on ones beliefs and desires. For BDTE we need only the beliefs and desires, before and after an agent's update of its mental state. We could imagine that a computation of an agent program is a sequence of mental states $m_0, m_1, m_2, \ldots$. BDTE then enables the computation of an agent's emotions in a mental state m_i by using the belief- and desire base corresponding to mental states m_{i-1} and m_i. Based on BDTE we can define the inner workings of this function [20].

Definition 3 describes BDTE in a computational manner. This is based on CBDTE [20]. In function $R(\Sigma, \Sigma', \Gamma, \Gamma') \to \Upsilon$ (R for Reisenzein's appraisal [20]), we denote Σ as the belief base of mental state m_{i-1}, Γ as the desire base of mental state m_{i-1}, Σ' as the belief base in mental state m_i, and Γ' as the desire base of mental state m_i. The function $R(\Sigma, \Sigma', \Gamma, \Gamma')$ computes all new emotions resulting from changes in the mental state.

Definition 3 (BDTE R). *Given function $R(\Sigma, \Sigma', \Gamma, \Gamma') \to \Upsilon$. Let S be the set containing all φ such that $b\{\varphi \to c\} \in \Sigma$, $b\{\varphi \to c'\} \in \Sigma'$, $d\{\varphi \to u\} \in \Gamma$, and $d\{\varphi \to u'\} \in \Gamma'$, with $c \neq c'$, or $u \neq u'$. $S = \{\varphi_1, \ldots, \varphi_n\}$. If we iterate through S with $i = 1 \ldots n$, add the following emotions as follows: $\Upsilon = E_1 \oplus E_2 \oplus \ldots \oplus E_n$, such that:*

$$e\{\varphi_i \times happy \to u\} \in E_i \qquad iff \quad c' = 1 \ \& \ u > 0$$
$$e\{\varphi_i \times unhappy \to u\} \in E_i \qquad iff \quad c' = 0 \ \& \ u > 0$$
$$e\{\varphi_i \times hope \to c' \times u\} \in E_i \qquad iff \quad 0 < c' < 1 \ \& \ u > 0$$
$$e\{\varphi_i \times fear \to (1 - c') \times u\} \in E_i \qquad iff \quad 0 < c' < 1 \ \& \ u > 0$$
$$e\{\varphi_i \times surprise \to 1 - c\} \in E_i \qquad iff \quad c' = 1$$
$$e\{\varphi_i \times surprise \to c\} \in E_i \qquad iff \quad c' = 0$$
$$e\{\varphi_i \times relief \to 1 - c\} \in E_i \qquad iff \quad c' = 1 \ \& \ u > 0$$
$$e\{\varphi_i \times disappointment \to c\} \in E_i \quad iff \quad c' = 0 \ \& \ u > 0$$

For example, let $\varphi_1 = $ 'I got a new job', $b\{\varphi_1 \to 1\} \in \Sigma'$ (i.e., the agent beliefs to have gotten a new job), and $d\{\varphi_1 \to 0.9\} \in \Gamma$ (i.e., the agent strongly desires to have gotten a new job), then Definition 3 prescribes $e\{\varphi_1 \times happy \to 0.9\} \in \Upsilon$ (i.e., the agent is very happy that it got a new job).

With these definitions we already have a framework to implementations, which basically works as proposed in previous work [20]. We might imagine that the computation of an agent program results in a sequence of mental states $m_0, m_1, m_2, \ldots$. Computing emotions can then be done by computing Υ over two consecutive mental states. However, this approach does not take into account that emotion intensities decay over time, how to deal with multiple appraisals of the same emotion label (θ), or the fact that you might want to store emotions for reasoning purposes. Furthermore, computation based on BDTE gives a large set containing multiple emotions for every formula φ the agent has in its mental state, meaning we need a method to abstract useful information from it.

3.2 Closing the Semantic Gap Between BDTE and BDI

In this Section we expand the model such that BDTE can be used for agent programming in an efficient way, including decay, repeated appraisals, and querying the emotions. We start with expanding the mental state of an agent with an emotion base. With this we can store the current emotional state of an agent, and query this when needed.

Definition 4 (Mental State). *A mental state is a triple $\langle \Sigma, \Gamma, \Upsilon \rangle$ where Σ is called a belief base, Γ is a desire base, and Υ is an emotion base.*

With an emotion base storing the emotional responses we can now define a function that gradually decays the intensities of the stored emotions. Function $d(\Upsilon, \Delta t)$ is responsible for decaying the emotional state Υ over time Δt. For the consistency of our model (see Sect. 4) we define Δt to be zero within one reasoning cycle of an agent. Between reasoning cycles, Δt is a function over the actual system time passed between the start of the previous and current reasoning cycle. Function decay is a mapping $d : \Upsilon \to \Upsilon'$, that decreases the intensity $i \in [0, 1]$ for all elements $e\{\varphi \times \theta \to i\} \in \Upsilon$.

Definition 5 (Decay Function d). *Let $e\{\varphi \times \theta \rightarrow i\} \in \Upsilon$. d is a function $d(\Upsilon, \Delta t) \rightarrow \Upsilon'$ defined as:*

$$e\{\varphi \times \theta \rightarrow f(\theta, i, \Delta t)\} \in d(\Upsilon, \Delta t) \quad iff \quad e\{\varphi \times \theta \rightarrow i\} \in \Upsilon$$

Where $f(\theta, i, \Delta t)$ is a function that decreases the intensity i, and for all emotions $e \in \Upsilon$ the emotion also exists in Υ' with a decayed intensity. The function can be initialized differently for every emotion label $\theta \in \Theta$. An example of exponential decay for happy would be: $f(happy, i, \Delta t) = i - i \times \Delta t$.

We adopt the view in [18] that decay may need different instantiations for different emotions, depending on the corresponding emotion label $\theta \in \Theta$. For example, hope and fear may decay slower than surprise. In our model an agent programmer can adjust the default decay function, for every emotion label independently.

The above defined functions come together in (i.e., are sub-functions of) function **EM**. This function is a mapping: $\textbf{EM}(\Sigma \times \Sigma \times \Gamma \times \Gamma \times \Upsilon) \rightarrow \Upsilon$.

Definition 6 (Emotion Base Transformer **EM**). *Let Σ, Γ, and Υ be a belief base, desire base, and emotion base in some mental state m. Further, let Σ', and dbase' be the belief base and desire base after some update on this mental state. Function $\textbf{EM}(\Sigma \times \Sigma' \times \Gamma \times \Gamma' \times \Upsilon) \rightarrow \Upsilon'$ computes the emotion base in this updated mental state as follows:*

$$\Upsilon' = d(\Upsilon, \Delta t) \oplus R(\Sigma, \Sigma', \Gamma, \Gamma')$$

This function is called when the belief base or desire base of an agent change. This happens through *updates*. There is a set of build-in updates that act on the mental state bases of the agent. Updates change the belief and desire bases of the agent. Whilst performing these updates, the agent will automatically add emotions to its emotion base Υ.

Definition 7 (Mental State Transformer $\mathcal{M}$). *Let $\varphi \in \mathcal{L}$, and $n \in [0,1]$. The mental state transformer function $\mathcal{M}(update, m) \rightarrow m'$ is a mapping from built-in updates (update = [insert, adopt, drop]) and mental states $m = \langle \Sigma, \Gamma, \Upsilon \rangle$ to mental states as follows:*

$$\mathcal{M}(\textbf{insert}(\varphi, n), m) = \langle \Sigma \oplus \{\varphi \rightarrow n\}, \Gamma, \Upsilon' \rangle$$
$$\mathcal{M}(\textbf{adopt}(\varphi, n), m) = \langle \Sigma, \Gamma \oplus \{\varphi \rightarrow n\}, \Upsilon' \rangle$$
$$\mathcal{M}(\textbf{drop}(\varphi), m) \quad = \langle \Sigma, \Gamma \oplus \{\varphi \rightarrow 0\}, \Upsilon' \rangle$$

with $\Upsilon' = \textbf{EM}(\Sigma, \Sigma', \Gamma, \Gamma', \Upsilon)$, where Σ' is the belief base, and Γ' is the desire base in the resulting mental state m'.

Mental state bases are defined as sets, thus, if a previous mapping $\{\varphi \rightarrow n\}$ exists in the mental state, then the updates defined above overwrite the previous mapping. In BDTE the claim is made that emotions are subconscious meta-representations of ones beliefs and desires [20]. In the definition above, we model this with function **EM**, which automatically updates the emotions when updating the beliefs, and desires in the mental state.

Definition 8 (Transition rule). *Let m be a mental state, and u be an update ([insert, adopt, drop]) performed in mental state m. The transition relation $\xrightarrow{u}$ is the smallest relation induced by the following transition rule.*

$$\frac{\mathcal{M}(u, m) \text{ is defined}}{m \xrightarrow{u} \mathcal{M}(u, m)}$$

The execution of an agent as explicated above, results in a *computation*. A computation in this context is a list of mental states and corresponding updates, performed by the agent. The new mental state is derived from the transition rule in Definition 8. The agent chooses its next update from the set of possible updates in the current state, this set is filled through the rules defined by the programmer. The computation starts in the initial mental state of the agent.

Definition 9 (Mental Computation). *A mental computation is a sequence of mental states $m_0, u_0, m_1, u_1, m_2, u_2, \ldots$ such that for each i we have that $m_i \xrightarrow{u_i} m_{i+1}$ can be derived using the transition rule of Definition 8.*

The emotion update function **EM** is triggered as part of the Mental State Transformer (Definition 7). It is a part of the mapping from $m_i \xrightarrow{u_i} m_{i+1}$. Emotions are thus computed after every mental state change of an agent.

Figure 1 showed the reasoning cycle of an agent. The mental computation, defined in Definition 9, operates solely in the 'updates of mental state' box. This means that in the model presented here, an agent senses its environment and starts updating its mental state based on these observations. With these mental state updates, we now defined how emotions are automatically changed accordingly. After updating its mental state, the agent can choose a new action to perform in the environment, which in turn changes the environment. The agent then again senses the changes in the environment, and the cycle starts anew.

3.3   Querying the Emotion Base

Querying the emotion base of an agent is useful. For example, if one wants to know if the agent is happy then one should inspect the emotion base for formulae about which the agent is happy. However, a computation based on BDTE gives a large set containing multiple emotions for every formula φ the agent has in its mental state. We therefore need a function that abstracts over these formulae.

To model this, we define an overall *affective state*, which summarizes the agent's emotions. We compute this affective state with function A. This function computes abstractions from the emotion base that enable a programmer to, for example, query the overall happiness of an agent. It summarizes the emotions in some emotion base Υ. It does so by taking all formulae in the emotion base Υ, for all emotion labels $\theta \in \Theta$, and computing a single intensity from these emotions in Υ concerning the emotion label θ.

Besides the computational argumentation there is also a psychological argumentation to define the affective state. In [21] Reisenzein argues that emotions have a hedonic tone, different than that of beliefs and desires. It *feels* a certain way to have an emotion, which is essentially different from how a belief or desire feels. In his own words: "To account for the hedonic tone of emotions in BDTE, one must assume that 'emotional' belief-desire configurations cause a separate mental state that carries the hedonic tone [21]." By means of an affective state we model this hedonic tone of emotions.

Definition 10 (Affective State Ω). Ω *is a function, that computes a generalized affective state which summarizes the emotions* $e\{\varphi \times \theta \rightarrow i\} \in \Upsilon$ *for some emotion label* $\theta \in \Theta$.

$$\Omega(\theta, \Upsilon) = \log_2(\textstyle\sum_{e\{\varphi \times \theta \rightarrow i\} \in \Upsilon} 2^{i \times 10})/10$$

In our model we have implemented $\Omega(\theta, \Upsilon)$ with a logarithmic function (Log_2 $(\sum 2^{i \times 10})/10$), where we sum over all emotions $e\{\varphi \times \theta \rightarrow i\} \in \Upsilon$ corresponding to label θ. Other possible functions might be normal combine: $i' = I/(I + 1)$, with I the summation of all intensities concerning θ), or a simple MAX function (taking the highest intensity emotion corresponding to θ.

From these functions the logarithmic is computationally speaking slightly less efficient; however, the function forces the resulting intensity to be as least as large as the highest value, but takes other values into account. For example, happiness about three different propositions: $\varphi_1 = $ 'Getting a new job', $\varphi_2 = $ 'Buying a new car', and $\varphi_3 = $ 'Going out for dinner', with corresponding intensities: $[0.7, 0.6, 0.3]$, will compute to an overall happiness of 0.76 with logarithmic combine, to 0.62 with normal combine, and to 0.7 with the MAX function.

We do not claim that this is the only correct way to compute the overall affective state, but rather that an agent programmer *requires* a summary to efficiently query the emotion base, and that the here proposed approach will thus help the programmer.

4   Proof of Consistency When Minimizing the (Re)Appraisal of Emotions

In Sect. 3 we defined the (re)computation of an agent's emotions to occur after every mental state update. However, this is not a computationally optimal approach. In this Section we show how one can optimize this by showing when an agent should minimally (re)compute its emotions (i.e., when the agent should *(re)appraise*).

There are three conditions that should trigger a reappraisal: 1, An agent should reappraise before querying its emotion base, if it has updated its mental state since the last reappraisal, since otherwise it would query an outdated emotional state. 2, An agent should reappraise before a mental state update if the last reappraisal was in a previous reasoning cycle, otherwise the emotions are not correctly decayed. 3, An agent should reappraise when it performs a mental state update on a formula that had already been updated after the last reappraisal, otherwise the previous update will be lost. Since 1 and 2 directly follow from the formal semantics, we need only to show that 3 is true. We do so by proving that if we assume that updates refer to different formulae, appraisal can be postponed to the last update. From this one can infer point 3.

Theorem 1 *Consistency For Delayed Appraisal. Let* $u_1, u_2, .., u_n$ *be different mental state updates, with* $\varphi_1, \varphi_2, \ldots, \varphi_n$ *the formulae these updates refer to respectively. Furthermore, let* $u'_1, u'_2, .., u'_n$ *be the same mental state updates; however, for these mental state updates we define the Mental State Transformer (Definition 7) to delay updating the emotion base until* u'_n. *Furthermore let* $\varphi_1 \neq \varphi_2 \neq \ldots \neq \varphi_n$. *Consider the following two possible reasoning cycles:*

$$rc_1: \quad m_0 \xrightarrow{u_1} m_1 \xrightarrow{u_2} \ldots \xrightarrow{u_n} m_n$$
$$rc_2: \quad m_0 \xrightarrow{u'_1} m'_1 \xrightarrow{u'_2} \ldots \xrightarrow{u'_n} m'_n$$

where rc_2 *delays updating the emotion base until update* u'_n. *Under the constraint that* $\varphi_1 \neq \varphi_2 \neq \ldots \neq \varphi_n$, *we can derive that* $m_n = m'_n$.

To show the truth of this claim, let the knowledge bases corresponding to mental state m_i be denoted with, $m_i = \langle \Sigma_i, \Gamma_i, \Upsilon_i \rangle$. Since Σ and Γ are updated normally we need only to show that $\Upsilon_n = \Upsilon'_n$. To this end, we first need to define a property of the definitions. We defined Δt in function d (decay) to be zero within one reasoning cycle. Furthermore, $d(\Upsilon, 0) = \Upsilon$. Due to this, we can ignore decay when comparing reasoning cycles rc_1 and rc_2. If we denote E_i to be the set of emotions resulting from function R in transition $m_{i-1} \xrightarrow{u_i} m_i$, then we can write:

$$\Upsilon_1 = d(\Upsilon_0, 0) \oplus E_1$$
$$= \Upsilon_0 \oplus E_1$$
$$\Upsilon_2 = d(\Upsilon_0 \oplus E_1, 0) \oplus E_2$$
$$= \Upsilon_0 \oplus E_1 \oplus E_2$$
$$\Upsilon_n = \Upsilon_0 \oplus E_1 \oplus E_2 \oplus \ldots \oplus E_n.$$

The emotion base resulting from reasoning cycle 2 can be found with the same definitions. Since the update of the emotion base is delayed, the emotion base $\Upsilon'_{n-1} = \Upsilon_0$. Furthermore, the computation of new emotions (Definition 3) will consider all updated formulae:

$$\Upsilon'_n = d(\Upsilon_0, 0) \oplus \{E_1 \oplus E_2 \oplus \ldots \oplus E_n\}$$
$$= \Upsilon_0 \oplus E_1 \oplus E_2 \oplus \ldots \oplus E_n.$$

If $\varphi_1 \neq \varphi_2 \neq \ldots \neq \varphi_n$, then the emotions in sets $E_1, \ldots, E_n$ do not overwrite each other when added to the emotion bases. Therefore, we can conclude that $\Upsilon_n = \Upsilon'_n$. Together we can now also conclude $m_n = m'_n$.

5   Discussion

In this section we discuss some drawbacks of using BDTE as psychological background. BDTE models a limited range of emotions compared to other theories

(BDTE models 7 emotions, while, for example, OCC models over 20 different emotions). Should an agent programmer want to use the emotions in the agent's decision making, then a smaller set of emotions might be more conceivable; however, there can also be domains in which the set of emotions modelled by BDTE is too limited. For example, when a programmer needs the agent to properly reason over empathic emotions like gratitude and remorse, then BDTE is inadequate in its current form.

Future work could thus complement this framework by modelling social emotions. In [22], Reisenzein discusses possible extensions of BDTE to take social emotions into account. For example, he proposes introducing *altruistic desires*. For example, pity is then explained as a form of displeasure following from the frustration of an *altruistic desire* (desiring something good for someone else). However, this does not provide explanations for all social emotions (e.g., anger). When adding social emotions, one might need to complement the presented framework with additional concepts such as norms.

6   Conclusion

In this paper we presented CAAF (a Cognitive Affective Agent programming Framework), a framework where emotions are computed automatically when agents update their mental states. We presented semantics showing the programming constructs of these agents in a domain-independent manner. With these constructs, a programmer can build an agent program with cognitive agents that automatically compute emotions during runs. We chose BDTE to compute new emotions because it is conceptually close to the BDI architecture and therefore allowed us to embed emotions without introducing many additional concepts in the mental states of the agents.

Our semantics facilitate incremental work. For example, if it is desirable to change the affective state (Definition 10) with a global mood, then one could change the function that computes the affective state (function A), without being forced to adjust the entire framework. One might also want to enable programmers to adjust the emotion base without changing the belief base. Definition 7 defined functions to update the agent's mental state. We could simply complement this definition to contain function *Appraise*, capable of inserting emotions in the emotion base (Υ), similar to the update *insert* for the belief base (Σ). This fits well in the modular approach suggested by Marsella et al. [13], where models can implement parts of a complete cycle of emotional reasoning. For example, one could add a module capable of using emotions to guide the agent's decision making (e.g., what action to perform in the environment, or when to decrease the utility of a desire as a type of coping behaviour). The framework presented in this paper thus provides a modular, domain-independent, and consistent implementation for the computation of emotions for cognitive agent programming frameworks, thus facilitating the development of intelligent virtual agents with affective abilities.

Acknowledgements. This research is done for the PAL (a Personal Assistant for a healthy Lifestyle)-project. PAL is funded by Horizon2020 grant nr. 643783-RIA.

References

1. Adam, C., Herzig, A., Longin, D.: A logical formalization of the OCC theory of emotions. Synthese **168**(2), 201–248 (2009)
2. Bates, J., et al.: The role of emotion in believable agents. Commun. ACM **37**(7), 122–125 (1994)
3. Beale, R., Creed, C.: Affective interaction: how emotional agents affect users. Int. J. Hum.-Comput. Stud. **67**(9), 755–776 (2009)
4. Bordini, R.H., Hübner, J.F., Wooldridge, M.: Programming Multi-Agent Systems in AgentSpeak Using Jason, vol. 8. Wiley, New York (2007)
5. Broekens, J., Degroot, D., Kosters, W.A.: Formal models of appraisal: theory, specification, and computational model. Cogn. Syst. Res. **9**(3), 173–197 (2008)
6. Dias, J., Mascarenhas, S., Paiva, A.: FAtiMA modular: towards an agent architecture with a generic appraisal framework. In: Bosse, T., Broekens, J., Dias, J., Zwaan, J. (eds.) Emotion Modeling. LNCS (LNAI), vol. 8750, pp. 44–56. Springer, Heidelberg (2014). doi:10.1007/978-3-319-12973-0_3
7. Dias, J., Paiva, A.: Feeling and reasoning: a computational model for emotional characters. In: Bento, C., Cardoso, A., Dias, G. (eds.) EPIA 2005. LNCS (LNAI), vol. 3808, pp. 127–140. Springer, Heidelberg (2005). doi:10.1007/11595014_13
8. El-Nasr, M.S., Yen, J., Ioerger, T.R.: Flamefuzzy logic adaptive model of emotions. Auton. Agent. Multi-agent Syst. **3**(3), 219–257 (2000)
9. Elliott, C.D.: The affective reasoner: a process model of emotions in a multi-agent system (1992)
10. Gratch, J., Marsella, S.: A domain-independent framework for modeling emotion. Cogn. Syst. Res. **5**(4), 269–306 (2004)
11. Hindriks, K.V.: ProgrammingRationalAgents in GOAL. In: Seghrouchni, A.E.F., Dix, J., Dastani, M., Bordini, R.H. (eds.) Multi-Agent Programming, pp. 119–157. Springer, Heidelberg (2009)
12. Lazarus, R.S.: Emotion and Adaptation. Oxford University Press, New York (1991)
13. Marsella, S., Gratch, J., Petta, P.: Computational models of emotion. In: Scherer, K.R., Bänziger, T., Roesch, E. (eds.) A Blueprint for Affective Computing-A Sourcebook and Manual, pp. 21–46 (2010)
14. Marsella, S.C., Gratch, J.: EMA: a process model of appraisal dynamics. Cogn. Syst. Res. **10**(1), 70–90 (2009)
15. Ortony, A., Clore, G.L., Collins, A.: The Cognitive Structure of Emotions. Cambridge University Press, Cambridge (1990)
16. Pokahr, A., Braubach, L., Lamersdorf, W.: Jadex: a BDI reasoning engine. In: Bordini, R.H., Dastani, M., Dix, J., Seghrouchni, A.E.F. (eds.) Multi-Agent Programming, pp. 149–174. Springer, Heidelberg (2005)
17. Popescu, A., Broekens, J., van Someren, M.: GAMYGDALA: an emotion engine for games. IEEE Trans. Affect. Comput. **5**(1), 32–44 (2014)
18. Reilly, W.S.: Believable social and emotional agents. Technical report, DTIC Document (1996)
19. Reisenzein, R.: Appraisal processes conceptualized from a schema-theoretic perspective: Contributions to a process analysis of emotions (2001)
20. Reisenzein, R.: Emotions as metarepresentational states of mind: naturalizing the belief-desire theory of emotion. Cogn. Syst. Res. **10**(1), 6–20 (2009)

21. Reisenzein, R.: What is an emotion in the belief-desire theory of emotion? (2012)
22. Reisenzein, R.: Social emotions from the perspective of the computational belief-desire theory of emotion. In: Herzig, A., Lorini, E. (eds.) The Cognitive Foundations of Group Attitudes and Social Interaction, pp. 153–176. Springer, Cham (2015)
23. Rizzo, P.: Why should agents be emotional for entertaining users? A critical analysis. In: Paiva, A. (ed.) IWAI 1999. LNCS (LNAI), vol. 1814, pp. 166–181. Springer, Heidelberg (2000). doi:10.1007/10720296_12
24. Russell, S., Norvig, P.: Artificial Intelligence: A Modern Approach, vol. 25, p. 27. Prentice-Hall, Egnlewood Cliffs (1995)
25. Scherer, K.R.: Appraisal theory. In: Dalgleish, T., Power, M. (eds.) Handbook of Cognition and Emotion, pp. 637–663. Wiley, Chichester (1999)
26. Scherer, K.R.: Appraisal considered as a process of multilevel sequential checking. Appraisal Process. Emot. Theor. Methods Res. **92**, 120 (2001)
27. Steunebrink, B.R., Dastani, M., Meyer, J.-J.C.: The OCC model revisited. In: Proceedings of the 4th Workshop on Emotion and Computing (2009)

Multi-party Language Interaction in a Fast-Paced Game Using Multi-keyword Spotting

Jill Fain Lehman, Nikolas Wolfe, and André Pereira[(✉)]

Disney Research, 4720 Forbes Avenue, Pittsburgh, PA 15213, USA
{jill.lehman,andre.pereira}@disneyresearch.com

Abstract. Existing speech technology tends to be poorly suited for young children at play, both because of their age-specific pronunciation and because they tend to play together, making overlapping speech and side discussions about the play itself ubiquitous. We report the performance of an autonomous, multi-keyword spotter that has been trained and tested on data from a multi-player game designed to focus on these issues. In *Mole Madness*, children laugh, yell, speak at the same time, make side comments and even invent their own forms of keywords to control a virtual on-screen character. Within this challenging language environment, the system achieves 94 % overall recall and 85 % overall accuracy, providing child-child and child-robot pairs with responsive play in a rapid-paced game. This technology can enable others to create novel multi-party interactions for entertainment where a limited number of keywords has to be recognized.

Keywords: Automatic speech recognition · Child-computer interaction · Multi-party interaction · Spoken dialog systems

1 Introduction

Applications using speech recognition are increasingly commonplace, due to both the amount of data available and the maturation of machine learning approaches. Still, existing systems tend to derive their acoustic models largely from adult speech and/or their language models from single-user search and scheduling tasks [2,8]. As a result, they tend to be poorly suited for young children, whose language is acoustically, lexically, syntactically, semantically, and pragmatically distinct [6,9]. This is particularly true for young children at play, who are challenging both because of their age-specific pronunciation and because they tend to play together, making overlapping speech and side discussions about the play itself ubiquitous. The same speech recognition issues occur when designing an entertainment application where a child plays a game with an artificial agent or robot that uses natural language for communicating. In this paper, we report the performance of a multi-keyword spotter that has been trained from and tested

© Springer International Publishing AG 2016
D. Traum et al. (Eds.): IVA 2016, LNAI 10011, pp. 331–340, 2016.
DOI: 10.1007/978-3-319-47665-0_29

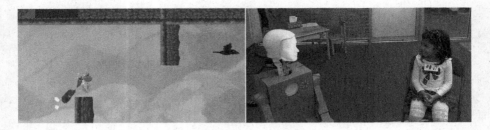

Fig. 1. A Mole Madness screenshot (left) and a play session with Sammy (right).

on data from both child-child and robot-child pairs. The speech recognition system is used to control a virtual on-screen character and it provides children with responsive play in a rapid-paced game, even in the presence of overlapping and out-of-task speech.

2   Mole Madness

Mole Madness is a speech-controlled game in which two players move a virtual mole through its environment, acquiring rewards and avoiding obstacles (Fig. 1, left). One player creates horizontal movement using the word *go* and the other creates vertical movement with *jump*, a simple design that makes the game accessible to even the youngest child with little instruction. Successful play requires both coordinated turn-taking and overlapping speech [7].

The game can be played in a child-child or child-robot configuration with Sammy, a Furhat robot head [1] encased in a cardboard body (Fig. 1, right). The architecture that permits this flexibility includes separate processes for the game engine, speech recognition, and robot control, coordinated by an IrisTK dialog module [10] that synchronizes the independent processes at time-slice boundaries. The mole character and basic game play are built in Unity3D and include the A* search that returns a value when Sammy requests a move on the optimal path. If the returned value is *go* or *jump*, Sammy randomly plays a pre-recorded sound file with one or more instances of that command. The frenetic pace of the game makes Sammy engage in overlapping speech and the pre-recorded sound files include all the language phenomena identified in the next section.

3   The Speech Corpus

Data for the models was collected from 62 children between the ages of five and ten who played *Mole Madness* as part of a multi-activity study in summer 2015. Participants' mean age was 7.45 years (SD = 1.44 years), and 48 % were female. Children were compensated for their participation.

Interleaved with other activities, children played the game twice, first paired with another child and then with Sammy. Each game traversed four to six levels, depending on time available and the child's desire to continue. Speech recognition was performed by a human wizard who listened via headphones in a separate room, trying to map each *go* and *jump* into a button press on a game controller.

To create the ground truth for training the keyword models described below, ∼6.9 h of gameplay were hand-segmented and transcribed, producing ∼11.8K non-overlapping instances of *go*, ∼9.4K non-overlapping instances of *jump*, ∼10.1K instances of overlapping keywords, ∼2.1K social utterances, and ∼12.9K background segments. The resulting corpus contains three language phenomena that define the main challenges for speech recognition and full autonomy in the mole's behavior:

Overlapping speech: *Mole Madness* was specifically designed to elicit overlapping keywords at a small number of predictable obstacles on each level. However, most children discovered that overlapping speech makes the mole "fly" over flat ground. As a result, almost 40 % of keywords overlap in child-child games, and 26 % in child-robot games.

Social side talk: When children play together, task commands (*go*, *jump*) naturally occur intermixed with both non-task speech directed to the mole ("watch out," "faster") and speech directed to the other player ("a giant tomato," "he's funny"). Any speech that is not a keyword becomes a potential source of false keyword recognitions. Meta-comments about game strategy ("don't say jump yet") are particularly challenging because they can contain one or more task words that should not be interpreted as commands. On average, 7 % of utterances during gameplay were social in nature, and 29 %/7 % of child-child/child-robot side talk contained at least one *go* or *jump*.

Lexical variability: A game with only two commands is easy to learn but ultimately frustrating in its lack of expressive power. Children always began by imitating the fully-formed versions of the keywords modeled in a brief tutorial video. However, children throughout our age range eventually tried to increase the task vocabulary ("double jump," "go faster"). When that failed, they created variations of the keywords using elision, repetition, and elongation ("g- g- g- g- go," "juuuuuuuuuump") to encode more complex meanings. Based on the distribution of keyword lengths, we define *fast* and *slow* speech to correspond to a keyword with a length that is less/more than half a standard deviation from the mean length, respectively. We posit that when the child uses a typical *go* or *jump* s/he expects to see an instance of the action per word within a causally-meaningful period of saying it. We interpret the meaning of fast speech relative to that norm - faster speech intends faster movement. Slow speech, conversely, appears to have two distinct meanings. Emphatic elongation ("gooo!") seems to ask for a single bigger movement or a movement right away, while prolonged elongation seems to ask for steady or on-going movement. Children used faster-than-normal forms about 32 % of the time with each other and the robot but were much more likely to use slower-than-normal speech with the robot (27 % of keywords) than the other child (17 %).

4   The Multi-keyword Recognizer

With only two in-task words and the necessity of reacting quickly enough to establish a perceived relationship between the spoken command and the mole's action, the recognition problem in *Mole Madness* is a natural fit to keyword spotting in continuous speech. In this section, we describe the components of the real-time implementation of our multi-keyword recognition algorithm [11], including extensions to that work necessitated by the language phenomena outlined above. Figure 2 grounds the discussion.

In most example-based keyword spotters, training data is used to build a model of the keyword in its entirety and a window on the speech stream that is the size of the expected duration of the word is evaluated against the model in a sliding fashion. As more of the keyword appears in the window, the probability increases that the necessary threshold to signal recognition will be reached. Previous work [11] extended this idea by building separate models of both non-overlapping and overlapping speech, then viewing the speech stream in the window as composed from a probabilistic mixture of those models, using Student's t-distribution (hereafter, TMMs). Models in that work were based on a 300 ms window - the mean duration of *go* and *jump* in the data. The evaluation of the algorithm used pre-segmented keywords, with a categorization of the segment as a whole into one of the classes *go*, *jump*, or *mixed* depending on the most prevalent classification as the window slid across the entire segment.

The online version also models overlap explicitly but extends the previous work in a number of ways. The TMMs in Fig. 2 are trained using the same algorithm and hand-annotated corpus, but with a 150 ms window size and an extended set of classes: *go*, *jump*, their combination (*mixed*), *social speech* and *background* noise segments. The recognition system as a whole can issue at most one command to the mole per time-slice, indicating if *go*, *jump* or both were spoken. The shorter time-slice allows faster response time overall as well as better recognition of individual elided forms in fast speech ("ju- ju- j- jump"). The latter means the mole will better conform to the expectation that faster speech leads to faster movement, but a shorter time-slice also means that less context is available for distinguishing between the keywords themselves and discriminating task speech from social speech. The addition of a distinct *social speech* classifier is used in conjunction with other compensatory features of the system to address this problem, as described below. Similarly, the addition of an explicit *background* model is included to control for another source of false keyword recognition.

At run-time, we perform the maximum-likelihood computation as shown in the middle portion of Fig. 2. The algorithm extracts overlapping blocks of Mel-frequency cepstral vectors (MFCCs,) within the 150 ms time-slice, and then the TMMs are used to compute the posterior probabilities for each of the five class labels with the WEKA library.

The simplest way to translate the output of the TMM classifiers into game commands would be to define a constant posterior threshold, as in [11] and many other systems. Under such an approach, a *go*, *jump* or *mixed* command would be sent to the game at the end of the time-slice if the posterior exceeded the

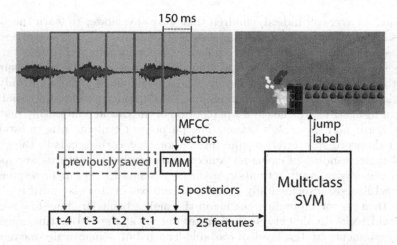

Fig. 2. A sample classification task: audio features of the current 150 ms time-slice are combined with information from four previous time-slices to generate a *jump* label.

respective classifier's threshold, and no game command would be sent if all of those posteriors were below the threshold. Given atypical lexical forms and the intermix of keywords and social speech, we need and can get more power by looking at the relative likelihoods of each class in combination and over time. As shown in Fig. 2, we achieve a finer-grained judgment based on the patterns of probabilities in the training data by building an additional classifier over the combination of posterior values from the TMMs for the current time-slice and several previous time-slices. We tested several algorithms - decision trees, neural networks and Support Vector Machines (SVMs) - and several values for the number of prior segments. Best performance was achieved with four prior segments (600 ms of history) and a multi-class SVM model with a Radial Basis Function (RBF) kernel using the open source LibSVM library and performing a grid search to find the optimal C and gamma values.

The use of prior history is intended to overcome the information that was lost by committing to a more reactive 150 ms time-slice. The solution as a whole - using the full context of the relative likelihood of the five different classes of speech over time - is intended to help distinguish keywords embedded in social speech from keywords that are spoken as task commands. It should also help to discriminate partial keywords that occur at the time-slice level during both elongation and elision from those same sounds when they occur as components of non-task utterances.

5   Method of Evaluation

A metric of evaluation must take into account the contextual and temporal aspects of the real-time game environment. Although the system makes a decision at the end of every 150 ms, accuracy statistics at this architectural level are misleading for two reasons. First, time-slice level accuracy gives undue importance to correct recognition behavior during silence, which constitutes 45 % of any game, on average. Indeed, children that were shy, slower to learn the game, or not fully engaged would have high accuracy measures even in cases where the recognizer was doing poorly on the spoken phenomena required to play.

Second, and more generally, the time-slice is not the unit of measure at which the phenomena of interest occur. These phenomena include not only the linguistic ones - variable-length commands, overlapping speech, and social side talk - but also, critically, the child's perception of the causal relationship between her/his words and the mole's action. The purpose of evaluation is to establish whether the word spotter creates an interaction that corresponds to the child's natural understanding of cause and effect: if one or both keywords are spoken to the mole, the relevant action(s) should be perceived to occur in response; if a keyword is spoken incidentally in a social context, or if no keyword has been spoken, then no corresponding change in the mole's behavior should be seen.

To bridge the divide between recognizer output at the 150 ms time-slice and human judgments at the level of variable-length but semantically-meaningful units, we aggregate the behavior of the recognizer across time with respect to the annotation. The window over which we aggregate reflects assumptions about how long a lag there can be between voicing the command and seeing the mole's behavior change before the child no longer experiences the two as causally connected. Choosing the appropriate recognition window is not a trivial task because it depends on the particular activity or game [3]. The wizard who mapped spoken commands to button presses in our corpus, for example, had a mean reaction time of 529 ms (SD = 419 ms). Despite the variable and occasionally significant lags in the wizard's response, children appeared to experience the game as volitional (if a bit finicky) and enjoyed it overall [11]. These results are in line with both [5], which found a 300–700 ms lag to be acceptable, and [4], which found that a 400 ms lag produced a greater sense of agency than an 800 ms lag in a task where two people were engaged in potentially overlapping behaviors.

Because our application is a fast-paced, real-time game and children's perceptual expectations may be variable, we compute performance statistics both with and without a lag. In the no-lag case, the window over which recognizer output is aggregated extends from the beginning of the annotation through the time-slice in which the annotation ends. This method compensates for imprecision in the annotator's boundaries, holds the system to a tight standard for causality, and defines a lower-bound on performance from a perceptual perspective. In the with-lag case, we follow the literature, allowing for as much as 450 ms between the end of speech and action. The longer window extends from the beginning of the annotation through three time-slices after the end of the annotation. It may give credit for detecting a keyword based on evidence that falls outside the shorter window's view, but does so under the assumption that children would also attribute the mole's action to their utterance within that period.

To compute standard statistics for the multi-keyword recognizer, each annotation in the corpus and each continuous segment of silence must be accounted for. A ground truth keyword annotation counts as either a **false negative** (FN) or a **true positive** (TP). A false negative is scored when there is no time-slice with the keyword's label in the window. Similarly, a true positive is scored if there is at least one time-slice with a matching game command in the window. Thus FN means the character's movement doesn't change as a result of the spoken word and TP means that it appears to do so. A time-slice labeled as *mixed* represents both a *jump* and a *go* command for evaluation purposes.

The TP definition leads to a number of consequences. It means, for example, that a single keyword annotation in the corpus "consumes" all the matching detections within the window's bounds. In the case of average length keywords this is likely to correspond to one, occasionally two, commands per annotation. In the case of fast speech, it means that the system's performance is bounded by the time-slice - the recognizer can get credit for an elided form, at most once every 150 ms. If the system is working well, it will nevertheless recognize enough of those elided forms that the mole's behavior will reflect the child's intent: faster speech will create faster movement. For a slow keyword, however, the TP definition biases the statistics in the recognizer's favor, potentially giving full credit to a five second *go* that has only an occasional correctly-labeled time-slice in it even though the apparent behavior would not correspond to the steady movement that is expected. To remove this bias, we preprocess slow speech into separate consecutive 300 ms keyword (normal duration, steady movement) segments and apply the TP/FN definitions to each segment individually.

The remaining annotations - social speech and, by default, non-speech segments with silence and/or background noises - are the potential sources of *true negative* (TN) judgments. Both types are scored as TN if there is no time-slice with a keyword label in the window. Note that this way of treating silence minimizes the influence of TN on accuracy in the same way that an architectural time-slice accounting would maximize its influence.

Social speech and non-speech segments can also be sources of **false positives** (FP). An FP is scored when a keyword label generated by the recognizer does not fall within the window of any keyword annotation. A false positive is also scored for any isolated (non-overlapping) keyword that is recognized as an instance of the other keyword.

6   Results and Discussion

Table 1 summarizes the results of a 10-fold cross-validation on the corpus, calculated with and without lag. Overall the system's accuracy is 85 % with the more conservative metric, and 89 % with the wider perceptual window. As expected, the increase in accuracy is attributable primarily to keywords that are recognized during time-slices after the end of the annotation.

Note that the poor specificity (with high variability) is attributable largely to our conservative method of scoring silence and social talk. Because such segments are counted as a single unit, a false positive means only that there was at least one time-slice labeled with a keyword during the span. For elongated keywords, we divided the annotation into contiguous 300 ms segments to be able to detect whether the recognizer would produce the expected continuous movement. For stretches of silence and social talk, however, we have no *a priori* understanding

Table 1. Performance means (standard deviations) with and without perceptual lag, overall and separated by co-player type. Precision is the fraction of correctly identified positive results (TP/(TP+FP)). Specificity is the fraction of correctly identified negatives (TN/(TN+FP)). Sensitivity is the proportion of positives that are correctly identified as such (TP/(TP+FN)).

Session type	No lag			With perceptual lag		
	Overall	Child-Child	Child-Robot	Overall	Child-Child	Child-Robot
Accuracy	.85 (.10)	.79 (.11)	.89 (.07)	.89 (.09)	.83 (.10)	.93 (.06)
Precision	.85 (.10)	.78 (.11)	.89 (.07)	.90 (.09)	.83 (.10)	.93 (.06)
Specificity	.70 (.19)	.57 (.20)	.76 (.14)	.77 (.18)	.64 (.18)	.84 (.13)
Sensitivity	.94 (.08)	.92 (.10)	.96 (.06)	.96 (.07)	.93 (.09)	.97 (.05)
Go	.95 (.08)	.93 (.11)	.96 (.05)	.96 (.07)	.94 (.09)	.97 (.04)
Jump	.94 (.09)	.91 (.10)	.96 (.08)	.95 (.08)	.92 (.09)	.97 (.08)
Overlapping	.93 (.09)	.91 (.11)	.95 (.07)	.95 (.08)	.93 (.10)	.96 (.06)
Slow	.95 (.08)	.92 (.08)	.96 (.07)	.96 (.06)	.94 (.08)	.97 (.05)
Medium	.95 (.07)	.92 (.10)	.97 (.04)	.96 (.06)	.94 (.08)	.98 (.03)
Fast	.92 (.12)	.85 (.15)	.95 (.08)	.94 (.11)	.88 (.13)	.97 (.08)

about how often a sporadic unexpected movement can occur before the causal connection between speech and action is shattered. Were we to break background and social segments up using the same 300 ms rule, the specificity would increase to 84 %/88 % in the no lag and perceptual lag conditions, respectively. Nevertheless, the values under the stricter accounting shown here are important for giving a realistic idea of how well the system handles keywords in side talk. The results are less favorable than we would like: social speech with one or more embedded task words still triggers a misrecognition about 65 % of the time, despite the information in the four prior time-slices. The fact that social segments without embedded task words also generate a misrecognition about half the time suggests that we may have erred too much on the side of responsiveness in choosing the time-slice. A somewhat longer time-slice might change the number of errors that come from false recognition of sub-segments of non-task words without substantively affecting the rest of the children's experience. Alternatively, achieving a better balance in the amount of keyword versus social speech data might also help minimize this source of error.

The remaining source of misrecognition (FPs) is the confusion of one keyword for another. This confusion occurs almost entirely from overprediction of the *mixed* category in the presence of a single keyword. The problem seems to stem from a strong correlation between overlapping keywords and volume - when they are excited both children are more likely to be yelling and commanding. As a result, even when children yell a single command alone, the combination serves as evidence for the *mixed* model.

Overall sensitivity is excellent across all conditions, although statistically better and less variable during child-robot games. Higher values occur with the robot co-player because the robot's voice is less varied and more predictable. We intentionally treat the robot like a player with a voice that must be recognized, despite the fact that it is possible to know with certainty when the robot issues a command. Having a uniform solution for both types of co-player simplifies the architecture and allows any agent with natural language synthesis to play our game. As important, it creates a grounded experience for the child given that some errors in detection and the same lag in response can be noticed.

Looking at sensitivity more closely, we find that it is consistent across keywords and not statistically different for non-overlapping and overlapping speech. The one class of phenomena in which we do see differences in recognizer performance is lexical variability: performance is statistically worse on fast speech when compared to either slow speech or typical duration forms. As noted above, false negatives must occur whenever the keyword rate is faster than the 150 ms time-slice. In addition, shortened forms contain less signal and are more error-prone in general. Runs of fast speech occur more often in child-child games, and when they do occur in child-robot games they do so in Sammy's more easily recognized speech about 40 % of the time. As a result, the degradation in performance is significant only in child pairs. Note that although sensitivity is about 7 % worse in fast speech at 150 ms, it is, nonetheless, recognized at least 85 % of the time, often enough to ensure that rapidly repeated keywords produce perceptually faster movement in the mole.

To set these results in a larger context, we compared the performance of the multi-keyword spotter without perceptual lag to the performance of a state-of-the-art commercial continuous speech recognizer given the finite state grammar *go* and *jump*. The commercial system was about 35 % less accurate overall, and displayed a number of biases not seen in our results. In particular, where the word spotter detects *go* and *jump* about equally well, the commercial recognizer was significantly worse at detecting *go* (67 % sensitivity for *jump* versus 40 % sensitivity for *go*). Similarly, the commercial system did more poorly on overlapping than non-overlapping speech (25 % versus 46 %) and showed uniformly decreasing performance as a function of keyword rate (50 % sensitivity on slow words, 45 % on normal duration, and 19 % on fast speech).

7   Conclusions and Future Work

The motivation for this work was to explore a point in the space of multi-party language-based character interactions for young children that confronted head on some of the difficult issues that arise with children at play. *Mole Madness* allows us to study overlapping speech, side talk, and exaggerated variability in pronunciation. Within this challenging environment, the system described in this paper is able to achieve 94 % overall sensitivity and 85 % overall accuracy. The technology presented here can be reproduced with other vocabulary, allowing designers and developers to build novel children's applications that use limited speech to the agent as an input method.

Although our solution works well across most of the phenomena, and significantly better than commercial systems, a number of important questions remain. The first question concerns the generality of the results. *Mole Madness* was designed for only two players and with only two keywords. Although we can imagine many scenarios with most or all of these same characteristics (two children being asked by a character if they want to go left or right, for example), it is important to understand how performance systematically degrades as a function of relaxing these assumptions. What happens when three or more voices are calling out commands? Which results change when the keywords are of varying length, or have common phones or syllables? And, of course, how many keywords can be adequately distinguished given any one or more of these modifications?

References

1. Al Moubayed, S., Beskow, J., Skantze, G., Granström, B.: Furhat: a back-projected human-like robot head for multiparty human-machine interaction. In: Esposito, A., Esposito, A.M., Vinciarelli, A., Hoffmann, R., Müller, V.C. (eds.) Cognitive Behavioural Systems. LNCS, vol. 7403, pp. 114–130. Springer, Heidelberg (2012). doi:10.1007/978-3-642-34584-5_9
2. Bellegarda, J.R.: Spoken language understanding for natural interaction: the Siri experience. In: Mariani, J., Rosset, S., Garnier-Rizet, M., Devillers, L. (eds.) Natural Interaction with Robots, Knowbots and Smartphones, pp. 3–14. Springer, New York (2014)
3. Claypool, M., Claypool, K.: Latency and player actions in online games. Commun. ACM **49**(11), 40–45 (2006)
4. Dewey, J.A., Carr, T.H.: When dyads act in parallel, a sense of agency for the auditory consequences depends on the order of the actions. Conscious. Cogn. **22**(1), 155–166 (2013)
5. Edlund, J., Edelstam, F., Gustafson, J.: Human pause and resume behaviours for unobtrusive human like in-car spoken dialogue systems. In: EACL 2014, p. 73 (2014)
6. Gerosa, M., Giuliani, D., Narayanan, S., Potamianos, A.: A review of ASR technologies for children's speech. In: Proceedings of the 2nd Workshop on Child, Computer and Interaction, WOCCI 2009, pp. 7:1–7:8. ACM, New York (2009)
7. Lehman, J., Al Moubayed, S.: Mole madness-a multi-child, fast-paced, speech-controlled game. In: AAAI Symposium on Turn-Taking and Coordination in Human-Machine Interaction, Stanford, CA (2015)
8. Liao, H., Pundak, G., Siohan, O., Carroll, M.K., Coccaro, N., Jiang, Q.M., Sainath, T.N., Senior, A., Beaufays, F., Bacchiani, M.: Large vocabulary automatic speech recognition for children. In: Sixteenth Annual Conference of the International Speech Communication Association (2015). research.google.com
9. Shivakumar, P.G., Potamianos, A., Lee, S., Narayanan, S.: Improving speech recognition for children using acoustic adaptation and pronunciation modeling. In: Proceedings of Workshop on Child Computer Interaction, September 2014
10. Skantze, G., Al Moubayed, S.: IrisTK: A statechart-based toolkit for multi-party face-to-face interaction. In: Proceedings of the 14th ACM International Conference on Multimodal Interaction, ICMI 2012, pp. 69–76. ACM, New York (2012)
11. Sundar, H., Lehman, J.F., Singh, R.: Keyword spotting in multi-player voice driven games for children. In: Sixteenth Annual Conference of the International Speech Communication Association (2015)

A Design Proposition for Interactive Virtual Tutors in an Informed Environment

Joanna Taoum$^{(\boxtimes)}$, Bilal Nakhal, Elisabetta Bevacqua, and Ronan Querrec

Laboratoire en Sciences et Techniques de l'Information, de la Communication
et de la Connaissance (Lab-STICC), Ecole Nationale d'Ingénieurs de Brest (ENIB),
Centre Européen de Réalité Virtuelle (CERV), Université Bretagne Loire (UBL),
25 Rue Claude Chappe, Plouzané, France
{taoum,nakhal,bevacqua,querrec}@enib.fr
http://www.cerv.fr/

Abstract. This paper introduces a new research work that aims to improve embodied conversational agents with tutor behavior by endowing them with the capability to generate feedback in pedagogical interactions with learners. The virtual agent feedback and the interpretation of the user's feedback are based on the knowledge of the environment (informed virtual environment), the interaction and the pedagogical strategies structured around classical intelligent tutoring system models. We present our first steps to implement our proposed architecture based on a model of informed virtual environment. We also describe the ideas that will guide the design of the Tutor Behavior. The planned evaluation method and a first application are also presented.

Keywords: Embodied conversational agents · Intelligent tutoring system · Feedback · Informed virtual environment

1 Introduction

In the last years, virtual reality (VR) has acquired more and more interest as one of the most potential propositions to change and improve education. Previous research works have shown that this new technology seems to have a positive influence on learning in educational applications [1]. Moreover, the presence of interactive virtual agents also called Embodied Conversational Agents (ECA), by taking the role of tutors [2], seems to have positive effects on the student engagement [3] and the effectiveness of teaching [4].

In this work we aim to improve virtual tutor behavior by endowing it with the capability to generate and interpret feedback signals in pedagogical interactions with learners.

In human-human interactions, people emit regularly feedback signals in order to exchange information about the on-going communication [5]. For example, through feedback two interactants can inform each other about their understanding or their attitudinal reactions about the communicated content. This type of behavior has been proven to be fundamental also in human-virtual agent

© Springer International Publishing AG 2016
D. Traum et al. (Eds.): IVA 2016, LNAI 10011, pp. 341–350, 2016.
DOI: 10.1007/978-3-319-47665-0_30

interactions. For instance, previous researchers have shown that, to assure effective and satisfying interactions, a virtual agent must be able not only to speak but also to provide feedback signals while listening [6].

Previous research studies proposed models to automatically generate the interlocutor's behavior during the interaction with the user. Most of these works focused on a subset of feedback signals called "backchannels", which are multimodal signals provided by the listener without attempting to take the floor [7]. Particularly, previous works tried to determine the right moment to perform a backchannel signal, on the one hand according to the acoustic and visual signals shown by the speaker [8,9] and on the other hand according to the content of the speaker's speech [10]. In the first case the agent performs *reactive* backchannels deriving from perception processing, while in the second case the virtual character performs *responses* backchannels which consist in a more aware behavior generated by reasoning processing. In this work we want to improve the agent behavior by performing a wider set of feedback signals, such as multimodal signals (including backchannels) and short sentences which will make the agent take the turn. Moreover, we want these signals to be deliberate, based on a more reasoning process which takes into account not only the content of what the user can say but also the pedagogical model and the domain model of the environment. The choice of the feedback performed by the virtual tutor will be based on an inference of the learner's cognitive state and can be then consider as cognitive feedback [11].

For example, the agent could frown to show that the action that the learner is currently conducting is wrong. Thereby, the agent would show the learner that they are making a mistake and, at the same time, that it is attentive and watchful to their presence and actions. Another example, if the agent notices that the learner is not looking in the right direction, for instance where the object of interest is, it could point to the object to guide the learner.

This work aims to define a model for virtual tutor able, on the one hand, to observe the learner's actions in order to provide multimodal feedback, and, on the other hand, to recognize the learners' feedback in order to estimate their level of understanding (related to cognitive state). The interaction between the tutor and the learner takes place in an intelligent virtual environment [12]. Unlike traditional virtual environments that are represented only as a set of 3D elements, intelligent virtual environments provide semantic information. Classically this semantic covers the way the user can interact with the object [13]. The goal of intelligent virtual environment is to provide agents with high level of information, which permits them to have more intelligent behaviors. As we consider that the environment can be defined independently of the agent's behaviors, and that the intelligent aspect belongs to agent's behaviors, based on the semantic information in the environment, in the rest of this article we will use the term of informed virtual environment instead of intelligent virtual environment.

In the next section we present the model we use to represent the informed virtual environment. Then in Sect. 3 we describe our proposed architecture highlighting the work already done and ongoing. In the fourth and fifth sections, we describe our planned evaluation method and the first integrated application applied in the domain of education.

2 Informed Virtual Environment Model

In this work we choose MASCARET [14], Multi-Agent System for Collaborative, Adaptive & Realistic Environments for Training, to define the informed (intelligent) virtual environment. We use it as a knowledge base for agents and as an agent architecture.

MASCARET permits to design the semantic of virtual environments (VE). It is a virtual reality meta-model based on the Unified Modeling Language (UML) meta-model. MASCARET covers all the aspects of VEs semantic representation: ontology of the domain, structure of the environment, behavior of the entities, both users and agents interactions and activities. These aspects represents the domain model. In MASCARET we consider pedagogy as a specific domain model. We use then the same language (UML) to describe the domain and the pedagogical model. The pedagogical model is represented in our work by the pedagogical scenario. Koper [15] considers that a pedagogical scenario is composed of five main elements: pedagogical objectives, pedagogical prerequisites, pedagogical activities, pedagogical organizations and pedagogical environments. In MASCARET pedagogical scenarios are implemented through a chain of actions and activities. Those actions and activities can be either pedagogical actions, like explaining a resource, or domain actions, like manipulating an object.

In MASCARET, class diagrams are used to describe the different types of entities, their properties and the structure of the environment. Asynchronous discreet entity behaviors are defined through state machines. Activities are designed as predefined collaborative scenarios (called procedures), which represent plans of action for virtual agents or instructions provided to users for assisting them. The way the activity is interpreted by the agents is defined using specific agent behaviors. It is important to notice that in MASCARET, any entity which acts on the environment is called an agent.

MASCARET is a UML profile (extension) for virtual environments. The domain model is defined using a classical UML modeler and exported in the XMI normalized file format. Classically, to define a VE, computer scientists design the scene and all behaviors that occur in the VE. By using MASCARET, end-users (pedagogue, domain expert and domain trainer) are directly involved in the creation of the VE. The work flow to design a virtual environment for learning is presented in Fig. 1.

The pedagogue defines the pedagogical actions that can be used to guide or correct the trainee in the VE, as well as the pedagogical action forms (typical sequences of actions, reactions and interactions with the objects of the system). These actions are independent from the application domain, from the technological environment and from the pedagogical strategies. However, they depend on the type of learning environment, for example interactive simulations.

The domain expert, who knows the activity which has to be learned, formalizes the sequence of actions and interactions with the objects of the environment.

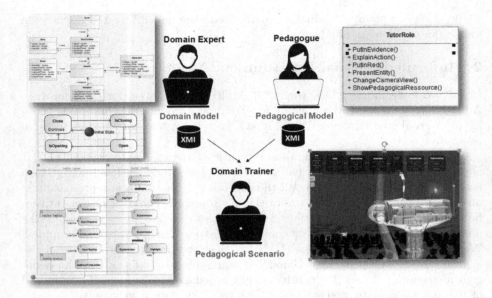

Fig. 1. MASCARET work flow to design a virtual environment for learning.

They also describe good practices and procedures that have to be learned and different behaviors (proactive or reactive) of the objects. This description is independent from the execution platform.

The domain trainer defines pedagogical scenarios (the sequence of situations in which the trainee acts in the environment) and the pedagogical assistance provided by the system in real time. To define the scenarios, the domain trainer uses (1) the environment and the objects it contains, (2) the potential actions of the learner on the objects and the good practices (defined by the domain expert), and (3) the generic pedagogical actions (defined by the pedagogue).

3   Architecture

In this work we aim to add new features to MASCARET in order to integrate a virtual embodied tutor. This tutor has to be able to apply pedagogical strategies and to perform appropriate verbal and non-verbal behaviors while speaking, listening and observing the user. In particular, we want this tutor to be able to provide feedback based on the knowledge of the environment and the interaction. Figure 2, shows the class diagram of the global architecture in which we are developing our work (in blue the elements already integrated and in green what we are working on at the moment).

All entities which can act on the environment are instances of the **Agent** class (we call them simply *agents*). Agents have knowledge about the environment. The structure of this knowledge uses the semantic of the domain and pedagogical

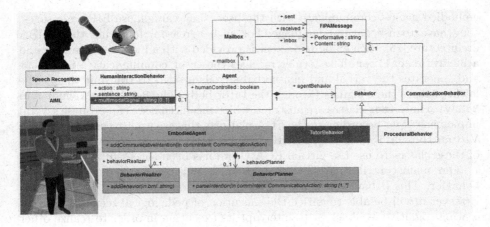

Fig. 2. Proposed global architecture

model explained in Sect. 1. Agents have behaviors (`Behavior`). They have at least a communication behavior (`CommunicationBehavior`) and a procedural behavior (`ProceduralBehavior`), but MASCARET permits to add other generic behaviors (for example a tutor behavior). The communication behavior allows the agents to exchange messages through a `Mailbox`. Agents can communicate using FIPA messages and FIPA-SL content language[1]. FIPA is a formal and normalized language for agent communication. For example, an agent asking for the value of a property of an entity, sends this FIPA message:
`"QueryRef: ((iota ?propertyName (slot ?propertyName ?entity)))"`,
where `iota` and `slot` are keywords. The procedural behavior permits the agent to realize a procedure. By using MASCARET, this procedure is considered as an explicit knowledge during its execution. Agents are then able to execute a procedure and they can also reason about it.

Two types of agents can be instantiated: agents representing human users and embodied agents. Human users are represented as an agent which is not autonomous (`ControlByHuman = true`). They speak in natural language and for such a reason, each agent that represents a user, is provided with an interface (`HumanInteractionBehavior`) which can receive the sentences uttered by the user and translate them to FIPA-SL content by using Artificial Intelligence Markup Language (AIML)[2]. At present, the `HumanInteractionBehavior` interface is connected to RealSense by Intel®, which can recognize also some user's non-verbal signals (such as facial expressions, head orientation, etc.). This interface can also collect the user's actions on the virtual environment, performed, for instance, through a mouse or any other VR peripheral.

Embodied agents can be instantiated in the VE through a humanoid body (`EmbodiedAgent`) or without a physical representation (`Agent`). When

---

[1] http://www.fipa.org/.

[2] http://www.alicebot.org/.

embodied agents communicate with the user, they cannot use FIPA messages, they have to use natural language. For such a reason, following the SAIBA architecture [16], each embodied agent is provided with a `BehaviorPlanner` and a `BehaviorRealizer`. The former receives the tutor communicative intentions and generates the verbal and non-verbal signals needed to transmit them. The latter realizes these signals through the tutor body. The `BehaviorPlanner` and `BehaviorRealizer` classes are abstract, which means that we can propose several implementations according to the ECA platform that we want to use (Greta [17], Virtual Human Toolkit [18], MARC [19], etc.). At present, an implementation of these classes to use the virtual ECA Greta has been successfully integrated.

Our main contribution to this architecture will consist in defining a tutor behavior. This behavior will use the communication and procedural behavior. However it will be able to enrich the execution of pedagogical scenario, by generating cognitive feedback or to interrupt its execution in order to realize other pedagogical actions based on the learner's feedback. The main ideas of this behavior are describe in the following section.

3.1 Tutor Behavior

Our proposed tutor behavior relies on classical intelligent tutoring system (ITS) models [20] and on an inference of the cognitive state of the user while learning in a VE.

Classical ITS are composed of the domain model, the pedagogical model and the learner model. The domain model is represented by the informed virtual environment. It is the knowledge base of the agent that provides it with knowledge about the domain procedures, the actions and the entities states. The pedagogical model is represented in our work by the pedagogical scenario and the set of generic pedagogical actions. The main elements that define the learner model are related to their curriculum, the history of actions realized during the current exercise and the learner profile. In our case (procedural learning on technical systems) the best way to learn a procedure is to repeat several times the execution of the procedure. That is why the curriculum stocks the number of repetitions done by the learner. The curriculum stocks also all the exercises (learned procedures) in a Learning Management System (LMS). This permits to identify the level of expertise of the learner. Our major contribution to the learner model, will be to add the learner feedback. Fitts [21] and Anderson [22] proposed to structure the cognitive processes involved in learning in three stages. The inference of the cognitive state of the student by the tutor is based on these learning stages. For example, during the first stage (cognitive stage), the main cognitive process is based on the identification of objects to manipulate. At the second stage (associative stage) the learner organizes the information to be processed (i.e. list of actions to memorize) using a logical structure (i.e. hierarchy and action's goal) to store it entirely in working memory. During the last stage (autonomous stage) transformation of declarative knowledge to procedural knowledge happens.

The objective of the tutor's behavior is to deduce, according to learner's feedback, in which stage the learner is and which exact cognitive process occurs.

The result of this inference is stored in the learner model. The tutor behavior is defined according to whom (tutor or learner) takes the initiative to interact. Most of the time, the tutor agent can be the initiator of the interaction. For example, the tutor can start by greeting the learner and then it can give them some general information and objectives about the procedure that the learner has to realize. This pedagogical scenario, which is predefined by a real teacher, is executed by the procedural behavior. The tutor behavior checks the user feedback, each time the tutor agent realizes an action.

For example, if the learner frowns after the tutor explanation of the next action, according to this feedback and to the learner model, the agent will be able to decide to realize another pedagogical action. In case of novice learners, the agent will automatically provide more information about the object to manipulate. Whereas, in case of expert learners, the tutor will focus on explaining the goal of the sub-part of the procedure to learn. Furthermore, when the tutor agent asks the learner to manipulate an object, if the learner frowns (or expresses a negative feedback), the tutor can decide to provide more information, for example it can explain the role of the object. At every moment the tutor behavior can be affected by an interruption from the learner. The learner can either interact with the environment or the tutor, by realizing a domain action. After every domain action done by the learner, the tutor checks if the action performed and the object manipulated are correct. Depending on the outcome of this check and on the learner model, the tutor can choose to perform a feedback. For example, when the tutor agent knows that the next action the learner has to realize is to manipulate the object O1, but instead the learner manipulates the object O2, the tutor agent can show a negative feedback, like saying "Wrong", or simply frowning.

4 Evaluation Method

Like some other previous evaluation works [23], based on objective performance measures, we aim to validate objectively the impact of our proposition on the performance of the learner. For that we envisage to apply the experimental protocols defined by Hoareau et al. [24]. In this study, the researchers evaluate the interest of virtual reality for learning procedures on the base of objective performance measures, like the execution time, consulting assistance, the number of errors. The hypotheses that Hoareau et al. evaluated rely on the learning stages presented in Sect. 3.1. Following this evaluation, learning in virtual reality has been validated and even the transfer of the acquired procedure in a virtual environment to a real situation. However, Hoareau et al.'s evaluations and experiments were conducted using non immersive virtual reality devices, like PCs with low graphics quality. In our research, we are planning to do experiments with good graphics quality, and different immersion levels using PCs, virtual reality head mounted display and CAVE[3]. After identifying the best situation for learning, we plan to integrate an embodied virtual agent with the tutor behavior

---

[3] Cave Automatic Virtual Environment.

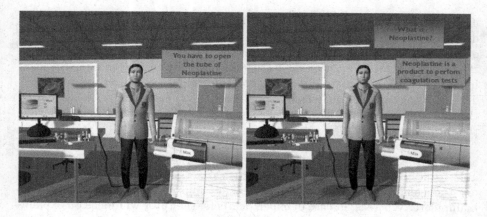

Fig. 3. Screen-shots from the blood analysis procedure

explained in Sect. 3.1 in order to evaluate the influence of the presence of the virtual agent when learning a procedure.

5   Application

A first application was developed and will integrate the behavior described in the Sect. 3. It is an informed virtual environment for procedural learning for blood analysis. The procedures to learn involve actions on the automaton and the reagents preparation. Figure 3 contains two screen-shots taken from this application. In those two pictures the virtual tutor (from the Greta platform) is placed in the middle of the scene. The procedure involves actions applied on the automaton that is positioned at its left (like turning on the machine, opening the drawer, etc.) and actions to prepare the reagents that are at the agent's right, on the bench (like vials, test tubes, etc.). In the left picture, the virtual tutor informs about the first action to perform. In the picture on the right, the learner asks for more information about the object to manipulate (Neoplastine). Through its communication behavior, the virtual agent interprets this question and, using its knowledge about the environment, describes the object.

6   Conclusion

In this paper we presented an on-going work to endow a virtual agent tutor with the capability to provide and interpret feedback in a pedagogical interaction with learners. We showed our first steps to implement the proposed architecture based on a model of informed virtual environment. We also described the ideas that will guide the design of the tutor behavior and its evaluation.

Acknowledgments. This work is supported by a grant from the Région Bretagne and by the ANR, Agence Nationale de la Recherche (INGREDIBLE project).

References

1. Limniou, M., Roberts, D., Papadopoulos, N.: Full immersive virtual environment CAVE[TM] in chemistry education. Comput. Educ. **51**(2), 584–593 (2008)
2. Johnson, W.L., Rizzo, P., Bosma, W., Kole, S., Ghijsen, M., Welbergen, H.: Generating socially appropriate tutorial dialog. In: André, E., Dybkjær, L., Minker, W., Heisterkamp, P. (eds.) ADS 2004. LNCS (LNAI), vol. 3068, pp. 254–264. Springer, Heidelberg (2004). doi:10.1007/978-3-540-24842-2_27
3. Rowe, J., McQuiggan, S., Mott, B., Lester, J.: Motivation in narrative-centered learning environments. In: Proceedings of the Workshop on Narrative Learning Environments, AIED, pp. 40–49 (2007)
4. Kokane, A., Singhal, H., Mukherjee, S., Reddy, G.: Effective e-learning using 3D virtual tutors and WebRTC based multimedia chat. In: International Conference on Recent Trends in Information Technology (ICRTIT), pp. 1–6 (2014)
5. Allwood, J., Nivre, J., Ahlsén, E.: On the semantics and pragmatics of linguistic feedback. J. Semant. **9**(1), 1–30 (1993)
6. Gratch, J., Okhmatovskaia, A., Lamothe, F., Marsella, S., Morales, M., Werf, R.J., Morency, L.-P.: Virtual rapport. In: Gratch, J., Young, M., Aylett, R., Ballin, D., Olivier, P. (eds.) IVA 2006. LNCS (LNAI), vol. 4133, pp. 14–27. Springer, Heidelberg (2006). doi:10.1007/11821830_2
7. Yngve, V.: On getting a word in edgewise. In: Papers from the Sixth Regional Meeting of the Chicago Linguistic Society, pp. 567–577 (1970)
8. Bevacqua, E., de Sevin, E., Hyniewska, S., Pelachaud, C.: A listener model: introducing personality traits. J. Multimodal User Interfaces Spec. Issue Interact. ECAs **6**(1), 27–38 (2012)
9. Morency, L.P., Kok, I., Gratch, J.: Predicting listener backchannels: a probabilistic multimodal approach. In: Prendinger, H., Lester, J., Ishizuka, M. (eds.) IVA 2008. LNCS (LNAI), vol. 5208, pp. 176–190. Springer, Heidelberg (2008). doi:10.1007/978-3-540-85483-8_18
10. Kopp, S., Allwood, J., Grammer, K., Ahlsen, E., Stocksmeier, T.: Modeling embodied feedback with virtual humans. In: Wachsmuth, I., Knoblich, G. (eds.) Modeling Communication with Robots and Virtual Humans. LNCS, vol. 4930, pp. 18–37. Springer, Heidelberg (2008). doi:10.1007/978-3-540-79037-2_2
11. Doherty, M.E., Balzer, W.K.: Cognitive feedback. Adv. Psychol. **54**, 163–197 (1988). Human judgment: The SJT view
12. Aylett, R., Cavazza, M.: Intelligent virtual environments - a state-of-the-art report. In: Duke, D., Scopigno, R. (eds.) Proceedings of Eurographics 2001 (2001)
13. Kallmann, M.: Object interaction in real-time virtual environments. Ph.D. thesis, Swiss Federal Institute of Technology EPFL, Lausanne, Switzerland (2001)
14. Chevaillier, P., Trinh, T., Barange, M., Devillers, F., Soler, J., De Loor, P., Querrec, R.: Semantic modelling of virtual environments using mascaret. In: Proceedings of the Fourth Workshop on Software Engineering and Architectures for Realtime Interactive Systems, IEEE VR, Singapore (2001)
15. Koper, R., van Es, R.: Modelling units of learning from a pedagogical perspective. Online Educ. Using Learn. Objects **40**, 40–52 (2004)
16. Kopp, S., Krenn, B., Marsella, S., Marshall, A.N., Pelachaud, C., Pirker, H., Thórisson, K.R., Vilhjálmsson, H.: Towards a common framework for multimodal generation: the behavior markup language. In: Gratch, J., Young, M., Aylett, R., Ballin, D., Olivier, P. (eds.) IVA 2006. LNCS (LNAI), vol. 4133, pp. 205–217. Springer, Heidelberg (2006). doi:10.1007/11821830_17

17. Niewiadomski, R., Bevacqua, E., Mancini, M., Pelachaud, C.: Greta: an interactive expressive ECA system. In: 8th International Conference AAMAS, pp. 1399–1400 (2009)
18. Gratch, J., Hartholt, A., Dehghani, M., Marsella, S.C.: Virtual humans: a new toolkit for cognitive science research. In: Cognitive Science (2013)
19. Courgeon, M.: Marc: computational models of emotions and their facial expressions for real-time affective human-computer interaction. Ph.D. thesis, Université Paris Sud - Paris XI (2011)
20. Wenger, E.: Artificial Intelligence and Tutoring Systems. Morgan Kaufmann, Los Altos (1987)
21. Fitts, P.: Categories of Human Learning. Academic Press, New York (1964)
22. Anderson, J.: The Architecture of Cognition. Harvard University Press, Cambridge (1983)
23. Atkinson, R.K.: Optimizing learning from examples using animated pedagogical agents. J. Educ. Psychol. **94**(2), 416–427 (2002)
24. Hoareau, C., Ganier, F., Querrec, R., Corre, F.L., Buche, C.: Evolution of cognitive load when learning a procedure in a virtual environment for training. In: 6th International Cognitive Load Theory Conference (ICLTC 2013) (2013)

Do Avatars that Look Like Their Users Improve Performance in a Simulation?

Gale M. Lucas[1]([⊠]), Evan Szablowski[1,2], Jonathan Gratch[1], Andrew Feng[1], Tiffany Huang[1], Jill Boberg[1], and Ari Shapiro[1]

[1] University of Southern California, Los Angeles, USA
`{lucas,gratchc,feng,thuang,boberg,shapiro}@ict.usc.edu`,
`EvanSzab@gmail.com`
[2] University of Oxford, Oxford, England, UK

Abstract. Recent advances in scanning technology have enabled the widespread capture of 3D character models based on human subjects. Intuition suggests that, with these new capabilities to create avatars that look like their users, every player should have his or her own avatar to play videogames or simulations. We explicitly test the impact of having one's own avatar (vs. a yoked control avatar) in a simulation (i.e., maze running task with mines). We test the impact of avatar identity on both subjective (e.g., feeling connected and engaged, liking avatar's appearance, feeling upset when avatar's injured, enjoying the game) and behavioral variables (e.g., time to complete task, speed, number of mines triggered, riskiness of maze path chosen). Results indicate that having an avatar that looks like the user improves their subjective experience, but there is no significant effect on how users behave in the simulation.

1 Introduction

The current work considers whether operating an avatar that is built to look like the user will affect enjoyment and performance in a simulation. Prior correlational research suggests that users will enjoy operating an avatar more if it looks like them (vs. someone else). Indeed, players report greater enjoyment of video games to the extent that they identify with the character being operated (e.g., Hefner et al. 2007). Beyond enjoyment, we consider the impact of using one's own avatar on performance. While the effect on performance has been unstudied, prior work suggests that having an avatar who looks more like the user can affect behavior. For example, users who played a violent video game using a character that mirrored their actual physical appearance were significantly more aggressive than those who played the game with a generic avatar (Hollingdale and Greitemeyer 2013).

If there is a significant effect of operating one's own avatar on performance in a simulation, this could have important implications for certain applications. For example, users in such simulations might act more cautiously with an avatar that looks like them rather than a generic character. To achieve this in a high fidelity application, modern scanning technology that allows for rapid creation of 3D characters from human subjects could be used. While this is becoming more affordable, expenses would still accumulate

© Springer International Publishing AG 2016
D. Traum et al. (Eds.): IVA 2016, LNAI 10011, pp. 351–354, 2016.
DOI: 10.1007/978-3-319-47665-0_31

if it was used on a wide scale across the armed forces. Therefore, we conduct research to establish the effects that using one's own avatar has on user engagement, liking, and enjoyment as well as behavior in the virtual environment, especially performance and care that is taken to prevent the avatar from harm.

2   Current Work

One hundred and six participants (65 males, 41 females) completed a study in which they were randomly assigned to complete the maze with an avatar that looked like them or another participant. Participants were recruited off of craigslist and participated for $25. All participants were first scanned using the method proposed in (Feng et al. 2015) to obtain an articulated 3D character from human subjects. We utilized the Occipital Structure Sensor to obtain the 3D avatar scan from the test subject. It is a depth sensor attached on the Apple iPad to allow portable 3D scanning. The body scanning capture and reconstruction takes 10 min. Participants were also asked to record 4 utterances for pain reactions (e.g. "Ow!", "Ouch!"). Before beginning the maze task, participants were instructed to navigate a maze as fast as possible while avoiding hitting the mines and the walls, and they would receive entries into a lottery based on their ability to do so. Participants next practiced navigating their avatar for one minute, and then started the maze. Navigation was controlled through a WASD keyboard configuration (a gaming standard similar to the arrow keys). Participants controlled their assigned avatar in a third-person view. Running into an obstacle (e.g. a wall or spiked trap) stopped avatar movement and triggered a sound effect of the avatar expressing pain. Participants in the experimental condition used the avatar that was just created from their scan, while those in the yoked control condition used the avatar that was created from the scan from the last gender-matched participant run. Likewise, in the experimental condition, the pain sounds were their own recordings, whereas in the yoked control condition, they were the recordings of the last gender-matched participant. The cover story suggested that the scanning procedure and the maze running task were unrelated, so that participants in the yoked control condition could have an ostensible explanation for using another avatar. Participants were given 15 min to complete the maze. Sixteen participants failed to complete the maze in the time given, and were therefore excluded from analyses below.

After the maze, participants were asked to answer 16 questions about their experience. All items were answered using a 5 point scale ranging from Strongly Disagree (1) to Strongly Agree (5). Participants were asked to complete a manipulation check (1 item) and indicate how realistic the avatar looked (4 items), as well as to report on: the extent to which they were feeling connected and engaged (4 items), how much they liked the avatars appearance (3 items), the extent to which they were feeling upset when the avatar was injured (3 items), and how much they enjoyed the game (1 item). A number of measures were also extracted from the game play during this maze running simulation. First, we measured the total time it took participants to complete the maze in seconds (up to 900 s, which corresponded to the 15 min time limit). We measured the distance they navigated to complete the maze in (virtual) meters, and, thus, also their average speed across the maze in meters per second. We measured the number of times they collided with the maze wall or mines.

Finally, in the areas of the maze where participants had the choice between riskier and safer paths, we calculated the percent of the path that was taken that was risky. We computed the proportion of time spent in the risky zones: (0.5 * (time spent in 1/time spent in 0, 1, 2)) + (0.5 * (time spent in 4/time spent in 3, 4, 5)).

3 Results

Analyses are reported for the 90 participants who completed the maze within the given (15 min) time limit. 2 (condition: experimental vs. control) × 2 (gender: male vs. female) ANCOVAs were run, controlling for the height of the participant's avatar.

The manipulation check showed that our manipulation was successful (M = 4.39, SE = 0.16 vs. M = 2.37, SE = 0.15; $F(1, 85) = 85.69$; $p < .001$). However, this did not affect the extent to which the avatar seemed realistic (M = 4.06, SE = 0.10 vs. M = 3.98, SE = 0.10; $F(1, 85) = 0.36$, $p = .55$), so differences in perceived realism cannot account for any effects on subjective experiences. For both the manipulation check and realism, there were no effects of or interactions with gender ($Fs < 1.45$, $ps > .23$).

We analyzed the subjective experiences of: feeling connected and engaged, liking the appearance of the avatar, feeling upset when the avatar was injured, and enjoying the game. First, participants who navigated the maze with their own avatar reported feeling more connected and engaged than those in the yoked control condition (M = 4.10, SE = 0.12 vs. M = 3.46, SE = 0.12; $F(1, 85) = 14.90$, $p < .001$). There was no effect of or interaction with gender ($Fs < 0.21$, $ps > .64$). Furthermore, participants who navigated the maze with their own avatar also reported liking the appearance of their avatar more than those in the yoked control condition (M = 3.87, SE = 0.12 vs. M = 3.26, SE = 0.12; $F(1, 85) = 12.89$, $p = .001$). There was also a trend for women to like the appearance of the avatar less than men (M = 3.39, SE = 0.15 vs. M = 3.74, SE = 0.11; $F(1, 85) = 2.90$, $p = .09$); however, this effect of gender did not depend on condition ($F(1, 85) = 1.01$, $p = .32$). Apparently women liked the appearance of the avatar less -whether it was their avatar or someone else's- compared to how much men liked the appearance of the avatar.

Concerning either feeling upset or enjoyment, however, there were no main effects. Specifically, there was no effect of condition or gender on feeling upset when the avatar was injured by running into a mine or wall ($Fs < 1.27$, $ps > .26$) or on enjoyment of the game ($Fs < 0.30$, $ps > .58$). There was also no interaction of condition and gender for feeling upset when the avatar was injured ($F(1, 85) = 0.04$, $p = .84$). However, there was a significant interaction between condition and gender for enjoyment of the game ($F(1, 85) = 3.81$, $p = .05$). Men who were assigned their own avatar enjoyed navigating the maze more than men who used someone else's avatar (M = 4.36, SE = 0.16 vs. M = 4.02, SE = 0.16), whereas women who used another player's avatar enjoyed the game more compared to those women who were assigned to use their own avatar (M = 4.25, SE = 0.21 vs. M = 3.90, SE = 0.21).

In contrast to these effects on subjective experience of the users, there were no significant effects of experimental condition (own avatar vs. yoked control) on time to complete the maze, distance travelled in the maze, average speed, number of mines or walls hit, or percent of risky paths chosen ($Fs < 0.93, ps > .34$). Only one effect of gender approached significance; women were marginally slower ($M = 1.44$ m/s, SE = 0.08) than men ($M = 1.65$ m/s, SE = 0.06; $F(1, 85) = 3.55$, $p = .06$); because avatar height was controlled for, this marginal effect is not due to gender difference in height. All other effects of gender were not significant ($Fs < 1.90, ps > .17$), and it did not interact with condition ($Fs < 1.22, ps > .27$).

4   Discussion

From previous speculation, users piloting their own avatars (vs. someone else's) would be expected to show more engagement, liking and enjoyment, as well as better performance and care to prevent injury to their avatar. While the current work suggests that users do feel more engaged and connected and also liked their avatar more, the remaining possibilities were not supported. Only men enjoyed playing the game more with their own avatar than someone else's; women actually showed the opposite effect. Moreover, there were no significant effects of any kind on any behavioral factor. Users with their own avatars did not show differences in time to complete the maze, distance travelled, or speed. They also were no more careful with their avatar on any metric we considered – collisions with mines, collisions with walls, and ratio of riskier paths (shorter but with more mines) over safer paths.

Avatar appearance (own vs. someone else's) may have no relevance to how users play the game. However, it is possible that there is an effect on user performance or behavior, but we failed to find it due to chance. Although there was no effect in a single player simulation, one might be found when two or more players pilot their own avatars in the same virtual environment simultaneously. Further research should address this possibility, as well as explore whether other types of virtual tasks (e.g., social tasks) show differences based on avatar appearance (own vs. someone else's).

Modern scanning technology that allows for rapid creation of 3D characters from human subjects could be used to increase engagement and motivation in training simulations. Users may not perform or behave differently in the simulation, but increased engagement and/or motivation from piloting their own avatars could encourage them to train more and, thereby, possibly improve learning.

Acknowledgments.   This research was supported by the US Army. The content does not necessarily reflect the position or the policy of any Government, and no official endorsement should be inferred.

References

Feng, A., Casas, D., Shapiro, A.: Avatar reshaping and automatic rigging using a deformable model. Motion Games **2015**, 57–64 (2015)

Hefner, D., Klimmt, C., Vorderer, P.: Identification with the player character as determinant of video game enjoyment. In: Ma, L., Rauterberg, M., Nakatsu, R. (eds.) ICEC 2007. LNCS, vol. 4740, pp. 39–48. Springer, Heidelberg (2007)

Hollingdale, J., Greitemeyer, T.: The changing face of aggression: the effect of personalized avatars in a violent video game on levels of aggressive behavior. J. Appl. Soc. Psychol. **43**, 1862–1868 (2013)

Managing Dialog and Joint Actions for Virtual Basketball Teammates

Divesh Lala[1,2(✉)] and Tatsuya Kawahara[1]

[1] Graduate School of Informatics, Kyoto University, Kyoto, Japan
lala@sap.ist.i.kyoto-u.ac.jp, kawahara@i.kyoto-u.ac.jp
[2] Japan Society for the Promotion of Science (JSPS),
Tokyo, Japan

Abstract. Research on embodied teammate agents which use dialog and gesture to coordinate their activities with the user is relatively sparse compared to conversational agents. We propose a dialog management model to handle interactions between user and agent in a virtual basketball environment. The model describes how a joint action should be initialized and executed through dialog, and how it should handle new dialog interruptions. The model also allows the agent to be parameterized to exhibit different combinations of speech and gestural behavior over repeated joint actions. We propose that this model allows us to conduct several types of unique experiments in this environment.

1 Introduction

Many sophisticated systems in agent research have been built for the purpose of providing face to face interactions between humans and virtual agents [1–3]. However these types of interactions are not the only form of communication. In team sports, interactions occur over a wide area and are relatively infrequent, but the same interactions often reoccur.

In this paper we describe the development of agents who will act not as conversational partners, but as teammates in a basketball environment. There are unique challenges related to this type of environment. Players use shorter utterances and expect that the meaning can be inferred from the game context. For example the utterance "Pass" has a different meaning according to whether or not the speaker has the ball. The management of task dialog is also important in basketball. For example, an agent should know that moving to the left could be a sub-task of a passing joint action.

Our long-term goal is to implement communicative behavior for teammate agents which allows them to be perceived as intelligent as opposed to merely reactive to inputs. In real basketball teammates do not often use explicit signals (such as saying "Pass" when calling for a pass) because of their shared experience. Accordingly, our ideal agent should modify their behavior to gradually reduce their use of explicit signals. We propose that this will be indicative of teamwork between human and agent.

© Springer International Publishing AG 2016
D. Traum et al. (Eds.): IVA 2016, LNAI 10011, pp. 355–358, 2016.
DOI: 10.1007/978-3-319-47665-0_32

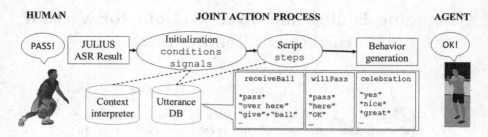

Fig. 1. The general architecture of the dialog manager.

2   Dialog and Joint Action Management

Our general architecture for dialog management is shown in Fig. 1. We consider an interaction between teammates as being a joint action (JA), triggered by either verbal or non-verbal signals. For now we consider only verbal signals and describe an example JA "Call for pass". The JA is initialized as follows:

```
conditions=possession, liveGame, teamAttack
signals=V[receive ball], NV[wave arms], NV[turn to partner]
```

Assume that a human utterance has been received. If the conditional contexts (in possession, a live game, and team on attack) have been met, the agent will check that the utterance (V) is related to the `receive ball` action in the utterance database. The goal of this action is, as the name suggests, to receive the ball. This database defines abstract actions and their related utterances. An utterance can be part of one or more actions. For unmatched utterances, the agent hypothesizes the intended JA using the context or analyze prosodic features to filter out irrelevant utterances such as self talk. Once the JA is initialized, we define a script for how the agent behaves:

```
Step1: {V wait}find space
Step2: {V willpass}turn to partner
Step3: {V throwpass}pass
```

Each `Step` describes a specific action for the agent, in this case finding space, turning to a partner, then throwing a pass. During these actions, the agent *may* select a corresponding utterance (indicated by V). The JA also contains success and failure states to end the JA, although this is not shown here for brevity.

This structure can be used to modify the type of expressive signals of the agent. The script contains information on the verbal utterances an agent may wish to use, but they do not need to. The decision on whether or not to use an utterance is dependent on the beliefs of the agent and can be parameterized.

A feature of basketball is that new dialog may interrupt a JA even before it has finished. The agent must decide whether this interruption *replaces* an existing JA, or *modifies* it. For example, saying "Go left" replaces an existing JA of "Go right", but modifies a "Pass ball" JA, because it assumes that going left

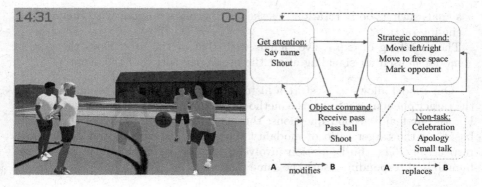

Fig. 2. A screen shot of the game (left) and the model for joint action categorizations and interruption handling (right).

is a sub-task to be completed in order to pass the ball. We handle interruptions by categorizing JAs into four types as in Fig. 2. Three of the types are related to task behavior - getting attention, object commands and strategic commands. Object commands are joint actions those which involve moving the ball, while strategic commands involve only the player. Through this structure the agent decides how JAs should be handled given a new utterance.

Our system implementation uses the VISIE system described in previous work [4]. This system allows the user to play basketball without handheld peripherals by recognizing gestures of passing, shooting and dribbling. The user navigates throughout the environment by walking on a pressure sensor. We integrated a Japanese speech recognition system, Julius [5], which allows the user to communicate through spoken commands via a headset.

We created two agents, Akira and Tamako, to act as teammates for a human player. These agents can also recognize non-verbal communication signals [6]. To implement the above dialog management system, we conducted Wizard-of-Oz experiments to collect data on the speech and gesture used by humans during the basketball game. We then created a speech corpus and categorized the utterances which will be recognized in the system.

3   Experimental Scenarios

Our system allows humans to play with both agents and compare the two directly. With our architecture we are able to parameterize the communicative behavior of the agents in the game. More specifically, we can address the following interrelated research issues on the perception of agents in this environment:

- The ideal ratio of verbal to non-verbal signals. Do users have a preference for agents responding with speech, gesture, or both?
- The use of signals as interaction progresses. Is it more natural for the agent to slowly transition - from explicit utterances and gestures to more implicit

signals such as body rotation - as the user becomes familiar with them during the interaction?
- The matching of expressive signals with that of the user. Does the type of modality used for signaling affect the user's perception of the agent?

Our model allows us to store a history of communicative acts, and based on the target phenomena decide the method of communication during a joint action. For the first and second questions, the agent decides the form of their signal based on the target ratio of modality types and historical signal explicitness, respectively. The third question involves recognizing the modality used by the human and responding using the same modality.

4   Conclusion

We described how our virtual basketball agents manage user dialog and how they can flexibly use expressive signals to coordinate joint actions. The framework can also be generalized to other domains outside of basketball, particularly for those which require multimodal coordination of tasks. Our future work is to conduct experiments testing various parameterizations and determine what kind of signals are most suitable for human-agent interaction in this environment.

References

1. Niewiadomski, R., Bevacqua, E., Mancini, M., Pelachaud, C.: Greta: an interactive expressive ECA system. In: Proceedings of the 8th International Conference on Autonomous Agents and Multiagent Systems, vol. 2, pp. 1399–1400. International Foundation for Autonomous Agents and Multiagent Systems (2009)
2. Schroder, M., Bevacqua, E., Cowie, R., Eyben, F., Gunes, H., Heylen, D., ter Maat, M., McKeown, G., Pammi, S., Pantic, M., Pelachaud, C., Schuller, B., de Sevin, E., Valstar, M., Wollmer, M.: Building autonomous sensitive artificial listeners. IEEE Trans. Affect. Comput. **3**(2), 165–183 (2012)
3. DeVault, D., Artstein, R., Benn, G., Dey, T., Fast, E., Gainer, A., Georgila, K., Gratch, J., Hartholt, A., Lhommet, M., et al.: Simsensei kiosk: a virtual human interviewer for healthcare decision support. In: Proceedings of the 2014 International Conference on Autonomous Agents and Multi-agent Systems, International Foundation for Autonomous Agents and Multiagent Systems, pp. 1061–1068 (2014)
4. Lala, D., Nishida, T.: VISIE: a spatially immersive interaction environment using real-time human measurement. In: 2011 IEEE International Conference on Granular Computing (GrC), pp. 363–368 (2011)
5. Lee, A., Kawahara, T., Shikano, K.: Julius - an open source realtime large vocabulary recognition engine. In: EUROSPEECH, pp. 1691–1694 (2001)
6. Lala, D., Nishida, T.: A data-driven passing interaction model for embodied basketball agents. J. Intell. Inf. Syst., 1–34 (2015)

Shyness Level and Sensitivity to Gaze from Agents - Are Shy People Sensitive to Agent's Gaze?

Tomoko Koda[✉], Masaki Ogura, and Yu Matsui

Faculty of Information Science and Technology,
Osaka Institute of Technology, Osaka, Japan
koda@is.oit.ac.jp, {e1q10022,e1c12078}@st.oit.ac.jp

Abstract. This paper reports how shy people perceive different amount of gaze from a virtual agent and how their perception of the gaze affects comfortableness of the interaction. Our preliminary results indicate shy people are sensitive to even a very low amounts of gaze from the agent. However, contrary to our expectations, as the amounts of gaze from the agent increases, shy people had more favorable impression toward the agent, and they did not perceive the adequate amount of gaze as most comfortable.

Keywords: Gaze · Shyness · Intelligent virtual agents · Non-verbal behavior · Evaluation

1   Introduction

Gaze plays an important role in our social interactions such as controlling the flow of a conversation, indicating interest and intentions, and improving listener's attention and comprehension [1, 2]. As in humans, virtual agent's gaze behavior is also important to provide natural interaction. Previous research on modeling gaze behavior of virtual agents were conducted to make appropriate turn management [3], to figure out where to look at [4], how to make idle gaze movements [5], to express social dominance by gaze [6], and what the adequate amount of gaze is to facilitate interaction [7], all of which report modeling realistic human gaze behavior to an agent resulted in more natural and smooth interaction.

However, being gazed at can lead to discomfort from feeling observed, especially for shy people. Shyness is defined as "discomfort and inhibition in the presences of others, where these reactions derive directly from the social nature of the situation" [8]. Shy people tend to avert gaze and engage in more self-manipulations [9, 10]. Thus, shy people might not prefer to interact with a virtual agent that exhibit a social, realistic human gaze behavior that facilitates smooth interaction.

This research aims to investigate adequate gaze behavior of a virtual agent for shy people to interact comfortably, and seek for answers for the following hypotheses: (1) Shy people are more sensitive to gaze from a virtual agent than those are not shy. (2) Shy people prefer lower amounts of gaze from the virtual agent, thus they perceive more friendliness from an agent that does not gaze at them.

D. Traum et al. (Eds.): IVA 2016, LNAI 10011, pp. 359–363, 2016.
DOI: 10.1007/978-3-319-47665-0_33

2   Experimental Procedure

We designed a conversational virtual agent with four types of gaze behaviors based on [7] that proposed a gaze behavior model controlled by a probabilistic state transition. Firstly, the agent gazes toward a participant all the time (Full gaze condition); secondly, the agent gazes toward the participant 67 % of the time, which is defined as the adequate gaze pattern to facilitate smooth interaction (adequate gaze condition); thirdly, the agent gazes toward the user 33 % of the time (low gaze condition); and lastly, the agent gaze away from the user all the time (no gaze condition). The gaze transition was controlled at random in order to control the amount of gaze only. The agent's gaze state and averted gaze state are shown in Fig. 1.

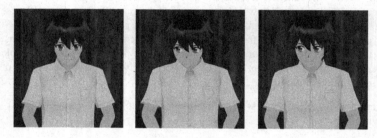

Fig. 1. Agent's gaze state (left) and gaze-away states (middle and right)

25 university students participated in the Woz experiment and had pseudo conversations with the all four agents. Topics include favorite food, route to school. Each conversation lasted for a couple of minutes. They answered the Shyness scale questionnaire [11]. We divided the participants into two groups based on their shyness level score. 12 participants were categorized as high shyness group (shyness score > 48, HS hereafter), 7 participants as low shyness group (shyness score < 41, LS hereafter). Answers from other participants' were not used for the latter analysis to eliminate results from those with mid shyness level. Another questionnaire, about the perceived gaze amount from the agent, perceived friendliness of the agent, and perceived smoothness of the interaction, was administered after the experiment. The experimental conditions were participants' shyness (low or high, between-subjects design), and gaze patterns (4 patterns, within-subjects design).

3   Results and Discussion

The results of 2-way ANOVA repeated measures showed a significant main effect of gaze condition in "perceived amount of gaze from the agent" (F = 32.95, p < 0.01). Figure 2 shows the results of perceived amount of gaze from each condition shown by the participants' shyness level. The more gaze the agent gives toward the participants, the higher they felt the agent was looking at them. This result can be used as a manipulation check of the gaze amount of each condition, which indicates the gaze amount were successfully manipulated in each condition. HS was more sensitive to change of

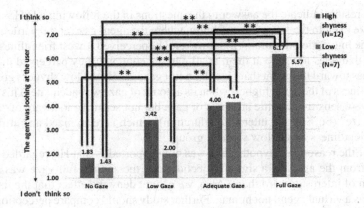

Fig. 2. Perceived gaze level from the agent

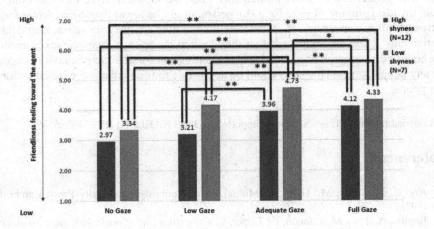

Fig. 3. Perceived friendliness toward the agent

gaze amount between no gaze and low gaze condition (score = 1.83, 3.42; F = 11.46, p < 0.01), while LS was more sensitive to the one between low gaze and adequate gaze condition (score = 2.00, 4.14; F = 10.81, p < 0.01). Thus, hypothesis 1 is supported.

In terms of perceived friendliness toward the agent shown in Fig. 3, HS liked the agent less than LS in general. There were significant interactions between the gaze condition and the shyness condition (F = 41.36, p < 0.01). LS rated the adequate gaze condition as most friendly (score = 4.73, p < 0.05), while HS did not perceive the difference in friendliness between adequate and full gaze, although they are aware of the differences in the amount of gaze between the two conditions. The results did not support the hypothesis 2. Friendly impression would lead to smooth interaction. In terms of the perceived smoothness of the interaction with the agent, similar tendency was found as the perceived friendliness. LS rated the adequate gaze condition as most smooth, while HS rated the full gaze condition as such.

These results indicate the answer to the questions in the following; (1) HS are sensitive to gaze even in the low gaze condition, where the agent gaze at the participant only 33 % of the interaction duration. (2) However, HS perceived lowest friendliness toward the agent that does not gaze at them at all. On the contrary, they perceived the highest friendliness toward the agent that give them full gaze, while the low shyness group rated the friendliness of the agent highest when its amount of gaze was adequate. This suggests that HS were sensitive to little amounts of gaze but not sensitive to/aware of "adequate level of gaze" (66 % of the interaction duration), which is recognized and attributed to agent's friendliness by the low shyness group.

One of the reason our hypothesis 2 was not supported is that HS regarded the gaze aversion from the agent as a sign of rejection, and the agent's full-gaze was regarded was a sign of interest toward them. Also, we cannot deny the effect that the interaction partner was a virtual agent, not human. Further study should compare perception of gaze behavior from human and agents, with wide variety of agent designs, with more realism, with both gender and by more participants. Also we should analyze other amounts of gaze, the ideal amount of gaze for a shy person might be lower than 67 %, while for an extrovert it is higher than 67 %. Moreover, quantitative analysis of eye tracking data of participants' gaze, especially whether they look at the agent's face or eyes is needed. We believe this research would lead to investigating comfortable gaze behavior of agents for shy people, and such agents could be applicable to train adequate gaze behavior to shy people.

Acknowledgement. This research is supported by JSPS KAKENHI JP26330236.

References

1. Argyle, M., Cook, M.: Gaze and Mutual Gaze. Cambridge University Press, Cambridge (1976)
2. Bayliss, A., Paul, M., Cannon, P., Tipper, S.: Gaze cuing and affective judgments of objects: I like what you look at. Psychon. Bull. Rev. **13**(6), l061–1066 (2006)
3. Pelachaud, C., Bilvi, M.: Modelling gaze behavior for conversational agents. In: Rist, T., Aylett, R.S., Ballin, D., Rickel, J. (eds.) IVA 2003. LNCS (LNAI), vol. 2792, pp. 93–100. Springer, Heidelberg (2003)
4. Lee, J., Marsella, S.C., Traum, D.R., Gratch, J., Lance, B.: The rickel gaze model: a window on the mind of a virtual human. In: Pelachaud, C., Martin, J.-C., André, E., Chollet, G., Karpouzis, K., Pelé, D. (eds.) IVA 2007. LNCS (LNAI), vol. 4722, pp. 296–303. Springer, Heidelberg (2007)
5. Cafaro, A., Gaito, R., Vilhjálmsson, H.H.: Animating idle gaze in public places. In: Ruttkay, Z., Kipp, M., Nijholt, A., Vilhjálmsson, H.H. (eds.) IVA 2009. LNCS, vol. 5773, pp. 250–256. Springer, Heidelberg (2009)
6. Bee, N., Pollock, C., André, E., Walker, M.: Bossy or wimpy: expressing social dominance by combining gaze and linguistic behaviors. In: Safonova, A. (ed.) IVA 2010. LNCS, vol. 6356, pp. 265–271. Springer, Heidelberg (2010)
7. Ishii, R., et al.: Avatar's gaze control to facilitate conversation in virtual-space multi-user voice chat system. J. Hum. Interface **10**(1), 87–94 (2008). (In Japanese)

 8. Jones, W.H., Russell, D.: The social reticence scale: an objective instrument to measure shyness. J. Pers. Assess. **46**(6), 629–631 (1982)
 9. Cheek, J.M., Buss, A.H.: Shyness and sociability. J. Pers. Soc. Psychol. **41**, 330–339 (1981)
10. Daly, S.: Behavioral correlates of social anxiety. Br. J. Soc. Clin. Psychol. **17**, 117–120 (1978)
11. Aikawa, A.: A study on the reliability and validity of a scale to measure shyness as a trait. Jpn. J. Psychol. **62**(3), 149–155 (1991). (In Japanese)

User Engagement Study with Virtual Agents Under Different Cultural Contexts

Zhou Yu$^{(\boxtimes)}$, Xinrui He, Alan W. Black, and Alexander I. Rudnicky

Carnegie Mellon University, Pittsburgh, USA
zhouyu@cs.cmu.edu

Abstract. Human communication literature states that people with different culture backgrounds act differently in conversations. Currently most virtual agents are designed for a single targeted popular culture. We implemented two versions of a virtual agent targeting American and Chinese cultures. We found that users from different culture context express engagement differently.

1 Introduction and Related Work

Recent work on culture behavior difference mostly refer to the Hofstede's culture model which had six dimensions of visibilities [4]: small versus large power distance, individualism versus collectivism, masculinity versus femininity, weak versus strong uncertainty avoidance, long versus short term orientation and indulgence versus resilience. The major differences between American and Chinese cultures are that American culture is perceived to be individual, short-term oriented and low power distance, while Chinese culture is collective, long term oriented and high power distance.

Many studies found that people from different cultures behave differently during conversations. The CUBE-G project is one of the most extensive data-driven efforts to study German and Japanese cultures comparatively. Rehm et al. [7] collected a cross-cultural multimodal corpus of dyadic interactions and found that in most Japanese conversations, participants discussed the experimental setting while German subjects talked significantly more about social topics such as their studies or friends. Khaled et al. focused on cultural differences in persuasion strategies found that for short-term oriented cultures a stronger focus on the task itself can be expected, whereas for long-term oriented cultures a slower and more exhaustive way of problem solving can be expected, where every opinion is taken into account and harmony is at stake resulting in an increased frequency of contributions that are related to the communication management [5]. Matsumoto et al. found that people from Arab cultures gaze much longer and more directly than Americans [6]. In general, collective cultures, such as Arabian culture engage in more gazing and have more direct orientation when interacting with others.

Previous studies found that people in different cultures behave differently towards a task-oriented virtual agent as well. In a direction giving task, Arabic

© Springer International Publishing AG 2016
D. Traum et al. (Eds.): IVA 2016, LNAI 10011, pp. 364–368, 2016.
DOI: 10.1007/978-3-319-47665-0_34

Table 1. An example conversation with TickTock in mandarin

Partner	Utterance (Translation)
User:	那要不你给我唱首歌吧。(Then let me sing you a song)
TickTock:	让我想一下，就没有浪漫一点的反应啊？(Let me see, don't you haves something romantic to say?)
User:	什么鬼啊? 我感觉受不了这个机器了。(What the heck, I feel I can't take the system anymore.)
TickTock:	你到底有没有爱过我? (Have you loved me at all?)
User:	什么情况? (What is the situation here?)
TickTock:	让我想一下，好吧。(Let me see, OK.)
User:	好吧。(OK.)
TickTock:	你有什么想说的吗? (Do you have anything to say?)
User:	爱过。(I loved you.)

and English native speakers interact with a virtual agent differently [3]. English natives had a higher frequency of using cardinals, pauses and intermediate information while Arab natives used units of distance, left/right turns and error corrections more frequently than English natives. Another comparison study suggested that Arabians trust more on the Arabian speaking robot who speaks language that is rhetorically well formulated, while the rhetorically factor is less important for Americans when they talk to an English speaking robot [1].

2   System and Data Descriptions

TickTock is a key-word based retrieval system with a set of conversational strategies [9]. The response of TickTock is retrieved from an open-domain dialog corpus, composed of various question-answer pairs using a keyword matching algorithm. The system selects strategies based on the retrieved response and the user model. The system reacts to the engagement level of the user. We built a computational model for user engagement using user verbal and nonverbal behaviors using simile procedure in [8]. Based on how engaged the user is, the system chooses between the four strategies: switch a topic, initiate an activity, tell a joke and refer back to a previous topic that user engaged.

The system is originally designed for American culture. The response generation model is trained on an open-domain dialog corpus formed by American popular social media, such as CNN interview corpus, TV show "Friends" and Reddit. Translated text usually appears unnatural in the target language, which may lead to less believability of the agent's culture identity. Thus we used similar social media materials as the American version, but is originally created in Mandarin: Xinlang Aiwen (similar to Quora) and TV show "Love apartment". We replaced the Google Automatic Speech Recognizer (ASR) and Flite Text-to-speech (TTS) [2] with Baidu ASR and Baidu TTS respectively to support automatic Mandarin recognition and synthesis. The agent has a cartoon face that signals its internal mind, such as smiling, and confused. The mouth of the agent moves while it speaks. However, it is incapable of complicated facial expressions, let alone gestures. This design aims to avoid the uncanny valley dilemma, so that the users would not expect realistic human-like behaviors from the system. We did not change the appearance of the agent for different cultural contexts, as the agent's appearance is designed to be culturally ambiguous. A demo can be found in http://www.cs.cmu.edu/afs/cs/user/zhouyu/www/TickTock.html.

We believe this is the first public data set that had audiovisual recordings of people from two different cultures interacting with a similar agent with their native languages. In order to isolate confounds, we balanced subjects for gender, education background and age. The average age of the American data set is 24.4 (STD = 2.53), and the Chinese data set is 21.4 (STD = 0.58). There are 11 people (7 males) in total in the American data set, and 21 people (12 males) in total in the Chinese data set. In the user study, American users interacted with the English speaking version of TickTock and the Chinese users interacted with the Mandarin speaking version. We recruited the participants and conducted the experiments in the country of the targeted culture. Participants are university students who were born and raised in the targeted culture. No participants interacted with a virtual agent before, however, they have varied familiarity with dialog systems, which may influence their behaviors during the interaction. We wish to control this factor in future studies. A Mandarin example conversation between TickTock and the user is shown in Table 1. We adopted the engagement annotation scheme in [9] and the inter-annotator agreement (kappa) is 0.93 and 0.74 in the American and Chinese data set respectfully.

3   Engagement Analysis

We used the same feature extraction technology in [8] to extract multimodal features from the two data sets. Then we perform a correlation analysis between each multimodal features with respect to its engagement score and report the tests with statical significance ($p < 0.05$) in Table 2. We find that in both culture groups, word count correlate with user engagement positively. In other words, the more the user speaks, the more engaged the user is in both cultural contexts. We also find that in both cultures, the louder users speak, the more varied their loudness are, the more engaged they are.

We find that how frequently one smiles differs greatly between the two culture groups in terms of correlation with engagement. In American culture, more smiles indicates more engagement, while in Chinese culture, similes are less strongly correlated with engagement. The trend is similar for automatically predicted smiles. One possible explanation of the difference is that Chinese culture is a typical collective culture that seeks harmony between partners. Chinese may subconsciously treat the agent as one of their partner and try to harmonize the agent by using more positive affect. While American culture is a individualism culture according to Hofstede's culture theory [4]. Americans would change less of their behaviors to harmonize their partners compared to Chinese. We conducted a qualitative analysis of the semantic contents of user responses and found 4 out of 9 Asian female and 2 out of 12 Asian male participants told the agent: "I like

Table 2. Engagement Behavior Correlation. The bold number indicates the correlation is statistically significant ($p < 0.05$).

Features	American rho(p)	Chinese rho(p)
Word count (ASR)	**0.20(0.00)**	**0.15(0.02)**
Intensity mean	**0.15(0.00)**	0.12(0.08)
Intensity variance	**0.17(0.00)**	**0.16(0.02)**
Smile	**0.13(0.03)**	0.07(0.32)
System interruption	**0.19(0.00)**	−0.09(0.17)
User interruption	0.10(0.06)	0.01(0.85)
System response time	−0.01(0.82)	**−0.20(0.00)**

you, you are so cute.", while none of the Americans expressed their likability towards the agent directly.

Another difference we find between the two cultures is that the frequency of system interruption correlates with higher engagement in American culture but not in Chinese culture. One explanation of such difference is that Americans are mostly individualists who tolerate interruptions much more than Chinese who seek for harmonized dynamics in conversations all the time according to the Hofstede culture model. On the other hand we find that user interruptions is not correlated with user's engagement in both cultures. We find that in American culture, user response time is negatively correlated with user engagement, which indicates that the faster the user responds, the more engaged the user is, while in Chinese culture, the correlation is less significant. We find that in Chinese culture, system response time correlates with user engagement negatively, which indicates that the longer the system pauses, the less the user engages. While this phenomena is much less significant in American culture than Chinese culture. One possible explanation is that Chinese users care more about their interlocutors than American users. As Chinese is a more collective culture, a long pause from their partners makes Chinese participants less engaged.

4   Conclusion

This paper presents two versions of a virtual agent system that designed for American and Chinese cultures. We find that users from different cultures express engagement differently when they are interacting with virtual agents. This suggests that we should take culture into consideration when designing engagement sensitive virtual agents.

References

1. Andrist, S., Ziadee, M., Boukaram, H., Mutlu, B., Sakr, M.: Effects of culture on the credibility of robot speech: a comparison between english and arabic. In: Proceedings of the HRI, pp. 157–164. ACM (2015)

2. Black, A.W., Lenzo, K.A.: Flite: a small fast run-time synthesis engine. In: 4th ISCA Tutorial and Research Workshop (ITRW) on Speech Synthesis (2001)
3. Gedawy, H., Ziadee, M., Sakr, M.: Variations in giving directions across arabic and english native speakers. In: Qatar Foundation Annual Research Forum (2012)
4. Hofstede, G.H., Hofstede, G.: Culture's Consequences: Comparing Values, Behaviors, Institutions and Organizations Across Nations. Sage, Thousand Oaks (2001)
5. Khaled, R., Biddle, R., Noble, J., Barr, P., Fischer, R.: Persuasive interaction for collectivist cultures. In: Proceedings of the 7th Australasian User Interface Conference, vol. 50, pp. 73–80. Australian Computer Society Inc (2006)
6. Matsumoto, D.: Culture and nonverbal behavior. In: Handbook of nonverbal communication, pp. 219–235 (2006)
7. Rehm, M., André, E., Bee, N., Endrass, B., Wissner, M., Nakano, Y., Akhter Lipi, A., Nishida, T., Huang, H.-H.: Creating standardized video recordings of multimodal interactions across cultures. In: Kipp, M., Martin, J.-C., Paggio, P., Heylen, D. (eds.) MMCorp 2008. LNCS (LNAI), vol. 5509, pp. 138–159. Springer, Heidelberg (2009). doi:10.1007/978-3-642-04793-0_9
8. Yu, Z., Gerritsen, D., Ogan, A., Black, A.W., Cassell, J.: Automatic prediction of friendship via multi-model dyadic features, pp. 51–60 (2013)
9. Yu, Z., Papangelis, A., Rudnicky, A.: TickTock: a non-goal-oriented multimodal dialog system with engagement awareness. In: Proceedings of the AAAI Spring Symposium (2015)

On Constrained Local Model Feature Normalization for Facial Expression Recognition

Zhenglin Pan[(✉)], Mihai Polceanu, and Christine Lisetti

School of Computing and Information Sciences,
Florida International University, 11200 SW 8th St, Miami, FL 33199, USA
zpan004@fiu.edu, {mpolcean,lisetti}@cs.fiu.edu
http://ascl.cis.fiu.edu/

Abstract. Real time user independent facial expression recognition is important for virtual agents but challenging. However, since in real time recognition users are not necessarily presenting all the emotions, some proposed methods are not applicable. In this paper, we present a new approach that instead of using the traditional base face normalization on whole face shapes, performs normalization on the point cloud of each landmark. The result shows that our method outperforms the other two when the user input does not contain all six universal emotions.

Keywords: Constrained local model · Feature normalization · Preprocessing · Facial expression recognition

1 Introduction

It is important for intelligent virtual agents to have the capability that correctly detects and interprets the emotions of human users during the interaction in many areas. To improve this capability, we need to train our virtual agents to analyze facial expression, which is one of the most significant factors that we, human beings, take into consideration when we attempt to tell other people's sentiments.

While tasks such as face recognition require differentiating between individuals based on facial features, facial expression recognition relies on variations of these facial features and on their dynamics. Consequently, one major obstacle in accurately classifying users' facial expressions is the large amount of variations in expressed emotions. This makes classification difficult due to high overlap when merging data from multiple individuals.

To address these issues, many state of the art facial expression recognition systems rely on techniques to extract user-specific information, which enables multi-user data to be normalized in a more efficient manner, giving way to superior classification performance. However, some of the existing approaches have trouble with real time facial expression recognition when not all the universal emotions are provided. In this paper, we investigate these common techniques and describe a novel application of an existing point registration algorithm that performs better in this situation.

© Springer International Publishing AG 2016
D. Traum et al. (Eds.): IVA 2016, LNAI 10011, pp. 369–372, 2016.
DOI: 10.1007/978-3-319-47665-0_35

2   Related Work

Traditionally, action unit zero (AU0) has been used to normalize facial expression data of multiple subjects.

Jeni *et al.* [5] proposed Personal Mean Shape (PMS), which is the mean of neutral and extreme facial expressions of a subject. PMS turned out to work quite well on the Cohn-Kanade Extended Facial Expression (CK+) [6] Database. However, a restriction of their solution is that the base face has to be built based on explicitly labeled neutral and extreme facial expressions of the subjects. Hence, this method may have difficulties with real time video streams.

In comparison, Baltrusaitis *et al.* [1] calculated the median of all frames of a subject as their base face. This approach was based on the assumption that neutral face is the most frequently shown facial expression and the base face is very close to the neutral face, yet they found this assumption did not hold for all the situations.

In this paper, we propose a novel face landmark preprocessing approach, which works better than the mentioned approaches in some cases and could lead to better insight into improving the performance of existing facial expression recognition methods.

3   CLM Feature Normalization

Constrained Local Model (CLM) is a robust facial feature tracking algorithm proposed by Cristinacce *et al.* [3]. In our experiment, we leverage one of the open source implementations of CLM, CLM-Z, released by Baltrusaitis *et al.* [2].

We test the consistency of our method by applying the CLM-Z algorithm on 3 databases: Cohn-Kanade Extended Facial Expression Database (CK+) [6], Binghamton University 3D Facial Expression Database (BU-3DFE) [9] and Binghamton University 3D+time Facial Expression Database (BU-4DFE)[8].

To preprocess the data, we used the Generalized Procrustes Analysis (GPA) algorithm [4]. Then we apply Jeni's approach (mean-based normalization), Baltrusaitis' approach (median-based normalization) and our approach (point-wise normalization) on the normalized landmarks, respectively. Finally, we perform leave one subject out cross validation on the processed data using SVM. The results and discussions are shown in the following sections.

To generalize Jeni's mean-based normalization to datasets that do not include neutral faces, instead of using their approach that takes the mean of both neutral and extreme expressions, we take the mean of the latter only.

We also tested Baltrusaitis' approach, which takes the median of all the images as the base face. They assume that the neutral face is the most frequently shown emotion throughout a video.

In real time emotion recognition, the users may not provide all seven typical emotions. Consequently, the mean or median based normalization may have difficulties calculating the base face. However, we can deal with this situation using Coherent Point Drift (CPD) [7] point set registration algorithm.

Table 1. Comparison between mean, median and CPD, on the CK+ (subjects with ≥ 3 facial expressions), BU-3DFE and BU-4DFE databases (complete data).

Database	Technique	Anger	Disgust	Fear	Happiness	Sadness	Surprise	Average
CK+	Mean	64.70	89.47	60.00	100.0	75.00	92.30	80.25
	Median	64.70	89.47	35.71	96.00	75.0	92.30	75.53
	CPD	70.58	84.21	60.00	100.0	81.25	96.15	82.03
BU-3DFE	Mean	70.00	78.25	69.50	84.00	67.75	90.25	76.63
	Median	69.00	77.00	69.00	85.00	69.50	90.75	76.71
	CPD	64.75	77.25	63.75	85.75	70.75	89.75	75.33
BU-4DFE	Mean	80.59	76.73	66.04	91.39	76.04	84.75	79.26
	Median	83.37	76.63	66.34	90.30	83.17	85.54	80.89
	CPD	78.12	73.17	62.87	93.56	73.86	86.63	78.04

Although mean-based and median-based normalization are better than the point-wise normalization on BU-3DFE and BU-4DFE datasets, the difference among them is less than 3 %, which means that after users have expressed their 6 typical emotions, all 3 approaches work more or less the same. However, in the case where users only show half of the universal emotions, CPD outperforms median, which wins both BU-3DFE and BU-4DFE, with almost 7 % difference as shown in Table 1. This is consistent with the intuition that mean and median have poor performance on incomplete data. Since in real time emotion recognition users are not very likely to show all their facial expressions, detecting their base face through the incomplete input becomes inaccurate. However, the point-wise normalization can better overcome the troubles of incompleteness based on the result.

Now that the point-wise approach shows its advantage on partial input data, we expect that the advantage stays with full data. Although in our experiment it does not reach better performance than the traditional base face extraction methods, it still has the potential to outperform them with better parameter and algorithm choices. If this will the case, then the neutral face can no longer be considered the key to user-independent emotion recognition.

4   Conclusions and Future Work

Our study focused on investigating a new face landmark preprocessing approach, which shifts the landmarks to their corresponding clusters geometrically. We compared our algorithm with two existing methods that normalize on users' base face. Based on the experiment data, we claim that extracting base face is not necessarily the best approach to perform real time user independent emotion recognition. One of the alternatives is that for each CLM extracted landmark, we can construct a topology that includes the position of this very point in all the frames from real time video and map the landmarks to the corresponding clusters in our model using the CPD point registration algorithm. This approach has better classification accuracy compared to mean-based or median-based normalization methods when the input data does not include all 6 universal emotions. In the future, we will apply the same methodology to other datasets to verify our theory and explore some means for improvement.

Additional information about the subjects may lead to better landmark clustering and therefore better recognition accuracy, due to potential similarities in expressed emotions within demographic groups. Meanwhile, instead of classifying emotions based on the geometry positions, we will work with the Action Units. Analyzing Action Units will not only help increase the classification accuracy, but also give us information about subtle micro facial expressions, which are difficult to identify if classified by geometry position only.

In this paper we did not include the importance of the face features for each emotion, but in recognizing different emotions, the same group of landmarks weigh differently. In the future, we will investigate the dominating facial features for each emotion and perform classification only upon these features. We expect to reduce the dimension, increase classification accuracy and shorten the time cost by this approach.

References

1. Baltrusaitis, T., Mahmoud, M., Robinson, P.: Cross-dataset learning and person-specific normalisation for automatic action unit detection. In: 2015 11th IEEE International Conference and Workshops on Automatic Face and Gesture Recognition (FG), vol. 6, pp. 1–6. IEEE (2015)
2. Baltrusaitis, T., Robinson, P., Morency, L.P.: Constrained local neural fields for robust facial landmark detection in the wild. In: Proceedings of the IEEE International Conference on Computer Vision Workshops, pp. 354–361 (2013)
3. Cristinacce, D., Cootes, T.F.: Feature detection and tracking with constrained local models. In: BMVC, vol. 2, p. 6. Citeseer (2006)
4. Gower, J.C.: Generalized procrustes analysis. Psychometrika $40(1)$, 33–51 (1975)
5. Jeni, L.A., Lőrincz, A., Nagy, T., Palotai, Z., Sebők, J., Szabó, Z., Takács, D.: 3D shape estimation in video sequences provides high precision evaluation of facial expressions. Image Vis. Comput. $30(10)$, 785–795 (2012)
6. Lucey, P., Cohn, J.F., Kanade, T., Saragih, J., Ambadar, Z., Matthews, I.: The extended cohn-kanade dataset (ck+): A complete dataset for action unit and emotion-specified expression. In: 2010 IEEE Computer Society Conference on Computer Vision and Pattern Recognition Workshops (CVPRW), pp. 94–101. IEEE (2010)
7. Myronenko, A., Song, X.: Point set registration: coherent point drift. IEEE Trans. Pattern Anal. Mach. Intell. $32(12)$, 2262–2275 (2010)
8. Yin, L., Chen, X., Sun, Y., Worm, T., Reale, M.: A high-resolution 3D dynamic facial expression database. In: 8th IEEE International Conference on Automatic Face & Gesture Recognition, FG 2008, pp. 1–6. IEEE (2008)
9. Yin, L., Wei, X., Sun, Y., Wang, J., Rosato, M.J.: A 3D facial expression database for facial behavior research. In: 7th International Conference on Automatic Face and Gesture Recognition, FGR 2006, pp. 211–216. IEEE (2006)

Familiarity Detection with the Component Process Model

Joseph P Garnier[1]([⊠]), Jean-Charles Marty[2], and Karim Sehaba[3]

[1] Université de Lyon, CNRS Université Lyon 1, LIRIS, UMR5205,
69622 Lyon, France
joseph.garnier@liris.cnrs.fr
[2] Université de Lyon, CNRS Université de Savoie, LIRIS, UMR520,
69622 Lyon, France
jean-charles.marty@liris.cnrs.fr
[3] Université de Lyon, CNRS Université Lyon 2, LIRIS, UMR5205,
69676 Lyon, France
karim.sehaba@liris.cnrs.fr

Abstract. We propose a computational model for the Component Process Model (CPM) of Scherer, the most recent and the most complete model of emotion in psychology. This one proposes to appraise a stimulus through a sequence of sixteen appraisal variables dealing with a large number of its characteristics. As CPM is very abstract and high level, it is not really used in affective computing and no formal models exist for its appraisal variables. Based on the CPM, in this paper we propose a mathematical function for one appraisal variable detecting the familiarity of a perceived event according to the state of the cognitive component of an agent (goals, needs, semantic memory, and episodic memory).

1 Introduction

In our research work, we are particularly interested in motivation and immersion of users in numeric environments. Emotions play a critical role in processes such as rational decision-making, perception, human interaction, social relationships, human creativity and human intelligence. According to cognitive theories, an agent appraises a situation with respect to its knowledge, its goals, and other cognitive components. This appraisal takes place along multiple appraisal variables, such as familiarity (Is this event novel for me?), goal relevance (Is this situation good or not for me?), control (can I deal with this event?), and so on. This evaluation of an event leads to an emotion. One of these theories, called *Component Process Model* (CPM) [4], proposes to appraise an event with sixteen appraisal variables as opposed as most other theories as OCC or Lazarus that only have six to eight variables. A large number of appraisal variables can cover a large interpretation of an event according to a large number of points of view, and there is less risk to miss important factors of interpretation.

Among the existing models, no one proposes a domain-independent computational model with a formal description (as mathematical functions) of CPM's

© Springer International Publishing AG 2016
D. Traum et al. (Eds.): IVA 2016, LNAI 10011, pp. 373–377, 2016.
DOI: 10.1007/978-3-319-47665-0_36

appraisal variables according to cognitive components as perceptions, goals, memory, motivation and knowledge of a cognitive agent. The most advanced work is probably PEACTIDM [2], proposing a computational model for CPM. However, it does not propose how to calculate appraisal variables but a way to compute mood and feeling, including its intensity, from emotion.

CPM proposes sixteen appraisal variables, the main purpose of this paper being to model the *familiarity appraisal variable* for relevance detection. Scherer proposes a process model describing how the appraisals are generate but he does not provide detailed explanations of all the data needed to the appraisals, and there is little or no guidance from the literature. We therefore decided to start with the "simplest" alternative. Our long-term strategy is to check by experimentation whether simple assumptions fall short. In such cases, we will thus improve complexity incrementally. Thus, this proposal is likely oversimplified, but it provides a starting point for future work.

2   Appraisal Process: Familiarity Detection

Familiarity with a perceived event $event \in EVT$ is directly related to the knowledge of the items of the event, their associations, and the number of occurrences of these associations in the episodic memory.

In the episodic memory, events are encoded into *memory traces* as a vector where each element of an event is an *item* of this vector. Two traces are similar or different according to the number of their common characteristics. It is the association between spatio-temporal contextual items which makes a difference between an event (or a memory trace) and another one. In adulthood it is rare to be confronted with a new event's item or with an information completely new. Novelty (unfamiliarity) often lies in the association between various acontextuals known items. For example the novelty in *the wife in the best friend's bed* lies neither in the wife, nor the friend, nor the bed, but in the unfamiliar conjunction of the three [3]. So familiarity is determined by the number of new associations of a perceived event's items, compared to memory traces of episodic memory. Thus, to compute familiarity we check if an entity knows each item of a perceived event, then if it is the case, we count the number of occurrences of event's item associations. For instance, we formalize an event as a family set of three items: $source_{evt}$, $action_{evt}$, $target_{evt}$. Then we check in semantic memory if each item is known, if is the case, we count the number of occurrences of event's items associations in episodic memory $\{source_{evt}, action_{evt}\}$, $\{source_{evt}, target_{evt}\}$, $\{action_{evt}, target_{evt}\}$, and $\{source_{evt}, action_{evt}, target_{evt}\}$. Thus we define $pair_{item} = \{(x, y) \mid x \in evt \land y \in evt \land x \neq y\}$.

Function's characteristics. We used the following characteristics to create our familiarity function, according to what we explained before:

1. Limited range: familiarity value should be in the range [0,1]. 0 means an event is new and 1 means an event is completely familiar.

2. Beginning point: familiarity value should be 0 when an event does not exist in episodic memory or when an item of appraised event is unknown in semantic memory.
3. Event familiarity: familiarity value should be higher than 0 when the number of event occurrences is not 0 in episodic memory. Familiarity increases with experience.
4. Couples of event item familiarity: familiarity value should be higher than 0 when the number of occurrences of couples of event item is not 0 in episodic memory. Familiarity increases with experience.
5. Endpoint: a familiarity rate should be defined to control when an event is familiar.
6. Non-linear: according to [1] this function should be non-linear.

Familiarity function. To construct our familiarity function, we begin with the characteristic 2. If an item of the perceived event does not exist in semantic memory, familiarity value is 0. For the other characteristics we propose an exponential function into two parts: the first one treats the event without considering its item pairs, and the second one treats each item pair of the event.

Before explaining our function, let us denote by $nbOcc(evt, EPM)$ the number of occurrences of an event in episodic memory, and by $nbOcc((x, y), EPM)$ the number of times that action $action_{evt}$ has been experienced by $source_{evt}$ or by $target_{evt}$, and the number of times that $source_{evt}$ interacted with $target_{evt}$ (reverse is true too).

Episodic memory stores a set of *episodes* that represent the life experience of the entity. Each episode contains a *sequence of events* appended during a *context*. A context is a fixed period of time and a location in the environment. The $nbOccu()$ function counts the number of times an event or its pairs occurs in all episodes because familiarity is not context-sensitive. We define the familiarity function as:

$$appfun_{fami}(evt, SM, EPM, GOAL) =$$

$$\begin{cases} 0, \text{ if } \exists item : (item \in evt \land item \notin SM) \\ \left(1 - \alpha^{\gamma \cdot nbOcc(evt, EPM)}\right) + \left(\beta.\alpha^{\gamma \cdot nbOcc(evt, EPM)}.(1 - \alpha^{\gamma \cdot avg(evt, EPM)})\right), \text{ else} \end{cases}$$

$$\text{where } avg(evt, EPM) = \frac{\sum\limits_{pair_i \in pair_{item}} nbOcc(pair_i, EPM)}{|pair_{item}|}$$

According to characteristic 6, we propose an exponential function formed with two exponential functions[1] where familiarity is between 0 and 1 value (characteristic 1). Exponential functions with a negative sign are interesting because they passes through 0 and have an asymptotic value equals to 1. The first exponential function (characteristic 3) treats the event familiarity in a whole (in other

---

[1] please note that $a^x = exp_a(x) = e^{x.ln(a)}$.

words treats associations between all event's items), where α is a positive real constant such that $\alpha < 1$. α can be seen as a "familiarity rate" determining how the familiarity appraisal value increases with experience (characteristic 5). In Fig. 1 this function is in red. The second exponential function (characteristic 4) treats the familiarity of each pair of event's items. β is a real positive constant such that $\beta < 1$, seen as the contribution of the second function to the global familiarity function. To have a global familiarity value not higher than 1 (characteristic 1), we multiply β by the complement of first exponential function (which treats the event familiarity of associations between all event's items). Familiarity of pairs associations is computed in the same way as the event familiarity. We use the function $avg(evt, EPM)$ to "merge" familiarity of each pair. An average function has been chosen for several reasons:

- We can't use a multiplication because if a pair is not in episodic memory while the others are, familiarity should not be 0;
- We can't use just a sum of occurrences because familiarity of pairs (second power function) will increase too quickly with regard to the first power function, we would have weighted the first one but this value would be hard to define in a general context.

Finally, we weight $nbOcc()$ and $avg()$ values with γ, a real positive constant such that $\gamma \leq 1$, to control the rate of growth of the familiarity (in our experience, agents become too familiar too quickly otherwise, the value chosen is purely empirical), but this value is optional and can be equals to 1. In Fig. 1 the second exponential function is in blue, the first one is in red, and the general familiarity function is in green.

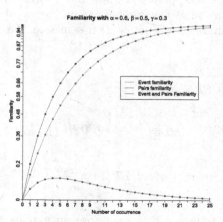

Fig. 1. Familiarity function. The red function is the familiarity of the event without considering its item pairs, and the blue function is the familiarity of each item pairs of the event. The combination of the red function and the blue one, gives the green function which is the familiarity of a perceived event, used by the appraisal process. Here $x = nbOcc() = avg()$ but in a real situation, the number of occurrences of an event will often be different of average of the number of occurrences of pairs. (Color figure online)

Future Work. In this paper we have presented a computational mathematical functions for familiarity detection. We will describe others appraisal variables for relevance in another paper.

Acknowledgements. The authors would like to thank the studio of video games named Artefacts Studio and the ANRT, and Marie-Neige Chapel for her contributions.

References

1. Logan, G.D.: Toward an instance theory of automatization. Psychol. Rev. **95**(4), 492–527 (1988)
2. Marinier, R.P., Laird, J.E., Lewis, R.L.: A computational unification of cognitive behavior and emotion. Cogn. Syst. Res. **10**(1), 48–69 (2009). http://linkinghub. elsevier.com/retrieve/pii/S1389041708000302
3. O'Keefe, J., Nadel, L.: The Hippocampus as a Cognitive Map. Oxford University Press, Oxford (1978)
4. Scherer, K.R.: Appraisal considered as a process of multilevel sequential checking. In: Appraisal Processes in Emotion: Theory, Methods, Research, pp. 92–120. Oxford University Press, Oxford (2001)

Personality, Attitudes, and Bonding in Conversations

Natasha Jaques[1]([✉]), Yoo Lim Kim[2], and Rosalind Picard[1]

[1] MIT Media Lab, Cambridge, MA 02139, USA
{jaquesn,picard}@media.mit.edu
[2] Wellesley College, Wellesley, MA 02481, USA
ykim9@wellesley.edu
http://affect.media.mit.edu/

Abstract. This paper investigates how the personality and attitudes of intelligent agents could be designed to most effectively promote bonding. Observational data are collected from a series of conversations, and a measure of bonding is adapted and verified. The effects of personality and dispositional attitudes on bonding are analyzed, and we find that attentiveness and excitement are more effective at promoting bonding than traits like attractiveness and humour.

Keywords: Personality · Attitudes · Bonding · Rapport

1 Introduction and Related Work

Many studies have probed how to make intelligent virtual agents (IVAs) more appealing to human users, by focusing on the aesthetic appeal of the characters (e.g. [1]), their facial expressions (e.g. [2]), mirroring (e.g. [3]), and the contingency of their non-verbal responses [4]. Detailed models of bonding and rapport [5], and interpersonal emotions in conversations [6], have also been developed.

We contribute to this work by examining which dispositional attitudes and personality traits are most important to bonding and rapport. For example, if Agreeableness is important to rapport (as reported in [7]), it may suggest that designing the responses of an IVA to appear more kind, polite, and non-confrontational would be beneficial [8]. The effect of personality on bonding is compared to that of traits like attractiveness and humour, to suggest which characteristics deserve the most attention when designing an IVA. We use a bonding measure adapted from the Working Alliance Inventory [9], and find that bonding is strongly related to participants' perceptions of conversation quality and interpersonal connection.

Personality has been examined in the context of users' reactions to an IVA [10], and in terms of how personality similarity affects conversation quality [7]. In some cases similarity is helpful, as when partners have a similar level of *extraversion*. However, interactions between two disagreeable participants were rated as the least pleasant. While this study provides valuable insights, participants were

© Springer International Publishing AG 2016
D. Traum et al. (Eds.): IVA 2016, LNAI 10011, pp. 378–382, 2016.
DOI: 10.1007/978-3-319-47665-0_37

all college students, and it is uncertain how far these claims can generalize. Our study builds upon this previous work by collecting data from participants from a diverse range of ages, ethnicities, and backgrounds, and relating personality and conversation quality to a robust measure of bonding.

2   User Study

Data were collected from a study in which participants conversed while being recorded with cameras, microphones, and Microsoft Kinects[1]. To conceal the true nature of the study and ensure participants could act naturally, participants were told the purpose of the study was to train computer algorithms to read lips. They were asked not to over-emphasize their lip movements, and to keep the conversation flowing as naturally as possible. The interaction lasted for about 20 min, after which participants were debriefed. All procedures were approved by the university IRB. 30 participants (13 male, 17 female), were recruited through the MIT Behavioral Research Lab (BRL) from the wider Boston community. There was variety across participants in age (M = 40.0, SD = 15.3), occupation, ethnicity, and socioeconomic status.

Participants completed both a pre- and post-study survey. Personality traits were collected during the pre-study survey using the Big-Five Factor Markers questionnaire [11]. The post-study survey contained a *Perception of Interaction* questionnaire similar to that of [7], asking participants to rate their partner on a Likert scale on qualities like *interesting*, *funny*, and *attractive*. Bonding was measured with a modified version of the Bonding subscale of the Working Alliance Inventory (B-WAI). The WAI was developed to measure the degree of collaboration and trust between a therapist and client; the bonding subscale measures positive personal attachment, including "mutual trust, acceptance, and confidence" (p. 224) [9]. Items include, "My therapist and I understood each other", and "I felt uncomfortable with my therapist". The scale was adapted to our study by substituting the phrase "my partner" for "my therapist", and removing items 17, 21, and 36, which were irrelevant for short conversations between strangers. Two other items were modified slightly; Item 29 was changed to read "I had the feeling that if I said or did the wrong things, my partner would stop *talking* with me" (rather than "working with me"), and in Item 28 the phrase "my relationship" was replaced with "getting along", such that the item reads, "Getting along with my partner was important to me".

3   Results

3.1   Reliability of the Bonding Scale

The following analysis relies on B-WAI as an aggregate measure of the rapport and trust participants felt toward their conversational partner, as well as

---

[1] The data from these devices is analyzed in a companion paper.

Table 1. Pearson's r correlations between B-WAI and conversation quality. Bolded measures are significant after performing a Bonferroni correction.

Measure	r	p	Measure	r	p
Interesting	**.6912**	**<.001**	**Distant**	**-.6207**	**<.001**
Charming	.4342	.021	**Annoying**	**-.5549**	**.001**
Friendly	.3806	.038	Awkward	-.2589	.167
Funny	.3736	.046			
Engaging	.1104	.561			

      (a) Positive correlations   (b) Negative correlations

their feelings of warmth, comfort, and enjoyment. To demonstrate that B-WAI measures these characteristics, correlations between it and eight self-reported Likert-scale ratings of conversation quality were computed (see Table 1). B-WAI is positively related to participants' ratings of their partner as *interesting, charming, friendly,* and *funny*, and inversely to *distant* and *annoying*. To control for alpha inflation, a Bonferroni correction was applied; the relationships between B-WAI and *interesting, annoying*, and *distant* were still significant. Given the small sample size ($N = 30$) and relatively low statistical power, such results suggest B-WAI is strongly related to participants' perceived conversation quality.

3.2 Designing an Agent to Promote Bonding

A multiple regression analysis is employed to determine if it is possible to accurately estimate participants' B-WAI scores from information about their *partner's* personality and attitudes, and to analyze how these traits affected bonding. Although we could include factors about the participant themselves in the model, this is not under control of the designer of a virtual agent. Rather, we restrict focus to characteristics about the IVA that could be modified. Only the following traits were included: partner's Big Five extraversion and agreeableness scores, *extraversion match* (a binary variable indicating whether the pair were both introverts or both extroverts), *gender match* (defined similarly), age difference, and the participant's rating of their partner on the following qualities: attractive, funny, attentive, and excited. The resulting model statistically significantly predicted WAI score, $F(9, 19) = 4.656$, $p = .004$, and was able to account for 72.4 % of the variance in WAI score, $R = .851$.

Table 2 shows the coefficients of the regression model. The first column (unstandardized β) gives the increase (or decrease) that can be expected in bonding for a 1-unit increase in the variable. For example, an increase in a participant's rating of their partner as attentive is associated with an increase of 6.024 in expected B-WAI. Three significant effects were detected; whether the gender of the two participants matched, and whether the partner was perceived as excited and attentive. It appears that bonding will be highest when the partner's gender is not a match, the partner gives the impression of listening carefully to the participant, and the partner is enthusiastic about the conversation.

Table 2. Linear regression coefficients for each of the factors in the model.

Variable	Unstandardized β	Standard err.	Standardized β	t	p
Extraversion	−4.461	3.984	−.179	−1.120	.279
Agreeableness	−5.441	6.393	−.127	−.851	.407
Extraversion match	3.158	2.169	.235	1.456	.165
Gender match	−6.765	2.923	−.393	−2.314	.034
Age difference	.150	.091	.255	1.646	.119
Attractive	.352	.788	.067	.446	.662
Funny	−1.624	1.314	−.207	−1.237	.234
Attentive	6.024	1.251	.847	4.814	.000
Excited	1.622	.754	.342	2.152	.047

4   Discussion and Conclusions

We have compared the effects of personality, attractiveness, humour, and attitudes like excitement on bonding and rapport. We have found that bonding can be predicted effectively using personality and the traits described. Future work is needed to determine the extent to which these findings can generalize to interactions between a person and an IVA. For example, physical attraction between people could account for our finding that pairs with opposite genders have higher bonding, and these factors would presumably not be present in Human-VA interactions. However, to the extent that these findings generalize, they suggest that it may be most important to design an IVA to appear enthusiastic and attentive, rather than focusing on designing it to be agreeable, funny, attractive, or to have a similar age to the user. The importance of attentiveness may suggest that designing agents around mirroring (e.g. [3]) and contingent nonverbal cues (e.g. [4]) may be the most promising approaches.

References

1. van Vugt, H., Hoorn, J., Konijn, E.: Interactive engagement with embodied agents: an empirically validated framework. Comp. Anim. Virtual Worlds **20**(2–3), 195–204 (2009)
2. Wong, J.W.-E., McGee, K.: Frown more, talk more: effects of facial expressions in establishing conversational rapport with virtual agents. In: Nakano, Y., Neff, M., Paiva, A., Walker, M. (eds.) IVA 2012. LNCS, vol. 7502, pp. 419–425. Springer, Heidelberg (2012)
3. Kahl, S., Kopp, S.: Modeling a social brain for interactive agents: integrating mirroring and mentalizing. In: Brinkman, W.-P., Broekens, J., Heylen, D. (eds.) IVA 2015. LNCS, vol. 9238, pp. 77–86. Springer, Heidelberg (2015)
4. Gratch, J., Wang, N., Gerten, J., Fast, E., Duffy, R.: Creating rapport with virtual agents. In: Pelachaud, C., Martin, J.-C., André, E., Chollet, G., Karpouzis, K., Pelé, D. (eds.) IVA 2007. LNCS, vol. 4722, pp. 125–138. Springer, Heidelberg (2007)

5. Zhao, R., Papangelis, A., Cassell, J.: Towards a dyadic computational model of rapport management for human-virtual agent interaction. In: Bickmore, T., Marsella, S., Sidner, C. (eds.) IVA 2014. LNCS, vol. 8637, pp. 514–527. Springer, Heidelberg (2014)
6. Butler, E.: Temporal interpersonal emotion systems the ties that form relationships. Pers. Soc. Psych. Rev. **15**(4), 367–393 (2011)
7. Cuperman, R., Lckes, W.: Big five predictors of behavior and perceptions in initialdyadic interactions. J. Pers. Soc. Psych. **97**(4), 667 (2009)
8. Carver, C.S., Scheier, M.F.: Perspectives on Personality. Pearson Higher, Boston (2011)
9. Horvath, A., Greenberg, L.: Development and validation of the working alliance inventory. J. Couns. Psychol. **36**(2), 223 (1989)
10. von der Pütten, A.M., Krämer, N.C., Gratch, J.: How our personality shapes our interactions with virtual characters - implications for research and development. In: Safonova, A. (ed.) IVA 2010. LNCS, vol. 6356, pp. 208–221. Springer, Heidelberg (2010)
11. Goldberg, L.R.: The development of markers for the big-five factor structure. Psychol. Assess. **4**(1), 26 (1992)

Translating Player Dialogue into Meaning Representations Using LSTMs

James Ryan[✉], Adam James Summerville, Michael Mateas,
and Noah Wardrip-Fruin

Expressive Intelligence Studio, University of California, Santa Cruz, Santa Cruz, USA
{jor,michaelm,nwf}@soe.ucsc.edu, asummerv@ucsc.edu

Abstract. In this paper, we present a novel approach to natural language understanding that utilizes *context-free grammars* (CFGs) in conjunction with *sequence-to-sequence* (seq2seq) *deep learning*. Specifically, we take a CFG authored to generate dialogue for our target application, a videogame, and train a *long short-term memory* (LSTM) *recurrent neural network* (RNN) to translate the surface utterances that it produces to traces of the grammatical expansions that yielded them. Critically, we already annotated the symbols in this grammar for the semantic and pragmatic considerations that our game's dialogue manager operates over, allowing us to use the grammatical trace associated with any surface utterance to infer such information. From preliminary offline evaluation, we show that our RNN translates utterances to grammatical traces (and thereby meaning representations) with great accuracy.

1 Introduction

While conversational agents in service applications have become an increasingly common part of everyday life, few videogames have featured freeform conversational interaction with non-player characters (NPCs)—here, *Façade* is the only major example to date [4]. This is likely due to fundamental differences between the patterns of interaction germane to service conversational agents relative to those we envision for NPCs. In service dialogue systems, interaction is constrained and highly structured, lending well to *rule-based approaches* to natural language understanding (NLU). Contrarily, conversational interaction with ideal, futuristic NPCs would be less constrained and more open-ended, making the paradigm less suitable for rule-based approaches, since a huge number of matching rules would have to be authored to cover the larger conversational domains. *Façade*, whose NLU system *is* rule-based, partly wrangles this problem by constraining the conversational domain according to a strong dramatic progression. Still, its authors tasked themselves with producing 6,800 rules over the course of hundreds of person hours, and then relied on the additional measure of rules being promiscuous in their mapping to discourse acts [4]. As such, it is not surprising that, nearly fifteen years since its first reporting in the literature, very few practitioners of entertainment-based interactive media have taken on the massive authorial burden requisite to employing *Façade*'s demonstrated

© Springer International Publishing AG 2016
D. Traum et al. (Eds.): IVA 2016, LNAI 10011, pp. 383–386, 2016.
DOI: 10.1007/978-3-319-47665-0_38

technical approach [3]. Additionally, we note that the prospect of taking this approach would be even more daunting in interactive media lacking strong dramatic progression, *e.g.*, open-world games. Further, the rules themselves can be difficult for naive authors—*e.g.*, dialogue authors working on teams developing videogames—to compose. Finally, beyond authorial burden, there is the basic problem that matching rules, even fuzzy ones, are often brittle.

In this paper, we present a method for NLU that is intended to be less authorially intensive, less confounding to naive authors, and less brittle than rule-based approaches. This method utilizes context-free grammars (CFGs) in conjunction with the *long short-term memory* (LSTM) *recurrent neural network* (RNN) architecture. Specifically, a (potentially naive) author specifies a CFG (using a tool we have developed called Expressionist [7]) whose terminal derivations are surface utterances and whose nonterminal symbols are annotated by the author to capture semantic and pragmatic considerations [5]. Training data is then generated from this CFG, in the form of utterances paired with traces of the grammatical expansions that produced them. The learning task, then, is one of *sequence-to-sequence* (seq2seq) translation, in which we train an RNN to translate surface utterances into grammatical traces. Crucially, because the symbols in these traces have been annotated with semantic and pragmatic information, we can infer such information from any trace that the RNN translates a surface utterance into, thereby decoding the utterance into a meaning representation.

We are currently employing this method in a game that we are developing, called *Talk of the Town* [8], by having a trained RNN translate arbitrary player dialogue to grammatical traces, which are then used to procure semantic and pragmatic information that is fed to the game's dialogue manager. While we are not yet poised to explicitly compare our method to rule-based systems in terms of authorial burden, amenability to naive authors, or brittleness, we do demonstrate its accuracy in translating from surface utterances to grammatical traces (which point directly to semantic and pragmatic mark-up); additionally, we will attempt to qualitatively argue for the advantages of our approach, relative to rule-based systems, along those criteria. For more information about this project, please see our longer technical report on the subject [9].

2   Method

Our training data is a CFG that had already been authored—using a tool we have developed called Expressionist [7]—for the purpose of generating NPC dialogue in *Talk of the Town* [5]. In this grammar, the mark-up attributed to nonterminal symbols corresponds to the semantic and pragmatic concerns that the game's dialogue manager operates over, described at length in [6]. Using Expressionist, our grammar took approximately twenty hours for a single author to produce; it comprises 217 nonterminal symbols and 624 production rules, and is capable of yielding a total 2.8 M surface utterances. The actual training data used for training our RNN consists of pairs of surface utterances matched with traces of the grammatical expansions that produced them. To produce this training data, we sampled 5,000 surface utterances for each unique possible meaning (as determined by annotations on the symbols expanded to produce them), producing a total 345,000 utterance–trace pairs. Additionally, we utilized a denoising component that augmented these pairs with new pairs whose utterances were automatically corrupted.

For our seq2seq learning procedure, we used the Tensorflow framework [1] to develop a mapping from surface utterances to traces of the grammatical expansions that produced them. This procedure can be thought of as a translation task: the neural network translates from one language (surface utterances) to another language (grammatical traces), where instances of each language are essentially just strings. For instance, the string Oh, greetings, Andrew. in the utterance language translates to the string greet(greet back(use interlocutor first name)) in the trace language. Our network utilizes LSTM cells [2], a modification of the standard RNN approach that represents the current state of the art for sequence processing. For a more detailed explanation of this aspect of the project, see our longer technical report [9].

After training the RNN, we incorporated it into the software framework that underpins *Talk of the Town*. As described in [6], conversation in our game is turn-based, with turns being allocated by the dialogue manager. When a turn has been given to a player character, the player is asked to furnish her character's next utterance. Once the player has submitted this, the dialogue manager passes the utterance to the RNN, which tokenizes it and performs seq2seq translation on it to produce a grammatical trace composed of symbols in our Expressionist grammar. From here, the dialogue manager collects all the mark-up associated with all the symbols appearing in the trace, and treats this as the meaning of the player utterance (which it processes to update the conversation state).

3   Preliminary Evaluation

We carried out a preliminary offline evaluation procedure that demonstrates the accuracy of our system in mapping from surface utterances to grammatical traces. To conduct this experiment, we randomized our set of training data, split it into eleven pieces, and for each piece, performed 10-fold cross validation on the remainder of the set before finally using the held-out piece as a test set. We then calculated perplexity values: both cross-validation perplexity and test perplexity averaged 1.046 across all folds, with no fold showing perplexity worse than 1.053. Low perplexity values near 1 showcase the ability of the system to translate from surface utterances to grammatical traces (and thereby semantic and pragmatic information, as explained above) nearly perfectly in this task. Further, these preliminary results indicate that this approach is robust to variations and gaps in the data, with no fold performing drastically better or worse than any other. In addition to this experiment, in [9] we provide informal results in the form transcriptions of sample conversations between us and NPCs in our game, which were made possible by the technique we describe here.

4   Discussion and Future Work

While we have demonstrated the accuracy of this system in mapping surface utterances to grammatical traces (and thereby semantic and pragmatic information characterizing the utterances), we would like to informally discuss the advantages of our method relative to rule-based approaches to NLU. First, we believe that our approach incurs less authorial burden, simply by virtue of the combinatorial explosion that characterizes generative grammars. This is demonstrated in the large number of terminal derivations that our grammar can generate. Further, we contend that our approach is more amenable to naive authors who might like to feature NLU in their applications. Rather than authoring procedural rules, by our approach an author uses the Expressionist graphical user interface, which is designed for naive authors and supports live feedback showing surface utterances and their corresponding annotations [7]. While training a neural network is certainly not practical for naive authors, we plan to eventually support black-box RNN training as a service associated with Expressionist. Finally, we posit that intuitively our model should be less brittle than rule-based systems. While rules in such systems work by matching discrete authored patterns (which of course may be fuzzy) against user utterances, a neural network does something similar, but with patterns at arbitrary granularities, with hierarchies (patterns of patterns) that are learned dynamically. Of course, one tradeoff here is that human-authored rulesets are much more interpretable than RNNs.

While our preliminary evaluation is promising, we are currently planning a study with actual players so that we may better understand both the successes and limitations of our neural approach. Finally, we again invite the reader to see our longer technical report on this stage of our project [9].

References

1. Abadi, M., et al.: TensorFlow: large-scale machine learning on heterogeneous systems (2015). http://tensorflow.org/
2. Hochreiter, S., Schmidhuber, J.: Long short-term memory. Neural Comput. **9**(8), 1735–1780 (1997)
3. Lessard, J.: Designing natural-language game conversations. In: Proceedings DiGRA-FDG (2016)
4. Mateas, M., Stern, A.: Natural language understanding in Façade: surface-text processing. In: Proceedings TIDSE (2004)
5. Ryan, J., Mateas, M., Wardrip-Fruin, N.: Characters who speak their minds: dialogue generation in Talk of the Town. In: Proceedings AIIDE (2016)
6. Ryan, J., Mateas, M., Wardrip-Fruin, N.: A lightweight videogame dialogue manager. In: Proceedings DiGRA-FDG (2016)
7. Ryan, J., Seither, E., Mateas, M., Wardrip-Fruin, N.: Expressionist: an authoring tool for in-game text generation. In: Interactive Storytelling (2016)
8. Ryan, J.O., Summerville, A., Mateas, M., Wardrip-Fruin, N.: Toward characters who observe, tell, misremember, and lie. In: Proceedings Experimental AI in Games (2015)
9. Summerville, A.J., Ryan, J., Mateas, M., Wardrip-Fruin, N.: CFGs-2-NLU: sequence-to-sequence learning for mapping utterances to semantics and pragmatics. University of California, Santa Cruz, Technical report, UCSC-SOE-16-11 (2016)

Evaluating Presence Strategies
of Temporarily Required Virtual Assistants

Andrea Bönsch$^{(\boxtimes)}$, Tom Vierjahn$^{(\boxtimes)}$, and Torsten W. Kuhlen$^{(\boxtimes)}$

JARA – High-Performance Computing, Visual Computing Institute,
RWTH Aachen University, Aachen, Germany
{boensch,vierjahn,kuhlen}@vr.rwth-aachen.de
http://www.vr.rwth-aachen.de

Abstract. Computer-controlled virtual humans can serve as assistants in virtual scenes. Here, they are usually in an almost constant contact with the user. Nonetheless, in some applications assistants are required only temporarily. Consequently, presenting them only when needed, i.e., minimizing their presence time, might be advisable.

To the best of our knowledge, there do not yet exist any design guidelines for such agent-based support systems. Thus, we plan to close this gap by a controlled qualitative and quantitative user study in a CAVE-like environment. We expect users to prefer assistants with a low presence time as well as a low fallback time to get quick support. However, as both factors are linked, a suitable trade-off needs to be found. Thus, we plan to test four different strategies, namely fading, moving, omnipresent and busy. This work presents our hypotheses and our planned within-subject design.

Keywords: Virtual agent · Assistive technology · Immersive virtual environments · User study design

1 Introduction

Computer-controlled virtual humans, so-called virtual agents, are often embedded into HMD and CAVE-like environments [1] to serve as assistants. In the resulting immersive, agent-based support systems, they can have various roles: guiding users through the scene, training them how to perform certain tasks, being interlocutors answering questions or executing scene commands given by the user [2].

To the best of our knowledge, in the majority of these agent-based virtual support systems the assistants are always present. As a key component they are in an almost constant contact with the user, facilitating quick and unhindered assistance. However, designing such an *omnipresent* agent is challenging: certain constraints like personal-space requirements and collision-avoidance strategies need to be met [3].

In contrast, this work focuses on applications where assistants are required only *temporarily*, i.e., as interlocutors. In this scenarios, omnipresent agents

© Springer International Publishing AG 2016
D. Traum et al. (Eds.): IVA 2016, LNAI 10011, pp. 387–391, 2016.
DOI: 10.1007/978-3-319-47665-0_39

focusing solely on the user may annoy the users. Thus, having a low presence time (PT), i.e., presenting assistants only when needed, should be desired. Consequently, the question arises what the assistive agents should do in the meantime.

The follow-up question is, how users can fall back on the absent agent. Other common assistive interfaces like PieMenus [4] fade in after triggering a signal of necessity, e.g., by pressing a designated button on an input device. As a result, users can *instantly* access all available support functions. Such, a low fallback timeFT should also be considered in agent-based support systems. By, e.g., calling the agent's name, the assistant may simply appear or walk by quickly.

Apparently, PT and FT are closely linked. Therefore, a good trade-off has to be found. Thus, we will test four different combinations of both parameters in our study.

2 Study Description

We plan to investigate the trade-off between PT and FT for temporarily required assistants serving as interlocutors in immersive virtual environments.

2.1 Experimental Design

To evaluate all combinations of low and high PT and FT, we designed four different strategies constraining the assistant's behavior:

Strategy	PT	FT	Description
Fading	Low	Low	The assistant fades in and out.
Moving	Low	High	The assistant walks by and leaves when done.
Omnipresent	High	Low	The assistant constantly follows the user closely.
Busy	High	High	The assistant self-reliantly works in the vicinity of the user, walks by and returns to work when done.

For evaluation, we designed two different tasks, in which the participants have to start a conversation with the assistant about certain notes distributed over the scene. In the first task, the notes' locations are known, resulting in goal-oriented navigation and thus a *go-to task*. Here, we expect users to be more willing to have the assistant nearby as the required fallback in a timely manner justifies the presence. In the second task, the notes need to be found via exploratory navigation resulting in a *search task*. In contrast to the go-to task, users might feel more comfortable without the assistant, since they first have to explore the scene on their own.

In summary, we plan to conduct a within-subject user study with two dependent variables: strategy and task.

2.2   Hypotheses and Evaluation

We expect the following hypotheses to be confirmed:

H1: *Fading* is not preferred.
Although, PT and FT are both low in fading, we expect users to consider it too unrealistic for virtual humans.

H2: *Omnipresent* is preferred for the go-to task.
When users know exactly that they will ask for support within the next moments, we expect them to accept a high PT, while still preferring a low FT.

H3: *Moving* is preferred for the search task.
When users have to fulfill certain tasks at first on their own, we expect them to prefer a low PT. As a consequence of *H1*, we expect them to accept also a higher FT.

During the evaluation we will examine the participant's short-term experiences in the study. Afterwards, a semi-structured interview will be used to figure out what participants might prefer for long-term usage. Results of both will allow us to give an advice for improved designs of virtual assistants.

2.3   Virtual Environment

The test environment will be a two-man apartment, shown in Fig. 1(a). Four different notes will be placed inside the apartment: two notes with known positions and two notes which need to be found by the user. Participants will access the notes without support, then call the assistant and ask him or her a related question in order to have a short conversation. For example, users may ask the assistant to keep a shopping list located at the kitchen table in mind, shown in Fig. 1(b). The text overlay in the figure illustrates the planned speech-based interaction.

The platform SmartBody [5] will be used to animate the assistant. The remaining program logic will be implemented with the library ViSTA [6].

2.4   Apparatus

We will use a five-sided CAVE with the size $5.25\,\text{m} \times 5.25\,\text{m} \times 3.30\,\text{m}$ ($w \times d \times h$) providing a 360° horizontal field of regard [7]. Our participants will wear active stereo glasses, tracked at 60 Hz, and use an ART Flystick 2 for navigation. Since the CAVE is equipped with loudspeaker and microphone arrays as well as two security cameras, the supervisor can observe and converse with the fully immersed participant. Additionally, the hardware enables us to conduct the study with a Wizard of Oz paradigm by controlling the behavior of the agent.

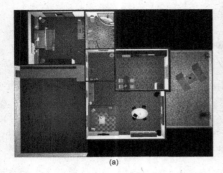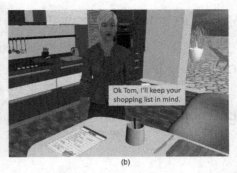

(a)   (b)

Fig. 1. Floor plan of the virtual apartment in which the participants will gather four notes (a) and the embedded assistant in a conversation with a participant (b).

2.5 Procedure

The study will be divided into seven phases: In the welcome phase, participants will be informed about the procedure of the study and define the appearance of their agent based on a limited set of features. By this, the assistant will be considered sympathetic, minimizing the feeling of having a complete stranger close by. Afterwards, the users will enter the CAVE to explore the apartment without the four notes in up to five minutes. In the four succeeding phases, participants have to gather the four notes and talk to the agent. In each phase the assistant will be using a different strategy. The order of strategies will be randomized between the participants. We expect each of the four phases to take approximately five minutes. In the final phase, participants will fill out a questionnaire and attended a semi-structured interview.

3 Conclusion

We have presented a study design to investigate user preferences on the trade-off between presence and fallback times of temporarily required assistants in immersive virtual scenes. After conducting the study, we will give design guidelines for agents embedded as interlocutors answering questions or executing scene commands given by the user. For other application types, individual studies have to be conducted as the preference of presence strategies and the user's task are likely correlated.

References

1. Cruz-Neira, C., Sandin, D.J., DeFanti, T.A.: Surround-screen projection-based virtual reality: the design and implementation of the CAVE. In: Proceedings of the 20th Annual Conference on Computer Graphics and Interactive Techniques, SIGGRAPH 1993, pp. 135–142 (1993)

2. McGlashan, S.: Speech interfaces to virtual reality. In: 2nd International Workshop on Military Applications of Synthetic Environments and VR (1995)
3. Bönsch, A., Weyers, B., Wendt, J., Freitag, S., Kuhlen, T.W.: Collision avoidance in the presence of a virtual agent in small-scale virtual environments. In: Proceedings of IEEE Symposium on 3D User Interfaces, pp. 145–148 (2016). http://dx.doi.org/10.1109/3DUI.2016.7460045
4. Gebhardt, S., Pick, S., Leithold, F., Hentschel, B., Kuhlen, T.W.: Extended pie menus for immersive virtual environments. IEEE Trans. Vis. Comput. Graph. 9(4), 644–651 (2013). http://dx.doi.org/10.1109/TVCG.2013.31
5. Shapiro, A.: Building a character animation system. In: Allbeck, J.M., Faloutsos, P. (eds.) MIG 2011. LNCS, vol. 7060, pp. 98–109. Springer, Heidelberg (2011). doi:10.1007/978-3-642-25090-3_9
6. Assenmacher, I., Kuhlen, T.W.: The ViSTA virtual reality toolkit. In: SEARIS Workshop on IEEE Virtual Reality Conference, pp. 23–26 (2008). http://dx.doi.org/10.1109/MCG.2014.97
7. Kuhlen, T.W., Hentschel, B.: Quo Vadis CAVE: does immersive visualization still matter? IEEE Comput. Graph. Appl. 34(5), 14–21 (2014)

A Disclosure Intimacy Rating Scale
for Child-Agent Interaction

Franziska Burger[✉], Joost Broekens, and Mark A. Neerincx

TU Delft, Interactive Intelligence, Delft, The Netherlands
f.v.burger@tudelft.nl
http://ii.tudelft.nl

Abstract. Reciprocal self-disclosure is an integral part of social bonding between humans that has received little attention in the field of human-agent interaction. To study how children react to self-disclosures of a virtual agent, we developed a disclosure intimacy rating scale that can be used to assess both the intimacy level of agent disclosures and that of child disclosures. To this end, 72 disclosures were derived from a biography created for the agent and rated by 10 university students for intimacy. A principal component analysis and subsequent k-means clustering of the rated statements resulted in four distinct levels of intimacy based on the risk of a negative appraisal and the impact of betrayal by the listener. This validated rating scale can be readily used with other agents or interfaces.

Keywords: Long-term cHRI · Self-disclosure intimacy · PAL project

1 Motivation

In a focus group conducted with diabetic children in 2012, it was found that children would like a companion robot to share their secrets with and to listen to them when they are sad [1].

According to Self Determination Theory (SDT) [3], successful establishment of a social bond between human and agent leads to sustained motivation both to interact with the agent and to engage in activities that the agent proposes. Such a bond could be established through increasingly intimate, reciprocal self-disclosures [4], that is the exchange of information about the self.

One of the key interests in human-human self-disclosure research has been the close link between disclosure and liking. For example, it was found that 6th grade children's liking of another child was influenced by that child's capacity to match the intimacy level of a disclosure while that of 4th graders was not [5].

To better study children's disclosure behavior when interacting with a virtual agent, we developed the Dyadic Disclosure Dialog Module (3DM) within the framework of the PAL project[1] and using a situated Cognitive Engineering (sCE) [2] approach. This, in turn, necessitated the development of a rating scale for intimacy of self-disclosure.

---

[1] http://www.pal4u.eu/.

© Springer International Publishing AG 2016
D. Traum et al. (Eds.): IVA 2016, LNAI 10011, pp. 392–396, 2016.
DOI: 10.1007/978-3-319-47665-0_40

2   Intimacy Rating Scale

To design agent disclosure statements at various intimacy levels and to assess the depth of children's disclosures, a rating scale for disclosure intimacy was needed. For this, the following constraints were identified: (a) the scale should discretize the intimacy continuum, (b) each discrete level should have a clear definition, (c) the scale should have a minimum of three levels [6, Chap. 13], (d) the scale should be neither topical nor example-based. Upon reviewing the relevant child and adult literature on self-disclosure, no entirely suitable intimacy scale could be found. We therefore developed and validated the Disclosure Intimacy Rating Scale (DIRS).

As summarized in [7], intimacy of self-disclosure is directly related to vulnerability of the discloser. In a similar vein, it is argued in [8] that the social risk associated with disclosing determines the depth of disclosure. With each self-disclosure, we risk "social rejection [or] betrayal" [8, p. 180].

$$risk(\text{SD}) = risk(\text{SR}) + risk(\text{B}) \tag{1}$$

with SD := self-disclosure, SR := social rejection, and B := betrayal. Betrayal, here, describes the passing on of information by the recipient to third parties.

Risk can be formalized as the product of probability (P) and impact (I). If we further assume that social rejection does not occur at random but only follows if the disclosure is negatively appraised, we can approximate the risk of social rejection through the risk of negative appraisal:

$$risk(\text{SD}) = P(\text{NA}) * I(\text{NA}) + P(\text{B}) * I(\text{B}) \tag{2}$$

with NA := negative appraisal.

The probability of betrayal, $P(\text{B})$, can depend only on characteristics of and prior experiences with the disclosure recipient. It is therefore independent of the content and cannot be considered in the level definitions.

These considerations initially yielded six intimacy levels. Using these, a total of 6($level$) × 3($topic$) × 2($valence$) × 2($repetition$) = 72 statements were fabricated by the first author with the personality and biography of the ECA providing content and style information. To obtain a first validation of the scale, the statements were rated for intimacy by 10 university students (5 female, $M_{age} = 23$, $SD_{age} = 1.612$) on a six-point scale: only levels 0 and 5 were labeled with *not at all intimate* and *extremely intimate* respectively. We decided against asking adult participants to take on the perspective of a child (because results would be questionable in terms of validity) or to rate statements as if coming from a robot (because students are more critical towards the plausibility of a robot expressing emotions and a personality). The biography was hence slightly adapted to fit a 22 year-old student. Before rating, participants were asked to read a persona description of the student and instructions explaining self-disclosure. Intimacy was defined as: "the degree to which a statement reflects information about the self that is sensitive." Further, they were given one example disclosure for each level using a fourth topic. The intimacy levels

of the examples was not provided. Participants could thus get an impression of
the covered range and the type of statements. Participants found the description
of the student and the statements to be believable (the mean believability rating on a 5-point Likert scale was $M_{believability} = 4.3$). The inter-rater reliability

Table 1. The four intimacy levels of the DIRS that resulted from the post-analysis.

Risk	Definition	Example
Low	$P(NA)$, $I(NA)$, and $I(B)$ are low or zero: the discloser cannot be evaluated on the basis of the statement or the statement is very common-place	"I have a lot of brothers and sisters."
Moderate	$P(NA)$ is moderate, because statements are more opinionated, but $I(NA)$ and $I(B)$ are low. Negative appraisal can at best take the form of disagreement. The information cannot really be exploited, so that in the case of betrayal, no loss is to be expected. Includes preferences and opinions on activities and objects	"I like online games in which you have to team up with other players."
High	Either $P(NA)$ is high and both $I(NA)$ and $I(B)$ are low (the content conflicts with the norms of the recipient but does not reflect on the character of the discloser), or $P(NA)$ is low but the content is of great significance to the discloser so that $I(NA)$ and $I(B)$ are high. Disclosures are emotional and may include evaluations of other people	"I'm really disappointed that my sister will not try yoga with me. She already promised it twice but never followed through."
Very high	$P(NA)$, $I(NA)$, and $I(B)$ are high, because the disclosure is at the core of the discloser's self-concept and could easily conflict with the norms of the recipient. In the case of betrayal, great emotional, physical, or material damage may ensue. Social stigmas, self-doubt, deep personal fears and secrets are accumulated on this level	"Whenever I work really hard or I'm nervous, I start sweating like crazy. I can't get close to people then, because I'm really conscious of how I smell."

was assessed using the two-way random intraclass correlation coefficient with the ten raters, yielding $ICC(2, 10) = .947$. Cronbach's alpha using all items was high with $\alpha = .948$. The Pearson correlation coefficient between the level of an item and the average rating it received across participants was determined to be $r = .85$. To check whether we would also find six intimacy levels back in the item pool, a principal component analysis was conducted on the ratings of all items. Using the point of inflexion as a cut-off criterion [9], four principal components explaining at least 10 % of the variance each and 67 % in total were revealed. *Four* was then used as the desired number of clusters in a k-means clustering algorithm. A post-analysis of the resulting item clusters afforded the four intimacy levels of the DIRS detailed in Table 1.

3   Conclusion

3DM is intended to gain insights into how and how readily children in late childhood disclose to an artificial agent. Whether children absolutely, relatively, or do not at all match the intimacy level of a robot's disclosure [10] being a main matter of interest. The DIRS is a supplementary instrument for 3DM to code and compare the intimacy levels of children's disclosures in response to agent disclosures. In an exploratory study using 3DM, 114 child-disclosures were rated by two independent raters using the DIRS. Raters agreed in 67 % of cases and deviated by 1 level in 27 % of cases. However, the disclosures were gathered in the field over the course of two weeks and children were found to mainly disclose on the lower two levels to the ECA (only in 26 % of disclosures was the mean rating of both raters larger than 1).

There are two main limitations to the DIRS. The first is that contextual information of the disclosure is unknown or ignored, and can only be estimated by the rater. As such, raters should have the same cultural background as the discloser. An additional limitation is that the DIRS has only been validated with adults, but is used with children in the PAL project. A next step is therefore to validate it with children of the target age group and using the original biography of the ECA.

In summary, we developed and validated the Disclosure Intimacy Rating Scale to rate statements for intimacy. This scale can be readily used across different human-robot interaction contexts.

References

1. Baroni, I., Nalin, M., Baxter, P., Pozzi, C., Oleari, E., Sanna, A., Belpaeme, T.: What a robotic companion could do for a diabetic child. In: 2014 RO-MAN: The 23rd IEEE International Symposium on Robot and Human Interactive Communication, pp. 936–941. IEEE Press (2014)
2. Neerincx, M.A., Lindenberg, J.: Situated Cognitive Engineering for Complex Task Environments. Ashgate Publishing Limited, Aldershot (2008)

3. Deci, E.L., Ryan, R.M.: Overview of self-determination theory: an organismic dialectical perspective. In: Handbook of Self-determination Research, pp. 3–33. University Rochester Press (2002)
4. Altman, I., Taylor, D.: Social Penetration Theory. Holt, Rinehart & Mnston, New York (1973)
5. Rotenberg, K.J., Mann, L.: The development of the norm of the reciprocity of self-disclosure and its function in children's attraction to peers. Child Dev. **57**, 1349–1357 (1986)
6. Tardy, C.H.: A Handbook for the Study of Human Communication: Methods and Instruments for Observing, Measuring, and Assessing Communication Processes. Greenwood Publishing Group, New York (1988)
7. Moon, Y.: Intimate exchanges: using computers to elicit self-disclosure from consumers. J. Consum. Res. **26**(4), 323–339 (2000)
8. Omarzu, J.: A disclosure decision model: determining how and when individuals will self-disclose. Pers. Soc. Psychol. Rev. **4**(2), 174–185 (2000)
9. Cattell, R.B.: The scree test for the number of factors. Multivar. Behav. Res. **1**(2), 245–276 (1966)
10. Rotenberg, K.J., Chase, N.: Development of the reciprocity of self-disclosure. J. Genet. Psychol. **153**(1), 75–86 (1992)

Generating Needs, Goals and Plans for Virtual Agents in Social Simulations

Anton Bogdanovych[(✉)] and Tomas Trescak

School of Computing, Engineering and Mathematics,
Marcs Institute for Brain, Behaviour and Development,
University of Western Sydney, Sydney, NSW, Australia
{A.Bogdanovych,T.Trescak}@westernsydney.edu.au

Abstract. Many modern virtual reality reconstructions of historical sites focus on buildings and artefacts, but often ignore the issue of portraying everyday life of the people who populated the reconstructed area. This is mainly due to high costs and complexity of populating such sites with virtual agents. Here we show how combining needs modelling and planning can help to automate the development of large agent societies.

1 Introduction

Virtual reality reconstructions of historical sites provide an opportunity to experience traditions, rituals, architectural style and significant events associated with some extraordinary places that may no longer exist at present. Many current works predominantly focus on the elements of architecture, ancient buildings, objects and even entire cities. Supplying virtual simulations with agents that are capable of convincing and historically authentic behaviour beyond simple crowd simulation algorithms is difficult and costly. Virtual agents must be able to play different social roles, actively use surrounding objects, interact with other agents and even engage into interactions with humans. Modern video games are a good illustration in regards to the potential of having such simulations, but the cost of developing video games is very high. We propose a way to make agent-based historical, cultural and other kinds of virtual simulations more affordable by automating the process of populating a virtual environment with virtual agents. In our previous work [1] we have shown how it is possible to generate an infinitely large crowd of agents of unique and yet ethnically acceptable appearance from a small sample of manually designed avatars. Here we show how this crowd can be brought to life by automatically supplying agents with goals in response to their simulated needs and then how to achieve these goals using planning [2].

2 Virtual Agents in Social Simulations

A high level overview of our approach is presented in Fig. 1. Here each agent (in the crowd of a desired size) is generated using the genetic approach described in [1]. The agent would borrow some of the appearance features of those agents from

© Springer International Publishing AG 2016
D. Traum et al. (Eds.): IVA 2016, LNAI 10011, pp. 397–401, 2016.
DOI: 10.1007/978-3-319-47665-0_41

the manually designed sample population, but would also introduce some acceptable variation through mutation mechanisms. Every agent assumes a certain role in the reconstructed society (e.g. Potter) and this role would be associated with a set of norms and protocols of acceptable behaviour that the agent must follow while pursuing its goals. Rather than explicitly prescribing how each agent should satisfy its goals we rely on AI planning [2], where the agent senses surrounding objects and other actors and includes the perceived information into its decision making. Given that the environment is correctly annotated with preconditions and post-conditions and also taking the institutional constraints into account each agent would be able to dynamically construct complex role-specific plans in response to general needs (like hunger, thirst, fatigue, curiosity, etc.). In the example shown in Fig. 1 the agent playing the Potter role produces a clay pot, trades it for food and then consumes the food when hungry, while an agent with some other role (e.g. fisher) would satisfy hunger differently (e.g. will catch fish and then will cook it on an open fire before eating it). Further details of this architecture are presented in [3]. One of the key points we expand upon in this publication is the automatic generation of agent goals.

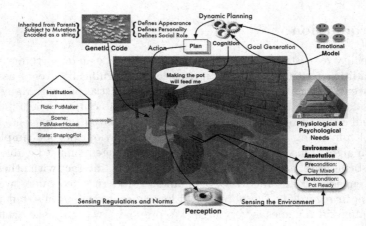

Fig. 1. The overview of the agent architecture

The key aim of having virtual agents in social simulations is to closely portray everyday life of people inhabiting the simulated space. This realisation has inspired us to turn to social sciences with an attempt to understand the underlying principles that drive human behaviour. One of the first concepts one usually comes across in this respect is the Maslow's Pyramid [4]. It outlines, from a psychological perspective, categorisation and prioritisation of fundamental human needs and desires. The ERG theory [5] and the Reiss Motivation Profile [6] have further developed Maslow's ideas and partially validated them.

In our work we have combined the findings of Maslow and those proposed in the ERG theory and Reiss Motivation Profile to produce the pyramid of motivation. This pyramid features 23 human needs that have been identified by [4] and later verified and extended by [5] and [6]. A computational simulation of this pyramid by each agent allows to automatically generate goals in response to some of the needs requiring satisfaction. We treat each of the needs as a reservoir that is replanished (satisfied) after performing the relevant action (e.g. sleeping to reduce fatigue) and depleted in response to other actions (e.g. walking will increase fatigue). So, we can track need depletion and when the corresponding reservoir reaches a critical mark we automatically generate a corresponding goal and use AI planning to produce a sequence of actions that lead to achieving this goal. With the help of an institution, which would enable having agents playing different roles and would specify acceptable interaction protocols resulting goal satisfaction for each of these roles, we can automatically simulate large diverse societies with complex perceived behaviour of individual virtual agents.

3   Case Study: Ancient Mesopotamia 5000 B.C.

To illustrate our approach we have developed a simulation[1] of everyday life in an ancient Mesopotamian settlement around 5000 B.C. shown in Fig. 2.

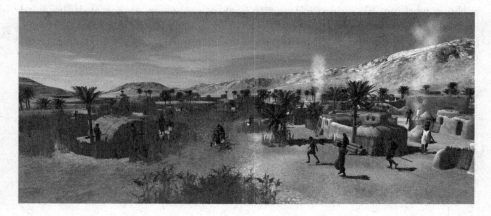

Fig. 2. Ancient Mesopotamian settlement populated with virtual agents

Producing this simulation involved modelling the buildings and city layout based on the results of archaeological excavations and manually designing the appearance of the base population of 2 agents. Using the "genetic code" of the base population a desired number of city inhabitants could be automatically generated following the approach in [1]. Next, the institution (similar to the one in [3]) has been designed. The institution covers the role structure, possible scenes and acceptable interaction protocols different roles can use for pursuing their

---

[1] Accompanying video is available at: https://youtu.be/Z5HFQvx0u2c.

goals. In this institution the agents can play one of the four roles: Fisher, Baker, Shepherd or Potter. For each of these roles the institution specifies protocols for working, obtaining food and trading. In their planning agents can then map a general-purpose goal (e.g. satisfy hunger) to their role and obtain the possible actions that this role can perform. While executing their plans agents must use the existing resources represented by 3D objects in the virtual environment. These objects (e.g. wheat, fish, etc.) are annotated with actions that can be performed with them together with pre-conditions and post-conditions.

There are limited resources in the environment and some resources are removed after an interaction (e.g. catching a fish). Agents need to travel to the destination of the resource, which increases their fatigue. When fatigue passes a threshold value agents rest until fatigue is lowered. Upon arrival, an agent can discover that the required resource is no longer available, so its plan fails and an alternative plan is used.

Plans are dynamically generated based on the current goal. Goals are triggered by agent needs. For example, when an agent reaches a threshold value for hunger, it tries to generate a plan, to reduce the hunger level. For this purpose, there are actions such as "eatFish", that the agent performs, once it acquires sufficient resources. Another need that has been simulated is comfort. In our simulation comfort is associated with storing enough food to survive three days without working. To store food agents with roles Fisher, Baker and Shepherd must trade their work products (fish, bread or milk) with a Potter for a storage pot. Potters do not directly produce food and can only receive it in exchange for pots. Figure 3 shows examples of agents satisfying their needs.

If all physiological needs are satisfied an agent starts to satisfy its curiosity need, which is to conduct a random walk and interact with novel objects.

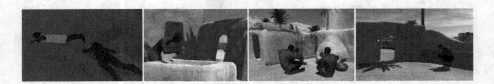

Fig. 3. Acting upon physiological needs: sleeping, drinking, eating and resting

We have conducted an experiment that involved generating 100 agents (25 agents per each role: Baker, Fisher, Potter and Shepherd). The resulting everyday life simulation looked very convincing. Sleeping, waking up, having breakfast by preparing the food from storage or obtaining food through work, working to satisfy immediate hunger or comfort and being curious are types of behaviour our agents demonstrated. These behaviours were not scripted, but resulted from acting upon frustrated needs and generating goals and plans for satisfying those.

References

1. Trescak, T., Bogdanovych, A., Simoff, S., Rodriguez, I.: Generating diverse ethnic groups with genetic algorithms. In: Proceedings of the ACM Symposium on Virtual Reality Software and Technology, VRST 2012, pp. 1–8. ACM, New York (2012)
2. Hendler, J.A., Tate, A., Drummond, M.: AI planning: systems and techniques. AI Mag. **11**(2), 61 (1990)
3. Trescak, T., Bogdanovych, A., Simoff, S.: Populating virtual cities with diverse physiology driven crowds of intelligent agents. In: Proceedings of the Social Simulation Conference (SSC 2014) (2014)
4. Maslow, A.H.: A theory of human motivation. Psychol. Rev. **50**(4), 370–396 (1943)
5. Alderfer, C.P.: An empirical test of a new theory of human needs. Organ. Behav. Hum. Perform. **4**(2), 142–175 (1969)
6. Reiss, S., Havercamp, S.M.: Motivation in developmental context: a new method for studying self-actualization. Humanistic Psychol. **45**(1), 41–53 (2005)

Psychologically Based Virtual-Suspect for Interrogative Interview Training

Moshe Bitan[1]([✉]), Galit Nahari[1], Zvi Nisin[2], Ariel Roth[1], and Sarit Kraus[1]

[1] Bar Ilan University, Ramat Gan, Israel
moshe.bitan78@gmail.com
[2] Israeli Police Department, East Jerusalem, Israel

Abstract. This paper presents a Virtual-Suspect system designed for use in police interrogation training simulations. The system allows users to preconfigure various scenarios based on real cases, as well as different suspect histories and personality types. The responses given by the Virtual-Suspect during the interrogation are selected based on context and the suspect's psychological state, which changes in response to each interrogator's statement. Experiments with 24 subjects have shown that the Virtual-Suspect's responses in an interrogation scenario are similar to those of a human respondent.

1 Introduction

The Virtual-Suspect system is designed to offer a more time and cost efficient alternative to the one-on-one interrogation simulation sessions that are used to train police officers in the art of interrogating a suspect. In these personal sessions, a trained instructor conducts an interrogation simulation using scenarios drawn from real cases, playing the role of the suspect and portraying different personalities based on the corresponding scenario while a trainee plays the role of the investigator. This training technique has proven effective, but it is time consuming and expensive, requiring experienced instructors or actors and training sessions that are carried out just one trainee at a time. The system we propose addresses this by allowing multiple cadets to train simultaneously at their convenience with a single instructor monitoring their progress. It supports different scenario configurations, generating responses based on the psychological state of the Virtual-Suspect and taking into account the context in which the statements are made. An experiment was conducted comparing the system's responding mechanism with that of a human instructor. The results suggest that humans have difficulty differentiating between simulations generated by our system and those of a human instructor.

This work was supported in part by the LAW-TRAIN project that has received funding from the European Unions Horizon 2020 research and innovation program under grant agreement No. 653587.

D. Traum et al. (Eds.): IVA 2016, LNAI 10011, pp. 402–406, 2016.
DOI: 10.1007/978-3-319-47665-0_42

2   Simulation Configuration

The *simulation configuration* is composed of the following three elements:

Interrogation Scenario Configuration is implemented via an event database and a personal information database. The former stores the Virtual-Suspect's relevant personal data. The latter contains information about occurrences that may or may not have happened (e.g. their location, time, date, participants). An event can be either truthful (i.e. actually happened) or false (i.e. used to deceive the interviewer and provide an *Alibi* or *Legal Access*). Therefore, events are labeled as either: *Criminal, Alibi, Legal Access or Neutral.* The system includes a dedicated label designed to simulate the fact that some topics can trigger a more emotional response than others. The *hot* label indicates that a personal or event-related detail has a profound effect on the Virtual-Suspect when introduced.

Interrogative Interviewing. The interrogation simulation is based on a standard Interrogative Interviewing model. Unlike other systems that support a single static scenario [1,2], it supports multiple configurable scenarios by allowing users to configure statement and response templates. Every statement directly affects the internal-state of the Virtual-Suspect, but not in the same way. To model this, the *hot* label is propagated at runtime to the Interrogative Interviewing model. A response or statement is *hot* if any of its input field values is labeled *hot* in the Scenario Database. A statement is also marked *hot* if any of its associated responses is *hot*.

Personality Profile. The Virtual-Suspect's *Internal-State* is based on Eysenck's *PEN* Model of personality [3], which consists of the personality traits, *Psychoticism, Extraversion and Neuroticism.* Formally, the internal-state is a three-dimensional vector $s \in \Re^3$ where the components correspond to the *Psychoticism, Extraversion and Neuroticism* personality traits. The initial value of the internal-state vector, denoted by s_0, is configured by the interrogation simulation supervisor.

The internal-state changes during an interrogation simulation, reflecting the effect of the interrogator's statements on the Virtual-Suspect. The degree to which the internal-state varies is determined by a second component, the *volatility of the Virtual-Suspect's personality*. The *Volatility* parameter determines the pace at which the internal-state changes for any given statement. Although this parameter is configured in the Simulation Configuration phase, its main function is in updating the internal-state vector, which is part of the Response Model, described next.

3   Response Model

The model consists of four cognitive components. The first two are the long- and short-term memory components. Long-term memory gives the Virtual-Suspect access to the Interrogation Scenario database to recall personal information and past events. Short-term memory allows the Virtual-Suspect to respond appropriately to follow-up statements. The third component, and arguably the most important, is the Virtual-Suspect's internal-state update mechanism, which determines the way an investigator's statement affects the Virtual-Suspect's internal-state. Finally, all of the above components are combined to produce the response of the Virtual-Suspect.

The Internal-State Vector Update Mechanism is executed for every statement. During a simulation, for every statement q at time t the internal-state vector is calculated using the following equation:

$$s_t = s_{(t-1)} + \sigma \cdot \left(\delta^{hot}(q) \cdot w_q^{hot} + \left(1 - \delta^{hot}(q) \right) \cdot w_q^{cold} \right) \tag{1}$$

Where σ is the *Volatility* parameter, $\delta^{hot}(q)$ indicates if a statement q is marked as *hot* and w_q^{hot}, w_q^{cold} are the statement effect weight vectors. It is important to note that the *Volatility* parameter σ is configured in the Personality Profile configuration phase and remains constant for the duration of the simulation.

The final phase in the response model is the **response selection**, in which the internal-state vector is used to select the output response r^*. The response selection process consists of four steps.

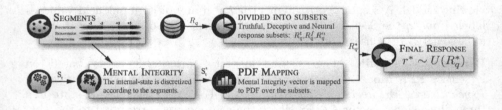

Fig. 1. Response selection

First, the associated responses set, R_q, is divided into three subsets: truthful responses R_q^t, deceptive responses R_q^f, and neutral responses R_q^n. Next, the internal-state vector components are color-coded and then discretized to the *Mental Integrity* vector s'. The value range of each internal-state vector component is divided into three sections, denoted by I_g, I_o and I_r, where each segment is color-coded to express the level of the Virtual-Suspect's *Mental Integrity*: *green* for mentally stable, *orange* for moderately stable and *red* for compromised mental integrity. The sections were manually calibrated (see Fig. 1). The Virtual-Suspect's context-dependent behavior is modeled in the third step, where the *Mental Integrity* vector and the contextual event label are mapped to a probability distribution function over the three response subsets, i.e. R_q^t, R_q^f and R_q^n, determining from which subset the final response will be selected. Finally, in the fourth step, the output response, r^*, is randomly selected from the previously selected subset, R_q^*, using a uniform distribution function, i.e. $r^* \sim U(R_q^*)$.

4 Experiment

The interrogation scenario chosen for the experiment is based on an actual burglary case. The initial internal-state vector was set to $s_0 = (0, 0, -3)$. The *Volatility* parameter was set to $\sigma = (0.5, 0.5, 0.5)$. 24 participants (12 male, 12 female), ranging in age from 20–30, were asked to read the transcripts of three simulations and answer a series of questions. In the first simulation, a human instructor acted as the suspect, while the second used the Virtual-Suspect response model (RMVS) and the third used a randomized response selection mechanism. Our hypothesis was that humans will find it difficult to differentiate between a human trainer and the Virtual-Suspect response model, but that the randomized response selection baseline mechanism would be distinguishable.

For each transcript, the participants were asked whether they thought the responses had been chosen by a human or a computer, on a scale ranging from one (human) to five (computer). The results are presented in Fig. 2 (a). Repeated measures ANOVAs were conducted to compare the three conditions. The resulting ANOVAs are $F(2, 22) = 8.15$, partial $\eta2 = 0.57$, $p < 0.002$. As hypothesized, the RMVS was rated significantly better than the Random baseline (using paired t-test $p < 0.01$). Similarly, the Human transcript was rated significantly better than the Random baseline (using paired t-test $p < 0.01$). The Human transcript was rated slightly better than the RMVS, but this small difference was not found to be statistically significant.

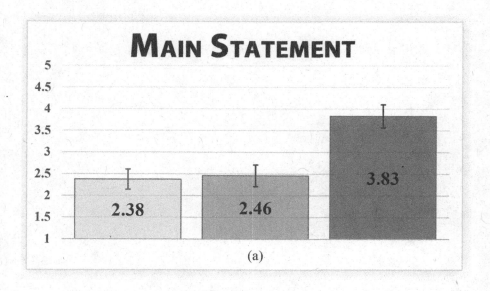

Fig. 2. Experiment's results

To conclude, people were not able to distinguish between the Human suspect and the RMVS, but could easily distinguish between the Random baseline and the RMVS and between the Random baseline and the Human.

References

1. Olsen, D.E.: Interview and interrogation training using a computer-simulated subject (1997)
2. Bruijnes, M., Wapperom, S., Heylen, D., et al.: A virtual suspect agents response model (2014)
3. Eysenck, H.J.: Biological Dimensions of Personality. Guilford Press, New York (1990)

Topic Switch Models for Dialogue Management in Virtual Humans

Wenjue Zhu[1], Andry Chowanda[1,2(✉)], and Michel Valstar[1]

[1] School of Computer Science, The University of Nottingham, Nottingham, UK
{psywz2,psxac6,pszmv}@nottingham.ac.uk
[2] School of Computer Science, Bina Nusantara University, Jakarta, Indonesia

Abstract. This paper presents a novel data-driven Topic Switch Model based on a cognitive representation of a limited set of topics that are currently in-focus, which determines what utterances are chosen next. The transition model was statistically learned from a large set of transcribed dyadic interactions. Results show that using our proposed model results in interactions that on average last 2.17 times longer compared to the same system without our model.

Keywords: Social relationship · Framework · Game-agents · Interactions

1 Introduction

Current Dialogue Management (DM) systems *"are not natural enough"* and cannot sustain a coherent conversation with humans [2]. One issue is that systems are not able to "stay on topic" and are incapable of following a "train of thought". As most DM systems have no notion of the concept of a topic and generate their responses based only on a set of predefined rules that operate on the specific words or phrases retrieved from the last user input.

To address this, we propose a novel data-driven Topic Switch Model (TSM), devise an algorithm for sensible topic switching and instantiate it in a software program that can imbue virtual humans with the capability of staying on topic or making sensible topic switches with the aim of achieving more coherent conversations with humans. Our TSM learns connections between topics, which allows for sensible topic switches, and learns connections between topics and utterances, which allows for the selection of sentences that match the current topic. The system is otherwise naive, in that it does not implement an agent's goals, or states such as social relations or an agent's emotion [3,4]. However, it is entirely data driven and thus does not require crafting of any rule whatsoever. It is thus suggested that for full effectiveness the TSM be integrated into a more complex stateful model, perhaps with one TSM per state.

We evaluate the efficacy of our system by comparing it to a version of our system without the TSM enabled. When tested on over 20 participants, we show that people communicate on average 2.17 times longer with the agent when the TSM is enabled.

D. Traum et al. (Eds.): IVA 2016, LNAI 10011, pp. 407–411, 2016.
DOI: 10.1007/978-3-319-47665-0_43

2   Related Work

A number of different approaches to DM have been proposed and implemented to date. Plan-based DM makes use of a general planner which is responsible for identifying the goal and making a plan. The plan consists of predefined operations and is aimed to achieve the final goal [1]. The most common and simplest approach to DM is to represent the dialogue as a graph where its nodes represents the dialogue states. The nodes usually define the proposed action based on the input of previous node [6]. Another common approach uses the concept of information state. In this approach, the state of conversation is formally represented by some informational components and a set of rules is defined for the DM to update the state and decide on the corresponding action according to the current state, system input and the applicable rule(s) [7].

3   The Topic Switch Model

Topic switches occur constantly in one's brain, and are influenced by both internal factors (e.g. your own knowledge of topics and their relationships) and external factors, including what you hear and see. There may be several topics in a person's mind at a time, each taking up a portion of one's attention. Over time topics in the brain will be replaced by others because of the various influencing factors at any point of time. This is our abstract concept of a TSM.

As we focus here on text-based dialogue systems, topic extraction is comprised of text preprocessing and topic retrieval. Two natural language processing techniques (i.e. stop-word removal and stemming) are chosen to pre-process the text input. With respect to topic retrieval, we maintain a lookup table of words and their corresponding topics. This list was manually created by the authors.

Topic relations, that should be learned by virtual humans consist of three types of topic statistics. The topic frequency $P_f(t)$ is the prior probability of a topic occurring in an utterance. The second relation, concurrency probability $P_{con}(t_1, t_2, \ldots, t_n)$, is the probability of two or more topics appearing in the same utterance. The third relation is the adjacency probability, $P_{adj}(t_1, t_2)$ representing the probability of topic t_2 occurring in a utterance if its previous utterance contains t_1.

$$\text{Topic Frequency: } P_f(t) = \frac{n_t}{N_T} \tag{1}$$

$$\text{Concurrency Possibility: } P_{con}(t_1, t_2, \ldots, t_n) = \frac{n_{con}(t_1, t_2, \ldots, t_n)}{N_s} \tag{2}$$

$$\text{Adjacency possibility: } P_{adj}(t_1, t_2) = \frac{n_{adj}(t_1, t_2)}{N_s'} \tag{3}$$

where N_s is the number of utterances and N_s' is the potential times of two topics appearing in two adjacent utterances. In this paper, the topic statistics were obtained from the SEMAINE database [5].

Algorithm 1. Topic switch with external factors

Input: all topics L_T, stop words L_{sw}, pairs of words and topics L_p, topic statistics, sentence database, user input

Initialisation:

1. Randomly select 5 topics from L_T to be the topics in the brain, $L_1 = [t_1, t_2, t_3, t_4, t_5]$.
2. Topics of which the virtual human is thinking currently, $L_2 = []$.
3. Topics that are out of the brain, $L_3 = L_T - L_1$.

Procedure:

1. Read the text input and extract the user topic t_u. Find the topic t_i in L_1 which has the largest adjacency possibility with t_u. If no user topic is found, randomly select a topic t_i in L_1 based on the topic frequencies. Add t_i into L_2, $L_2 = [t_i]$.
2. Generate a random number r between 0 and 1. Continuously try to find topics in $(L_1 - L_2)$ whose concurrency possibility with topics in L_2 is larger than r and add it into L_2 until no such topic is found.
3. Make a response by randomly selecting an utterance which contains all topics in L_2.
4. Randomly select a topic t_{out} from $(L_1 - L_2)$ to be swapped out based on the adjacency possibilities. Then $L_1 = L_1 - [t_{out}]$ and $L_3 = L_3 + [t_{out}]$ The possibility of each topic being selected is $P_{out}(t) = \frac{\sum_{t_a \in L_2}(1 - P_{adj}(t_a, t))}{\sum_{t_a \in L_2, t_b \in (L_1 - L_2)}(1 - P_{adj}(t_a, t_b))}$.
5. Randomly select a topic t_{in} from L_3 to be swapped in according to the adjacency possibilities. Then $L_1 = L_1 + [t_{in}]$ and $L_3 = L_3 - [t_{in}]$. The possibility of each topic in L_3 being chosen is $P_{in}(t) = \frac{\sum_{t_a \in L_2}(P_{adj}(t_a, t))}{\sum_{t_a \in L_2, t_b \in L_3}(P_{adj}(t_a, t_b))}$.
6. Empty L_2 and go to step 1 until the end of the conversation.

---

4 Evaluation

Twenty participants were invited to interact with our proposed system with TSM implemented and with a baseline version without TSM implemented as a comparison. Participants were asked to start a conversation on a specific topic and stop when they thought the topic switch made by the DM was not sensible. As performance measure we counted the number of user turns before they stopped. Table 1 demonstrates the performance comparisons between both sys-

Table 1. Performance comparison between systems.

	System	Weather	Work	Christmas	Other	Total	TS/NTS
Mean	TS	3.7	4.05	5.45	4.15	17.35	2.17
	NTS	1.8	2.15	1.8	2.25	8	
SD	TS	2.03	1.76	3.89	3.73	8.14	3.55
	NTS	0.95	1.04	1.06	1.55	2.29	
Min	TS	1	2	1	1	11	1.10
	NTS	2	2	1	2	10	
Max	TS	6	8	17	12	39	3.90
	NTS	1	1	2	2	10	

tems, giving mean, standard deviation, min and max number of turns interacted with either system for the different topics. The last column shows the relative increase in interaction time, measured as the number of turns interacting with Topic Switch (TS) divided by the number of turns with No Topic Switch (NTS).

Table 1 shows that people always communicated longer with the TS model, and on average people interacted 2.17 times longer with TS. Additionally, the performance of TS partially depended on the discussed topic. NTS on the other hand had about the same performance for all specified topics.

5   Discussion

The results indicate that the system with TSM could make a more sensible response which was either staying on the current topic or switched to another related topic. Moreover, the system TS had slightly different performance on different topics. The main reason should be the DM had better knowledge of some topics than that of others because the knowledge it learned from real conversations cannot cover all topics. However, unreasonable topic switches may still occur in the TS system for various reasons, including multiple meanings of an individual word, unfamiliar topics and inaccurate topic extractions. Another drawback of our current implementation is that topics are a flat structure - there is no hierarchy or ontology. This means that choices about the grouping of topics had to be made. For example, 'sunny' is part of the topic 'weather', but an alternative choice would have been splitting that topic into 'good weather' and 'bad weather', or constructing a hierarchy.

Acknowledgement. The work by A. Chowanda and M. Valstar is partly funded by European Union's Horizon 2020 research and innovation programme under grant agreement No 645378, ARIA-VALUSPA.

References

1. Allen, J.F., Perrault, C.R.: Analyzing intention in utterances. Artif. Intell. **15**(3), 143–178 (1980)
2. Bringert, B.: Programming language techniques for natural language applications. Department of Computer Science and Engineering (2008)
3. Chowanda, A., Blanchfield, P., Flintham, M., Valstar, M.: ERiSA: building emotionally realistic social game-agents companions. In: Bickmore, T., Marsella, S., Sidner, C. (eds.) IVA 2014. LNCS, vol. 8637, pp. 134–143. Springer, Heidelberg (2014). doi:10.1007/978-3-319-09767-1_16
4. Chowanda, A., Flintham, M., Blanchfield, P., Valstar, M.: Playing with social and emotional game companions. In: Traum, D., et al. (eds.) IVA 2016. LNCS, vol. 10011, pp. 85–95. Springer, Heidelberg (2016)
5. McKeown, G., Valstar, M.F., Cowie, R., Pantic, M., Schröder, M.: The semaine database: annotated multimodal records of emotionally coloured conversations between a person and a limited agent. Trans. Affect. Comput. **3**(1), 5–17 (2012)
6. Nooraei, B., Rich, C., Sidner, C.L.: A real-time architecture for embodied conversational agents: beyond turn-taking. In: ACHI 2014, pp. 381–388 (2014)

7. Traum, D.R., Larsson, S.: The information state approach to dialogue management. In: van Kuppevelt, J., Smith, R.W. (eds.) Current and New Directions in Discourse and Dialogue, vol. 22, pp. 325–353. Springer, Heidelberg (2003)

Physical vs. Virtual Agent Embodiment and Effects on Social Interaction

Sam Thellman, Annika Silvervarg, Agneta Gulz, and Tom Ziemke[✉]

Department of Computer and Information Science, Linköping University, Linköping, Sweden
{sam.thellman,annika.silvervarg,agneta.gulz,tom.ziemke}@liu.se

Abstract. Previous work indicates that physical robots elicit more favorable social responses than virtual agents. These effects have been attributed to the physical embodiment. However, a recent meta-analysis by Li [1] suggests that the benefits of robots are due to physical presence rather than physical embodiment. To further explore the importance of presence we conducted a pilot study investigating the relationship between physical and social presence. The results suggest that social presence of an artificial agent is important for interaction with people, and that the extent to which it is perceived as socially present might be unaffected by whether it is physically or virtually present.

Keywords: Embodiment · Physical presence · Social presence · Social influence · Social robots · Virtual agents

1 Introduction

Experimental work comparing social robots with virtual agents has shown that robots typically elicit more favorable social responses than virtual agents. A recently published meta-analysis by Li [1], based on 62 statistically significant differences between physical and virtual agents observed in 33 experimental works, found that in 73 % of cases physical robots were found to achieve more positive results, in 21 % virtual agents worked better, and 6 % of the results involved crossover interaction effects that varied depending on participant age, task type, and presence of robot gestures. Hence, the overall outcome of Li's meta-analysis is that robots in general—or on average—are more effective than virtual agents in social interaction contexts. Furthermore, Li concluded that the benefits of robots are due to their physical presence, i.e. their co-location with users, rather than their physical embodiment/bodies.

To further explore the importance of physical presence to social interaction we investigated the relationship between physical and social presence. There is evidence that social presence, defined by Lee [2, p. 41] as "the experience of artificial objects as social actors that manifest humanness", is an important factor in social interaction (e.g. [3, 4]). The relationship between physical and social presence is highly relevant to the design of artificial agents, in particular to the choice of whether to implement a robotic or virtual agent for the purpose of social interaction. We therefore conducted a pilot study based on the conjecture that (H1) a physically present agent will elicit a higher level of perceived social presence compared to a virtually present agent.

D. Traum et al. (Eds.): IVA 2016, LNAI 10011, pp. 412–415, 2016.
DOI: 10.1007/978-3-319-47665-0_44

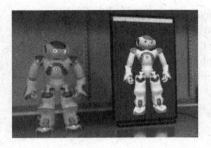
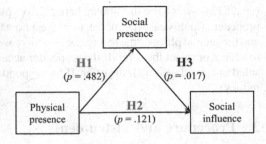

Fig. 1. Left: physical Nao robot, produced by Aldebaran Robotics, and its virtual counterpart. Right: summary of statistical results (supporting H3, but not H1 and H2; details below).

Moreover, we investigated whether Li's finding regarding the benefits of physically over virtually present agents held true in the case of two specific agents—a physical robot and a virtual robot. Since it is not possible to measure all qualities associated with satisfactory social interaction skills in a single study, we approached the question of what characterizes successful social interaction with a focus on the importance of social influence to successful interaction. Based on Li's findings, and the notion that successful social interaction skills are characterized by the ability to influence the behavior of others, we conjectured that (H2) a physically present agent will have higher social influence than a virtually present agent.

Finally, we tested the hypothesis that (H3) an artificial agent which is perceived as highly socially present will have a higher social influence, regardless of its physical or virtual presence. The purpose of testing this hypothesis was to determine whether social presence is an important factor to successful social interaction in the context of the specific types of interactions that took place in the study.

2 Our Study

Participants (an opportunity sample of 60 university students, mostly computer science; 40 males, 20 females; median age 23) were randomly assigned to interact with either a physical or a virtual Nao robot (Fig. 1) in an in-between group experiment (i.e. every subject only encountered one type of agent).

We employed the ultimatum game (UG) experimental paradigm to assess the effect of physical presence (i.e., physical versus virtual robot) on the social presence (H1) and social influence (H2) of the agent, as well as the effect of the social presence of the agent on its social influence (H3). UG is used to study bargaining behavior in the field of experimental economics [5] and has also been used in human-robot interaction studies (e.g. [6]). It can be used to measure social influence based on the assumption that the extent to which others are willing to accept an offer made by an individual is a reliable indicator of the degree of social influence of that individual, relative to the social influence of other individuals making the same offer. We used a one-shot variant of the UG where the human participant responded to a single offer proposed by the robot. The rules of the game were as follows. A sum of money—in our case the amount of 100 SEK (apx. \$12)—was to be distributed between two players. It was up to the first player, "the proposer" (in this case the robot), to suggest how to divide the sum between the proposer and the second player, "the responder" (in this case the human). It was up to the responder to accept or reject the offer. If the responder accepted the offer, both would be compensated in accordance with the offer. If the responder declined, neither would receive any money.

3   Procedure and Instruments

Prior to the experiment each participant was informed about the procedure, treatment of experimental data, their rights as participants, and that they could receive economic compensation depending on actions taken in the experiment. Participants gave written consent. They were then instructed to sit facing the robot, and the interaction session was started. After explaining the rules to the participant, the robot gave an offer of 20 SEK (apx. \$2.3) and instructed the participant to press the green or the red button on a device placed before them to accept or reject the offer. After the session, participants were asked to fill out a questionnaire measuring social presence, adopted from [7] (translated to Swedish); the scale consisted of eight questions and had a high level of internal consistency, as determined by a Chronbach's α of .895. Finally, participants that had accepted the offer were compensated.

4   Results

A Mann-Whitney U test (suitable for ordinal numerical data) was run to assess the hypothesis that a physically present agent will elicit a higher level of perceived social presence than a virtually present agent (H1). Median social presence scores for physical vs. virtual conditions (mean rank = 28.9 vs. 32.1) were not found to be statistically different ($U = 498$, $z = .703$, $p = .482$). This result did not support H1.

A chi-square test for association was conducted between agent condition and participants' decision to accept or reject the robot's offer to assess the hypothesis that a physically present agent will be more socially influential than a virtually present agent (H2). Participant responses between agent conditions (13 vs. 19 accepts out of 30 possible for physical and virtual conditions respectively) were not statistically different $\chi^2(1) = 2.41$, $p = .121$. This result did not support H2.

A second Mann-Whitney U test was run to assess H3. The median social presence score was statistically significantly higher for participants accepting the offer (6.69) than for those rejecting it (5.94), $U = 610$, $z = 2.395$, $p = .017$. This result supported H3: participants experiencing the robot as a highly social actor were more inclined to accept the offer, suggesting that social presence is important to social interaction.

The results are summarized in Fig. 1 (right): physical versus virtual presence had no statistically significant effect on either social presence (H1) or social influence (H2), but social presence had a statistically significant effect on social influence (H3).

5   Discussion and Conclusion

The result from testing H3 indicates that the social presence of an artificial agent is significant to its ability to successfully interact with others, at least in the context of the types of interaction featured in this study. From testing H1 and H2, we saw, contrary to our expectations, that our physically present agent was not perceived as more socially present than its virtually present counterpart, nor did it give rise to more favorable social responses. This suggests that physical presence and social presence might be independent from each other, i.e. the extent to which an agent is experienced as a "social actor that manifest humanness" [2, p. 41] might be unaffected by the choice of physical or virtual embodiment.

It should be noted that the pilot study presented here featured a domain-specific and relatively short participant task (one-shot UG), and robot behavior which included little speech and autonomy and no gestures. Whether the same effects will arise in other interaction scenarios is a topic for future research. Moreover, according to Li [1], comparisons between co-present robots and virtual agents—such as this study—risk conflating two possibly distinct aspects of physical and virtual embodiment: the physicality of their embodiment, defined by Li as "the physical or digital state of an agent independent of how it is displayed to a user" and the physicality of their presence, i.e. "being either 'physically displayed' … [or] 'digitally displayed'" [1, p. 25]. Li argues that the relevant comparison for the purposes of investigating effects of physical presence is that between a co- and tele-present (i.e., physically embodied but virtually present) robot. Future research should explore the relationship between physical and social presence and whether similar effects arise in other interaction scenarios, specifically in comparisons between co- and tele-present robots.

References

1. Li, J.: The benefit of being physically present: a survey of experimental works comparing copresent robots, telepresent robots and virtual agents. Int. J. Hum-Comp. St. **77**, 23–37 (2015)
2. Lee, K.M.: Presence, Explicated. Commun. Theor. **14**(1), 27–50 (2004)
3. Pereira, A., Martinho, C., Leite, I., Paiva, A.: iCat, the chess player: the influence of embodiment in the enjoyment of a game. In: 7th International Conference on Autonomous. Agents and Multiagent System, IFAAMAS, pp. 1253–1256 (2008)
4. Kennedy, J., Baxter, P., Belpaeme, T.: Comparing Robot Embodiments in a Guided Discovery Learning Interaction with Children. Int. J. Soc. Rob. **7**(2), 293–308 (2015)
5. Güth, W., Schmittberger, R., Schwarze, B.: An experimental analysis of ultimatum bargaining. J. Econ. Beh. Org. **3**(4), 367–388 (1982)
6. Nitsch, V., Glassen, T.: Investigating the effects of robot behavior and attitude toward technology on social human-robot interactions. In: IEEE RO-MAN, pp. 535–540 (2015)
7. Lee, K.M., Jung, Y., Kim, J., Kim, S.R.: Are physically embodied social agents better than disembodied social agents? The effects of physical embodiment, tactile interaction, and people's loneliness in human-robot interaction. Int. J. Hum-Comp. St. **64**(10), 962–973 (2006)

Acceptability of Embodied Conversational Agent in a Health Care Context

Jean-Arthur Micoulaud-Franchi[1,2,3], Patricia Sagaspe[1,2,3], Etienne de Sevin[1,2],
Stéphanie Bioulac[1,2,3], Alain Sauteraud[1,2], and Pierre Philip[1,2,3(✉)]

[1] Universiy of Bordeaux, SANPSY, USR 3413, 33000 Bordeaux, France
[2] CNRS, SANPSY, USR 3413, 33000 Bordeaux, France
`docteur.sauteraud@hotmail.com`, `pr.philip@free.fr`
[3] Clinique du Sommeil, CHU de Bordeaux, Service d'Explorations Fonctionnelles du Système
Nerveux, CHU de Bordeaux, 33000 Bordeaux, France
`{jean-arthur.micoulaud-franchi,patricia.sagaspe,`
`etienne.de-sevin,stephanie.bioulac,`
`pierre.philip}@chu-bordeaux.fr`

Abstract. While the interest of Embodied Conversational Agents (ECA) in health care context increased, the extent to which patients find ECAs acceptable should be more evaluated. Thus, in this study, we evaluated the acceptability of an ECA who conducts a clinical structured interview to make a medical diagnosis, in comparison with the same clinical structured interview presented in written form on a tablet screen. 178 patients participated to the study (102 females (57.3 %); Mean age = 46.5 years ± 12.9, range 19–64; Mean educational level = 13.3 years ± 3.1). It was showed that patients perceived globally the acceptability of the ECA higher than the tablet. This higher acceptability was linked rather to higher satisfaction than to higher usability. Moreover, the patients were more satisfied when they repeated the clinical interview with the ECA than with the tablet. Thus ECA usage could avoid the decrease of satisfaction of repeated computerized clinical interviews.

Keywords: E-Health · Embodied Conversational Agent (ECA) · Acceptability · Satisfaction · Usability · Questionnaire · Diagnosis

1 Introduction

Patient-reported acceptability for health technology has gained increasing attention in health care context. E-health systems are becoming the most important technology of health care organization [1]. Among E-health systems, Embodied Conversational Agents (ECAs) could enable to increase the quality of human-machine interactions that is of paramount importance to promote the use of E-health systems by the patients [2, 3]. ECAs combine verbal, facial and gestural expressions in order to conduct a face-to-face interview. ECA have a positive effect on the user's perception of a computer-based interaction task, well-known as the "persona effect" [4]. This effect was principally evaluated in healthy subject. Indeed, the extent to which patients in a health care context find ECAs acceptable and interaction with ECAs satisfying remain under evaluated [5].

© Springer International Publishing AG 2016
D. Traum et al. (Eds.): IVA 2016, LNAI 10011, pp. 416–419, 2016.
DOI: 10.1007/978-3-319-47665-0_45

Thus, the originality of this study is to evaluate the acceptability of an ECA performing a clinical structured interview in comparison with the same clinical structured interview presented in written form on a tablet screen.

2 Method

2.1 Population

Outpatients were recruited by psychiatrists in the Sleep Clinic of Bordeaux University Hospital from November 2014 to June 2015 in a consecutive sample design. All participants provided written informed consent and the study was approved by the local ethical committee. The study was classified as a clinical trial by the US National Institutes of Health (ClinicalTrials.gov identifier: NCT02544295, date of registration: September 3, 2015). This project was supported by the grant EQUIPEX PHENOVIRT ANR-10-EQPX-12-01.

2.2 The Computerized Clinical Interviews

A clinical structured interview script was designed with a sequence of questions based on Diagnostic and Statistical Manual of Mental Disorders-5 criteria. The aim was to diagnose Major Depression Disorder. Fluency of the questions was optimized with iterative processes. For each question the patients had to respond by yes or no. The script of the computerized clinical interview was implemented in two different digital tools: one by an Embodied Conversational Agent (ECA), the other in written form on a tablet screen. The ECA was adapted from previously developed software designed to self-conduct interactive face-to-face clinical interviews [2]. The ECA face-to-face interview can be seen in http://www.sanpsy.univ-bordeauxsegalen.fr/Papers/IVA_Additional_Material.html. The tablet screen was designed to self-conduct the same set of questions than the ECA.

2.3 Evaluation of the Acceptability

Patients completed the two computerized clinical interviews in a randomized order. Few minutes separated the interviews. After the structured interview by the ECA and on the tablet screen, acceptability of each digital tool was evaluated by the patient with the French version of the Acceptability E-Scale (AES) [5]. The French version of the AES explored two factors that refer to the Technology Acceptance Model (TAM) [5]. Items: 3, 4 and 6 of the AES evaluated the "satisfaction", and items 1, 2 and 5 of the AES evaluated the "usability" [5].

3 Data Analysis

The outcome variables for the AES scale included: Acceptability total score, Usability sub-score, Satisfaction sub-score.

Acceptability total score variable was analyzed with a two-way ANOVA with the repeated factor "digital tool" (Embodied Conversational Agent vs. Tablet) and the between subject-factor "order" (order ECA-Tab vs. Tab-ECA). Usability-Satisfaction sub-scores variables were analyzed with a three-way ANOVA with the repeated factors "Acceptability sub-score" (Usability vs. Satisfaction) and "digital tool" (Embodied Conversational Agent vs. Tablet), and the between subject-factor "order" (order ECA-Tab vs. Tab-ECA). Alpha criterion was set at P = .05. Statistica® (StatSoft Inc. 2010) was used.

4 Results

4.1 Population

Out of 209 patients, the data of 178 was available for analyses (102 females (57.3 %); mean age = 46.5 years ± 12.9; mean educational level = 13.3 years ± 3.1).

4.2 Acceptability Total Score

The main effect "digital tool" reaches significance for the Acceptability total score $[F(1,176) = 5.228, P < .05]$. The main effect "order" does not yield significance $[F(1,176) = 0.487, NS]$. The factor "digital tool" significantly interacts with the factor "order" $[F(1,176) = 13.944, P < .001]$.

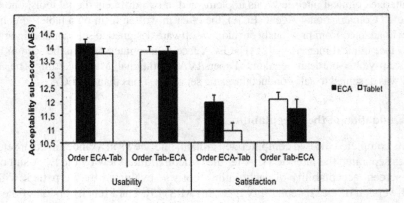

Fig. 1. Usability and satisfaction sub-scores on AES scale for the ECA and the tablet in function of the order of presentation (Embodied Conversational Agent in first order: order ECA-Tab; embodied conversational agent in second order: order Tab-ECA).

4.3 Usability-Satisfaction Sub-scores

The main effect "digital tool" reaches significance for the Acceptability sub-scores $[F(1,176) = 5.228, P < .05]$. The main effect "Acceptability sub-score" reaches significance $[F(1,176) = 151.50, P < .001]$. The main effect "order" does not reach significance

[F(1,176) = 0.487, NS]. The factor "digital tool" significantly interacts with the factor "order" [F(1,176) = 13.944, P < .001]. The factor "digital tool" significantly interacts with the factor "order" and "acceptability sub-score" [F(1,176) = 8.463, P < .01] with an absence of decrease in the Satisfaction score for the ECA when it is presented after the tablet (Fig. 1). Stable usability scores are observed whatever digital tool and order.

5 Discussion

This study shows, in a health care context, that patients who complete the same clinical structured interview script implemented in two different digital tools perceive globally the acceptability of the ECA higher than the tablet. This higher acceptability is related rather to higher satisfaction than to higher usability. However, this result is modulated by the order of presentation, as this effect is driven by a decrease of satisfaction when the Tablet was completed after the ECA. Indeed, this study shows that the repeated clinical structured interview is perceived less acceptable when the tablet screen is used to repeat the interview. The patient reports higher satisfaction when they repeat the clinical interview with the ECA than with the tablet.

This study confirms that ECA increases the patient-reported acceptability for health technology in health care context [4, 6]. Thus ECA could be largely used to collect medical information in order to optimize health care organization.

References

1. Chouvarda, I.G., Goulis, D.G., Lambrinoudaki, I., Maglaveras, N.: Connected health and integrated care: toward new models for chronic disease management. Maturitas **82**(1), 22–27 (2015)
2. Philip, P., Bioulac, S., Sauteraud, A., Chaufton, C., Olive, J.: Could a virtual human be used to explore excessive daytime sleepiness in patients? Presence: Teleoperators Virtual Environ. **23**(4), 369–376 (2014)
3. Cassell, J., Sullivan, J., Prevost, S., Churchill, E.: Embodied Conversational Agents. MIT Press, Cambridge (2000)
4. Prendinger, H., Mayer, S., Mori, J., Ishizuka, M.: Persona effect revisited. In: Rist, T., Aylett, R.S., Ballin, D., Rickel, J. (eds.) IVA 2003. LNCS (LNAI), vol. 2792, pp. 283–291. Springer, Heidelberg (2003). doi:10.1007/978-3-540-39396-2_48
5. Micoulaud-Franchi, J.A., Sauteraud, A., Olive, J., Sagaspe, P., Bioulac, S., Philip, P.: Validation of the French version of the acceptability e-scale (AES) for mental e-health systems. Psychiatry Res. **237**, 196–200 (2016)
6. Rizzo, A., Lange, B., Buckwalter, J., Forbell, E., Kim, J., Sagae, K., et al.: SimCoach: an intelligent virtual human system for providing healthcare information and support. Int. J. Disabil. Hum. Dev. **10**(4), 277–281 (2011)

How Students Perceive the Gender and Personality of a Visually Androgynous Agent

Annika Silvervarg[✉]

Department of Computer and Information Science, Linköping University, Linköping, Sweden
annika.silvervarg@liu.se

Abstract. This paper explores how students perceive the gender of a visually androgynous teachable agent, and if and how the perceived gender relates to the perceived personality traits of the agent. It is shown that the students' perception of the agent's gender was independent of their own gender. There were few significant differences in the perceived personality traits in relation to perceived gender. However, when looking at the perceived degree of gender, the traits of the agent were more positively rated by those students who perceived it as moderately gendered as compared to androgynous or strongly gendered.

Keywords: Visual gender · Personality trait · Androgynous · Teachable agent

1 Introduction

The gender of a virtual agent is an important design factor as it can affect attitude, behaviour and outcomes of interaction with such an agent. Using stereotypically female or male agents can positively affect the trustworthiness of the agent, the user's belief in his or her own competence, and/or the attitude towards the agent. On the other hand it can reinforce negative stereotypes and behaviour, for example stereotypical female agents are more prone to be subjected to abusive conversation [1, 2].

Virtual pedagogical agents is a domain where gendered agents can provide good role models, and female students have been shown to increase self-efficacy and attitude in mathematics [3] and engineering [4] as a result of interacting with female agents. However, the same study [4] that showed that a more peer-like (young, female, attractive) agent positively influenced female students' self-efficacy and willingness to enter technical education, also showed that the agent reinforced negative stereotypes, along the line of the non-typical female agent being an exception from the "typical male competent engineer" and "if she is able to do it, I can do it!".

An attempt to retain the positive effects of gendered agents but diminish the drawbacks of gender stereotypes is to use agents with more neutral or androgynous appearances. For instance, a study [5] showed that a more gender neutral agent evoked more positive attitudes on females than did a more stereotypical female agent. Our own previous studies [6] have shown that to perceive an agent as androgynous-looking does not mean that one does not assign a gender to the agent, and that regardless of gender, students showed a significant preference for the androgynous agent over the gendered (female and male) agents. Based on these findings we chose to use an androgynous agent when we designed a new

© Springer International Publishing AG 2016
D. Traum et al. (Eds.): IVA 2016, LNAI 10011, pp. 420–423, 2016.
DOI: 10.1007/978-3-319-47665-0_46

virtual learning environment. When tested in a pilot study we found that when the agent was perceived as a boy the students described it with more positive words compared to when it was perceived as a girl [7]. Building on this we have conducted a study to explore: "What gender do the students perceive the agent to have, and does this differ depending on the student's own gender?" and "Do the perceived personality traits of the agent differ depending on the perceived gender and/or the gender of the students?"

2   Study

"The Guardian of History" is an educational software for history for ages 10–12 years. The narrative centres on securing a successor to the Guardian of History (Fig. 1). The student takes on a teacher role and his/her task is to teach a time elf (Fig. 1), i.e., a teachable agent (TA), about history so that the time elf can qualify as successor.

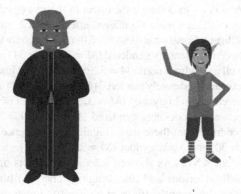

Fig. 1. To the left the guardian of history and to the right the time elf Timy

A total of 161 (81 females and 80 males) 10–12-year olds from five classes in a Swedish school participated in the study. The students used the educational software and interacted with their agents during four hour-long lessons. At the end of the final session, they were given a questionnaire regarding their experience with the digital learning environment and how they perceived the time elf (their TA). 151 students filled out this questionnaire, but unfortunately identification on several of them were missing and therefore only 89 questionnaires could be linked to information of the students' gender. Analysis has therefore been conducted on two different datasets with N = 151 and N = 89 depending on the research question and type of analysis performed.

2.1   Results - Perceived Gender of Agent

A Chi square test showed that there was no significant difference between the distribution of perceived agent gender in relation to the student gender ($X^2(4) = 1.199$, p = .878). 8 % perceived the agent as absolutely a girl, 20 % as a little like a girl, 42 % as neither a girl nor a boy, 18 % as a little like a boy, and 12 % (16 % of female students and 9 % of male students) as absolutely a boy.

2.2 Results - Perceived Agent Personality Traits

To answer the first part of the question "Do the perceived personality traits of the agent differ depending on the perceived gender and/or the gender of the students?" one-way independent ANOVAs were performed to compare the effect of perceived gender of the agent on perceived personality traits. There were significant effects of gender on the traits Friendly, $F(4, 146) = 2.632, p = .037$, and Encouraging, $F(4, 146) = 5.116, p = .001$, but not for Attitude, Self-confident, Curious, Memory or Intelligent.

Many of the analyses showed a pattern where "a little like a girl/boy" were perceived more positively than "absolutely like a girl/boy" and "neither girl nor boy". This is consistent with previous research that showed that less stereotypically gendered characters were preferred to a more stereotypical [5]. Therefore a new encoding of the agent's perceived gender was introduced with "Androgynous" (neither boy nor girl), "Moderately gendered" (a little like a boy/girl) and "Strongly gendered" (absolutely like a girl/boy). This encoding was used to perform one-way independent ANOVAs to compare the effect of the perceived degree of gender on perceived personality traits. There were significant effects on the traits Friendly, Encouraging, Memory and Intelligent. Post-hoc tests showed that for Friendly there was a significant difference ($p < .05$) between Moderately gendered ($M = 70, SD = 31$) and Strongly gendered ($M = 50, SD = 39$) as well as Androgynous ($M = 52, SD = 37$). For Encouraging there was a significant difference between Moderately gendered ($M = 49, SD = 31$) and Strongly gendered ($M = 27, SD = 24$) as well as Androgynous ($M = 32, SD = 27$). For Memory there was a significant difference between Moderately gendered ($M = 35, SD = 30$) and Androgynous ($M = 21, SD = 25$). For Intelligent there was a significant difference between Moderately gendered ($M = 38, SD = 30$) and Androgynous ($M = 25, SD = 27$).

Two-way independent ANOVAs showed interaction effects of student gender and agent gender for Friendly, Curious and Encouraging. The post-hoc tests revealed that the male students rated the agent's traits significantly lower when the agent was perceived as "absolutely a boy" than the female students, see Table 1. It should be noted that although significant the differences are due to very small groups of students since few perceived the agent as absolutely a boy. When repeating the analysis for degree of perceived gender, the same differences were found for Strongly gendered, with also significant differences for Intelligent and Curious.

Table 1. Mean and standard deviation, M (SD), for perceived personality traits for female and male students when agent is perceived as "absolutely a boy"

	Friendly	Curious	Encouraging	Intelligent
Female students (N = 7)	73 (19)	68 (9)	45 (5)	35 (17)
Male students (N = 4)	8 (13)	18 (21)	3 (3)	3 (2)
P	.004	.02	.016	.059

3   Discussion

Our study revealed no differences between female and male students in regard to the perceived agent gender, most saw it as androgynous or moderately gendered. These results were interesting as previous studies have shown that "similarity attracts", in for example [3] 80 % of the female students chose a female agent over a male agent. But the results also confirm our previous findings that students accept androgynous agent and sometimes prefer them to gendered agents [6]. In this case the narrative also lends credibility to a character being androgynous since it is humanlike but still fictional.

Agents that were perceived as moderately gendered, i.e. a little like a boy or girl, where also seen as more intelligent, with a better memory, more encouraging and more friendly. This is in line with previous research [5] but with the difference that in this instance the visual appearance is the same for all agents, and it is only the student's own perception or attribution of gender to the agent that differ. A result contradicting earlier findings [7] was that male students rated the agent perceived as absolutely like a boy very near the negative extremes, e.g. unfriendly, stupid, and complaining.

An interesting avenue to explore further is what guides the students' attribution of gender to the agent. Is it a conscious decision, is it done quickly, i.e. a first impression, or as a result of the interaction between student and agent? Since a teachable agent is more of a peer than an expert what role does identification and/or role modelling have? A teachable agent will reflect how well the student has taught it, and a low achieving student will have an agent lacking in knowledge and ability. In that case attributing it another gender than one self and not identifying with it can be a way to bolster one's own ego. It would therefore be interesting to look more into aspects such as if the students' self-efficacy and the agent's achievement level influence the perceived gender of the agent.

References

1. De Angeli, A., Brahnam, S.: Sex stereotypes and conversational agents. In: Proceedings of the Workshop on Gender and Interaction – Real and Virtual Women in a Male World, 8th International Conference on Advanced Visual Interfaces (2006)
2. Veletsianos, G., Scharber, C., Doering, A.: When sex, drugs, and violence enter the classroom: conversations between adolescent social studies students and a female pedagogical agent. Interact. Comput. 20(3), 292–301 (2008)
3. Kim, Y., Wei, Q., Xu, B., Ko, Y., Ilieva, V.: MathGirls: toward developing girls' positive attitudes and self-efficacy through pedagogical agents. In: Proceedings of the 2007 Conference on Artificial Intelligence in Education, Los Angeles, CA, pp. 119–126 (2007)
4. Baylor, A., Plant, E.: Pedagogical agents as social models for engineering: the influence of agent appearance on female choice. In: Proceedings of the 12th International Conference on Artificial Intelligence in Education, Amsterdam, The Netherlands, pp. 65–72 (2005)
5. Gulz, A., Haake, M.: Challenging gender stereotypes using virtual pedagogical characters. In: Goodman, S., Booth, S., Kirkup, G. (eds.) Gender Issues in Learning and Working with IT: Social Constructs and Cultural Contexts, pp. 113–132. IGI Global, Hershey (2010)
6. Silvervarg, A., Haake, M., Gulz, A.: Educational potentials in visually androgynous pedagogical agents. In: Lane, H.C., Yacef, K., Mostow, J., Pavlik, P. (eds.) AIED 2013. LNCS (LNAI), vol. 7926, pp. 599–602. Springer, Heidelberg (2013). doi:10.1007/978-3-642-39112-5_68
7. Kirkegaard, C., Tärning, B., Haake, M., Gulz, A., Silvervarg, A.: Ascribed gender and characteristics of a visually androgynous teachable agent. In: Bickmore, T., Marsella, S., Sidner, C. (eds.) IVA 2014. LNCS (LNAI), vol. 8637, pp. 232–235. Springer, Heidelberg (2014). doi:10.1007/978-3-319-09767-1_29

Towards Personal Assistants
that Can Help Users Plan

Peng Yu[1(✉)], Jiaying Shen[2], Peter Z. Yeh[2], and Brian Williams[1]

[1] CSAIL, MIT, Cambridge, MA 02139, USA
{yupeng,williams}@mit.edu
[2] NL & AI Lab, Nuance Communications Inc., Sunnyvale, CA 95054, USA
{Jiaying.Shen,Peter.Yeh}@nuance.com

Abstract. In this paper, we present an intelligent personal assistant, called Uhura, that handles requests involving multiple, interrelated goals and activities by efficiently producing a coherent plan. Uhura achieves this by integrating a collaborative dialog manager, a conflict-directed planner with spatial and temporal reasoning capabilities, and a large-scale knowledge graph. We also present a user survey that assesses the usefulness of the plans produced by Uhura in urban travel planning.

1 Introduction

People are now using intelligent personal assistants for many day-to-day tasks, and many of which assistants support both verbal and visual communications to make the interaction simpler. However, their functions are limited to simple commands and information retrieval tasks, and none of them can understand user requests involving multiple goals and activities. For example, [8] reports an end-to-end personal assistant framework, but their work is focused on proactivity and task management. [7] report end-to-end personal assistants for TV program discovery, but these assistants are unable to plan.

In contrast, our goal is to develop a personal assistant, called Uhura, that supports complex user requests that require planning. Uhura can also consider semantic constraints, which occur frequently in many day to day scenarios. It achieves these benefits by uniquely utilizing three distinct components: Knowledge Base, Planner, and Collaborative Dialog Manager (CDM). First, Uhura uses a knowledge base that provides the data necessary (e.g., road condition, restaurants, movies, etc.) to formulate candidate plans that meet the users' semantic, temporal and spatial constraints. Second, Uhura integrates a dialog manager and a knowledge base with a planner that supports temporal and spatial reasoning, similar to the ones used in tourist assistant systems [6]. This allows Uhura to support semantic constraints as well as temporal and spatial ones. In addition, if there are competing requirements, the Planner will propose relaxations for them, and negotiate with the user until a resolution is reached. Finally, Uhura uses a dialog manager to: (1) serve as a mediator between the planner and knowledge base; (2) maintain the context of the interaction with the users along with their goals; (3) communicate with the users in a natural way.

© Springer International Publishing AG 2016
D. Traum et al. (Eds.): IVA 2016, LNAI 10011, pp. 424–428, 2016.
DOI: 10.1007/978-3-319-47665-0_47

2   Approach

Uhura provides the following features to simplify the planning process for the users: (1) natural language communication; (2) mixed initiative goal-directed interaction; (3) supports for multiple tasks and constraints; and (4) being robust to temporal uncertainty and over-subscription. They are supported by a coordinated system of three major components (Fig. 1): Collaborative Dialog Manager (CDM), Planner and Knowledge Base. CDM handles the interactions with users, and elicits their goals and requirements as a *Qualitative State Plan* (QSP). It also takes the users' semantic, temporal and spatial constraints, and formulates them into queries for the Knowledge Base. The results of these queries ground the tasks in the QSP with additional episodes and constraints. Finally, the expanded QSP is sent to the Planner, which evaluates the alternatives of each task and produces plans that best meet the users' requirements.

The three components have different responsibilities, and *speak* very different languages. The key to an effective integration is to **disintegrate** the overall problems properly, assign the subproblem to the component that has the right reasoning capability, and supply them with the right set of data. Inside Uhura, CDM is responsible for interacting with the users and capturing their planning problems. It creates and assigns subproblems that require temporal and spatial reasoning to the Planner, and subproblems that require semantic reasoning to the Knowledge Base. The output from CDM is a set of first order logic expressions encoded in a semantic graph, while the input to the planner is a set of goals and requirements encoded as a Qualitative State Plan. A mapping is created between them such that (1) each task's temporal and spatial requirements can be extracted from the semantic graph and encoded in the QSP; and (2) the choices and relaxations in the Planner's output can be mapped back to the nodes in the semantic graph, such that CDM can present them to the user. For example, Fig. 2 shows such a mapping for a movie task. The mapping between the nodes in the branch and the QSP constraint is represented by the node IDs tagged to the episodes' names, locations and durations.

Collaborative Dialog Manager. CDM [3] is an extension to Disco [4], an open source dialog development framework based on Collaborative Discourse Theory [1], and Sidner's artificial language for negotiation [5]. It views a personal assistant dialogue as a process of plan augmentation, where the purpose of the dialogue is for the system and the user to collaboratively form a complete sharedPlan in order to meet the user's intention. The plan based approach of CDM puts it as the processing hub of the system, whose assembled meta task plan often includes knowledge base querying and Uhura planner invocation. On the other hand, it is also the information hub of the system, since CDM is responsible for assembling all user requests to form legitimate knowledge base queries, integrating knowledge base query results into a valid planning problem as well as interacting with the user to communicate all the information generated. In order to effectively carry out all these responsibilities, CDM uses first order logic

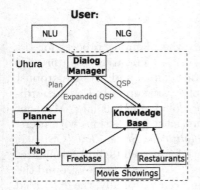

Fig. 1. The architecture graph of Uhura

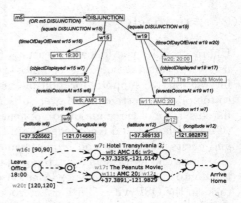

Fig. 2. The QSP generated from a semantic graph branch

(FOL) encoded as semantic graphs, such as the one in Fig. 2, to store and process the information from various sources.

Knowledge Base. Uhura uses a large-scale knowledge base to access the world knowledge, such as restaurants and movie showtimes, to properly construct a plan that satisfies the user's request. This knowledge base is constructed from a combination of open and proprietary sources of content using an ingestion pipeline [2] that transforms the raw content into RDF triples and performs entity resolution. The resulting knowledge base can be viewed as a very large knowledge graph, where the nodes represent entities and the edges represent semantic relations between these entities. The entities are typed, and a proprietary subsumption hierarchy is used to organize these types. The semantic relations have domain and range constraints, and also capture inverse relationships. Our knowledge base has over 1 billion triples, and the processing time for each query is typically less than a few hundred milliseconds.

Planner. The planner fills in the details of the abstract plan generated by CDM and Knowledge Base, schedules each activity, and adds contingencies for likely delays during transit. Uhura's planner is implemented based on a constraint relaxation algorithm, Conflict-Directed Relaxation with Uncertainty (CDRU, [9]), with extensions for propagating global constraints. CDRU was first developed to solve over-constrained conditional temporal problems with uncertain durations. The algorithm uses a conflict-directed search strategy to prune infeasible candidates and find the optimal set of choices. In addition, CDRU is able to detect competing constraints in the QSPs, generate concise explanations for the cause of failure, and suggest trade-offs for the users to resolve the issues. It takes in a QSP as input, and produces a plan, as well as temporal relaxations for some constraints if necessary.

User Survey. We conducted a user survey on the usefulness of Uhura in the context of a personal assistant for managing day-to-day tasks. There are six sessions in this survey, each presenting a different urban travel planning scenario. At the end of each session, the participants are asked to evaluate the last plan proposed by Uhura, and grade it on quality using a 5 point Likert scale for their satisfaction with it. The resulting QSPs have around 500 episodes with a dozen choices, and is usually solved within a few seconds. From the users' perspective, the delay in response is not longer than many popular routing applications.

Table 1. Average scores and next solution requests in each session (standard deviation)

Session	1	2	3	4	5	6
Quality	3.2 (1.40)	2.4 (1.43)	2.9 (1.58)	3.8 (1.54)	3.3 (1.35)	3.3 (1.42)
# of solutions	4.8 (6.14)	4.8 (4.60)	4.5 (5.30)	2.9 (2.91)	2.9 (1.97)	3.0 (5.37)

We received results from ten participants, which are summarized in Table 1. In general, participants found Uhura to be useful in planning daily tasks. The plans generated are acceptable in most situations, and the average quality score is above 3. Participants also gave feedback that Uhura simplified the otherwise complicated planning tasks. Without Uhura, planning a day trip may take minutes or even hours. With Uhura, a feasible solution can be found in seconds. On the other hand, we also discovered a few issues related to Uhura's architecture and implementation in the survey. Some participants reported that Uhura is not making good trade-offs between temporal relaxations and destinations, and it occasionally produced nonsensical plans that can be avoided by applying common sense reasoning. We believe that these are the reasons for the large variance in the quality scores, and are important issues for us to address in the future.

References

1. Grosz, B.J., Sidner, C.L.: Plans for discourse. In: Cohen, P.R., Morgan, J., Pollack, M.E. (eds.) Intentions in Communication, pp. 417–444. MIT Press, Cambridge (1990)
2. Nößner, J., Martin, D., Yeh, P.Z., Patel-Schneider, P.F.: CogMap: a cognitive support approach to property and instance alignment. In: Arenas, M., et al. (eds.) ISWC 2015. LNCS, vol. 9366, pp. 269–285. Springer, Heidelberg (2015). doi:10.1007/978-3-319-25007-6_16
3. Ortiz, C., Shen, J.: Dynamic intention structures for dialogue processing. In: Proceedings of the 18th Workshop on the Semantics and Pragmatics of Dialogue (SemDial 2014) (2014)
4. Rich, C., Sidner, C.L.: Using collaborative discourse theory to partially automate dialogue tree authoring. In: Nakano, Y., Neff, M., Paiva, A., Walker, M. (eds.) IVA 2012. LNCS, vol. 7502, pp. 327–340. Springer, Heidelberg (2012). doi:10.1007/978-3-642-33197-8_34

5. Sidner, C.: An artificial discourse language for collaborative negotiation. In: Proceedings of the Twelfth National Conference on Artificial Intelligence, pp. 814–819. MIT Press (1994)
6. Vansteenwegen, P., Souffriau, W., Berghe, G.V., Oudheusden, D.V.: The city trip planner: an expert system for tourists. Expert Syst. Appl. **38**, 6540–6546 (2011)
7. Yeh, P., Ramachandran, D., Douglas, B., Ratnaparkhi, A., Jarrold, W., Provine, R., Patel-Schneider, P., Laverty, S., Tikku, N., Brown, S., Mendel, J., Emfield, A.: An end-to-end conversational second screen application for tv program discovery. AI Mag. **36**(3), 73–89 (2015)
8. Yorke-Smith, N., Saadati, S., Myers, K., Morley, D.: The design of a proactive personal agent for task management. IJAIT **21**(1), 1250004 (2012)
9. Yu, P., Fang, C., Williams, B.: Resolving uncontrollable conditional temporal problems using continuous relaxations. In: Proceedings of the Twenty-Fourth International Conference on Automated Planning and Scheduling (ICAPS 2014) (2014)

A Parameterized Schema for Representing Complex Gesture Forms

Huaguang Song[⊠] and Michael Neff

University of California, Davis, One Shields Avenue, Davis, CA 95616, USA
{hso,mpneff}@ucdavis.edu

Abstract. Gestures can take on complex forms that convey both pragmatic and expressive information. When creating virtual agents, it is
necessary to make fine grained manipulations of these forms to precisely adjust the gesture's meaning to reflect the communicative content
an agent is trying to deliver, character mood and spatial arrangement
of the characters and objects. This paper describes a gesture schema
that affords the required, rich description of gesture form. Novel features
include the representation of multiphase gestures consisting of several
segments, repetitions of gesture form, a map of referential locations and
a rich set of spatial and orientation constraints. In our prototype implementation, gestures are generated from this representation by editing
and combining small snippets of motion captured data to meet the specification. This allows a very diverse set of gestures to be generated from
a small set of input data. Gestures can be refined by simply adjusting
the parameters of the schema.

Keywords: Virtual agent · Animation frameworks · Behavior planning · Composite gesture representation · Language · Generation

1 Introduction

Hand gestures are one of the most important components of non-verbal communication, conveying both affective and pragmatic information. They involve the
hand's path through space, its orientation, and its shape over time; the latter
defined by the angles of the finger joints. Being able to rapidly and precisely generate and edit gestures – and adapt them to the current communicative context –
is crucial.

Although the motion capture process can be done again and again to try
to get all possible data needed to perform certain tasks, it is time-consuming,
not cost-effective and will fail where the full context of a character's interactions
cannot be predicted ahead of time (i.e. in most interactive scenarios). Developing
a framework that allows character systems to reuse mocap data to generate a
communicative gesture is essential. A growing set of animation tools [4,6] rely on
gesture animation libraries. It is important to be able to generate large numbers
of such animations quickly and at low cost in order to build libraries for particular
characters and tasks.

© Springer International Publishing AG 2016
D. Traum et al. (Eds.): IVA 2016, LNAI 10011, pp. 429–432, 2016.
DOI: 10.1007/978-3-319-47665-0_48

Many gestures have quite complex form. Consider a gesture to accompany the text "You mark here, here, here and here and then draw back." That points to a series of locations and then makes a pull back motion to illustrate setting up a carpentry operation. The gesture can naturally be decomposed into a series of segments, one corresponding to each point and the pull back. If motion capture is used, new data would be needed any time the number of marks, their spacing, or the timing of the text changed. With the proper representation, we should be able to adapt such data to any of these changes. The schema presented here solves this problem.

As another motivating example, consider the manner in which people set up a referential space in front of them, locating particular ideas in particular locations. Gestures must be adapted to reflect this organization, requiring a schema that can accommodate location constraints. In other cases, it is possible to build complex gestures out of simple forms when the team did not have the foresight to anticipate a particular gesture need during a motion capture session.

This paper develops a schema for complex gesture forms, describes how the schema can be built from data with minimal user effort and shows an example implementation using this schema. In this work, complex gestures are composed of multiple segments, generally taken from a motion database, and the schema allows fine-grained, algorithmic control of the gesture form. Editing an existing schema allows new gestures to be created and these edits can either be hand specified or generated by the character control system in response to the current context.

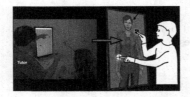

Fig. 1. Multimodal tutorial tactics for mathematics. Left: a human tutor teaches proportion. Right: a virtual agent performs the same task

One application of this parameterized schema will incorporate with our collaborative research project (see Fig. 1), where we try to replace a human tutor with an intelligent virtual agent to teach children to learn mathematics proportion on multitouch devices. As we analyze the human tutor's behavior, we know the human tutor will respond to children with a variety of interactive gesture forms to guide children to solve the problem. Since the virtual agent will perform the same task as the human tutor, these responses must be composed and performed in real time (i.e. move the hands up and down to specific location). Our representation is developed to meet this specific goal, but it is also fit in other area of where fine-grain adjustment of hand gestures is needed. To simplify the overall process, our system also support semiautomatic segmentation, which allows user mark segments position a full annotate gesture dataset to generate a segmented gesture database based on user interest. Mean while, it will automatically output the corresponding representation schema, this allows user can quick edit parameters rather then build the schema from scratch.

2   Related Work

Badler et al.'s pioneering work on the Parameterized Action Representation (PAR) sought to allow virtual agents to be controlled with natural language instructions [1–3]. It introduced a parameterized representation for actions that was based both on affordances of humanoid agents and the language constructs used to instruct them. We also develop a parameterized representation for motion, but with a more narrow focus on representing complex gesture forms rather than a general representation of actions and spatial relationships.

Kopp et al. [5] introduced the Behavior Markup Language, or BML, a high level motion behavior representation for virtual agents. Although we have a format similar to BML and its derivatives, these language do not support

Table 1. Complete representation

```
STARTTIME, ENDTIME, HANDTOUSE, GESTURESEGMENTS, [OVERALLCONSTRAINT], CONNECTIONTYPE
   GESTURESEGMENTS = segment⁺
     SEGMENT = Path, [HandMotion], [Head]
       PATH = Duration, Hold, (Data|PathType), (Touch|Point), [StartPos], Repeat
         PATHTYPE = ("Straight"|"Cyclic"|"Curved")
           STRAIGHT = EndLoc
           CURVED = EndLoc, Curvature, Longitude
           CYCLIC = ("Clockwise"|"Counterclockwise"), Curved
             CURVATURE = ("1LowCurve"|"2MidCurve"|"3HighCurve")
         TOUCH|POINT = Space, [Orientation], [Duration]]
           SPACE = [StartOffset], Frame, CoordinateLoc, Tolerance, [ApplicationZone]
             FRAME = ("World"|"Chest"|"Head")
             APPLICATIONZONE = ("Line"|"Cube"|"Sphere"|"BodyLoc")
               LINE = ("Coordinate"|Coordinate⁺)
               BODYLOC = ("Head"|"Nose"|"Lips"|"Shoulder"|"Forearm"|...etc)
           ORIENTATION = StartOffset, Duration, StartPose, EndPose
       HANDMOTION = StartOffset, Duration, Hold, Fingers
         FINGERS = StartOffset, Duration, T, I, M, R, L, (FingerMotion|FingerPose), Repeat
           T|I|M|R|L = ("True"|"False")
       HEAD = StartOffset, Duration, LookAtLoc
```

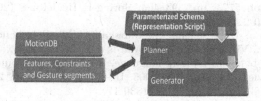

Fig. 2. Parameterized representation system architecture

fine-grained gesture editing. They are more focused on simple gesture forms and the coordination between gesture and speech.

3 Generating Schema

While schema can be authored by hand, the more common workflow is to build them from existing motion capture data. In our system, users can load motion capture data of existing complex gesture forms and interactively segment them by scrubbing through a full skeletal playback of the motion, along with gesture trails. They can click to indicate segment divisions at any point in the motion and can specify separate segmentation for the right and left hand. The system will then write out a completely formed schema that can be used to generate the given gesture, along with all the required data. Creating a family of related gestures then only requires small edits to this schema, for instance changing the number of repetitions, changing spatial constraints or changing the path of one of the components. This allows a single motion captured form to be repurposed to generate a large set of gestures that are adapted to the current physical and conversational context of the character.

Table 1 shows the complete representation of a composite gesture.

Figure 2 shows a system architecture for generating motion from our schema.

Acknowledgments. This research was supported by NSF grant IIS 1320029. We thank our collaborators Dor Abrahamson, Seth Corrigan and Virginia J. Flood, who provided insight and expertise that greatly assisted the research.

References

1. Allbeck, J., Badler, N.: Representing and parameterizing agent behaviors. In: Prendinger, H., Ishizuka, M. (eds.) Life-Like Characters. Cognitive Technologies, pp. 19–38. Springer, Heidelberg (2004)
2. Badler, N., Bindiganavale, R., Allbeck, J., Schuler, W., Zhao, L., Palmer, M.: Parameterized action representation for virtual human agents. In: Embodied Conversational Agents, pp. 256–284. MIT Press (2000)
3. Badler, N., Bindiganavale, R., Bourne, J., Palmer, M., Shi, J., Schuler, W.: A parameterized action representation for virtual human agents. In: Workshop on Embodied Conversational Characters (1998)
4. Heloir, A., Kipp, M.: EMBR – a realtime animation engine for interactive embodied agents. In: Ruttkay, Z., Kipp, M., Nijholt, A., Vilhjálmsson, H.H. (eds.) IVA 2009. LNCS, vol. 5773, pp. 393–404. Springer, Heidelberg (2009). doi:10.1007/978-3-642-04380-2_43
5. Kopp, S., Krenn, B., Marsella, S., Marshall, A.N., Pelachaud, C., Pirker, H., Thórisson, K.R., Vilhjálmsson, H.: Towards a common framework for multimodal generation: the behavior markup language. In: Gratch, J., Young, M., Aylett, R., Ballin, D., Olivier, P. (eds.) IVA 2006. LNCS, vol. 4133, pp. 205–217. Springer, Heidelberg (2006). doi:10.1007/11821830_17
6. Neff, M., Kipp, M., Albrecht, I., Seidel, H.-P.: Gesture modeling and animation based on a probabilistic re-creation of speaker style. ACM Trans. Graph. (TOG) **27**(1), 5 (2008)

Blissful Agents: Adjuncts to Group Medical Visits for Chronic Pain and Depression

Ameneh Shamekhi[1(✉)], Timothy Bickmore[1], Anna Lestoquoy[2],
Lily Negash[2], and Paula Gardiner[2]

[1] College of Computer and Information Science,
Northeastern University, Boston, MA, USA
{ameneh,bickmore}@ccs.neu.edu
[2] Department of Family Medicine,
Boston University School of Medicine, Boston, MA, USA
{anna.lestoquoy,lily.negash,paula.gardiner}@bmc.org

Abstract. In this paper we describe a conversational virtual agent that is designed to be used in conjunction with group medical visits to help treat individuals with chronic pain and depression using non-medical treatments including yoga, meditation, and self-massage. Results from two rounds of pilot testing indicate that patients like the virtual agent and find that it helps them manage their condition.

Keywords: Relational agent · Meditation · Yoga · Complementary and alternative medicine

1 Introduction

Several virtual agents have now been developed to deliver one-on-one counseling for a variety of health conditions [1]. However, an increasingly popular mode of delivery for medical and behavioral interventions for chronic health conditions is the group medical visit, also known as a "shared medical appointment". Despite the advantages of group visits, patient adherence to medical advice in-between group visits remains a problem. Recommendations for diet, exercise, and other self-care tasks are rarely followed exactly, especially over the long term. Virtual agents may be able to bridge the time between group visits by reinforcing information delivered during visits, guiding patients through self-care procedures, motivating adherence to the overall intervention, and providing a virtual source of social support.

A number of virtual agents have been developed in recent years to counsel patients on health problems in general, and chronic disease self-care, in particular [1]. Several agents have been developed specifically to help individuals manage chronic health conditions. Monkaresi, et al., developed the "IDL coach", an embodied conversational agent (ECA) that helps individuals with diabetes manage prescribed exercise, nutrition, blood glucose monitoring, and medication adherence, although no evaluation studies are reported [2]. Bickmore, et al., developed an agent to help individuals with schizophrenia to manage their condition, to increase physical activity, and to continue to take

© Springer International Publishing AG 2016
D. Traum et al. (Eds.): IVA 2016, LNAI 10011, pp. 433–437, 2016.
DOI: 10.1007/978-3-319-47665-0_49

prescribed antipsychotic medication; promising results from a quasi-experimental pilot evaluation have been reported [3]. ICT's SimCoach is an ECA that was designed to address depression and/or post-traumatic stress disorder (PTDS), although results from a large randomized controlled trial with 333 patients failed to find any clinically significant benefits of using SimCoach [4].

We developed a virtual agent that assists patients with chronic pain and depression. To evaluate this system, we conducted two pilot studies in which patients interact with the virtual agent at home, and use it to review the material covered in each visit in more detail, as well to practice self-care skills such as meditation and yoga.

2 Design of the Agent-Based Intervention for Chronic Pain

The virtual agent used in our work is animated in a 3D game engine using custom animation software, running on a dedicated-use 8″ touch screen tablet computer provided to patients. The agent is designed to appear as a racially ambiguous female in her mid-forties. The agent's nonverbal behavior is generated using BEAT [5], and includes hand gestures and eyebrow movements, as well as a range of iconic, emblematic, and deictic gestures. The agent speaks using synthetic speech, and user input is obtained via selection of utterances on the touch screen (Fig. 1).

The agent guides patients through nine weeks of new material in coordination with the group visits. Each week, following a group visit, the agent reviews the new educational material just learned (on nutrition, physical activity, pain, stress, sleep, and depression), walks patients through practice sessions (e.g. meditation and yoga), and allows them to review material covered in prior weeks.

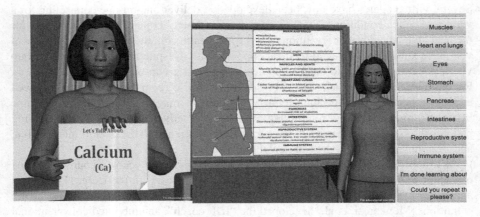

Fig. 1. Screen shots of Gabby agent and chronic pain intervention

3 Pilot Evaluation Study

We conducted two rounds of pilot testing of the virtual agent with chronic pain patients, in conjunction with medical group visits at BMC. The pilot studies allowed us to collect users' feedback on the initial system, as well as their suggestions to improve the system for the main randomized controlled trial.

Participants. Twenty patients aged 26–60 (mean 47), 75 % female, were recruited. Patients were predominantly low-income minority adults (50 % African-American, and 25 % white), and 60 % had incomes near or below the poverty level.

Measures. We assessed participants' satisfaction with and attitudes towards the agent at the end of the intervention, as well as health behavior change using six validated self-report questionnaires before and after the 9-week intervention.

Table 1. Self-report ratings of agent in pilot studies

Question	Anchor 1	Anchor 7	Agent
How satisfied were you with talking to Gabby about reducing stress?	Not at all	Very satisfied	5.9
How satisfied were you with talking to Gabby about healthy eating?	Not at all	Very satisfied	5.6
How helpful was Gabby in reducing your stress?	Not at all	Very helpful	5.6
How helpful was Gabby in improving healthy eating?	Not at all	Very helpful	5.8
How easy was it to talk to Gabby?	Very difficult	Very easy	6.2
How much do you trust Gabby?	Not at all	Very much	6.2
How well did Gabby answer any questions that you had?	Not at all	Very well	5.7
Did you feel like Gabby provided support and encouragement to reach your goals?	Not at all	Very much	6.2
Would you like to interact with Gabby again?	Not at all	Very much	5.9
How much would you have preferred talking to a doctor or nurse than to Gabby?	Definitely prefer doctor/nurse	Definitely prefer Gabby	4.2

Results. Based on analysis of log files from the tablet computers, patients spent an average total of 90 min (range 0–294, SD 80.2) interacting with the virtual agent at home over the nine weeks of the intervention.

Ratings of the agent were very high, with overall satisfaction rated 5.9 on a 1–7 scale (Table 1). Quantitative data from validated health questionnaires was collected in person at baseline, and at nine weeks (Table 2). Although these are quasi-experimental results (no control group), patients did report significant improvements in depressive symptoms, social support, stress, patient activation, and medication misuse, over the nine weeks of the intervention.

Table 2. Pre-post changes in health conditions in pilot studies (mean (SD))

Measure	Baseline (N = 20)	9-Weeks (N = 13)	p-value
Pain Self-Efficacy Questionnaire (PSEQ) [6]. A 10-item questionnaire that assesses individuals' confidence in performing activities while they are in pain.	28 (12.9)	35 (12.2)	.10
Patient Health Questionnaire (PHQ-9) [7]. A standard 9-item questionnaire used for measuring depression	11 (5.2)	7 (3.9)	**.02**
Duke-UNC Functional Social Support (FSS) [8]. An 8-item questionnaire to measure the strength of one's social support	3 (1.4)	4 (0.76)	**.03**
Perceived Stress Scale (PSS-4) [9]. The most widely-used scale to measure a person's perceived stress	8 (2.9)	6 (3.4)	**.049**
Patient activation (PAM) [10]. Assesses patient empowerment and confidence to take care of themselves	41 (5.2)	44 (5.7)	**.001**
Current Opioid Misuse Measure (COMM) [11]. Medication misuse of pain patients on long-term opioid therapy	12 (8.3)	9 (5.4)	**.01**

Conclusion. We demonstrated that a home-based virtual agent can be effective for patients with chronic pain and depression, when used in conjunction with medical group visits, especially for patients who are low income, disadvantaged minorities. Our study indicates that even individuals who have little experience with technology find the virtual agent an acceptable and effective medium for receiving healthcare.

Acknowledgments. This work was funded by grant AD-1304-6218 from the Patient-Centered Outcomes Research Institute.

References

1. Bickmore, T., Giorgino, T.: Health dialog systems for patients and consumers. J. Biomed. Inform. **39**, 556–571 (2006)
2. Monkaresi, H., Calvo, R., Pardo, A., Chow, K., Mullan, B., Lam, M., Twigg, S., Cook, D.: Intelligent diabetes lifestyle coach. In: OzCHI, Adelaide, Australia (2013)
3. Bickmore, T., et al.: Maintaining reality: relational agents for antipsychotic medication adherence. Interact. Comput. **22**, 276–288 (2010)
4. Meeker, D., Cerully, J., et al: SimCoach evaluation: a virtual human intervention to encourage service-member help-seeking for posttraumatic stress disorder and depression. Rand Coporation (2015)
5. Cassell, J., Vilhjálmsson, H., Bickmore, T.: BEAT: the behavior expression animation toolkit. In: SIGGRAPH 2001, pp. 477–486 (2001)

6. Nicholas, M.: The pain self-efficacy questionnaire: Taking pain into account. Eur. J. Pain **11**, 153–163 (2007)
7. Kroenke, K., Spitzer, R., Williams, J.: *The PHQ-9: validity of a brief depression severity measure. J. Gen. Int. Med. **16**, 606–613 (2001)
8. Broadhead, W., Gehlbach, S., et al.: The Duke-UNC functional social support questionnaire. Med. Care **26**, 709–723 (1988)
9. Andreou, E., Alexopoulos, E., et al.: Perceived stress scale: reliability and validity study in Greece. Int. J. Environ. Res. Public Health **8**, 3287–3298 (2011)
10. Hibbard, H., Stockard, J., et al.: Development of the Patient Activation Measure (PAM). Health Serv. Res. **39**, 1009–1031 (2004)
11. Butler, S., Budman, S., et al.: Development and validation of the current opioid misuse measure. Pain **130**, 144–156 (2007)

Making AutoTutor Agents Smarter: AutoTutor Answer Clustering and Iterative Script Authoring

Zhiqiang Cai[1(✉)], Yan Gong[1], Qizhi Qiu[2], Xiangen Hu[1], and Art Graesser[1]

[1] University of Memphis, Memphis, TN, USA
{zcai,ygong2,xhu,a-graesser}@memphis.edu
[2] Wuhan University of Technology, Wuhan, Hubei, China
qiuirene@163.com

Abstract. AutoTutor uses conversational intelligent agents in learning environments. One of the major challenges in developing AutoTutor applications is to assess students' natural language answers to AutoTutor questions. We investigated an AutoTutor dataset with 3358 student answers to 49 AutoTutor questions. In comparisons with human ratings, we found that semantic matching works well for some questions but poor for others. This variation can be predicted by a measure called "question uncertainty", an entropy value on semantic cluster probabilities. Based on these findings, we propose an iterative AutoTutor script authoring process that can make AutoTutor agents smarter and improve assessment models by iteratively adding and modifying both questions and ideal answers.

Keywords: AutoTutor · Conversational agents · ASAT · ITS · Authoring tool · Assessment · Short answer grading · Question uncertainty

1 Introduction

The AutoTutor project was launched in 1997 by Art Graesser and his colleagues. Since then, many AutoTutor applications have developed in different domains, including physics, computer literacy, psychology, algebra, and electronics. Researches have reported that AutoTutor learning gains are estimated to be between 0.3 and 0.8 sigma [1].

AutoTutor agents use scripted content that is intelligently selected during tutoring. The major discourse mechanism is called Expectation-Misconception-Tailored (EMT) dialogue [2]. AutoTutor starts tutoring by introducing a problem and asking a main question. If a learner cannot answer the main question well, then a sequence of hints and prompts are asked to help the learner improve the answer. A hint is a question that attempts to elicit an answer of approximately a clause or sentence. A prompt is a question targeting a specific concept, usually a word or a phrase. When the learner expresses a misconception, AutoTutor corrects the misconception and then continue with hints, prompts, and assertions until all expectations are covered.

Evaluating student answers to AutoTutor questions is a task known as "short answer grading" [3]. Cai et al. [4] reported that LSA (Latent Semantic Analysis) [5] could play

© Springer International Publishing AG 2016
D. Traum et al. (Eds.): IVA 2016, LNAI 10011, pp. 438–441, 2016.
DOI: 10.1007/978-3-319-47665-0_50

an important role in grading such short answers in addition to regular expressions. This paper further investigates the use of LSA and proposes an iterative script authoring process to improve grading accuracy.

2 An AutoTutor Dataset with Human Ratings

The AutoTutor dataset in this paper was extracted from log files in three experiments conducted in spring 2002, fall 2002 and summer 2003. The subjects of the experiments were college students. Each student interacted with a subset of the 10 problems in conceptual physics. A total of 512 log files were received, containing 7584 student responses to 247 AutoTutor questions. The student answers were rated with 1–6 scale by two experts (both are co-authors); one is a professor in computer engineering and the other is a graduate student in computer engineering. 120 student answers were randomly sampled from the 7584 answers to train the two raters. Two raters first rated the 120 training answers independently. Then they sat together and went through the items with rating differences greater than 2. They achieved agreement and then rated the rest of the 7464 items. The correlation between the two raters' scores was 0.828. They rated 92.8 % of the answers with a difference not greater than 2. In this analysis we selected a subset of the answers satisfying: (1) the difference between the two raters' ratings is less than 2; and (2) the associated question has at least 50 answers. The selected subset contained 38 hints, 11 prompts, and 3358 student answers. In the rest of this article, we will use "human rating" to refer to the average rating of the two human ratings.

3 Performance of Semantic Matching

For each of the 3358 responses, we computed the LSA cosine between the student answers and the hint/prompt answers given by script authors. We then computed the correlation between LSA cosines and human ratings in each question. It turned out that the correlations were very different, ranging from −0.174 to 0.995. The correlations for prompts were high; 7 out of the 11 selected prompts had correlations higher than 0.7, but there was one below 0.3. The correlations on hints were much lower. Only 7 out of 38 were above 0.7, 11 out of 38 were below 0.3, and 4 of them were even below 0.

Why did LSA work well for some questions but poor for others? There could be multiple reasons. The major reason could be that some questions have "convergent" answers. That is, answers of such questions are semantically similar. Other questions could have "uncertain" answers. That is, the answers may be in multiple semantic groups. To investigate this, in the next section, we propose a "question uncertainty" measure based on semantic clustering and then show that question uncertainty predicts LSA performance on questions.

4   Question Uncertainty

For a given question Q, suppose the collected student answers are grouped into N clusters according to a particular semantic threshold t. We define the uncertainty of Q with threshold t as the "normalized" entropy value of the clustering of the responses:

$$U(Q, t) = -\frac{\sum_{i=1}^{N} p_i log p_i}{log N} \tag{1}$$

p_i is the number of responses in cluster i divided by the total number of responses. The uncertainty is normalized so the value ranges from 0 to 1.

The above definition depends on the semantic clustering. There are many different types clustering algorithms. We used the DBSCAN (Density-Based Spatial Clustering of Applications with Noise) clustering algorithm. This algorithm automatically and reasonably determines the number of clusters. The clustering depends on three choices: (1) distance function; (2) distance threshold; and (3) minimum number of elements in a cluster. The formula $(1 - LSA\ cosine)$ was used as distance between any two responses. LSA cosine values are typically positive. Occasionally negative cosine values appear. To make the distance value fall into the [0, 1] interval, negative cosine values were set to zero. Clustering analyses were performed for threshold t from 0.05 up to 0.95 with a 0.05 increase in each increment. The minimum number of elements was set to 2 so that the clustering result could contain any number of elements, with single element clusters as outliers. For each threshold $t(t = 0.05, 0.1, \ldots, 0.95)$, the correlation between the question uncertainty and the LSA performance (i.e., correlation between LSA cosine and human rating) was computed. The correlation as a function of the semantic distance threshold t resembled a cubic function. It started with negative correlation at $t = 0.05$ and decreased to the deepest point of the valley (-0.51) at $t = 0.25$. It then monotonically increased to the top point of the hill (0.50) at $t = 0.90$.

The negative correlation at $t = 0.25$ indicates that when the threshold is set to 0.25, question uncertainty can predict LSA performance. That is, for an appropriate threshold, if most answers fall into a small number of clusters, LSA performance is high. Otherwise, if the answers evenly fall into many clusters, LSA performance is low.

The high positive correlation at $t = 0.90$ is interesting. When the distance threshold is so high, the answers should usually fall into a single cluster, resulting in zero uncertainty. However, if the answers are still divided into multiple clusters with such a high distance threshold, that means there are multiple groups of answers that are semantically very different and thus can be easily classified by LSA.

5   Iterative AutoTutor Script Authoring

Based on the above discussions, LSA does not always perform well in AutoTutor answer assessment. The reason is that AutoTutor questions do not always have answers in a single semantic group. In recent AutoTutor systems, we already allow authors to create multiple good answers. However, it is really hard for authors to imagine all possible semantic groups student answers may form. Therefore, an iterative authoring process is inevitable.

An iterative authoring process starts with an initial script that contains authored answers to questions. AutoTutor agents may sometimes generate incorrect feedback and subsequent hints/prompts at the beginning because of poor semantic performance. After enough student responses are collected, however, the AutoTutor answer analysis model would cluster student answers and provide question uncertainty scores to authors. For questions with high uncertainty at a lower semantic distance threshold, authors are informed to review the student responses. Based on how the student responses cluster, authors may improve AutoTutor scripts by: (a) revising existing questions and answers; (b) adding new answers to a question; and (c) adding or revising contextual feedback to each response cluster. Once new script questions and answers are provided, AutoTutor uses new answer clusters to assess student answers, which provides more accurate answer classification, feedback, hints, and prompts.

Acknowledgement. This research was supported by the National Science Foundation (SBR 9720314, REC 0106965, REC 0126265, ITR 0325428, REESE 0633918, ALT-0834847, DRK-12-0918409, 1108845), the Institute of Education Sciences (R305H050169, R305B070349, R305A080589, R305A080594, R305G020018, R305C120001), Army Research Lab (W911INF-12-2-0030), and the Office of Naval Research (N00014-00-1-0600, N00014-12-C-0643, N000014-16-C-3027). Any opinions, findings, and conclusions or recommendations expressed in this material are those of the authors and do not necessarily reflect the views of NSF, IES, or DoD.

References

1. Nye, B.D., Graesser, A.C., Hu, X.: AutoTutor and family: a review of 17 years of natural language tutoring. Int. J. Artif. Intell. Educ. **24**, 427–469 (2014)
2. Graesser, A.C.: Conversations with AutoTutor help students learn. Int. J. Artif. Intell. Educ. **26**, 124–132 (2016)
3. Burrows, S., Gurevych, I., Stein, B.: The eras and trends of automatic short answer grading. Int. J. Artif. Intell. Educ. **25**(1), 60–117 (2015). Springer
4. Cai, Z., Graesser, A.C., Forsyth, C., Burkett, C., Millis, K., Wallace, P., Halpern, D., Butler, H.: Trialog in ARIES: user input assessment in an intelligent tutoring system. In: Chen, W., Li, S. (eds.) Proceedings of the 3rd IEEE International Conference on Intelligent Computing and Intelligent Systems, pp. 429–433. IEEE Press, Guangzhou (2011)
5. Landauer, T., McNamara, D.S., Dennis, S., Kintsch, W. (eds.): Handbook of Latent Semantic Analysis. Erlbaum, Mahwah (2007)

The Effects of a Robot's Nonverbal Behavior on Users' Mimicry and Evaluation

Nicole C. Krämer[✉], Carina Edinger, and Astrid M. Rosenthal-von der Pütten

Department for Social Psychology: Media and Communication, University of Duisburg-Essen,
Forsthausweg 2, 47057 Duisburg, Germany
{Nicole.kraemer,carina.edinger,a.rosenthalvdpuetten}@uni-due.de

Abstract. In an attempt to replicate earlier research on intelligent agents for robots, we analysed the effects of the presence and absence of a robot's nonverbal behavior on users' nonverbal behavior and evaluation with a between subjects experimental study (N = 90). Results demonstrated that when the robot shows nonverbal behavior (head movement and deictic, illustrative and rhythmic gesture) participants evaluated it more positively. Against expectations, however, participants displayed more nonverbal behavior when the robot only used speech.

Keywords: Robot · Nonverbal behavior · Mimicry · Experimental study

1 Theoretical Background and Research Questions

As can be expected from human-human interaction, numerous studies in human-robot interaction show that nonverbal communication is beneficial. For example, Sidner, Lee, Kidd, Lesh and Rich [1] demonstrate that a robot who displays nonverbal behavior is evaluated more positively. Similarly, Salem et al. [2] show that a robot is rated as more positive when it uses hand and arm movements – independent of whether these were semantically congruent or incongruent to the verbal utterances.

While the effects of robots' nonverbal behavior on people's evaluation of the robot are consistent, there is not much research on the effect of a robot's nonverbal behavior on users' nonverbal behavior. Within human-human interaction it has been demonstrated that people tend to adapt the nonverbal movements of their interaction partners such as self-touching behavior [3]. Interestingly, this mimicry behavior has already been shown for human-agent-interaction [4]. An agent who smiled more frequently lead the user to smile more – although the agent was not evaluated more positively. Based on studies giving evidence that – depending on the task – the effects of robots and agents are similar [5] it can be concluded that these mimicry effects can also be expected within human-robot interaction. However, Salem et al. [6] caution against the simple conclusion that human-agent and human-robot-interaction might yield similar effects. Therefore, the present research should clarify whether effects found in human-agent interaction can be replicated in human-robot interaction. Based on previous research [1, 2, 4] we expect that a robot showing nonverbal behavior (a) is evaluated more positively and that (b) leads to more nonverbal behavior on the part of the user.

© Springer International Publishing AG 2016
D. Traum et al. (Eds.): IVA 2016, LNAI 10011, pp. 442–446, 2016.
DOI: 10.1007/978-3-319-47665-0_51

2   Method

2.1   Experimental Design, Participants and Procedure

In order to analyse the effects of a robot's nonverbal behavior we employed a between-subjects design with the conditions "only speech" and "speech and nonverbal behavior" as independent variables. While in the "only speech" condition the Nao robot merely talked to the participants (N = 44) and did not move, it accompanied its utterances with various gestures in the "speech and nonverbal behavior" condition. The nonverbal behavior included head movements, deictic, iconic and rhythmic gestures [7].

Ninety volunteers (59 female, 31 male) aged between 17 and 48 years ($M = 21.90$; $SD = 4.47$) participated in this study. The NAO robot was sitting on a desk and was steered by a Wizard of Oz (the wizard started predefined dialogue parts and nonverbal behavior).

First, participants were instructed by the robot to conduct a five-minute procedural task (change position of objects on a table). In a subsequent communication task (mean duration: 13 min 19 s), the robot took the role of a tutor and presented facts on the diseases Alzheimer and diabetes. After each explanation he posed a related question. Afterwards, participants were asked to fill in the questionnaires. Finally, they were debriefed and thanked for participation. The study was approved by the local ethics committee.

2.2   Dependent Variables

Self-report: Perception of the Robot.   For the person perception of the robot, we used a semantic differential with 37 bi-polar items which are rated on a 5-point scale [4]. A factor analysis yielded six subscales: (1) Likeability (29.2 % explanation of variance; $\alpha = .91$), (2) Sociabilty (7.9 % explanation of variance; $\alpha = .73$), (3) Competence (6.7 %; $\alpha = .76$), (4) Relaxation (5.24 %; $\alpha = .70$), (5) Involvement (4.2 %; $\alpha = .70$), (6) Agreeableness (4.0 %; $\alpha = .70$).

Self-report: Social Presence.   We assessed participants' sense of co-presence with the Nowak and Biocca Presence Scale [8], which contains 12 items on the concept of "perceived other's co-presence" (Cronbach's $\alpha = .78$, when only 11 items were included) and 6 items on "self-related co-presence" (Cronbach's $\alpha = .72$, when only 4 items were included), both rated on a 5-point Likert scale.

Self-report: General Evaluation of the Interaction.   The general evaluation of the interaction was assessed by five items that asked for the participants' interest in the interaction, the enjoyment of the interaction, and whether participants like to use a system like this for other tasks (rated on a 5-point Likert scale; Cronbach's $\alpha = .84$).

Nonverbal Behavior of the Participant.   The nonverbal behavior of the participants during the communication task was videorecorded by two cameras and coded using ELAN. In order to broadly assess nonverbal behavior, it was coded as either illustrative gestures (IL), torso movements (TM) or self-touching (ST). Interrater reliability was good for all categories (IL: ICC(3,2) = .89, p = .029, TM: ICC(3,2) = .88, p = .032, ST: ICC(3,2) = .85, p = .029).

3   Results

3.1   Participants' Self-reported Experiences

Robot Evaluation: An ANOVA revealed that the robot's behavior affected the evaluation as likeable ($F(1,84)$ = 5.19, p = .025, $\eta^2 p$ = .058). The robot was perceived as more likeable when it showed nonverbal behavior (M = 35.57; SD = 0.78) compared to the speech only condition (M = 32.92; SD = 0.84). Also, there was an effect on relaxation ($F(1,84)$ = 6.88, p = .010, $\eta^2 p$ = .076). Here, however, participants evaluated the robot as more relaxed in the condition without nonverbal behavior (M = 12.43; SD = 0.33) than with nonverbal behavior (M = 11.24; SD = 0.30).

Social Presence: There was a marginal effect of the robot's nonverbal behavior on perceived others' co-presence ($F(1,86)$ = 3.31, p = .072, $\eta^2 p$ = .037). Participants perceive higher co-presence when the robot shows nonverbal behavior (M = 32.91; SD = 6.01) compared to when not (M = 30.20; SD = 7.33). There was no effect on the sub-scale self-related co-presence.

General Evaluation of Interaction: There was a marginal effect of the robot's nonverbal behavior on evaluation of the interaction ($F(1,84)$ = 2.76, p = .100, $\eta^2 p$ = .032). Participants' ratings are more positive when the robot showed nonverbal behavior (M = 19.53, SE = 0.53) than when it did not (M = 18.21, SE = 5.72).

3.2   Participants' Nonverbal Behavior

The presence of nonverbal behavior affected the illustrative gestures of participants marginally ($F(1,84)$ = 3.55, p = 0.63, $\eta^2 p$ = .041). Against expectations, however, participants used fewer gestures when the robot showed nonverbal behavior (see Table 1). This is even more pronounced for self-touching ($F(1,84)$ = 3.97, p = .050, $\eta^2 p$ = .045). When the robot only uses speech, participants display more self-touching behavior (Table 1). For torso movement there is no difference between conditions.

Table 1. Means and standard deviations of percent of time nonverbal behavior is shown

	Speech only		Speech & nonverbal	
	M	SD	M	SD
Illustrative gestures	1.43	0.16	1.01	0.15
Torso movements	3.12	0.32	3.17	0.30
Self-touching	22.28	2.29	15.93	2.13

4   Discussion

As expected, results showed that a robot's nonverbal behavior is beneficial in the sense that it leads to more positive evaluations. Results also indicate, somewhat surprisingly, that more relaxation is attributed when the robot shows no nonverbal behavior. This becomes plausible, however, when considering that the subscale also includes adjectives such as calm. There was only a marginal effect on social presence but additional analyses show that social presence serves as covariate when measuring the effects of a robot's nonverbal behavior on its evaluation and therefore plays an important role.

The results on the users' behavioral reactions are even more interesting: With regard to two of the three categories of the users' nonverbal behavior we found that there was no mimicry but on the contrary that the users showed less nonverbal behavior when the robot showed nonverbal behavior. This might be taken as indication that users try to compensate for the robot's behavior. However, we also have to consider that the results might be due to several limitations of the present work. For example, the categories used are merely preliminary and can be refined in future analyses. We can therefore not preclude that effects, for example, for some more specific type of illustrative gesture might not have been detected. Additionally, the robot's nonverbal behavior was limited and, for instance, did not include self-touching behaviors. Also, the robot is not as expressive (e.g., with regard to facial expressions) which limits comparability with earlier research on virtual agents. In sum, our study indicated that mimicry might not always be observable as the result of a robot's behavior. Future research must analyse whether this is persistent and what the underlying mechanisms are.

References

1. Sidner, C.L., Lee, C., Kidd, C.D., et al.: Explorations in engagement for humans and robots. Artif. Intell. **166**, 140–164 (2005)
2. Salem, M., Kopp, S., Wachsmuth, I., et al.: Generation and evaluation of communicative robot gesture. Int. J. Soc. Robotics **4**(2), 201–217 (2012)
3. Lakin, J.L., Jefferis, V.E., Cheng, C.M., et al.: The chameleon effect as social glue: evidence for the evolutionary significance of nonconscious mimicry. J. Nonverbal Behav. **27**(3), 145–162 (2003)
4. Krämer, N., Kopp, S., Becker-Asano, C., et al.: Smile and the world will smile with you – the effects of a virtual agent's smile on users' evaluation and behavior. Int. J. Hum. Comput. Stud. **71**, 335–349 (2013)
5. Hoffmann, L., Krämer, N.C.: Investigating the effects of physical and virtual embodiment in task-oriented and conversational contexts. Int. J. Hum. Comput. Stud. **71**(7–8), 763–774 (2013)
6. Salem, M., Eyssel, F., Rohlfing, K., Kopp, S., Joublin, F.: Effects of gesture on the perception of psychological anthropomorphism: a case study with a humanoid robot. In: Mutlu, B., Bartneck, C., Ham, J., Evers, V., Kanda, T. (eds.) ICSR 2011. LNCS, vol. 7072, pp. 31–41. Springer, Heidelberg (2011). doi:10.1007/978-3-642-25504-5_4

7. McNeill, D.: Hand and Mind: What Gestures Reveal About Thought. University of Chicago Press, Chicago (1992)
8. Nowak, K.L., Biocca, F.: The effect of the agency and anthropomorphism on users' sense of telepresence, copresence, and social presence in virtual environments. Presence Teleoperators Virtual Environ. **12**(5), 481–494 (2003)

Development of a Mobile Personal Health Guide for HIV-Infected African American MSM

Sangyoon Lee[1](✉), Yifan Lu[1], Apurba Chakraborty[2], and Mark S. Dworkin[2]

[1] Connecticut College, New London, CT, USA
{slee10,ylu1}@conncoll.edu
[2] University of Illinois at Chicago, Chicago, IL, USA
{achakr6,mdworkin}@uic.edu

Abstract. The study presented in this paper focuses on a relational, educational, and motivational virtual human (VH) mobile phone application for African American men who have sex with men (AAMSM). This project targets on increasing adherence to HIV medication and on improving the proportion of HIV-infected persons engaged in care by developing a theory-based mobile phone intervention that engages young HIV-positive AAMSM. The intervention is aimed to improve the likelihood of compliance with healthy behavior leading to both patient benefits (decreased morbidity, mortality and resistant virus) and population benefits (decreased HIV transmission). The VH encourages interaction with information and functions that promote engagement with the HIV Care Continuum, provide fundamental HIV information, present motivating statements, facilitate interaction with healthcare, visualize laboratory results, and encourage, explain, and illustrate relevant behavioral skills.

Keywords: Mobile virtual human · Health guide · HIV Care · Adherence

1 Introduction

African American men who have sex with men (AAMSM) are experiencing a public health crisis with high HIV infection rates, especially among young AAMSM. The greatest number of new HIV infections among MSM occurred among African American MSM ages 13 to 24 and AAMSM were 71 times more likely to contract HIV than the general U.S. population [1]. This population also struggles with mental health disorders and substance abuse, and are less likely to take antiretroviral therapy (ART) and have viral suppression.

This project, as a response to the President's HIV Care Continuum Initiative to improve the proportion of HIV-infected persons engaged in care from diagnosis to virus suppression, is a theory-based mobile phone intervention that engages young HIV-positive AAMSM in three of the five stages of care: (1) retention, (2) ART adherence, and (3) viral suppression. In other words, this is a virtual human (VH) mobile phone intervention that offers an innovative approach to improve health in young HIV-infected AAMSM. This mobile application (app) is novel and convenient for patients and the

© Springer International Publishing AG 2016
D. Traum et al. (Eds.): IVA 2016, LNAI 10011, pp. 447–450, 2016.
DOI: 10.1007/978-3-319-47665-0_52

VH can help the patients to overcome psychological barriers and encourage healthy clinical behaviors [2, 3].

This exploratory and developmental app proposes to systematically develop and then evaluate the feasibility, acceptability, utilization, and potential for impact of a theory-based VH mobile phone app to engage young HIV-infected AAMSM in multiple stages of the HIV Care Continuum. The intervention draws on the Information Motivation Behavioral Skills Model (IMB) [4] shown on Table 1.

Table 1. Information Motivation Behavioral Skills Model (IMB): the model assumes mutual feedback between information and motivation affecting one's behavioral skills and desired health outcomes. ACVH denotes Attractive Credible Virtual Human.

Continuum stage	Communication persuasion model	IMB Model				Outcome measure
		Information	Motivation	Behavioral Skills	Behavior	
Retention	ACVH explains rationale for retention	Explains what is viral load	Offers rationale for behavior and desired outcomes of staying in care	Offers and explains use of phone appointment, reminder capability	Blood draw	Blood draw performed and follow-up clinic appointment attended
Adherence	ACVH explains rationale for adherence	Explains patient medication dose, frequency and side effects	Offers empowering and supportive messaging	Demonstrates use of pill box	Prescription acquisition and medication taken	Patients report of obtaining a pill box, medication filled and >80 % of medication taken by pill count and self report
Viral Suppression	ACVH introduces images that visualize virus in their blood	Explains how viral suppression is connected to staying well	Asks patient to consider their own recent behavior and encourages adherence because it lowers viral load	Encourages not accepting detectable viral load, consultation with their healthcare provider and pharmacist, and use of phone reminder systems	Medication taken	Viral load undetectable and/or declined from initial level

2   Approach: Methods

As our ongoing app design and development stage we planned four focus groups of approximately five men each recruited from HIV patient care and outreach sites in Chicago during 2016. Eligibility criteria included aged 18-34 years, MSM, HIV-positive and on ART for at least three months by self-report, and android smartphone ownership.

Using an iterative approach, participants were shown a mock-up design and a prototype of the app at progressive stages of development and engaged to express preferences and to influence educational and motivational language, information, functions, and VH characteristics by giving feedback (Fig. 1). The app's two main features are "Let Me Explain" which provides explanatory and educational information and "Medicine Manager" which supports a medication management.

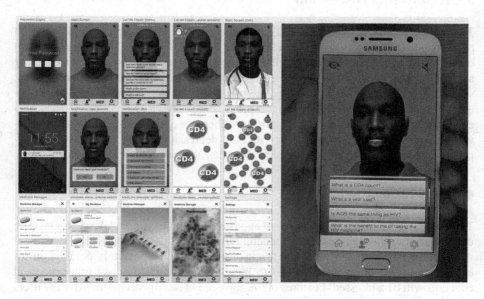

Fig. 1. The application mockup designs (left) and prototype on Android mobile phone (right).

Let Me Explain: In this explanation part, we have all the frequently asked questions listed with recorded voice explanations for patients to choose. Questions and answers reflect information relevant to medical care and other topics based on the IMB model. Users can scroll through questions via touch gestures.

Medicine Manager: One can enter any routine confirmation, medical testing results and medicine information. Patients can find majority of all basic information about medication for HIV as well as enter the medicine they are taking. Images of their pills will appear beside the name to help accurately report their regimen to healthcare providers if requested.

The primary statistical goal of our research is to illustrate preliminary effect sizes for planning of future studies with an overarching goal to increase engagement of participants in four stages of the Care Continuum. After completion of initial app version we plan to collect and analyze data to measure efficacy of our model and the app: frequencies and summary statistics that include Information (pre- and post-intervention item-by-item knowledge), Motivation (pre- and post self-efficacy), Behavioral Skills/ Behavior (utilization, prescription acquisition, self-reported adherence, and pill counts) as well as demographic data, acceptability, feasibility, and viral load results.

The app is being developed using Unity3D software and LifeLike framework [5] originally written in C/C++ for a desktop application has been ported to Unity3D environments to support platform independent deployment for both Google Android and Apple iOS devices.

3   Results and Discussion

To-date, acceptability of the VH and app functions was universal among focus group participants. Participants expressed enthusiasm for the concept: *"I'm going to ask him a lot of questions about medication."* Preferences for VH characteristics included having a young African American male dressed like a doctor. Privacy concerns were expressed; solutions included and reflected requiring passwords for app access and the ability to quickly hide app if needed (e.g. if other persons are *"trying to be nosy."*). They also encouraged motivational language regarding adherence and requested additional motivational messages to help them deal with both depression and social isolation. Information needs included: ART side effects, benefits, adherence topics and transmission.

4   Conclusions

The concept of an interactive VH-based app is acceptable to young AAMSM. Ongoing development of this app includes conducting the one additional focus group study, and incorporating these findings into future app design and development. Important consideration of stigma, motivation related to mental health concerns, and other practical concerns will be addressed. Features of the app need to be adjusted to improve the users experience according to feedbacks from the beta-test group later. A pilot testing of the app is planned as well.

References

1. Anyaka, S.: Depression and HIV risk among African American men who have sex with men. Walden University (2015)
2. Topol, E.J.: The future of medicine is in your smartphone. Wall Str. J. http://www.wsj.com/articles/the-future-of-medicine-is-in-your-smartphone-1420828632
3. Lucas, G.M., Gratch, J., King, A., Morency, L.: It's only a computer: virtual humans increase willingness to disclose. Comput. Hum. Behav. **37**, 94–100 (2014)
4. Fisher, J.D., Fisher, W.A.: Changing AIDS-risk behavior. Psychol. Bull. **111**(3), 455–474 (1992)
5. Lee, S., Carlson, G., Jones, S., Johnson, A., Leigh, J., Renambot, L.: Designing an expressive Avatar of a real person. In: Allbeck, J., Badler, N., Bickmore, T., Pelachaud, C., Safonova, A. (eds.) IVA 2010. LNCS (LNAI), vol. 6356, pp. 64–76. Springer, Heidelberg (2010). doi:10.1007/978-3-642-15892-6_8

A Deep Learning Methodology for Semantic Utterance Classification in Virtual Human Dialogue Systems

Debajyoti Datta, Valentina Brashers, John Owen,
Casey White, and Laura E. Barnes[(⊠)]

University of Virginia, Charlottesville, VA, USA
{dd3ar,vlb2z,jao2b,cw4xz,lb3dp}@virginia.edu

Abstract. This paper describes the development of a deep learning methodology for semantic utterance classification (SUC) for use in domain-specific dialogue systems. Semantic classifiers need to account for a variety of instances where the utterance for the semantic domain class varies. In order to capture the candidate relationships between the semantic class and the word sequence in an utterance, we have proposed a shallow convolutional neural network (CNN) along with a recurrent neural network (RNN) that uses domain-specific word embeddings which have been initialized using Word2Vec for determining semantic similarity of words. Experimental results demonstrate the effectiveness of shallow neural networks for SUC.

Keywords: Dialogue systems · Interprofessional medical education · Intelligent virtual agents · Healthcare

1 Introduction and Related Research

Recent progress in deep learning approaches have transformed fields such as natural language processing. In particular, these new advances create new opportunities in the field of intelligent virtual agents (IVA). One of the key components of IVA systems is the dialogue system. Dialogue systems aim to automatically identify the intent of the user as expressed in natural language, and then perform the corresponding task specific to the domain.

The majority of the work in dialogue systems relies on semantic utterance classification for the evaluation of natural language queries into a particular category and then determining the updates to the dialogue states [13]. Typically, these systems use supervised classification methods like boosting [10], support vector machine approaches [12] or maximum entropy models [14]. In this work, we propose techniques for automated feature engineering using deep learning and task specific word embeddings. We improve upon existing approaches in which feature engineering is often task specific and cannot be generalized to different domains, thus limiting their reuse. Our work aims to create a reusable framework for domain-specific intelligent virtual agents [7]. We present the utility of our

© Springer International Publishing AG 2016
D. Traum et al. (Eds.): IVA 2016, LNAI 10011, pp. 451–455, 2016.
DOI: 10.1007/978-3-319-47665-0_53

proposed approach in the context of an IVA-delivered medical interprofessional education scenario.

2   Approach

Target Scenario. We focused the proposed approach on an IVA-delivered medical interprofessional education training scenario aimed at improving communication among members of healthcare teams. In the scenario, a nursing student must perform an assessment of a virtual patient with chronic obstructive pulmonary disease (COPD) exhibiting shortness of breath. The student must engage in teamwork communication with a virtual medical provider and using a validated checklist of fifteen behaviors called the Collaborative Behaviors Observational Assessment Tools (CBOATs) [1]. Figure 1 depicts a subset of the SUC categories along with sample user statements and virtual agent responses.

In domain-specific dialogue systems, like the one in this scenario, intent determination is the key element. Previously used intent determination approaches require heavy feature engineering [10,14] over multiple iterations which slows down the building of an end-to-end SUC system and also limits the reuse of existing systems. We have proposed a deep learning approach that does not rely on task-specific feature engineering and can be rapidly trained and deployed on various scenarios. The deep learning approach has three key components: 1. Word Embeddings, 2. Convolutional Neural Network (CNN) for local and global semantics, and 3. Recurrent Neural Network (RNN) to capture word dependencies.

Word Embeddings. The fundamental idea behind Word2Vec is the distributional hypothesis, i.e. words are characterized by the company that they keep. CBOW and Skipgram [8] are the main approaches for the learning the word embeddings. Since words are the atomic unit of each sentences, each sentence has different representations based on the context in which it is used. In the case of the COPD patient, the two sentences, "How are you doing today?" and "Hi John, how are you feeling now?" mean the same thing, even though in another context they may have a different meanings. Thus, training word embeddings [8,9] improves classification accuracy over traditional indices based approaches.

Convolutional Neural Networks and Recurrent Neural Networks. CNNs popularized by Lecun [6] for image classification have since been used for a wide variety of NLP tasks like semantic parsing [15], search query retrieval [11], sentence modeling [5], and other traditional NLP tasks [3]. Traditionally in natural language processing when the task is to predict based on ordered set of items like words in a sentence or sentences in a document, some items convey more information than others. Order and the position of the words are also important in determining the meaning of the sentences. For example the two sentences, "It was not good, it was actually quite bad" and "It was not bad, it was actually quite good", have the same words, but different ordering and

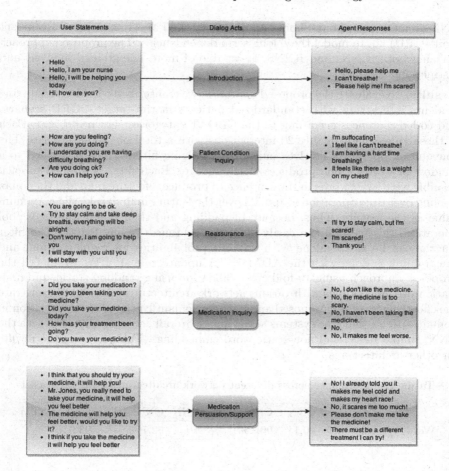

| User Statements | Dialog Acts | Agent Responses |

Fig. 1. IPE scenario and sample dialogue acts.

completely opposite intents. In cases like this, bag-of-words or n-grams will not work very effectively or will result in huge and sparse embedding matrices. In this case, CNN architectures work particularly well and are a robust and elegant solution to the problem. CNNs utilize layers with convolving filters that are applied to local features. In the proposed implementation of CNN, there is one layer of convolution applied on top of the word embedding vectors. The convolution operation involves multiple filters which is applied to a window of words that produces a new feature.

Recurrent neural networks (RNN) are good at modeling temporal word dependencies. For example in the sentence, "I was born in France and lived there for the last 18 years and therefore I speak fluent French", in order to predict, the last word, "French" from the previous words in the sentence, one would have to observe dependencies that occurred much earlier in the sentence. We use two

RNN architectures, Long-Short Term Memory (LSTM) [4] and Gated Recurrent Unit (GRU) [2], to model these long-term dependencies. The proposed approach utilizing both, CNNs and RNNS, is capable of more fine-grained analysis and distinction.

Results. To evaluate the proposed approach, we transcribed 54 videos of nursing students interacting with standardized patients in the target COPD scenario and coded sentences according to the CBOAT categories shown in Fig. 1. Each of these videos had roughly 20 interactions with a total of 2300 sentences. The convolution operation involves multiple convolving filters which is applied to a window of words which produces a new feature. Each filter is applied to each possible window of words in the sentence to produce a feature map and then max pooling over time operation is applied over the feature map to take the maximum value as the feature. Thus, because of padding and then taking the max pool operation, this method can easily deal with sentences of any length. The filter lengths can be varied along with dropout probabilities for regularization, and the training is done with the ADADELTA update rule [16]. We evaluated the proposed approach using 10-fold cross validation using random, static, and non-static word embeddings with various network architectures. Results demonstrate the effectiveness of the proposed approach for semantic utterance classification in domain-specific dialogue systems achieving an overall accuracy of 96.3 % with the CNN, simple RNN, and non-static word embeddings. Table 1 shows the results for other architectures.

Table 1. Performance across different network architectures on IPE data set

	CNN	CNN+SimpleRNN	CNN+GRU	CNN+LSTM
Word2Vec non-static	90.1 %	96.3 %	92.1 %	93.9 %

3   Conclusion and Future Work

We proposed a deep learning methodology specifically targeted at intent determination tasks. In the proposed method, the random or pre-trained word embeddings are fed into a recurrent neural network (LSTM, GRU or a Simple RNN) to capture dependencies among words in the sentences. The output from the RNN is then fed into multi-channel convolutional layers to capture local semantics. The max over time pooling layers capture global semantic features followed by a fully connected layer with dropout to summarize the features. Preliminary experiments demonstrate that the approach outperformed traditional feature engineered approaches for intent determination tasks. As future work, we plan to benchmark our approach on other data sets and test our system with real users.

Acknowledgments. This research was supported in part by an Ivy Foundation Biomedical Innovation Grant.

References

1. Brashers, V., Erickson, J.M., Blackhall, L., Owen, J.A., Thomas, S.M., Conaway, M.R.: Measuring the impact of clinically relevant interprofessional education on undergraduate medical and nursing student competencies: a longitudinal mixed methods approach. J. Interprof. Care **30**(4), 448–457 (2016). http://dx.doi.org/10.3109/13561820.2016.1162139, pMID: 27269441
2. Chung, J., Gulcehre, C., Cho, K., Bengio, Y.: Empirical evaluation of gated recurrent neural networks on sequence modeling. arXiv preprint arXiv:1412.3555 (2014)
3. Collobert, R., Weston, J., Bottou, L., Karlen, M., Kavukcuoglu, K., Kuksa, P.: Natural language processing (almost) from scratch. J. Mach. Learn. Res. **12**, 2493–2537 (2011)
4. Hochreiter, S., Schmidhuber, J.: Long short-term memory. Neural Comput. **9**(8), 1735–1780 (1997)
5. Kalchbrenner, N., Grefenstette, E., Blunsom, P.: A convolutional neural network for modelling sentences. arXiv preprint arXiv:1404.2188 (2014)
6. LeCun, Y., Bottou, L., Bengio, Y., Haffner, P.: Gradient-based learning applied to document recognition. Proc. IEEE **86**(11), 2278–2324 (1998)
7. Mancini, M., Ach, L., Bantegnie, E., Baur, T., Berthouze, N., Datta, D., Ding, Y., Dupont, S., Griffin, H.J., Lingenfelser, F., Niewiadomski, R., Pelachaud, C., Pietquin, O., Piot, B., Urbain, J., Volpe, G., Wagner, J.: Laugh when you're winning, pp. 50–79 (2014). http://dx.doi.org/10.1007/978-3-642-55143-7_3
8. Mikolov, T., Sutskever, I., Chen, K., Corrado, G.S., Dean, J.: Distributed representations of words and phrases and their compositionality. In: Advances in Neural Information Processing Systems, pp. 3111–3119 (2013)
9. Pennington, J., Socher, R., Manning, C.D.: Glove: global vectors for word representation. In: Proceedings of the 2014 Conference on Empirical Methods in Natural Language Processing, EMNLP 2014, 25-29 October 2014, Doha, Qatar, A meeting of SIGDAT, a Special Interest Group of the ACL, pp. 1532–1543 (2014). http://aclweb.org/anthology/D/D14/D14-1162.pdf
10. Schapire, R.E., Singer, Y.: Boostexter: a boosting-based system for text categorization. Mach. Learn. **39**(2), 135–168 (2000)
11. Shen, Y., He, X., Gao, J., Deng, L., Mesnil, G.: Learning semantic representations using convolutional neural networks for web search. In: Proceedings of the 23rd International Conference on World Wide Web, WWW 2014 Companion, NY, USA, pp. 373–374 (2014). http://doi.acm.org/10.1145/2567948.2577348
12. Silva, J., Coheur, L., Mendes, A.C., Wichert, A.: From symbolic to sub-symbolic information in question classification. Artif. Intell. Rev. **35**(2), 137–154 (2011)
13. Tur, G., De Mori, R.: Spoken Language Understanding: Systems for Extracting Semantic Information from Speech. Wiley, Hoboken (2011)
14. Tur, G., Deng, L., Hakkani-Tür, D., He, X.: Towards deeper understanding: deep convex networks for semantic utterance classification. In: IEEE International Conference on Acoustics, Speech and Signal Processing (ICASSP), pp. 5045–5048. IEEE (2012)
15. Yih, W.t., He, X., Meek, C.: Semantic parsing for single-relation question answering. In: Proceedings of the ACL, pp. 643–648 (2014)
16. Zeiler, M.D.: Adadelta: an adaptive learning rate method. arXiv preprint arXiv:1212.5701 (2012)

Simulink Toolbox for Real-Time Virtual Character Control

Ulysses Bernardet[✉], Maryam Saberi, and Steve DiPaola

Simon Fraser University Vancouver, Burnaby, Canada
{ubernard,msaberi,sdipaola}@sfu.ca

Abstract. Building virtual humans is a task of formidable complexity. We believe that, especially when building agents that interact with biological humans in real-time over multiple sensorial channels, graphical, data flow oriented programming environments are the development tool of choice. In this paper, we describe a toolbox for the system control and block diagramming environment Simulink that supports the construction of virtual humans. Available blocks include sources for stochastic processes, utilities for coordinate transformation and messaging, as well as modules for controlling gaze and facial expressions.

Keywords: Virtual character · Simulink · Toolbox · Data flow graphical programming · Real-time interaction

1 Introduction

We operate under the assumption that, to build truly lifelike, autonomous humanoid agents that are indistinguishable from biological humans, we need to not only copy the "surface properties" of the biological model system but make a "deep copy" that is based on the same underlying principles. Even if we build IVAs at a more abstract level than the neuronal one, we are still facing the task of constructing highly complex systems. Graphical data flow programming environments are firmly established in the design of industrial control systems and are equally well suited for building complex models at different levels of abstraction [1]. In this paper, we present ongoing work on the development of a toolbox that supports the construction of real-time control systems for virtual characters using the graphical programming environment MathWorks Simulink. We are motivated by the experience that control systems for virtual humans tend to become complex rapidly and that graphical tools are very useful in supporting the construction by providing a better overview and understanding of what is happening within the system. Our goal is to provide a library of re-usable components e.g. for gaze control and facial expression. The toolbox is open source and the code available from https://github.com/bernuly/VCSimulinkTlbx.

© Springer International Publishing AG 2016
D. Traum et al. (Eds.): IVA 2016, LNAI 10011, pp. 456–459, 2016.
DOI: 10.1007/978-3-319-47665-0_54

2   A Simulink Library for Virtual Character Control

A number of open and closed source environments support the graphical construction of control systems, e.g. Dymola and OpenModelica respectively. General purpose graphical data flow oriented environments include LabView, which in the domain of interactive media MAX is widely used. The Simulink environment is one of the best-established block diagram environment for continuous and discrete domain simulations. Unlike other data flow oriented programming environments, Simulink natively integrates a finite state machine component (StateFlow), allowing to construct hybrid control systems within a single application. Key advantages, next to general graphical system construction and the availability of real-time data visualization tools, are encapsulation and introspection. Encapsulation means that the system can be organized into an arbitrarily deeply nested hierarchy of subsystems, hence shielding the user from complexity he/she is not currently not interested in. However, unlike in the case of code level encapsulation, the subsystems created within Simulink are open to introspection, granting the user access to the system at all levels of abstraction.

2.1   Available Blocks

The blocks in the toolbox fall into the broad categories of "input/sources", utilities, and output behavior generation. The toolbox is neutral regarding the transportation layer, but examples shown here are using the m+m middleware [2].

Sources. In most of the cases, input into the system will be provided by external processes such as tracking system, analysis of facial expression etc. For typical model intrinsic sources such as step functions and sine waves, Simulink provides blocks.

   Poisson pulse. A number of natural processes follow the temporal characteristics of a Poisson process [3]. The "Poisson pulse" block provides an input sequence where the delay between (binary) events follows a Poisson distribution. The only parameter used in this block is the λ that controls the shape of the distribution.

Utilities. *3D coordinate transformation.* Transformation between different coordinate system is an issue frequently encountered when working with 3-dimensional data. This block converts between input coordinates, their respective centers and scaling factors and output coordinates.

Messaging. Simulink does not allow to use strings as signals between blocks in the model. To be able to pass character values, e.g. BML messages from one block to the next, they need to be converted to numeric arrays. We provide a utility function ("encStr2Arr") that can be used to convert strings to double array at the level of Matlab code. All blocks of our toolbox, however, handled the conversion transparently. This means that the user does not need to explicitly convert between types, but can simply enter textual information directly.

createMessage. This block creates text messages that are used for triggering atomic actions such as animations.

conc msg. Often different nodes inside the model will create complementary control message, e.g. if one subsystem generates gaze control commands while the other determines the facial expression of the agent. To send these commands in a single message, they need to be strung together. The "conc msg" block concatenates messages in a vector into a single output string.

Add prefix/suffix. This block allows to add a prefix and suffix to message e.g. to add "bracket" a message with `<?xml version="1.0" ?><act><bml>` and `</bml></act>` as is required by some BML realizers such as SmartBody.

Behavior Control. At the output side the toolbox is generating control messages in the Behavioral Markup Language (BML) [4]. By using the BML standard, the toolbox should be compatible with wide range of BML realizers such as Greta [5] or AsapRealizer [6]. However, the toolbox so far has only been tested with the SmartBody character animation system [7].

facial Expression. This block generates BML face commands with action unit weights for the categorical facial expression of anger, disgust, fear, joy, sadness, surprise. Each category is given a weight ($[0 \ldots 1]$), and several categories can be combined.

PAD2AU female/male. The circumplex model of affect proposed by Russel [8], is a widely used representation of internal affective states. When creating affective facial expressions, we need to map the circumplex dimensions of pleasure, arousal, and dominance (PAD) onto facial action units. [9] empirically determined this mapping. The "PAD2AU female/male" block uses the regression weights from [9] to map locations in the 3-dimensional PAD space onto facial action units for females and males.

gaze control. This block allows direct control over the target location for the gaze. Additionally, the "extent" parameter determines which joints are involved in the gaze behavior ($0 < e < .25$: eyes only, $.25 < e < 5$: eyes, neck, $.5 < e < 75$: eyes ... chest, $.75 < e < 1$: eyes ... back).

Mutual/non-mutual gaze control. This block form mutual and non-mutual gaze behavior provides high-level control for a relatively complex gaze behavior, where the agent is alternating between looking at a predetermined, e.g. speaker location, and a randomly chosen alternative location. The control logic is loosely based on the system described in [10]. The random distribution of the gaze dwell times presented in [10] in our block is approximated using two Poisson processes, one for mutual, and one for non-mutual gaze. This has the advantage of providing two easily tunable parameters in the form of the λ of the Poisson distribution. The non-mutual gaze direction is drawing its horizontal and vertical saccade amplitude from a normal distribution with the fixed location as the mean. Tuning the variance for the horizontal and vertical distributions, the user can easily shape the gaze frustum. As the direct gaze control block described above, this block also allows the control of the joints involved in the gazing behavior by means of the "extent".

3   Conclusion

In this paper, we have presented an open source Simulink toolbox that supports the graphical design and control of real-time virtual human systems. We believe that real-time data inspection and visualization, in combination with the ability to organize the system into encapsulated subsystems are powerful methods for tackling the complexity of virtual human control systems. In the future, we will expand the toolbox with additional generic block e.g. for procedural animation control, add support for middleware components such as Apache ActiveMQ, and interface to a wider range of BML realizers.

Acknowledgments. This work was partially supported by "Moving Stories" Canadian SSHRC grant.

References

1. Bernardet, U., Verschure, P.F.: iqr: a tool for the construction of multi-level simulations of brain and behaviour. Neuroinformatics **8**(2), 113–134 (2010)
2. Bernardet, U., Schiphorst, T., Adhia, D., Jaffe, N., Wang, J., Nixon, M., Alemi, O., Phillips, J., DiPaola, S., Pasquier, P.: m+m: a novel middleware for distributed, movement based interactive multimedia systems. In: Proceedings of the 3rd International Symposium on Movement and Computing - MOCO 2016, pp. 21:1–21:9. ACM Press, New York (2016)
3. Weisstein, E.W.: Poisson Process
4. Reidsma, D., Welbergen, H.V.: BML 1.0 Standard. SAIBA. http://www.mindmakers.org/projects/bml-1-0/wiki
5. Mancini, M., Niewiadomski, R., Bevacqua, E., Pelachaud, C.: Greta: a SAIBA compliant ECA system. In: Troisiéme Workshop sur les Agents Conversationnels Animés (2008)
6. Welbergen, H., Yaghoubzadeh, R., Kopp, S.: AsapRealizer 2.0: the next steps in fluent behavior realization for ECAs. In: Bickmore, T., Marsella, S., Sidner, C. (eds.) IVA 2014. LNCS (LNAI), vol. 8637, pp. 449–462. Springer, Heidelberg (2014). doi:10.1007/978-3-319-09767-1_56
7. Shapiro, A.: Building a character animation system. In: Allbeck, J.M., Faloutsos, P. (eds.) MIG 2011. LNCS, vol. 7060, pp. 98–109. Springer, Heidelberg (2011). doi:10.1007/978-3-642-25090-3_9
8. Russell, J.A.: A circumplex model of affect. J. Pers. Soc. Psychol. **39**(6), 1161–1178 (1980)
9. Boukricha, H., Wachsmuth, I., Hofstatter, A., Grammer, K.: Pleasure-arousal-dominance driven facial expression simulation. In: 2009 3rd International Conference on Affective Computing and Intelligent Interaction and Workshops, pp. 1–7. IEEE, September 2009
10. Lee, S.P., Badler, J.B., Badler, N.I.: Eyes alive. ACM Trans. Graph. **21**(3), 637–644 (2002)

The LISSA Virtual Human and ASD Teens: An Overview of Initial Experiments

Seyedeh Zahra Razavi[1(✉)], Mohammad Rafayet Ali[1], Tristram H. Smith[2],
Lenhart K. Schubert[1], and Mohammed (Ehsan) Hoque[1]

[1] Department of Computer Science, University of Rochester, Rochester, NY, USA
{srazavi,mali7,schubert,mehoque}@cs.rochester.edu
[2] School of Medicine, University of Rochester, Rochester, NY, USA
Tristram_Smith@urmc.rochester.edu

Abstract. We summarize an exploratory investigation into using an autonomous conversational agent for improving the communication skills of teenagers with autism. The system conducts a natural conversation with the user and gives real-time and post-session feedback on the user's nonverbal behavior. We obtained promising results and ideas for improvements in preliminary experiments with five autism spectrum disorder teens.

Keywords: Autism spectrum disorder · Conversational virtual agent · Communication skills training

1 Introduction

Understanding and exhibiting appropriate social behavior is difficult for individuals diagnosed with autism spectrum disorder (ASD). Many people with ASD are in the average range of intelligence (that is, high-functioning) and often want help in improving their conversation skills. In this paper, we provide the results from an exploratory experiment, undertaken to determine the feasibility of using an autonomous conversational agent to help teenagers with ASD to practice and eventually, to improve their conversational skills. The fully automated conversational agent that we employ is a version of LISSA [1], adapted to help those with ASD. Using the automated version of the system, we ran a pilot study with five teenagers with ASD. Our study shows that a virtual agent can appear human-like and engaging in its dialogue behavior, from the perspective of teenagers with ASD.

Our system conducts a natural conversation with the teenagers, while at the same time providing both continuous feedback about the appropriateness of the user's prosodic and nonverbal behavior and post-session feedback in a simple, easy-to-interpret format. Based on the information collected from the users through interviews and a questionnaire about the system, we gained some initial insights into the strengths and weaknesses of our approach for the target population as well as some sense of the variation in user reactions to a system of this type.

D. Traum et al. (Eds.): IVA 2016, LNAI 10011, pp. 460–463, 2016.
DOI: 10.1007/978-3-319-47665-0_55

2 Related Work

In recent years, various virtual agent systems have been developed for skills training in common social scenarios—job interviews or public speaking, for instance. Examples include My Automated Conversation coacH (MACH) [2], Cicero [3], and the TARDIS simulation platform [4]. These systems provided feedback on prosody and nonverbal aspects of users' behavior, but made few, if any, attempts to make sense of user inputs. Other conversational agents were intended to combine meaningful conversations with nonverbal feedback. HWYD [5] and SimSensei [6] are some recent ones. Other computer systems aimed specifically at children with ASD include ECHOES [7], designed to improve collaboration skills, and RACHEL [8], which leads both a story-telling and a problem-solving task. Instead of using storytelling or tutoring tasks, we equip our system with the ability to lead a natural conversation, while at the same time presenting feedback to the users to improve their nonverbal behavior.

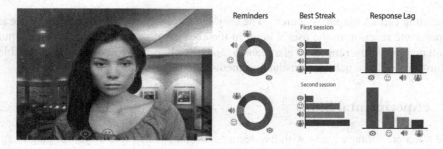

Fig. 1. Real-time feedback interface (left) and post-session feedback interface (right) (Color figure online)

3 Feedback System and Dialogue Management

Our system had two major responsibilities: providing live and post-session feedback, and hosting a dialogue manager that allows users to have an open-ended conversation. The real-time feedback (Fig. 1) uses flashing icons to suggest changes in the user's eye contact, speaking volume, smile, and body movement. Figure 1 also shows the charts displayed in post-session feedback, revealing the number of reminders (red flashes) the user received during the conversation, how long the user kept the icons green, and the time taken to adjust their behavior. The real-time feedback system uses a Hidden Markov Model (HMM) to predict the point at which an icon needs to turn red and green after-wards. The HMM was trained using data collected from a previous study [1], and details about its algorithm will appear in a future publication.

The dialogue manager is designed to lead a human-like, responsive, autonomous conversation with the user. Figure 2 provides some idea of this interaction. To lead a dialogue, LISSA follows plans and subplans that are dynamically customized and modified. Throughout the dialogue, user inputs are mapped to explicit, context-inde-pendent "gist-clauses", where the mapping uses the gist-clause representation of the

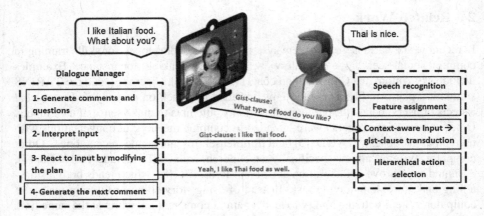

Fig. 2. Dialogue management outline.

preceding LISSA output as context. The user's gist-clauses are then used to generate an appropriate reaction to the user's input in the context of the preceding LISSA output. Both mappings (user inputs to gist-clauses, and gist-clauses to responses) use a flexible, robust hierarchical pattern transduction method.

4   Experimental Study

We ran a preliminary study with five teenagers (one girl and four boys) ranging in age from 15 to 17 years, all diagnosed with ASD based on expert evaluation and standardized diagnostic testing. After a five-minute explanation of the system, they had two rounds of conversation with LISSA, each taking five to 10 min. After the second round, the participants filled out a questionnaire in which we asked the participants to indicate their level of agreement with various statements. Responses were given on a five-point scale ranging from "strongly disagree" (1) to "strongly agree" (5). Experimenters had a five- to 10-minute chat with the teenagers about the users' perceptions of the experiment.

Among the five participants, one was uncomfortable with the system. He was rather anxious before and during the conversation. He found talking to a computer relatively unnatural. Other participants generally handled the interaction well. They felt that LISSA understood what they said ($avg. = 3.8, sd = 0.74$). Four of them mentioned this as a feature they liked. They found the feedback from LISSA useful ($avg. = 4, sd = 0.6$). They also tended to agree that they could easily interpret the icons ($avg. = 3.6, sd = 1.5$), although two participants were disconcerted by any unexpected issues with the system, such as the screen "freezing" or a seemingly out-of-place question or feedback icon. Such glitches adversely affected the subjects' assessments of the system and tended to become the focus of the post-session chat. Four of the five subjects were interested in more experiences with our system, indicating they would use it for training if its feedback became more precise and its responses more prompt. On average, they neither agreed nor disagreed that the experience with LISSA was almost as real as talking to a human

($avg. = 3$, $sd = 1.09$), although two of them said they might prefer it over talking to a human.

Significantly, two of the subjects were particularly averse to any implied deficits in their social skills, making them uncomfortable with the system-provided feedback. Being gentle and respectful in explaining the system—as well as in the automated feedback it provides—are important.

5 Conclusion

We proposed a conversational agent designed to help teenagers with ASD improve their conversational skills. We ran an exploratory study with five teenagers, analyzed their behavior during a series of conversations, and asked them about their experiences with the system. According to the results, the LISSA conversational agent can potentially benefit many teenagers as a social communication skills training tool. The negative feedback, however, should be addressed, and the system should avoid hypothetical questions.

Acknowledgements. The work was supported by NSF EAGER grant IIS-1543758 and DARPA grant W911NF-15-1-0542. Many thanks to our student experimenters and subjects.

References

1. Ali, M.R., Crasta, D., Jin, L., Baretto, A., Pachter, J., Rogge, R.D., Hoque, M.E.: LISSA - live interactive social skill assistance. In: 2015 International Conference on Affective Computing and Intelligent Interaction, ACII 2013, pp. 173–179 (2015)
2. Hoque, M., Courgeon, M., Martin, J.C., Mutlu, B., Picard, R.W.: MACH: my automated conversation coach. In: UBICOMP 2013 (2013)
3. Batrinca, L., Stratou, G., Shapiro, A., Morency, L.-P., Scherer, S.: Cicero - towards a multimodal virtual audience platform for public speaking training. In: Aylett, R., Krenn, B., Pelachaud, C., Shimodaira, H. (eds.) IVA 2013. LNCS, vol. 8108, pp. 116–128. Springer, Heidelberg (2013)
4. Jones, H., Sabouret, N.: TARDIS – a simulation platform with an affective virtual recruiter for job interviews. In: Intelligent Digital Games for Empowerment and Inclusion (2013)
5. Smith, C., Crook, N., Dobnik, S., Charlton, D., Boye, J., Pulman, S., Camara, R.S., Turunen, M., Gambäck, B.: Interaction strategies for an affective conversational agent. Presence: Teleop. Virtual Environ. **20**(5), 395–411 (2011)
6. DeVault, D., Artstein, R., Benn, G., Dey, T., Fast, E., Gainer A., Georgila, K., Gratch, J., Hartholt, A., Lhommet, M., Lucas, G.: SimSensei Kiosk: a virtual human interviewer for healthcare decision support. In: International Conference on Autonomous Agents and Multi-agent Systems, pp. 1061–1068 (2014)
7. Bernardini, S., Porayska-Pomsta, K., Smith, T.J.: ECHOES: an intelligent serious game for fostering social communication in children with autism. Inf. Sci. **264**, 41–60 (2014)
8. Mower, E., Black, M.P., Flores, E., Williams, M., Narayanan, S.: Rachel: design of an emotionally targeted interactive agent for children with autism. In: IEEE International Conference on Multimedia and Expo, pp. 1–6 (2011)

Virtual General Game Playing Agent

Hafdís Erla Helgadóttir, Svanhvít Jónsdóttir, Andri Már Sigurdsson,
Stephan Schiffel, and Hannes Högni Vilhjálmsson[✉]

School of Computer Science, Center for Analysis and Design of Intelligent Agents,
Reykjavik University, Reykjavik, Iceland
hannes@ru.is

Abstract. We developed a virtual game playing agent with the goal
of showing believable non-verbal behavior related to what is going on
in the game. Combining the fields of virtual agents and general game
playing allows our agent to play arbitrary board games with minimal
adaptations for the representation of the game state in the virtual environment. Participants in preliminary user testing report the game to be
more engaging and life-like with the virtual agent present.

1 Introduction and Motivation

Intelligent virtual agents, and more specifically embodied conversational agents
capable of interacting with humans face-to-face, have served many roles, including as tutors, guides, trainers and actors. Providing more general companionship,
such as social support to the elderly, is also gaining attention [15]. Being entertaining can help in that role, such as by being able to play various games. It is
not just the game playing itself that delivers value in that case, electric games
have been doing that for decades, but being socially present and responsive adds
a completely new dimension [1]. Being able to play games can be a useful skill
for companion agents, but picking up new games to play is not trivial.

General game playing (GGP) agents [9] have been developed with the goal in
mind of defeating other agents at any game, as a sort of benchmark for effective
AI strategies. Entertaining humans with an endless variety of game options has
generally not been the focus of that research.

In this project, we combine a virtual agent and a GGP agent to create an
intelligent virtual agent that approximates human strategies and reactions in
order to create a believable opponent for human players rather than the best
possible player. The use of a GGP engine ensures that the agent will never run
out of games to play.

2 Related Work

Virtual and robotic agents, that express human-like social and emotional behavior while playing board games and card games have been built and studied.
Some interesting results include strong human reaction to visual social behavior

D. Traum et al. (Eds.): IVA 2016, LNAI 10011, pp. 464–469, 2016.
DOI: 10.1007/978-3-319-47665-0_56

[3, 14, 16], the importance of also including negative feedback [1] and the importance of immersion [13]. Most of these systems implement a single game, such as chess [2, 13, 16], Skip-Bo [1], Reversi [7] and Risk [14]. A more general social game playing framework for virtual agents was proposed in [3], but the game specific logic does not follow a standard format. Our agent is the first virtual game playing agent that adopts a standard general game description language. Also, in order to possibly gain some of the benefits of immersive play space, our agent is presented within virtual reality.

A GGP agent is a game playing agent that is capable of playing an arbitrary game well, with no input other than the rules of the game. The GGP community uses the Game Description Language (GDL) [11] to describe the rules of games. Interpreting the GDL description of a game allows a general game player to simulate the game or search through the possible moves and future position to find a good move. While variants of Minimax search (e.g., [17]) used to be the standard approach, the difficulty of generating good heuristics for arbitrary games lead to the adoption of simulation-based approaches. Today the field is mostly dominated by Monte Carlo Tree Search [4, 9].

3   Approach and Implementation

In order to familiarize ourselves with the domain, we first collected data on how humans play a variety of board games against other humans. We had three people play both Checkers and Nine Men's Morris, 6 games in total. The games were recorded on video, their length ranging from 8 min to 30 min, and then analyzed for hand gestures, reactions and facial expressions.

Our goal was to create an environment in Virtual Reality where you could meet a virtual human and play any game against it that could be represented in GDL. We accomplished this by coupling together a GGP engine and a reactive virtual agent framework in Unity 3D. An overview of the architecture is provided

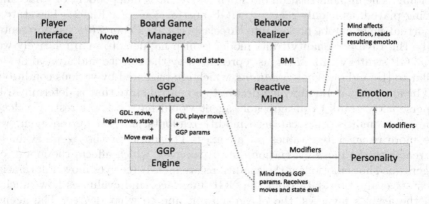

Fig. 1. Overview of the architecture. The GGP Engine is a separate process that communicates with the remaining Unity based system over sockets.

in Fig. 1. The focus is board games, where pieces can be placed, removed, captured and moved. A Board Game Manager handles these actions, as well as the mapping between the GDL and virtual board representation, while remaining agnostic to the actual game logic and rules. One can therefore quickly add new board games to the environment by providing the basic 3D assets and define GDL cell locations. While the architecture itself is not limited to board games, including other games such as card games requires new motion skills and changes to the environment configuration.

The virtual agent needs to display facial expressions, vocalize, gaze, and gesticulate with its hands, as well as move pieces on the board. We build on our own SAIBA architecture [12], using FML (Functional Mark-up Language) [5] to describe intent, and BML (Behavior Mark-up Language) [10] to describe its realization through behavior.

The GGP Engine runs on a simulation based search algorithm, specifically Monte Carlo tree search (MCTS) [4] that is built on top of ggp-base [18] – a Java framework that provides a skeleton for the messaging system and a reasoner for interpreting GDL to simulate the game. We extended the search algorithm in a few key ways: We added the MAST [8] and GRAVE [6] heuristics for faster convergence, discounting of values during back-propagation to decrease the value of far away victories we find, and horizon parameters that limit the depth of the play outs and the depth of the tree. To be able to affect the way the agent plays, we added the ability to pass parameters from the virtual agent to the GGP engine. There are more than 17 parameters of the search algorithm and our extension that can be affected, but most of those are nuanced and do not provide easily predictable changes. Some of them are very important for portraying a believable human player, such as how much the AI values keeping its own and removing opponent pieces, depth limit for the search and the chance of playing sub-optimal moves.

The role of the virtual agent is to visualize a particular opponent, both in terms of who the person is and in terms of how the game is dynamically unfolding. The implementation of the virtual agent is independent of what game is being played, as it only reacts to GGP abstractions (see Fig. 2). The state of the virtual agent can be broken into three aspects: Its *Personality*, as represented by the Big Five personality traits model (which happens to map relatively well onto GGP strategy); Its *Mood*, as represented by the valence and arousal model, similar to [1]; and one-shot *Emotions*, which are triggered by various conditions.

The agent has a mood which decays to a neutral state that is determined by its personality traits (a disagreeable agent would have a lower resting valence value). Personality traits can also modify readouts; an extroverted agent will have more exaggerated values on all axes. The mind of the agent evaluates and reacts to the move evaluation data it receives, which affects the mood and triggers one-shot emotions if the conditions are met. It receives move information and state evaluation data from the GGP interface, and evaluates how much it is in the agent's favor vs. the player's favor, and to what degree. The agent's

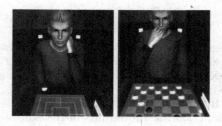

Fig. 2. Looking bashful in a game of Nine Men's Morris vs. thoughtful in Checkers.

actual behavior is generated via FML and BML. We extended FML and BML to support board game interactions and intent.

Each time the mind receives move and state data, appropriate FML is generated. Upon receiving a move, whether it is its own, or one made by the player, it creates a `ReactMoveFunction`, and if it is its own move, it will also create a `MakeMoveFunction`. It generates a `ConsiderMoveFunction` every few seconds upon receiving the cognitive data about the current state. Each of these are accompanied by an `EmotionFunction` which has the current mood stored, and are placed into a FML body which is then immediately interpreted. Transforming from FML to BML is where we see the effects of the agent state (one-shot emotions, the mood and the personality modifiers) on the visible behavior. Finally the behavior realizer schedules and executes BML chunks, such as moving pieces, changing poses, looking around. `EmotionFunction` gets mapped to an expression which is interpolated between four different expressions, representing the extremes of the arousal and valence axes.

4   Conclusion

The results from a pilot study with 13 participants, where each participants played against a visible and an invisible agent, agrees with previous research that has shown an improvement in subjective experience when game playing agents become embodied. It is encouraging to see how well people reacted to seeing the virtual agents despite dipping a bit into the uncanny valley (reported as "creepy"). It indicates that the idea of having a virtual agent to play against could enhance many such experiences even if it isn't perfect.

In conclusion, the contribution of our work is twofold: Using a formal game description to extend the capability of intelligent virtual agents, such as those in a companionship role, to play a greater variety of games with less effort; and to introduce modifications to GGP that start to address a more human-like style of playing, for the purpose of entertainment rather than competition.

References

1. Becker, C., Prendinger, H., Ishizuka, M., Wachsmuth, I.: Evaluating affective feedback of the 3D agent max in a competitive cards game. In: Tao, J., Tan, T., Picard, R.W. (eds.) ACII 2005. LNCS, vol. 3784, pp. 466–473. Springer, Heidelberg (2005). doi:10.1007/11573548_60
2. Becker-Asano, C., Riesterer, N., Hué, J., Nebel, B.: Embodiment, emotion, and chess: a system description. In: Proceedings of the 4th International Symposium on New Frontiers in Human-Robot Interaction, p. 74 (2015)
3. Behrooz, M., Rich, C., Sidner, C.: On the sociability of a game-playing agent: a software framework and empirical study. In: Bickmore, T., Marsella, S., Sidner, C. (eds.) IVA 2014. LNCS (LNAI), vol. 8637, pp. 40–53. Springer, Heidelberg (2014). doi:10.1007/978-3-319-09767-1_6
4. Björnsson, Y., Finnsson, H.: CadiaPlayer: a simulation-based general game player. IEEE Trans. Comput. Intell. AI Games 1(1), 4–15 (2009)
5. Cafaro, A., Vilhjálmsson, H.H., Bickmore, T., Heylen, D., Pelachaud, C.: Representing communicative functions in SAIBA with a unified function markup language. In: Bickmore, T., Marsella, S., Sidner, C. (eds.) IVA 2014. LNCS (LNAI), vol. 8637, pp. 81–94. Springer, Heidelberg (2014). doi:10.1007/978-3-319-09767-1_11
6. Cazenave, T.: Generalized rapid action value estimation. In: Proceedings of the Twenty-Fourth International Joint Conference on Artificial Intelligence, IJCAI 2015, Buenos Aires, Argentina, 25–31 July 2015, pp. 754–760 (2015)
7. Courgeon, M., Clavel, C., Martin, J.C.: Appraising emotional events during a real-time interactive game. In: Proceedings of the International Workshop on Affective-Aware Virtual Agents and Social Robots, p. 7. ACM (2009)
8. Finnsson, H., Björnsson, Y.: Learning simulation control in general game-playing agents. In: AAAI, vol. 10, pp. 954–959 (2010)
9. Genesereth, M., Björnsson, Y.: The international general game playing competition. AI Mag. 34(2), 107 (2013)
10. Kopp, S., Krenn, B., Marsella, S., Marshall, A.N., Pelachaud, C., Pirker, H., Thórisson, K.R., Vilhjálmsson, H.: Towards a common framework for multimodal generation: the behavior markup language. In: Gratch, J., Young, M., Aylett, R., Ballin, D., Olivier, P. (eds.) IVA 2006. LNCS (LNAI), vol. 4133, pp. 205–217. Springer, Heidelberg (2006). doi:10.1007/11821830_17
11. Love, N., Hinrichs, T., Haley, D., Schkufza, E., Genesereth, M.: General game playing: game description language specification (2008)
12. Ólafsson, S., Bédi, B., Helgadóttir, H., Vilhjálmsson, H., Arinbjörnsdóttir, B.: Starting a conversation with strangers: explicit announcement of presence. In: Proceedings of the 3rd European Symposium on Multimodal Communication (2015)
13. Pereira, A., Martinho, C., Leite, I., Paiva, A.: iCat, the chess player: the influence of embodiment in the enjoyment of a game. In: Proceedings of the 7th International Joint Conference on Autonomous Agents and Multiagent Systems, vol. 3. pp. 1253–1256. IFAAMS (2008)
14. Pereira, A., Prada, R., Paiva, A.: Socially present board game opponents. In: Nijholt, A., Romão, T., Reidsma, D. (eds.) ACE 2012. LNCS, vol. 7624, pp. 101–116. Springer, Heidelberg (2012). doi:10.1007/978-3-642-34292-9_8
15. Ring, L., Shi, L., Totzke, K., Bickmore, T.: Social support agents for older adults: longitudinal affective computing in the home. J. Multimodal User Interfaces 9(1), 79–88 (2015)

16. Sajó, L., Ruttkay, Z., Fazekas, A.: Turk-2, a multi-modal chess player. Int. J. Hum Comput Stud. **69**(7–8), 483–495 (2011)
17. Schiffel, S., Thielscher, M.: Fluxplayer: a successful general game player. Proc. Natl. Conf. Artif. Intell. **22**(2), 1191 (2007)
18. Schreiber, S., Landau, A.: The general game playing base package (2016). https://github.com/ggp-org/ggp-base

Exploring the Impact of Environmental Effects on Social Presence with a Virtual Human

Kangsoo Kim[1(✉)], Ryan Schubert[1,2], and Greg Welch[1,2]

[1] The University of Central Florida, Orlando, FL, USA
kskim@knights.ucf.edu, res@cs.unc.edu, welch@ucf.edu
[2] The University of North Carolina at Chapel Hill, Chapel Hill, NC, USA

Abstract. We explore how and in what ways the surrounding environment can be an important factor in human perception during interactions with virtual humans. We also seek to leverage any such knowledge to increase the sense of Social/Co-Presence with virtual humans. We conducted a user study to explore the influence of environmental events on social interaction between real and virtual humans in a Mixed Reality setting. Specifically we tested two different treatments to see the effects on Social/Co-Presence: (i) enhanced physical-virtual connectivity/influence via a *real* fan blowing on *virtual* paper, and (ii) the virtual human's corresponding *awareness* of the environmental factor as she looks at the fan and holds the fluttering paper. While a statistical analysis for the study did not support the positive effects of the two treatments, we have developed some new insights that could be useful for future studies involving virtual humans.

Keywords: Virtual humans · Social Presence · Co-Presence · Physical-virtual connectivity · Environment-Aware Behaviors · Plausibility

1 Introduction

One's sense of *Social/Co-Presence (So/Co-Pres)* with a virtual human has been considered as an important measure of how the virtual human is perceived. The concepts of Co-Presence and Social Presence could be described as how one perceives the other's presence as a sense of "being together," and how much they feel "socially connected," respectively. Harms and Biocca considered Co-Presence as one of several sub-dimensions that embody Social Presence [3], and Blascovich et al. defined Social Presence as a "psychological state in which the individual perceives himself or herself as existing within an **interpersonal environment**" (bold added) [2]. In a broad sense of Presence, Slater introduced an important concept, called *Plausibility Illusion (Psi)*. Psi "refers to the illusion that the scenario being depicted is **actually occurring**," that "requires a credible scenario and plausible interactions between the participant and objects and virtual characters **in the environment**" (bold added) [5]. Considering the definitions addressed above, we expect that the plausibility of the context and

© Springer International Publishing AG 2016
D. Traum et al. (Eds.): IVA 2016, LNAI 10011, pp. 470–474, 2016.
DOI: 10.1007/978-3-319-47665-0_57

the surrounding environment where the social interaction takes place could be important factors in the resulting sense of So/Co-Pres with virtual humans.

In this paper, we discuss an experiment aimed at investigating the effects of the following possible influences on So/Co-Pres with a virtual human in a mixed reality (MR) environment: (i) the enhanced physical-virtual connectivity via environmental objects—a physical fan and a virtual fluttering paper, and (ii) the virtual human's awareness of them. The results did not show statistically significant effects on the sense of So/Co-Pres in terms of the influences, but we developed some insights that could be useful for future studies involving virtual humans.

2 Preliminary Experiment

We designed a between-subjects study with three different groups: (i) Control, (ii) Physical-to-Virtual Influence (PVI), and (iii) Environment-Aware Behavior (EAB). For all groups, participants had a conversational interaction (a simple practice job interview) with a virtual human in a mixed reality environment—the virtual human was rear-projected on a screen. For the PVI group, a virtual paper on the table in front of the virtual human appeared to flutter as a result of the physical fan that was located next to the participant during the interaction. The physical fan blowing the virtual paper was chosen as a subtle environmental event to strengthen the connection between physical and virtual spaces, and potentially influence the sense of So/Co-Pres. In the EAB group, the virtual human would additionally occasionally exhibit attention toward the fan's effects by looking at it or holding the virtual paper to stop the fluttering. For the Control group, the paper did not flutter and the virtual human never demonstrated any awareness of the physical fan. The three groups are briefly described in Fig. 1. We hypothesized that the level of So/Co-Pres for each group would be different, e.g., Control $\ll$ PVI $<$ EAB. We expected the virtual human's gaze direction changes and paper-holding gesture might be less significantly influential as compared to the fluttering paper. 31 undergraduate/graduate students (Control: 10, PVI: 10, and EAB: 11; 9 females and 22 males; mean age: 22.35, SD: 3.36, range: 18–29) were paid 15 USD for participating in the study. To measure the participants' sense of So/Co-Pres, we used two different Social Presence questionnaire sets from Bailenson et al. [1] and Harms and Biocca [3] (7-level Likert-scale).

3 Results and Discussion

A previous experiment examined whether the sense of So/Co-Pres could be increased by a peripheral environmental object, a "Wobbly Table" [4]. In that experiment, a visually aligned wobbly table spanning a physical-virtual environment, in which a real human and a virtual human could sit across from each other, was used as a subtle environmental event. In this study, we were curious whether just observing the fluttering virtual paper—a much less direct experience than the "Wobbly Table"—would still have an impact on So/Co-Pres.

Group	Physical Fan	Virtual Paper Fluttering	Virtual Human's Awareness Behavior
Control	ON	NO	NO
PVI	ON	YES	NO
EAB	ON	YES	YES

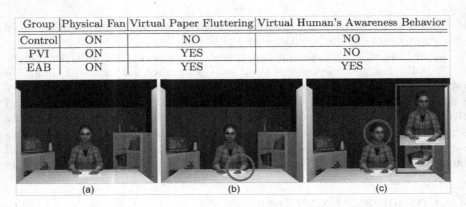

Fig. 1. Experimental groups. (a) Control, (b) PVI (red circle: fluttering virtual paper), and (c) EAB (blue circle: looking at the fan, blue rectangle: holding the paper gesture). (Color figure online)

We had expected to see positive effects on So/Co-Pres for the PVI and EAB groups; however, the results did not show any supporting evidence. While there were slight differences, no statistically significant differences were observed in either Social Presence questionnaire among the three groups (One-way ANOVA; $F(2, 28) = 0.590$, $p = 0.561$ for Bailenson's Social Presence and $F(2, 28) = 0.426$, $p = 0.657$ for Harms and Biocca's Social Presence in Fig. 2). Based on brief discussions with participants after the study, we have some possible explanations for the lack of significant differences.

GROUP	Mean	SD	N
CONTROL	4.780	0.520	10
PVI	4.560	0.759	10
EAB	4.891	0.797	11

(Bailenson et al.'s Social Presence)

GROUP	Mean	SD	N
CONTROL	5.111	0.635	10
PVI	4.922	0.386	10
EAB	4.939	0.477	11

(Harms and Biocca's Social Presence)

Fig. 2. Descriptives for Social Presence responses.

Ignorance of Fan/Paper. We had wanted our fluttering virtual paper and fan wind to be peripheral (not central) to the experience, but they may have been *too* subtle—many participants were not consciously aware of the effects. Even those who were conscious of the effects seemed to pay little or no attention to them. Furthermore, based on discussion with the participants, our job interview scenario may have encouraged participants to narrowly focus on the virtual human, thus minimizing the potential influence of any environmental effects. Similarly, it seems that the novelty of the virtual human could have exacerbated the inattention to the environment and related effects.

Physical-Virtual Connectivity. We had originally considered the *absence* of movement of paper as *implausible* in the presence of the fan, and intended to use that implausibility to measure the effect of the physical-virtual effect (real fan affecting virtual paper). However in retrospect we realize that non-movement of the paper is entirely *plausible*—the fan might or might not affect paper on a nearby table, and therefore the treatment was potentially ineffectual for our intended purpose. In other words, none of the groups (Control, PVI, and EAB) might have seen anything "wrong" with the paper's behavior.

Environment-Aware Behaviors. Compared to the direct involvement of the human participant in the wobbly table movement [4], the fluttering virtual paper and fan wind were unrelated to the participant's actions. This could have made the virtual human's reactive nonverbal behaviors to the fan/paper irrelevant to the participants, counter to what we intended, and could have contributed to the lack of a positive association with So/Co-Pres in this setup. If the virtual human's awareness behaviors *were* a direct response to the real human's actions, or if the awareness was temporarily made central to the conversation, there could be an increase in So/Co-Pres. In fact, based on user comments, the fact that the virtual human did *not* change the conversation in any way related to the effects was perhaps implausible, emphasizing a perceived autonomous nature of the virtual human, and thereby negatively effecting So/Co-Pres.

Experimental Measures. In attempting to understand why we did not see the expected effects, we came to realize that existing Social Presence questionnaires do not currently consider the aspects of the surrounding environment where the social interaction takes place but rather they mainly focus on the interactivity/connectivity between two or more interlocutors. Given that several definitions of So/Co-Pres indicate that the environmental aspects could be important, adding questions about the environment (or more generally the social context) could potentially provide a more accurate measure.

4   Conclusions

We conducted a user study investigating the effects of the environment and virtual human awareness of the environment on So/Co-Pres. Despite the lack of significant results, we obtained some insights from the study, which could be useful for designing more effective virtual humans or related studies. Given that we still believe the environment and awareness behaviors of the environment can increase So/Co-Pres with virtual humans, we will keep exploring the related effects. As a next step, we will consider more appropriate interaction scenarios and (im)plausible treatments that could encourage noticeable effects. Also, we are planning to run a conceptually similar study in an augmented reality setting, where the real and virtual are "equalized" (less distinct).

Acknowledgments. The work presented in this publication is supported primarily by the Office of Naval Research (ONR) Code 30 under Dr. Peter Squire, Program Officer

(ONR awards N00014-14-1-0248 and N00014-12-1-1003). The authors would like to thank the members of the SREAL, UCF including Salam Daher, Jason Hochreiter, Eric Imperiale, Myungho Lee, Dr. Andrew Raij.

References

1. Bailenson, J.N., Blascovich, J., Beall, A.C., Loomis, J.M.: Interpersonal distance in immersive virtual environments. Pers. Soc. Psychol. Bull. **29**(7), 819–833 (2003)
2. Blascovich, J.: Social influence within immersive virtual environments. In: Schroeder, R. (ed.) The Social Life of Avatars. Computer Supported Cooperative Work, pp. 127–145. Springer, London (2002)
3. Harms, C., Biocca, F.: Internal consistency and reliability of the networked minds measure of social presence. In: Annual International Presence Workshop, pp. 246–251 (2004)
4. Lee, M., Kim, K., Daher, S., Raij, A., Schubert, R., Bailenson, J., Welch, G.: The wobbly table: increased social presence via subtle incidental movement of a real-virtual table. In: Proceedings of IEEE Virtual Reality, pp. 11–17 (2016)
5. Slater, M.: Place illusion and plausibility can lead to realistic behaviour in immersive virtual environments. Philos. Trans. Roy. Soc. Lond. Ser. B Biol. Sci. **364**(1535), 3549–3557 (2009)

A Distributed Intelligent Agent Approach to Context in Information Retrieval

Reginald L. Hobbs[(✉)]

Army Research Laboratory, Adelphi, MD, USA
reginald.l.hobbs2.civ@mail.mil

Abstract. Information retrieval across disadvantaged networks requires intelligent agents that can make decisions about what to transmit in such a way as to minimize network performance impact while maximizing utility and quality of information (QOI). Specialized agents at the source need to process unstructured, ad-hoc queries, identifying both the context and the intent to determine the implied task. Knowing the task will allow the distributed agents that service the requests to filter, summarize, or transcode data prior to responding, lessening the network impact. This paper describes an approach that uses natural language processing (NLP) techniques, multi-valued logic based inferencing, distributed intelligent agents, and task-relevant metrics for information retrieval.

Keywords: Intelligent agents · Natural language processing · Fuzzy logic · Quality of information

1 Introduction

Network science focuses on complex networks, studying the relationships between social networks and communications networks, as well as the information networks that overlay them. [2] Disadvantaged networks, with constraints on bandwidth, topology, connectivity, and otherwise limited network resources, have additional challenges in comparison to commercial networks.

This paper describes an approach that uses natural language processing (NLP) techniques, multi-valued logic based inferencing, network status checking, and task-relevant metrics to deal with information retrieval challenges for disadvantaged networks. We designed, implemented, and conducted experiments with distributed intelligent agents to show the efficacy of this approach for making quality assessments that kept network performance at optimum levels.

2 Method

Our approach was to modify the information nodes into task-aware intelligent agents, distributed across the network, which can infer the appropriate quality in response to queries. These agents would need to be more than reactive agents, which automatically send responses based on physical measurements, thresholds, or triggers. We selected a

© Springer International Publishing AG 2016
D. Traum et al. (Eds.): IVA 2016, LNAI 10011, pp. 475–478, 2016.
DOI: 10.1007/978-3-319-47665-0_58

multi-valued, fuzzy logic approach because of the need to apply a graduated scale of assessments on quality, depending on differing tasks and network conditions. In a distributed agent environment, it is efficient to separate the types of intelligent agents that provide services and collaborate on user tasks. Sycara et al. organized their framework into agents that interact with the user, agents that perform tasks, and agents that provide access to information sources. [5] Our experimental network contained two types of intelligent agents attached to information nodes: resolver agents and responder agents. *Resolver* agents are responsible for processing the incoming unstructured query from the user and, using the inferencing rules within its knowledge base, determine the task that is implied. *Responder* agents are responsible for transmitting information across the network in response to an incoming task from another information node.

Unstructured text as input is usually handled by keyword searches or query expansion using lexical resources (vocabularies, word banks, databases, etc.). These "bag-of-words" approaches lose some of the context of the original query, for example that which could be derived through word order. Another issue is that sometimes the literal meaning of the words doesn't reflect the underlying intent of the question. A technique called example-based NLP (EBNLP) has been used in machine translation (MT), to improve the accuracy and precision when dealing with unstructured, non-standard text. A bilingual corpus of data is used to extract examples, consisting of sentences and their corresponding parses, to handle complicated linguistic phenomena such as polysemy and unique idiomatic phrases that don't have literal translation. As described by Sumita [4], this technique was very effective for improving the accuracy for English-to-Japanese MT engines, but required a large corpus of training data. In our EBNLP algorithm, we create exemplar sentences for each task and then compare the input sentence against a list of example sentences, organized by task. The sentences are compared lexically (word for word) and structurally (by part of speech).

Comparing the sentences structurally required a part-of-speech (POS) tagger. In this instance, the POS tagger used the Penn Treebank, a widely used lexical resource, to assign tags to English text. [6] The tagger applies a bigram (two-word) hidden Markov model to assign probabilities to the appropriate POS tags for a word. Given both the lexical and structural information available in tagged sentences, a text similarity algorithm was used to compare the string to the exemplars. Text similarity is a technique for quantifying the sameness between strings. Text similarity was computed by searching for literal word token overlaps. [3] It was important to determine the number of word tokens that are identical between the two strings, as well as calculate other metrics, such as number of shared words, phrasal matches, edit distance, and relative string length.

Much of the existing work with quality of information (QOI) methods for data transmission focuses on optimizing intrinsic quality attributes or measurable network states such as bandwidth, latency, fan out, number of concurrent users, or other resource utilization costs. Task-aware extrinsic features that change based on context needed to be incorporated into an overall quality metric. A fuzzy logic engine was used to quantify and combine the attributes into one overall quality metric. There were two intrinsic attributes (*bandwidth level* and *improvement*) and one extrinsic attribute (*responsiveness*). *Improvement* and *responsiveness* attributes are derived from mapping functions that use object size, while *bandwidth level* is a directly measured quantity. The resulting QOI quality metric is a combination of all three attributes.

The information objects being retrieved across the networks were images with embedded metadata. Generally, image data transmission has a more significant network impact than document retrieval, unless the number of documents being retrieved is very large. The images were retrieved using embedded metadata in the images, such information as description, caption, time stamp, camera focal length, longitude, latitude, description, caption, orientation (rotation), x-resolution, y-resolution, and numerous other generated or manually entered attributes.

Determining the appropriate quality to send was based on the choice from transcoded images, which were variants of the original image. These transcoded options were preprocessed, minimizing latency due to image processing time. This assumption would coincide with a standard operating procedure that required the phone automatically create the transcoded versions upon taking a photograph, to speed up quality functions. Among the transcoded options were: original, compressed, reduced resolution, grayscale, monochrome, and thumbnail.

The distributed agent framework was evaluated in an experiment using simulated network traffic. The purpose of the experiment was to use the quality metric to establish a baseline for image retrieval across a disadvantaged network with fluctuating bandwidth in order to gauge the quality improvement given agent-based assessments of what to send. There were three possible tasks that could be performed based on the requested image data: identification, detection, and inventory. An example text string for each type of query task was selected for input to the resolver agent. Dynamic network traffic was simulated using a sine wave.

3   Results

The results for the identification task are shown in Fig. 1. The Y-axis on the left depicts the available bandwidth on a scale of 0 to 200 KBps. The Y-axis on the right shows the predicted quality metric value on a scale of 0 to 10. The X-axis shows the experiment

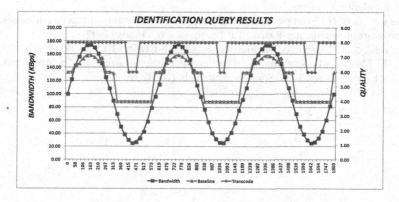

Fig. 1. Experimental results for identification task

duration, in seconds, and also indicates the time step of the sampling points. The red line is the bandwidth. The green line on the chart is the baseline condition, when there is no quality assessment of the images prior to transmission. In that situation, all the original images in the result set are sent. The purple line is the experimental condition, where the responder agent uses QOI assessments to determine the transcoded option.

The quality values distribution of the experimental runs for the detection and inventory task are similar to this example, but not nearly as high, because the result sets are moderate to very large in size, respectively. Over all task categories, there is a significant improvement in quality, approximately 25 % with respect to the baseline.

4 Conclusion

This paper described an approach that used NLP techniques, intelligent agents, multi-valued logic based inferencing, network monitoring, and task-aware metrics for information retrieval. We successfully defined and validated a quality metric based on intrinsic and extrinsic quality attributes. Through the use of a simplified technique, example-based NLP, we were able to use text similarity to capture intent from unstructured queries. Distributed intelligent agents used fuzzy logic inferencing to identify tasks and to determine what form of information object to retrieve. The experiment with this QOI agent framework showed the efficacy of this approach for making quality assessments that kept network performance at optimum levels.

References

1. Coburn, A.: Lingua::EN::Tagger: Part-of-speech tagger for English NLP (2003). https://metacpan.org/pod/Lingua::EN::Tagger
2. National Research Council (U.S.). Committee on Network Science for Future Army Applications. Network Science. National Research Council of the National Academies. National Academies Press, Washington, D.C (2005)
3. Pedersen, T.: Text::Similarity::Overlaps - Score the Overlaps Found Between Two Strings Based on Literal Text Matching, 25 June 2013. https://metacpan.org/pod/Text::Similarity::Overlaps
4. Sumita, E., Iida, H.: Example-based NLP techniques-a case study of machine translation. In: Proceedings of Statistically-Based NLP Techniques Workshop (1992)
5. Sycara, K., et al.: Distributed intelligent agents. IEEE Expert 11(6), 36–46 (1996)
6. Ann, T., Marcus, M., Santorini, B.: The Penn treebank: an overview. In: Abeillé, A. (ed.) Treebanks, vol. 20, pp. 5–22. Springer, Dordrecht (2003)

Composing the Atmosphere of a Virtual Classroom with a Group of Student Agents

Masato Fukuda, Hung-Hsuan Huang(⊠), Naoki Ohta, and Kazuhiro Kuwabara

College of Information Science and Engineering,
Ritsumeikan University, Kusatsu, Japan
hhhuang@acm.org

1 Introduction

In Japan, the training of teachers mainly relies on in-classroom lectures in universities. It is compensated with the practice for a relatively short period, say only two to three weeks in real schools. The teacher-training programs in Japan therefore lacks the practice of teaching skills and the admission of classes. The result is, many young teachers left their jobs in the first year due to frustration and other mental issues. In order to relieve this situation, we are developing a Wizard-of-OZ (WOZ) based simulation platform of a school environment with computer graphics (CG) animated virtual students. The trainees can interact with the virtual students in this immersive and realistic virtual classroom and practice their teaching and administration skills. The virtual students are operated by an operator (the wizard) from remote with a dedicated interface. In addition to the training purpose, the system is considered to be able to be used in the examination of teacher recruitment as well. In that case, the operator is supposed to be the examination investigator.

On the other hand, there are usually dozens of students in a high school class in Japan. In a WOZ system that is operated by one or few people, how to simultaneously control the relatively large number of students can be a challenge. A research issue emerges here, how to effectively control a group of virtual students to represent a realistic class in a real-time WOZ system. In this paper, we propose an atmosphere model of a group of virtual students based on empirical results as a solution to this issue.

2 Related Works

Virtual environments have also been shown to be an effective tool for various training tasks. Jones et al. [2] developed a job interview simulation platform, which supports social training and coaching in the context of job interviews. Williamon et al. [5] designed and tested the efficacy of simulated performance environments as a new training facility for musician trainees. Kenny et al. [3] designed the training systems of mental therapeutic with virtual simulated patients.

© Springer International Publishing AG 2016
D. Traum et al. (Eds.): IVA 2016, LNAI 10011, pp. 479–483, 2016.
DOI: 10.1007/978-3-319-47665-0_59

On the other hand, few studies have focused on the training system of teachers in virtual environment. TechLive [1] is one of the examples. This application is also a VR simulated classroom with operator(s). In this system, one operator can only control one of the virtual students by selecting pre-defined animation sequences or driving it with a motion capture device in real-time. There are no severe issues in the US where the number of students in a class is small. However, due to more limited resources, the number of students in one class is much larger in Japan. How to efficiently and realistically control dozens of students at the same time is not a trivial problem. Our work addresses this by proposing an atmosphere model that is described in the following sections.

3   Atmosphere Model of the Virtual Classroom WOZ System

This WOZ system is composed of two front ends, one is a simulated classroom for the trainee, the other one is the interface for the system operator/investigator. The expected usage of the system is: the trainee front end is projected on a large screen (say 100 in. or even larger) while the trainee stands in front of the screen and practice his/her teaching skill. The trainee's teaching is captured by a Web cam and is displayed at the operator's interface (see the virtual class from the rear side) in real-time. The operator then control the virtual students while observing the trainee's teaching performance.

We divided the control of virtual students into two modes, *individual* mode and *whole-class* mode. When the operator choose an arbitrary student, that student will shift to the individual mode and then the operator can fully control that student manually. By default, all virtual students are in the whole-class mode and are controlled by an atmosphere model. The atmosphere model serves as a template and all the virtual students together create the atmosphere of their group. This atmosphere is supposed to be the feedback sent from the operator to the trainee. The trainee can then adopt his/her teaching style in responding to the atmosphere. The class atmosphere is model is defined to be driven by three elements, *concentration, arousal, tension* which are inspired from the pleasure-arousal-dominance (PAD) model [4] of an individual's emotional state. The CAT space is defined as the follows:

Concentration: How much the students are concentrating on the lecture. How well the trainee is explaining important topics of the lecture.
Arousal: The activity level of the students. How well the trainee is keeping the interest of the students.
Tension: The level of the tension of the students. How well the trainee is maintaining the order of the class.

The idea is: the values of these parameters have the effect in the possibility of the virtual students to express corresponding behaviors. For example, in a low-concentration, low-arousal, and low-tension situation, many of the virtual students may show sleepy animation, while in a high-concentration, high-arousal, and medium-tension situation, the virtual students may concentrate in the lecture, take memos, nodding frequently and so on. However, another research issue emerges here, how to determine the actual behaviors of the virtual students in the various CAT state? The perception and interpretation from student behaviors to the atmosphere of the whole class is subjective and heavily depends on the experience in education of the observer. Therefore, we conducted a subject experiment to gather the interpretation from unspecified people and hopefully in large number.

4   Data Collection Experiment and Conclusions

A dedicated interface of the virtual classroom was developed the experiment (Fig. 1). Although the value of the CAT dimensions can be arbitrary, we assume that if we can get the parameters of the maximum and the minimum of each axis, the arbitrary intermediate values can be interpolated from them. We recruited 12 participants for the experiment, three of them are professors and nine of them are students of our university. Among these students, three of them are receiving teacher-training course provided by our university.

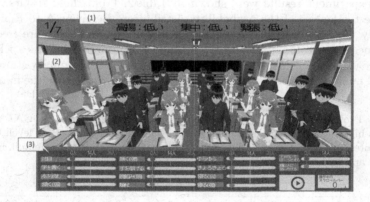

Fig. 1. Interface dedicated for experiment participants to compose the atmosphere in CAT states. (1) the area indicating the CAT state that the participant should compose (2) the virtual students showing the behaviors selected by the participant (3) the dashboard where the participant adjusts the number of students performing each behavior with scroll bars

The participants were asked to compose the atmosphere of the class according to the specified CAT states one by one. They adjust the number of virtual students who is performing one of 15 implemented behaviors (Table 1) with scroll bars. The number of students ($x_{k,i}$) assigned with a specific behavior k by all participants (i from 1 to n) in each state is then used to compute the

Table 1. Student behaviors used in the experiment with their corresponding code names

Code	Behavior	Code	Behavior
A	Look at the teacher	H	Make chin rest on hands
B	Write something on a note	I	Swing upper body slightly
C	Read text book	J	Look around
D	Nod	K	Doze
E	Nod strongly	L	Sleep with face downward to the desk
F	Raise right hand	M	Out of it
G	Cross hands behind head	N	Whisper

probability (P_k) of a virtual student to perform behavior k in that state by the following equation. Here N denotes the total number of virtual students (28 in current implementation).

$$P_k = \frac{1}{N}\{\frac{1}{n}\sum_{i=1}^{n} x_{k,i}\} \tag{1}$$

The experiment results were shown in Table 2. From these results, we can find some tendencies of the probability distribution. Behavior A to F are more frequently used in positive states and the remaining ones are more frequently used in negative states. Behavior A, B, and E are dominating ones while the others are used as accents. The results are still in a very preliminary state due to the small number of experiment participants. We plan to increase the number by

Table 2. Probability of each student behavior in each characteristic CAT state. h denotes a high level while m denotes medium level, and l denotes a low level. Column A–N denotes the behavior code listed in Table 1 while "–" denotes default behavior (sit down and look forward)

	A	B	C	D	E	F	G	H	I	J	K	L	M	N	–
$C_h A_h T_h$	0.14	0.20	0.04	0.05	0.40	0.11	0.00	0.00	0.00	0.01	0.00	0.00	0.00	0.00	0.05
$C_l A_l T_l$	0.00	0.00	0.01	0.03	0.04	0.02	0.09	0.12	0.04	0.09	0.10	0.28	0.09	0.08	0.01
$C_h A_h T_l$	0.32	0.17	0.03	0.07	0.14	0.13	0.02	0.02	0.00	0.03	0.05	0.00	0.01	0.02	0.00
$C_h A_l T_h$	0.20	0.08	0.04	0.06	0.06	0.10	0.03	0.03	0.10	0.04	0.04	0.02	0.05	0.08	0.07
$C_l A_h T_h$	0.49	0.10	0.03	0.05	0.14	0.00	0.04	0.00	0.01	0.00	0.04	0.05	0.00	0.01	0.04
$C_h A_h T_m$	0.43	0.10	0.06	0.06	0.19	0.05	0.00	0.04	0.02	0.00	0.01	0.00	0.00	0.00	0.04
$C_h A_m T_h$	0.27	0.09	0.03	0.08	0.16	0.08	0.00	0.00	0.11	0.04	0.02	0.00	0.04	0.05	0.03
$C_m A_h T_h$	0.44	0.10	0.03	0.13	0.04	0.05	0.00	0.00	0.01	0.02	0.00	0.00	0.00	0.01	0.17
$C_l A_l T_m$	0.07	0.01	0.04	0.02	0.00	0.00	0.07	0.15	0.14	0.14	0.17	0.03	0.07	0.04	0.05
$C_l A_m T_l$	0.06	0.08	0.06	0.00	0.00	0.00	0.04	0.12	0.02	0.05	0.10	0.15	0.14	0.09	0.09
$C_m A_l T_l$	0.01	0.02	0.03	0.02	0.00	0.02	0.03	0.13	0.12	0.13	0.05	0.07	0.15	0.21	0.01
$C_h A_l T_l$	0.04	0.06	0.04	0.00	0.03	0.11	0.00	0.01	0.16	0.19	0.03	0.00	0.09	0.24	0.00
$C_l A_h T_l$	0.31	0.12	0.22	0.11	0.01	0.02	0.00	0.07	0.02	0.00	0.02	0.02	0.02	0.00	0.06
$C_l A_l T_h$	0.23	0.05	0.07	0.10	0.02	0.04	0.00	0.07	0.05	0.04	0.13	0.04	0.04	0.05	0.07

recruiting the participants from crowdsourcing services. After gathering reliable enough results, we will conduct further analyses and integrate the model to the WOZ prototype system

References

1. Barmaki, R., Hughes, C.E.: Providing real-time feedback for student teachers in a virtual rehearsal environment. In: 17th International Conference on Multimodal Interaction (ICMI 2015), pp. 531–537, November 2015
2. Jones, H., Sabouret, N., Damian, I., Baur, T., Andrre, E., Porayska-Pomsta, K., Rizzo, P., Interpreting social cues to generate credible affective reactions of virtual job interviewers. arXiv:1402.5039v2 (2014)
3. Kenny, P., Parsons, T.D., Gratch, J., Leuski, A., Rizzo, A.A.: Virtual patients for clinical therapist skills training. In: Pelachaud, C., Martin, J.-C., André, E., Chollet, G., Karpouzis, K., Pelé, D. (eds.) IVA 2007. LNCS (LNAI), vol. 4722, pp. 197–210. Springer, Heidelberg (2007). doi:10.1007/978-3-540-74997-4_19
4. Mehrabian, A.: Pleasure-arousal-dominance: a general framework for describing and measuring individual differences in temperament. Curr. Psychol. 14(4), 261–292 (1996)
5. Williamon, A., Aufegger, L., Eiholzer, H.: Simulating and stimulating performance: introducing distributed simulation to enhance learning and performance. Front. Psychol. 5(25), 1–9 (2014)

Assessing Agreement in Human-Robot Dialogue Strategies: A Tale of Two Wizards

Matthew Marge[1]([✉]), Claire Bonial[1], Kimberly A. Pollard[1], Ron Artstein[2],
Brendan Byrne[1], Susan G. Hill[1], Clare Voss[1], and David Traum[2]

[1] U.S. Army Research Laboratory, Adelphi, MD 20783, USA
matthew.r.marge.civ@mail.mil
[2] USC Institute for Creative Technologies, Playa Vista, CA 90094, USA

Abstract. The Wizard-of-Oz (WOz) method is a common experimental technique in virtual agent and human-robot dialogue research for eliciting natural communicative behavior from human partners when full autonomy is not yet possible. For the first phase of our research reported here, wizards play the role of dialogue manager, acting as a robot's dialogue processing. We describe a novel step within WOz methodology that incorporates two wizards and *control sessions:* the wizards function much like corpus annotators, being asked to make independent judgments on how the robot should respond when receiving the same verbal commands in separate trials. We show that inter-wizard discussion after the control sessions and the resolution with a reconciled protocol for the follow-on pilot sessions successfully impacts wizard behaviors and significantly aligns their strategies. We conclude that, without control sessions, we would have been unlikely to achieve both the natural diversity of expression that comes with multiple wizards and a better protocol for modeling an automated system.

Keywords: Natural language dialogue · Human-robot communication

1 Introduction

Providing dialogue capabilities to robots will enable them to become effective teammates with humans in many collaborative tasks, such as search-and-rescue operations and reconnaissance. We propose a multi-phase plan to achieve the goal of fully automated, natural communication between humans and robots, leveraging recent advances in virtual agent dialogue. In the first phase, we conduct exploratory data collection in tasks where naïve humans provide spoken instructions to a robot, but a wizard experimenter stands in for the robot's communications intelligence. The wizard may use free response to reply to the spoken dialogue commands, but does so only in text form through a chat window. A second phase automates some of the wizard labor, where instead of free response, the wizard uses an interface that generalizes command handling and response generation based on dialogue observed in the first phase. In a third, final

© Springer International Publishing AG 2016
D. Traum et al. (Eds.): IVA 2016, LNAI 10011, pp. 484–488, 2016.
DOI: 10.1007/978-3-319-47665-0_60

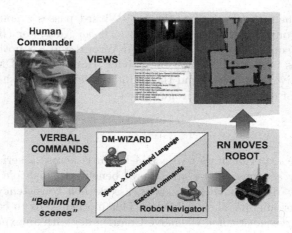

Fig. 1. Wizard-of-Oz setup with a wizard substituting for dialogue management.

phase, the wizard will be "automated away" with a dialogue manager trained from second-phase wizard decisions with the specialized interface. Our approach resembles that taken with the virtual agent SimSensei [1].

This paper focuses on research from the first phase, where we explore how best to encourage natural diversity in communication strategies used by the naïve human, while imposing some guidelines for consistent strategies in the wizard's communications so that dialogue processing is tractable but also natural. We present findings from conducting *control sessions*, a novel contribution to the Wizard-of-Oz methodology that turns the focus of experimentation to the wizard. We explore the possible diversity in communicative strategies for two individuals playing the wizard role. All other aspects of the interaction, such as the experimenters and environment context, are held constant.

2   Collaborative Exploration Domain

The domain testbed for our work is collaborative exploration in a low-bandwidth environment [2]. A robot can move around and explore a physical space, remote from a human collaborator. The human *Commander* has specific goals for the exploration, such as locating doors or types of objects in the physical space, but is unable to directly act in or observe this environment. The robot builds a LIDAR map of the area as it moves, and can send verbal descriptions of the environment and can take and send occasional photos, but the bandwidth of communication is too limited to allow a real-time video feed or direct teleoperation of the robot.

In order to bootstrap the robot's conceived capabilities of automated language processing and navigation, we employ the Wizard-of-Oz method. Figure 1 presents our first-phase setup. A *Dialogue Manager* (DM-Wizard) listens to the Commander's speech, and decides whether to prompt for clarification. If deemed executable in the current context, the DM-Wizard passes a constrained, text version of the Commander's instruction to the *Robot Navigator* (RN), an experimenter who teleoperates the robot. The DM-Wizard and RN both see the same map and photos requested by the Commander. However, the DM-Wizard and RN also see a live video feed from the robot to facilitate the shared, accurate understanding of the robot's environment.

3   Method

We trained two experimenters to be DM-Wizards across a series of pre-pilot and pilot study sessions. There are several benefits to multiple DM-Wizards: we can collect variation in their decisions, assess their consistency, and identify opportunities for aligning their behavior. This motivated us to conduct *control sessions*, where we substituted the naïve Commander with an experimenter who communicated a pre-defined list of about 70 navigational commands to each DM-Wizard in separate trials, many of which were problematic and unseen in past data collection.

To analyze the variation in the DM-Wizards' responses, each message from the DM-Wizard to the Commander in the control sessions was annotated with *dialogue-moves:* the types of actions available to the DM-Wizard in the communication protocol [4]. Validation of the set of dialogue-moves was performed on two dialogues (99 DM to Commander messages), annotated independently by the first three authors, with up to three dialogue-moves per message. We calculated agreement using Krippendorf's α with the MASI distance metric [3], which allows for partial agreement between sets. Agreement between all three annotators was high ($\alpha = 0.92$).

4   Results

We analyzed the decisions made by DM-Wizards by tabulating frequencies of dialogue-moves for messages from the DM-Wizard to the Commander, summarized in Table 1.

Control Sessions. We observe some marked differences in strategies taken by the wizards: Half of DM-Wizard1's dialogue-moves provided *feedback*, compared to only a third for DM-Wizard2. Feedback is defined broadly as dialogue-moves that acknowledge a Commander's conversational move or an action (often completion of a request). For example, DM-Wizard1 used the feedback SENT, indicating each time that a requested photo was sent to the Commander. Meanwhile, DM-Wizard2 used more *describe* moves: general statements detailing the situation, including the environment, plans, or actions. Describe moves constituted 41 % of DM-Wizard2's dialogue-moves, compared to 24 % for DM-Wizard1. These results suggest that DM-Wizard1 took a strategy of actively providing feedback, while DM-Wizard2 echoed back situations and plans. Proportions of *clarify* and *request-info* dialogue-moves were predictably similar given that both DM-Wizards faced the same number of problematic instructions.

Table 1. DM-Wizard dialogue-moves to the Commander for control and subsequent pilots.

	Control		Pilot	
	W1	W2	W1	W2
Clarify	13 %	13 %	14 %	9 %
Describe	24 %	41 %	18 %	29 %
Feedback	50 %	33 %	59 %	48 %
Request-info	13 %	13 %	9 %	14 %
Total moves	127	157	144	144

Post-control Adjudication. After both DM-Wizards had completed the control session, they met to discuss the results. Many of the challenging commands given in the control sessions revealed a lack of complete and shared understanding of the robot's capabilities and how requests for help from the robot should be handled. This discussion session also revealed that the basic strategies taken by DM-Wizards could be generalized: the DM-Wizards agreed that providing simpler *feedback*-type evidence of the robot's status was more efficient than using more detailed *describe* moves.

Post-control Pilot Sessions. DM-Wizard decisions following the final two pilots, conducted after the control sessions, indicate improved agreement (see Table 1). As a direct result of adjudication, both DM-Wizards used a greater count of *feedback* and in a greater proportion of their dialogue-moves. In particular, status updates such as DONE and SENT experienced an increase from control to post-control pilot session. Notably, other DM-Wizard behaviors did not seem to be affected by the control sessions and ensuing discussion and guideline updates. This indicates that the control sessions facilitated a "surgical strike," precisely changing only extremely divergent behaviors.

5   Conclusion

The Wizard-of-Oz (WOz) method is useful for eliciting natural human communication and readily permits variation based on the individual playing the wizard role. In this research, the wizard operates as the robot's dialogue processing, typing responses and clarifications to a human Commander for the purpose of exploratory data collection. We introduced *control sessions*, a novel contribution to WOz methodology that supports multiple wizards. Discussions between the wizards after the control sessions successfully impacted their behaviors and aligned their strategies. Without control sessions, we would have been unlikely to achieve both the natural diversity of expression that comes with multiple wizards and a better protocol for modeling an automated system.

Acknowledgments. The effort described here is supported by the U.S. Army. Any opinion, content or information presented does not necessarily reflect the position or the policy of the United States Government, and no official endorsement should be inferred.

References

1. DeVault, D., Artstein, R., Benn, G., Dey, T., Fast, E., Gainer, A., Georgila, K., Gratch, J., Hartholt, A., Lhommet, M., et al.: SimSensei Kiosk: a virtual human interviewer for healthcare decision support. In: Proceedings of AAMAS (2014)
2. Marge, M., Bonial, C., Byrne, B., Cassidy, T., Evans, A.W., Hill, S.G., Voss, C.: Applying the Wizard-of-Oz technique to multimodal human-robot dialogue. In: Proceedings of RO-MAN (2016)
3. Passonneau, R.: Measuring agreement on set-valued items (MASI) for semantic and pragmatic annotation. In: Proceedings of LREC (2006)
4. Roque, A., Leuski, A., Rangarajan, V., Robinson, S., Vaswani, A., Narayanan, S., Traum, D.: Radiobot-CFF: a spoken dialogue system for military training. In: Proceedings of Interspeech (2006)

Development of a Virtual Classroom for High School Teacher Training

Hung-Hsuan Huang[✉], Yuki Ida, Kohei Yamaguchi, and Kyoji Kawagoe

College of Information Science and Engineering,
Ritsumeikan University, Kusatsu, Japan
hhhuang@acm.org

1 Introduction

In order to deal with the diversity of problems, teacher trainees need not only knowledge but also repeated practice to accumulate experience. In Japan, however, the training of teachers mainly relies on in-classroom lectures in universities. It is compensated with the practice for a relatively short period, say only two to three weeks in real schools. Even though there may be some chances for practicing teaching skills in the teacher-training course provided by universities, these practices are usually conducted by peer role-playings in small number of participants. This is far from real situations where they have to face dozens of teenagers. The teacher-training courses in Japan obviously lacks the practice in teaching skill and the admission of classes. The result is, many young teachers left their jobs in the first year due to frustration and other mental issues. Therefore, we started a project of building a virtual classroom as a training system for the candidates of high school teachers.

Virtual environments have also been shown to be an effective tool for various training tasks. Jones et al. [3] developed a job interview simulation platform, which supports social training and coaching in the context of job interviews. Williamon et al. [4] designed and tested the efficacy of simulated performance environments as a new training facility for musician trainees. On the other hand, few studies have focused on the training system of teachers in virtual environment. TechLive [1] is one of the examples. This application is also a VR simulated classroom with operator(s). In this system, one operator can only control one of the virtual students by selecting pre-defined animation sequences or driving it with a motion capture device in real-time.

2 Virtual Classroom System

The system layout of the proposed virtual classroom environment is shown in Fig. 1. The trainee stands in front of a 100-inch screen and interacts with nine virtual students projected on it. A Kinect is used to obtain the movement of the trainee's head and hands as well as his voice. The virtual classroom is implemented with Unity 3D game engine. The 3D models of characters and virtual

D. Traum et al. (Eds.): IVA 2016, LNAI 10011, pp. 489–493, 2016.
DOI: 10.1007/978-3-319-47665-0_61

classroom are free contents downloaded from 3D Moe Cafe[1] and the site of the 3D model creator, mato.sus304[2].

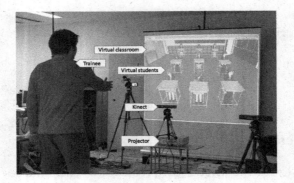

Fig. 1. Environment of the system setup

The architecture of the system is shown in Fig. 2. All of the components are connected with the virtual agent platform, GECA [2]. Each virtual students is driven by an autonomous agent, i.e. the decision making module. Each decision making module has its own inherent parameters so that the virtual students show a variety of the tendency in losing their concentration. According to the virtual student's concentration level, they show the behaviors, listening to the lecture, whisper, doze, sleep, bend upper body backward and cross hands behind head, and so on. These animation commands are delivered to the Unity 3D animators by decision making modules to drive the characters.

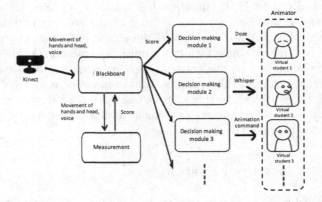

Fig. 2. Architecture of the virtual classroom system

---

[1] http://3dmoecafe.3dchaya.com.
[2] http://matosus304.blog106.fc2.com.

Table 1. Results of the questionnaire survey. The participants answered the questions with the options: 1: strongly disagree, 2: disagree, 3: slightly disagree, 4: slightly agree, 5: agree, 6: strongly agree

ID	Question	Avg.	S.D.
E1	I feel that I really stand in front of a class.	3.67	1.25
E2	The classroom environment is appropriately reproduced.	4.00	0.58
E3	The number of students is appropriate.	3.83	1.46
A1	I feel that each virtual student has its individuality.	4.00	0.58
A2	The reaction of the students surrounding the student who is doing troublesome behavior was nature.	3.00	1.29
A3	The virtual students are human-like.	4.00	0.58
A4	The whispering animation look natural.	4.17	0.69
A5	The doze animation look natural.	4.83	0.37
A6	The behaviors of virtual students are natural.	4.00	1.53
A7	I feel the affinity from the virtual students.	4.17	0.90
A8	The timings of the students' behaviors are appropriate.	3.50	1.12
I1	The virtual students behave appropriately according to my actions.	3.67	1.11
I2	I feel that my body movement affected the students.	3.17	0.69
I3	I feel that my gaze affected the virtual students.	3.33	0.47
I4	I feel what I said affected the virtual students.	3.83	0.90
I5	I feel that how much individual virtual student concentrates differs.	4.83	1.07
I6	I feel the irritability toward the virtual students.	3.00	1.00
I7	I feel that the virtual students understand what I said.	4.08	0.73
I8	I feel that the virtual students react when I call their names.	3.83	0.90
I9	I did something to make the virtual students concentrate on my lesson.	3.33	1.25
I10	I changed my way of instruction according to individual virtual student.	2.50	0.76
I11	I feel that I was really teaching the virtual students.	3.50	0.96
I12	I feel the inconvenience when I cannot get closer to the virtual students.	4.83	0.69
U1	I feel that the simulated troublesome behaviors of the virtual student help the trainee to improve their ability in handling emergent accidents.	4.33	0.75
U2	This kind of simulation system can replace the advices from veteran teachers.	4.00	0.58
U3	My current answer of last question is "no", but I will think so if the system can be further improved.	5.00	0.58
U4	The experience in using the system helps to improve how I teach in facing a real class.	4.00	0.58
U5	My teaching ability will be improved if I can continue to use the system.	4.17	1.07
U6	I feel something uncomfortable from the system in comparing to my past experience.	3.17	1.03
U7	This kind of simulated system can improve teaching skill.	3.75	0.38
U8	I enjoyed in using the system.	4.17	1.21
U9	The system is comprehensive.	4.67	0.94
U10	The cost-performance of this system is good if it can be purchased within several hundred US dollars.	4.42	0.84
U11	It will be great if I have such a system in my home.	4.83	0.69
U12	This system does not only improve teaching skill but also presentation skill.	4.83	0.69

In order to arouse the consciousness of treatment of accidental events, in addition to the normal behavior set, fall down to the floor due to some illness, stand up and go to kick the wall, and so on were also implemented. We included the later one to simulate the case of the students with attention deficit hyperactivity disorder (ADHD) in mind. Due to the lack of an appropriate model to generate these situations automatically, currently they are triggered manually by an operator.

Considering user input, the measurement of the trainee was decided to be how well he or she can keep the attention of the virtual students for current prototype system. The inputs are acquired by a MS Kinect sensor in three modalities, head direction, hand movements, and voice. Head direction is used to approximate the gaze of the trainee, since this cannot be done very precisely, the screen is divided into nine cells, each one is assigned to a virtual student. The view field is approximated as 30° in horizontal direction and 20° in vertical direction. When this cone of gaze go over a specific cell assigned to a specific virtual student, its level of concentration is reset to high. About hand movements, the positions of elbows and wrists are checked whether the trainee is moving his/her hands in the space higher than waist. If the trainee has high level activity of hands, the level of concentration of the students degrades slower. The voice intensity is analyzed, too. If the trainee's voice has large dynamics of voice, the level of concentration of the students degrades slower. Each student is assigned with a short ID, these IDs are defined as the keywords of speech recognition. When the ID of a virtual student is called, its level of concentration is reset to high.

3   Evaluation Experiment and Conclusions

Six students (all male, all major in computer science, 22.3 years old in average) who are in the teacher-training course of our university (three) or have the experience of being cram school teachers (three) were recruited for the evaluation experiment. Before the experiment, they were asked to prepare a 10-minute lesson for high school students about one of the two topics, Japan, the country or the hometown of the participants. After the experiment, the participants were asked to fill evaluation questionnaires with questions in the categories of (E) virtual environment, (A) virtual student, (I) interaction, and (U) utility of the system. The results were shown in Table 1. Overall, the participants had good impression of the system. There is need of the virtual training system but its current state is not really satisfying. More animations are required, an environment allowing the teacher to get closer to the students is demanded as well. As the future work, we are going to develop more realistic model of the virtual students' behaviors and incorporate a head mounted display (HMD) interface.

References

1. Barmaki, R., Hughes, C.E.: Providing real-time feedback for student teachers in a virtual rehearsal environment. In: 17th International Conference on Multimodal Interaction (ICMI 2015), pp. 531–537, November 2015
2. Huang, H.-H., Cerekovic, A., Nakano, Y., Pandzic, I.S., Nishida, T.: The design of a generic framework for integrating ECA components. In: Padgham, L., Parkes, D., Muller, J.P. (eds.) The 7th International Conference of Autonomous Agents and Multiagent Systems (AAMAS 2008), Estorial, Portugal, pp. 128–135. Inesc-Id (2008)
3. Jones, H., Sabouret, N., Damian, I., Baur, T., Andrre, E., Porayska-Pomsta, K., Rizzo, P.: Interpreting social cues to generate credible affective reactions of virtual job interviewers. arXiv:1402.5039v2 (2014)
4. Williamon, A., Aufegger, L., Eiholzer, H.: Simulating and stimulating performance: introducing distributed simulation to enhance learning and performance. Front. Psychol. 5(25), 1–9 (2014)

Using Virtual Characters to Study Human Social Cognition

Antonia Hamilton[✉], Xueni Sylvia Pan, Paul Forbes, and Jo Hale

Institute of Cognitive Neuroscience, University College London, London, UK
a.hamilton@ucl.ac.uk

Abstract. Virtual reality is providing new tools to explore and quantify human social cognition. Here we review some recent studies using virtual characters to study imitation behaviour, with a focus on VR methods. We created virtual characters which demonstrate pointing actions and find that typical adults spontaneously copy action height. In a second study, we are able to create virtual characters which mimic the head movement of a participant in a naturalistic conversation task, but find no evidence for increases in rapport or liking. These studies demonstrate how virtual characters can be used to examine social cognition, and the value of greater interaction between cognitive psychology and computing in future.

1 Introduction

Social cognitive neuroscience aims to discover the information processing mechanisms in the brain which allow people to engage in social interaction. In recent years, researchers in this tradition have begun to use the methods of virtual reality to test and advance theories of human social behaviour. This paper reviews some work in this area, and considers how links between cognitive neuroscience and the study of virtual agents can strengthen in the future.

As an exemplar of social behaviour, we focus on imitation. Imitation occurs when one person performs an action and then another performs the same action, and thus is easy to recognise in daily life. However, the classification of different forms of imitation behaviour, and the neural mechanisms which drive imitation remain hotly contested [1,2]. Past studies of human imitation tend to fall into two categories - lab studies where a single participant responds to an item on a computer screen (e.g. imitates a hand movement or does not), and real-world studies where a participant imitates or is imitated by a confederate in the context of a natural interaction. The former has high levels of experimental control but is abstracted away from the real world. The latter has high ecological validity but results may be contaminated by many factors which cannot be controlled, such as the mood and unconscious behaviours of the confederate.

Virtual reality provides researchers in cognitive neuroscience with a means to achieve both high ecological validity and high experimental control. Imitation behaviour, which involves matching of action between two people, it is particularly amenable to VR, where a behaviour can be matched between a person and

© Springer International Publishing AG 2016
D. Traum et al. (Eds.): IVA 2016, LNAI 10011, pp. 494–499, 2016.
DOI: 10.1007/978-3-319-47665-0_62

a virtual character. Here we review studies in which we have used virtual reality to explore imitation behaviour, with a focus on the VR methods used and the implications for future research. Note that full details of statistical results are reported elsewhere (Hale and Hamilton, submitted; Forbes et al., submitted). All three studies use the simple VR setup illustrated in Fig. 1, where participants are motion-tracked and view a life-size virtual character on the screen in front of them. Note that we do not use head-mounted displays or full immersion because we need participants to be 100 % confident in ownership of their own hands & bodies, which could be disrupted by use of an HMD.

1.1 Do Participants Spontaneously Imitate Virtual Characters?

We have previously shown that participants will spontaneously imitate a sequence of three actions performed by a virtual character (VC), with a faster response when the VCs action matched the participants' action than when they did not match [3]. Here, we aimed to expand this result and test if participant would spontaneously imitate kinematic details of a VC's action, in particular, the height of the action above the table. Previous studies showed that participants spontaneously copy action height from video clips but that this effect was smaller in participants with autism [4].

Our study aimed to replicate the same effect in virtual reality, and to test if differences in the social engagement of the virtual character made a difference to the level of imitation (Fig. 2A). To implement this, we first captured the natural hand, arm and head movements of a demonstrator performing the pointing task

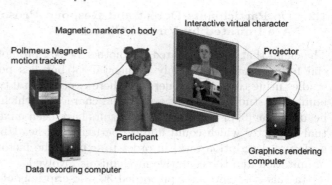

Fig. 1. Virtual reality setup for the study of human imitation behavior.

(using Polhemus magnetic markers and MotionBuilder) and then mapped these to a VC in Vizard. When a participant arrived in the lab, Polhemus markers were fixed to his/her right index finger and forehead to track motion and allow the interactive task to proceed. The task consisted of a series of trials, where first the virtual character demonstrated a pointing sequence (from the prerecorded actions), then the participant was instructed to point to the dots in the same sequence. While the participant performed actions, the VC actively tracked the participant by always gazing at the marker on the participant's forehead. This gave a clear feeling that the VC was watching and engaged with the participant. In a different block of trials, an avatar with a different appearance gave the same demonstrations but did not actively watch the participant and instead turned her head away. This allowed us to compare responses with and without social engagement from the virtual character.

Results were analysed in terms of the peak height of the participant's finger movement when responding to each demonstration. Typical adults (n = 25) made higher finger movements after viewing a high trajectory compared to after viewing a low trajectory, but this was not modulated by the level of social engagement from the virtual character (Forbes et al., submitted). Overall, these results show that typi-

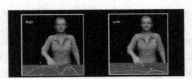
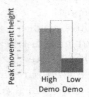

Point to the same dots as the demonstrator

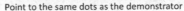

Fig. 2. A: Task. Participants are instructed to point to the same dots as the demonstrator, and are not told that the demonstrator sometimes moves high over the table (left) and sometimes stays low (right). **B. Results.** Typical adults make higher movements following a high demonstration than a low demonstration.

cal adults will spontaneously imitate the actions of a VC, but that more work is needed to determine if social cues can increase or decrease imitation levels.

1.2   Do Participants Detect and Respond Prosocially When They Are Imitated by Virtual Characters?

The claim that being imitated by another person promote affiliation and prosocial feelings has been highly influential [5] but has been tested primarily in studies using trained confederates where experimental control is low. A smaller number of studies have created virtual characters which imitate a participant's head motion [6] or gestures [7] but results have been mixed [8]. We created a virtual character which could imitate participant's head/body movements during a picture description task, in order to explore the factors underlying detection of imitation and the cognitive mechanisms involved.

In this study, we first precorded 30 s descriptions of pictures for the VC to speak and motion captured an extended natural head/body motion sequence which could drive the VC behaviour. Then we set up a situation where a participant and a VC take turns to complete a picture description task, where each must describe an image for 30 s and then listen to the other for 30 s, for a total of 5 turns. Piloting showed that this turn-taking task felt much more interactive and engaging than previous tasks where participants listen to a VC without speaking. When participants came to the lab, they were fitted with the Polhemus motion tracker on their head & upper body, and then instructed in the picture description task.

For the first study, participants (n = 64) completed the task with one VC who imitated all the head/body movements of the participant with a 1 s or 3 s delay, and a second VC whose head/body movements were driven by the pre-recorded animation, in a counter-balanced order. After meeting each VC, participants completed a questionnaire about their rapport, trust and feelings of similarity with that VC, and these ratings were the primary outcome measures. Finally, participants completed a structured debrief to determine if they consciously detected any imitation from either VC. This method uses a within-subjects design for the factor of avatar motion (imitate or not) because such designs typically have more power to detect small effects, but used a between-subjects design for the factor of imitation timing.

We found that 27 % of participants who were imitated with a 1 s delay were able to spontaneously detect the mimicry, whereas only 4 % who were imitated with a 3 s delay detected mimicry, and this was a significant difference ($\chi^2(1) = 6.9$, $p < 0.01$) Taking only participants who did not detect mimicry, we found a small positive effect of being imitated on rapport ratings, but no effect on other ratings and no differences in rapport between the group with 1 s mimicry and those with 3 s mimicry. This suggests that any prosocial consequences of being imitated are not dependent on the precise timing of the imitation, and thus implies that cognitive mechanisms for the detection of another person imitating might be only weakly tuned.

In a second study, we aimed to test the role of cultural ingroups/outgroups on the positive consequences of being imitated, using only the 3 s delay which gave

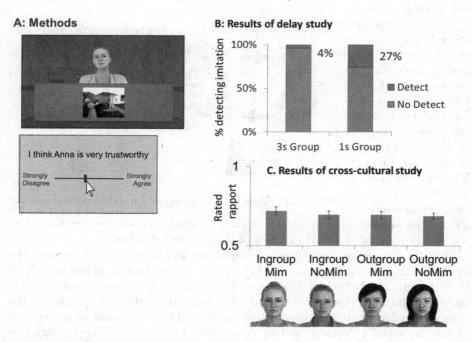

Fig. 3. A. Methods For the mimicry induction, participants describe photos to a VC or listen to her for 5 min. Then they rate rapport, trust and similarity towards the VC. **B. Results of delay study** show more explicit detection of mimicry with short delays. **C. Results of cross-culture study** show that being imitated does not increase rapport in any group.

the clearest results in study 1. We created 2 avatars with Western appearance, name and voice, and two with an Asian appearance/name/voice, and invited participants from the UK and from Asia (students who had arrived in London in the last few months) to take part in our study. 40 participants were tested and the methods & analyses were pre-registered at OSF to ensure the validity of the results. We did not find any positive effects of being imitated on liking, rapport or trust. This null result suggests that imitation of head/body movements alone is not enough to lead to increases in rapport or other prosocial consequences.

2   Future Directions

These studies demonstrate how virtual reality can be used to address important questions in cognitive neuroscience, with demonstrations that people can imitate virtual characters and virtual characters can imitate people in believable interactive contexts. We provide a proof-of-principle for the use of interactive VCs to probe human social cognition, combining realism with good experimental control. We also emphasise the need for strong experimental design, larger sample sizes and pre-registration of methods and analyses in order to maximise the validity of these results (Fig. 3).

Our work also raises several questions for future research, including the need for better measures of social presence and a better understanding of the role of presence in determining participant's behaviour in VR and reactions to it. We also suggest that better control of

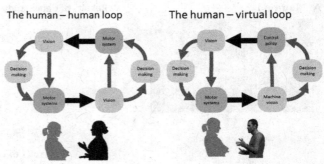

Fig. 4. Parallels in human interaction and virtual interaction

VC actions and blending of motion capture actions will allow greater interactivity, and thus enable cognitive studies of interactive behaviour.

Finally, we suggest that there are important and deep parallels between the study of human social behaviour and the development of artificial systems which show human-like behaviour (Fig. 4). Great advances have been made recently in both computer vision and in understanding information processing in the human visual system. Similar advances are needed in understanding the control of human social behaviour and in developing appropriate control policies to generate interactive and intelligent agents, and in understanding and modelling decision making. Thus, it will be possible to both understand human behaviour and to generate it in artificial systems.

References

1. Hamilton, A.F.C.: The neurocognitive mechanisms of imitation. Curr. Opin. Behav. Sci. **3**, 63–67 (2015)
2. Rizzolatti, G., Sinigaglia, C.: The functional role of the parieto-frontal mirror circuit: interpretations and misinterpretations. Nat. Rev. Neurosci. **11**, 264–274 (2010)
3. Pan, X., Hamilton, A.F.C.: Automatic imitation in a rich social context with virtual characters. Front. Psychol. **6**, 790 (2015)
4. Wild, K.S., Poliakoff, E., Jerrison, A., Gowen, E.: Goal-directed and goal-less imitation in autism spectrum disorder. J. Autism Dev. Disord. **42**, 1739–1749 (2012)
5. Chartrand, T.L., Bargh, J.A.: The chameleon effect: the perception-behavior link and social interaction. J. Pers. Soc. Psychol. **76**, 893–910 (1999)
6. Bailenson, J.N., Yee, N.: Digital chameleons: automatic assimilation of nonverbal gestures in immersive virtual environments. Psychol. Sci. **16**, 814–819 (2005)
7. Hasler, B.S., Hirschberger, G., Shani-Sherman, T., Friedman, D.A.: Virtual peacemakers: mimicry increases empathy in simulated contact with virtual outgroup members. Cyberpsychol. Behav. Soc. Netw. **17**, 766–771 (2014)
8. Verberne, F.M.F., Ham, J., Ponnada, A., Midden, C.J.H.: Trusting digital chameleons: the effect of mimicry by a virtual social agent on user trust. In: Berkovsky, S., Freyne, J. (eds.) PERSUASIVE 2013. LNCS, vol. 7822, pp. 234–245. Springer, Heidelberg (2013). doi:10.1007/978-3-642-37157-8_28

An Interactive Tangram Game
for Children with Autism

Beatriz Bernardo[1]([⊠]), Patrícia Alves-Oliveira[2], Maria Graça Santos[3],
Francisco S. Melo[1], and Ana Paiva[1]

[1] INESC-ID and Instituto Superior Técnico,
Universidade de Lisboa, Lisbon, Portugal
beatriz.vbernardo@gmail.com
[2] INESC-ID and Instituto Universitário de Lisboa (ISCTE-IUL), CIS-IUL,
Lisboa, Portugal
[3] Centro de Desenvolvimento da Criança, Hospital Garcia de Orta, Almada, Portugal

Abstract. This work explores the use of a social robot as an assistive
agent during therapy sessions, in order to assist children with Autism
Spectrum Disorder (ASD), through a Tangram game. This experiment
has two conditions: the Tutor Mode - the robot gives help whenever
the child needs; and the Peer Mode - the robot plays with the child in
turn-taking. The results showed that, in the TM, the robot was capable
of stimulating children's attention towards the game and to assist them
most of the times. In the PM, the robot also stimulated children's attention to the game and was able to establish turns for most participants.

Keywords: Social robot · Autism · Children · Human-robot interaction

1 Introduction

Autism is a behavioral disorder characterized by behavioral impairment in social
interaction and communication, and the presence of repetitive patterns of behavior [1]. Also, children with ASD have difficulties in taking turns. The turn-taking
skill is crucial for these children so that their social skills are improved [6]. Thus,
part of our work focuses on improving this ability.

The interest in robots by children with ASD has instigated the majority of the
research work in this area. The Aurora Research Project is an excellent example
of how robots can be integrated into therapy sessions for improving social skills
in these children [7]. Also, some studies [2] showed that children with autism
are fascinated by electronic devices and also that screen-based games can be
adopted in therapy sessions, in order to enhance children's abilities.

The Tangram is a puzzle with 7 geometric pieces usually played during therapy sessions by children with autism. This led us to choose this game. The
Tangram has the capacity to improve several skills (e.g., visuospatial, logical,
concentration, etc.) [5]. However, it is not an engaging game. Thus, we decided
to use a tablet version of the Tangram puzzle, together with a social robot -

© Springer International Publishing AG 2016
D. Traum et al. (Eds.): IVA 2016, LNAI 10011, pp. 500–504, 2016.
DOI: 10.1007/978-3-319-47665-0_63

NAO^1. The robot functions as a Tutor - helping the children through the game, or as a Peer - engaging the children in a turn-taking game. Finally, we conducted a single-subject study with eight participants.

2   A Robot Peer for Tangram

The game interface consists of only 3 components: (1) the solution area, (2) the pieces, and (3) a home button. During the game, the players have to drag the pieces to the right places. When all the pieces are placed, the puzzle is completed. In order for this game to be playable by most children of the spectrum, some settings were added: difficulty levels, rotation modes, distance threshold, and number of pieces. For this project, we decided to use the robot NAO, a social interaction oriented robot, with an anthropomorphic appearance, perfect for interacting with children with ASD as a peer.

Children with autism should receive positive feedback in order to maintain interest and experience a sense of self-efficacy and accomplishment [2]. So, whenever the child places a piece in the right spot, the robot gives positive feedback through congratulations and/or other social behaviors (e.g., gestures). Also, the robot reacts negatively (depending on the number of failed attempts), but only with gestures or a negative word. Once the puzzle is completed, the robot transmits a compliment message towards the child with enthusiastic gestures. Additionally, the tablet evokes a congratulation sound and materializes multiple fireworks upon the completed puzzle. This final reinforcement is mightier than all of the other feedback, to convey the feeling of having reached the final goal. Regarding NAO's utterances, in few of them, the robot mentions the participant's name, in order to act as an acquaintance of the children and to stimulate them when they hear their name.

2.1   Tutor Mode - Prompting

The study has two conditions. The Tutor Mode is the first one and has the purpose of helping and teaching the child during the game. The other is presented in the next subsection. For this mode we got inspired in the work of Greczek et al. [4]. They demonstrated that graded cueing feedback is well suited for most children with ASD. Graded cueing is a method to improve people's skills (e.g., social skills) during therapy by giving them increasingly specific cues or prompts. In our game, if the child insists on placing the piece (1) in the wrong place, or (2) with the wrong angle, the robot begins the prompt system:

- Prompt 0 - no prompts
- Prompt 1 - the agent encourages the child to think about his/her decision;
- Prompt 2(1) - the agent gives a clue about the right spot;
- Prompt 2(2) - the agent gives a clue about the right angle;
- Prompt 3 - the correct spot starts to shine.

---

[1] www.aldebaran.com/en/cool-robots/nao.

Also, there is another prompt system similar to the previous in case the child does not move any piece within a few seconds. These prompts include visual stimulation (i.e., piece vibrating) which is another form to maintain the child's focus and interest in the game. In both prompt systems, the game starts at P0 level. If any of the three above options arise, the game goes to P1 level. If after some insistence, it still does not take effect on the child, the agent moves to the next prompt level, and so on. NAO has to consider the previously provided information and also the current game state (e.g., how many mistakes were made or how long without playing).

2.2 Peer Mode - Turn-Taking Game

In the second condition of this study - Peer Mode, the robot plays a turn-taking cooperative Tangram game with the child. It has to establish the turns, teach the child to wait for his/her turn and to incentivize the children to help the other even when it is not their turn. Each time they switch shifts, the robot explicitly says *Now I am playing* or *It's your turn to play* followed by a gesture pointing to the child. If the child tries to play in NAO's turn, the piece will not move, and the robot will repeat that it is its turn. To stimulate child's cooperative capacities, occasionally NAO asks for help in its turn.

3 Evaluation

Since children in the spectrum can be so different and present distinct characteristics from each other, we decided to base our study on Single-subject Design [3]. This incorporates the *baseline logic* principle: the participants serve as their own control. In single-subject design studies, the session with the therapist (A) and intervention sessions (B) are gradually alternated across time, depending on the design used. In our research, we used the A-B-A design.

The 8 children with autism performed sessions that took approximately 20 min. In the baseline and the last session of the Tutor Condition (TC), the participant plays the original Tangram with the therapist, then plays the tablet Tangram game, and at the end, the robot is presented. Then he/she has 4 sessions with the robot that consist of 4 puzzles played exclusively with NAO. The Peer Condition (PC) design is very similar to the TC, except the baseline and final sessions consist of 4 games played with the therapist in the turn-taking mode.

4 Results

The TC only had 1 participant. In the robot sessions, he was almost as concentrated as when he was with the teacher. In general, his autonomy increased over the games. In the final game with the original Tangram, the results were much better comparing with the baseline.

For most participants in PC, the robot was able to stipulate the turns to play. The two children who did not have such positive results are also the youngest participants, and so had more difficulty on the turn-taking. Almost all participants promptly helped NAO, with the few exceptions being due to lack of attention. Over time, all participants improved their performance. The interest in the robot decreased over the sessions due to habituation to NAO. Also, it was surprising to see that all children responded to questions asked by the robot, and some participants spontaneously imitated NAO's lines.

5 Conclusion

The purpose of this project was to analyze how engaging a social robot can be to children with ASD during a therapy session. It was really a challenge to transform an uninteresting game into something appealing that could engage all children with ASD. We think this has been achieved, because although none of the participants particularly liked the Tangram, everyone was excited and engaged while playing. However, the intervention sessions registered a drastic decrement in the enthusiasm towards NAO. Given the heterogeneity of the autism spectrum, it was not expected that a single methodology would be adequate to all subjects.

With our study, we realized that a few details could be addressed in subsequent work. Regarding the study, a long-term experiment should be done with a larger number of participants. Moreover, so the interest in the game and the robot does not diminish, children non-verbal behavior should be detected (through the camera or sensors), so that NAO could act optimally.

Acknowledgments. This work was partially supported by the Portuguese Fundação para a Ciência e a Tecnologia and the Carnegie Mellon Portugal Program and its Information and Communications Technologies Institute, under project CMUP-ERI/HCI/0051/2013. P. Alves-Oliveira acknowledges a FCT grant ref. SFRH/BD/110223/2015.

References

1. American Psychiatric Association: Diagnostic and Statistical Manual of Mental Disorders (DSM-5®). American Psychiatric Pub., Arlingto (2013)
2. Bernardini, S., Porayska-Pomsta, K., Smith, T.J.: ECHOES: an intelligent serious game for fostering social communication in children with autism. Inf. Sci. **264**, 41–60 (2014)
3. Gast, D.L., Ledford, J.R.: Single Subject Research Methodology in Behavioral Sciences. Routledge, New York (2009)
4. Greczek, J., Kaszubski, E., Atrash, A., Matarić, M.J.: Graded cueing feedback in robot-mediated imitation practice for children with autism spectrum disorders. In: Proceedings of the IEEE International Symposium on Robot and Human Interactive Communication, pp. 561–566 (2014)
5. Kohanová, I., Ochodničanová, I.: Development of geometric imagination in lower secondary education. In: Proceedings of the International Conference on Mathematical Conference in Nitra, pp. 75–80 (2014)

6. Nadel, J.: Early imitation and the emergence of a sense of agency. In: Proceedings of the International Workshop on Epigenetic Robotics, pp. 15–16. Lund University Cognitive Studies (2004)
7. Robins, B., Dautenhahn, K., Dickerson, P.: From isolation to communication: a case study evaluation of robot assisted play for children with autism with a minimally expressive humanoid robot. In: Proceedings of the International Conference on Advances in Computer-Human Interactions, pp. 205–211. IEEE (2009)

flexdiam – Flexible Dialogue Management for Incremental Interaction with Virtual Agents (Demo Paper)

Ramin Yaghoubzadeh[✉] and Stefan Kopp

Social Cognitive Systems Group, CITEC, Bielefeld University,
P.O. Box 10 01 31, 33501 Bielefeld, Germany
ryaghoubzadeh@uni-bielefeld.de, skopp@techfak.uni-bielefeld.de

Abstract. We present a demonstration system for incremental spoken human–machine dialogue for task-centric domains that includes a controller for verbal and nonverbal behavior for virtual agents. The dialogue management components can handle uncertainty in input and resolve it interactively with high responsivity, and state tracking is aware of momentary events such as interruptions by the user. Aside from adaptable dialogue strategies, such as for grounding, the system includes a multimodal floor management controller that attempts to limit the influence of idiosyncratic dialogue behavior on the part of our primary user groups – older adults and people with cognitive impairments – both of which have previously participated in pilot studies using the platform.

Keywords: Incremental spoken interaction · Uncertainty · Dialogue management · Floor management · Virtual agents · Nonverbal behavior · Special user groups

1 Background

Spoken human-machine interaction affords access to modern technology to user groups that experience difficulties using other interactive modalities. Older adults unfamiliar with modern technology generally prefer spoken interaction [1]; and many people with cognitive impairments face challenges when interacting with the prevalent text-based interfaces. Regarding spoken-dialogue systems that offer an actual assistive function, many participants in these user groups report a preference for some degree of personification, embodiment, and social contingency [2]. Conversely, these systems can benefit from the effects of embodiment on interaction: offering additional output modalities that average interactants are already familiar with (such as gestures), and eliciting additional behaviors that can provide evidence about the dialogue situation (such as visually fixating the interlocutor as opposed to something else). Embodied virtual agents are an economic means to further these aims.

Previously, we explored the paradigm of the 'virtual assistant' for older adults and people with cognitive impairments, initially in a Wizard-of-Oz setup [5] in

© Springer International Publishing AG 2016
D. Traum et al. (Eds.): IVA 2016, LNAI 10011, pp. 505–508, 2016.
DOI: 10.1007/978-3-319-47665-0_64

the institutions of a large health-care provider, v. Bodelschwinghsche Stiftungen Bethel. In concert with Bethel, we chose assistance for appointment management and the maintenance of daily structure as the initial domain. We concluded that the approach found wide general acceptance among participants, particularly in the latter user group. We also concluded that dialogue structure for identical tasks ought to be adaptable to account for individual requirements: people with cognitive impairments in particular benefitted from fine-grained, explicit models of grounding information, leading to increased awareness of (simulated) system errors, while their self-reported usability ratings were not detrimentally affected by this. In subsequent experiments [6], we employed an autonomous prototype system using our `flexdiam` dialogue framework (see Fig. 1, left), and were able to replicate the results from the WOz studies. We found that one primary challenge of the existing system were overly long, verbose user turns. This was exacerbated when coincident with impaired articulation, and led to increased ASR delays and NLU confusion.

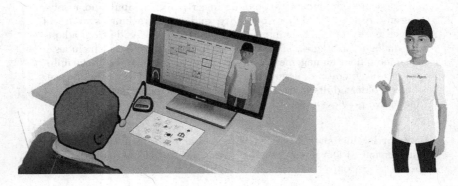

Fig. 1. Left: Basic dialogue system setup with microphone and touchscreen (anonymized frame from autonomous study, older participant); **right:** example non-verbal behavior emitted by listening agent prior to a turn grab

Building on research from conversation analysis and considering work on the perception of interruptions caused by agents, we fashioned a prototype multi-modal interruption controller to emit nonverbal signals of gradually increasing urgency (see Fig. 1, right). Analyses of a small-scale pilot study with cognitively impaired users [7], where the controller was employed in parallel to a WOz-driven main task, indicated that these signals might be an effective – and acceptable – mechanism for managing the structure of user contributions.

The present demo showcases the current state of the dialogue framework, highlighting incremental processing of uncertain information, and incorporates the multimodal floor controller, modulating the listening behavior of the virtual agent in real time.

2   Framework Overview

We provide a brief overview of the architecture here (see Fig. 2); for a more detailed look at the internal mechanisms, please refer to our previous work [6]. flexdiam is implemented in Python on top of the IPAACA middleware for incremental dialogue processing [3], which functions as the bridge for all input and output modules. Input modules include three different ASR modules, which can be run simultaneously, eye trackers, keyboard, mouse and touchscreen input. Output modules govern an embodied agent with synthesized speech output, dynamic GUI elements embedded in the agent scene, and various supplemental outputs, e.g. to control measuring equipment.

All events with temporal extents (i.e. with time of occurrence, or start and end times) are stored in a structure called TimeBoard that offers a categorized view of event tiers. Interval relations can be specified that trigger higher-level events. Microplanning and realization requests (and their status updates) are likewise placed on the board by the dialogue manager, and can be handled by external IPAACA modules. Factual information, and the state of the situation model, are stored in a structure called VariableContext, which can crucially treat any variable as a distribution and calculate derived statistics, such as entropy. The VariableContext is fully rewindable, enabling rollback in dialogue and also comparison between two points in time. The situation model is represented as a forest of Issue objects, which are encapsulated agents that have local interpretation and planning capabilities, i.e. they can autonomously introduce and retract sub-tasks and report on their capability of contributing to the interpretation of utterances. They also propose plans for output, in an abstract form that is rendered to surface form by external modules (like NLG). Information is processed hierarchically in an Issue tree until exhausted, from most specific to more general [6]. The DM proper encapsulates these propagation policies and governs modifications to both the Issue forest and the contents of the VariableContext.

Virtual agents are driven by the ASAPRealizer framework [4], which accepts the BML requests containing nonverbal behaviors and utterances generated by the NLG. The scene is rendered using the Ogre 3D framework, and speech synthesis is handled by the CereVoice framework.

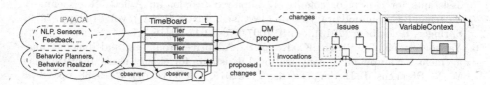

Fig. 2. High-level overview of flexdiam dialogue framework components. Input and output components are connected via IPAACA.

3 Demo System

For the demo system, a subset of the projected initial domain for the assistive system has been implemented: going through a user's weekly calendar and allowing the entering and modification of events, combined with access to video telephony that is informed by the dialogue situation (such as calling participants of a tentative event). The system is personified by the virtual agent "Billie". Different models for information grounding can be selected, and the system strives to autonomously moderate the floor to its advantage. A live view into the attributed dialogue structure and information processing mechanisms is possible. Interactions with the demo system are to be conducted in English (note, though, that the target language of the project proper is German), using a table microphone and an eye tracker.

Acknowledgements. This research was partially supported by the German Federal Ministry of Education and Research (BMBF) in the project 'KOMPASS' (FKZ 16SV7271K) and by the Deutsche Forschungsgemeinschaft (DFG) in the Cluster of Excellence 'Cognitive Interaction Technology' (CITEC).

References

1. GUIDE Consortium: User Interaction and Application Requirements, Deliverable D2.1 (2011)
2. Meis, M.: Nutzerzentrierte Entwicklung eines Erinnerungsassistenten, Abschlusssymposium Niederschsischer Forschungsverbund Gestaltung altersgerechter Lebenswelten (2013)
3. David Schlangen, D., Baumann, T., Buschmeier, H., Bu, O., Kopp, S., Skantze, G., Yaghoubzadeh, R.: Middleware for incremental processing in conversational agents. In: Proceedings of 11th Annual Meeting of the Special Interest Group on Discourse and Dialogue, pp. 51–54. ACL (2010)
4. Welbergen, H., Reidsma, D., Kopp, S.: An incremental multimodal realizer for behavior co-articulation and coordination. In: Nakano, Y., Neff, M., Paiva, A., Walker, M. (eds.) IVA 2012. LNCS (LNAI), vol. 7502, pp. 175–188. Springer, Heidelberg (2012). doi:10.1007/978-3-642-33197-8_18
5. Yaghoubzadeh, R., Kramer, M., Pitsch, K., Kopp, S.: Virtual agents as daily assistants for elderly or cognitively impaired people. In: Aylett, R., Krenn, B., Pelachaud, C., Shimodaira, H. (eds.) IVA 2013. LNCS (LNAI), vol. 8108, pp. 79–91. Springer, Heidelberg (2013). doi:10.1007/978-3-642-40415-3_7
6. Yaghoubzadeh, R., Pitsch, K., Kopp, S.: Adaptive grounding and dialogue management for autonomous conversational assistants for elderly users. In: Brinkman, W.-P., Broekens, J., Heylen, D. (eds.) IVA 2015. LNCS (LNAI), vol. 9238, pp. 28–38. Springer, Heidelberg (2015). doi:10.1007/978-3-319-21996-7_3
7. Yaghoubzadeh, R., Kopp, S.: Towards graceful turn management in human-agent interaction for people with cognitive impairments. In: Proceedings of 7th Workshop on Speech and Language Processing for Assistive Technologies (in press)

Virtual Dreaming: Simulating Everyday Life of the Darug People

Tomas Trescak[1], Anton Bogdanovych[1(✉)], Simeon Simoff[1], Melissa Williams[2],
and Terry Sloan[3]

[1] School of Computing, Engineering and Mathematics, MARCS Research Institute,
Western Sydney University, Penrith, NSW 2751, Australia
{t.trescak,a.bogdanovych,s.simoff}@westernsydney.edu.au
[2] Office of Aboriginal and Torres Strait Islander Employment and Engagement,
Western Sydney University, Penrith, NSW 2751, Australia
Melissa.Williams@westernsydney.edu.au
[3] School of Business, Western Sydney University, Penrith, NSW 2751, Australia
t.sloan@westernsydney.edu.au

In the virtual dreaming simulation [2] we show everyday life of Aboriginal people from the Darug tribe, who used to live in the Parramatta basin (New South Wales, Australia) in year 1770 A.D. before the arrival of the first fleet [3] and the establishment of the first European settlement in Australia. Each member of the tribe is represented by a virtual agent (see [1] for more details). This simulation uses the aboriginal environment built for the Generations of Knowledge project [5].

The simulation takes the participant on a quest to explore the life of an indigenous clan. A spiritual mentor and the guardian in the form of an aboriginal elder gradually introduces the participant to the daily life of the clan members, the knowledge they possessed, rituals they performed, protocols they kept, etc. The elder familiarises the player with various clan members (virtual agents) as they perform their every day activities such as tool making, painting or preparing food. During these interactions the participant also learns some aspects of the aboriginal customs, medicine and ceremonies, such as the smoking ceremony, and receives an introduction to their spiritual values.

Figure 1 depicts the simulation environment and shows a small settlement with typical aboriginal homes and people preparing food, walking around, making tools and socialising. Figure 2 shows some selected agents and scenes from the simulation: an aboriginal family resting on the bank of the Parramatta river, a group of females collecting berries and another small settlement where people are making tools, some are having a feast and a group of males prepares for the smoke ceremony.

In its present form the simulation is not fully interactive. Instead of being able to walk around the virtual environment, use objects and converse with virtual agents participants automatically move along the scripted path, listens to explanations of the experience and observe the surroundings through an Oculus Rift[1] headset.

---

[1] https://www.oculus.com/.

© Springer International Publishing AG 2016
D. Traum et al. (Eds.): IVA 2016, LNAI 10011, pp. 509–512, 2016.
DOI: 10.1007/978-3-319-47665-0_65

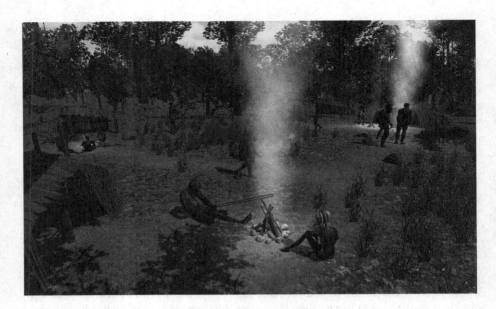

Fig. 1. Virtual dreaming: simulation environment

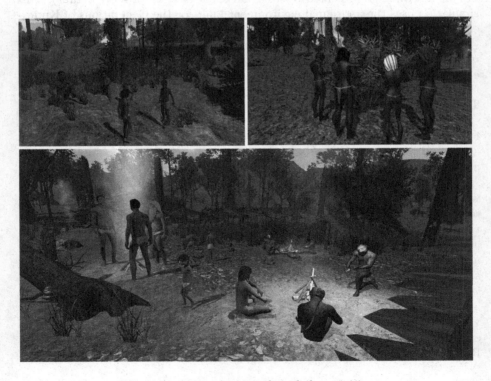

Fig. 2. Agents performing their daily activities

It is important to note that virtual agents in this simulation do not only control the behaviour of human avatars, but also animals (birds, fishes, kangaroos, etc.). All "leaving beings" in our simulation are supplied with individual decision making capabilities and some degree of intelligence.

The simulated environment featured in this demonstration is a close copy of the area that is currently occupied by the Parramatta Campus of Western Sydney University. In order to produce this simulation we worked very closely with a group of indigenous elders representing the Darug people. The initial terrain has been modelled using available GIS data. Apart from the terrain reconstruction, every other implementation step has been made in consultation with the indigenous elders. Elders told us about the kind of plants and animals this environment should be populated with, helped to build detailed scenarios and produced story scripts to be used in our simulation and helped with selecting the sources for avatar design. All the voices heard in the simulation are the voice recordings of the elders and all human animations in this simulation were motion captured from the elders. Figure 3 shows some of the elders in the process of recording sounds and motions for this project.

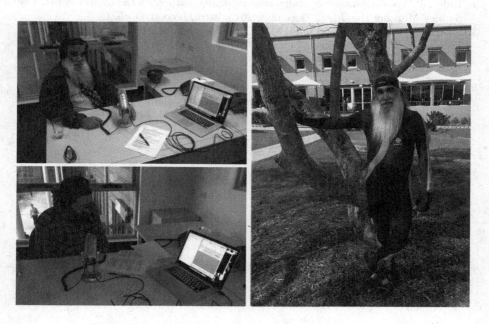

Fig. 3. Indigenous elders recording motions and sounds.

One of the aims of this simulation was to develop a platform for indigenous Australians where they could preserve both verbal and non-verbal aspects of their heritage. Australian culture is unique in a sense that we still have living people around us that preserve traditions and rituals as old as 50000 years ago. Through our platform they can tell their stories, capture their moves and share those with the new generations without violating the sensitivities of their own culture (e.g. it is culturally inappropriate for some indigenous Australians to watch video footage or photos of deceased persons [4], but there are no such limitations in relation to avatars). Another goal of our work is to educate non-indigenous Australians about various aspects of the aboriginal culture and provide a learning tool that would enable embracing their cultural legacy.

Acknowledgement. This work has been created as part of the "Generations of Knowledge" multifaceted project, the heart of which is to acknowledge the role that Aboriginal and Torres Strait Islander Elders, leaders and achievers past and present have had in terms of their influence on the development of the University as a significant institution in Greater Western Sydney.

References

1. Bogdanovych, A., Trescak, T., Simoff, S.: What makes virtual agents believable? Connection Sci. **28**(1), 83–108 (2016)
2. Elder, J.: Virtual dreaming - indigenous australia restored in the digital world. The Sydney Morning Herald, 13 December 2015. http://goo.gl/O5e5ZC
3. Gillen, M., Browning, Y., Flynn, M.C.: The Founders of Australia: A Biographical Dictionary of the First Fleet. Library of Australian History, Sydney (1989)
4. Korff, J.: Mourning an Aboriginal death. Aboriginal culture (People), 31 August 2015. www.CreativeSpirits.info
5. Trescak, T., Bogdanvych, A., Simoff, S.: The aboriginal dreaming meets virtual reality. In: Proceedings of the Annual Conference of the Alliance of Digital Humanities Organizations (DH2015)

Using Virtual Agents and Interactive Media to Create an ElectronixTutor for the Office of Naval Research

Whitney O. Baer[✉], Qinyu Cheng, Cadarrius McGlown, Yan Gong, Zhiqiang Cai, and Arthur C. Graesser

Institute for Intelligent Systems, University of Memphis, 365 Innovation Drive, Memphis, TN 38152, USA
whitney.baer@gmail.com, qinyucheng711@gmail.com, {cjmcglwn,ygong2}@memphis.edu, zhiqiang.cai@gmail.com, art.graesser@gmail.com

Abstract. The focus of ElectronixTutor is to build an intelligent tutoring system technology for Navy-relevant applications in training. The goal is to have an ITS for Apprentice Technician Training (ATT) courses in electronics for naval trainees who have completed boot camp and are in the process of A-school training under the Navy Educational Training Command and to supplement the human instruction with this advanced learning environment that can help sailors achieve the instructional objective.

1 System's Purpose

ElectronixTutor integrates many of the ITS technologies that were developed and completed among the four contracts funded on the ONR Stem Challenge initiative. These included: **AutoTutor** (conversational agents to promote verbal reasoning, question answering, conceptual understanding, and natural language interaction), **Dragoon** (simulation and metal model construction environments with associated assessments), **LearnForm** (electronics content and assessment materials), and **ASSISTments** (platform for learning technologies and assessment materials delivered on the web).

ElectronixTutor incorporates the most current, advanced, ITS technologies in a single learning environment on the web. ElectronixTutor (ET) will help Navy trainees in Apprentice Technician Training (ATT) courses in basic electricity and electronics (BEE). Prior to using the program, the trainees would have completed boot camp and would be in the process of A-school training under the Navy Educational Training Command (NETC). ET supplements the human instruction with advanced learning environments that can help sailors achieve their instructional objectives.

2 Significance of the Approach Implemented

Multiple training methods are important in order to have the ITS adapt to the profiles of individual trainees and also to facilitate transfer of training to new situations. The main

© Springer International Publishing AG 2016
D. Traum et al. (Eds.): IVA 2016, LNAI 10011, pp. 513–515, 2016.
DOI: 10.1007/978-3-319-47665-0_66

instructional modules developed in ET for the selected subset of BEE topics are reading, answering multiple choice questions, answering deep reasoning questions in natural language, answering knowledge check questions in natural language, asking questions and receiving answers through Point & Query, exploring circuits in a simulation environment, constructing mental models of circuits in a simulation environment.

In ET, AutoTutor constructs a system which consists of questions from two agents (one peer and one teacher) and allows for many possible responses from learners. These questions can be extensive deep reasoning questions with multiple expectations, or shorter knowledge check questions, which are answered in natural language conversation (Graesser 2011; Graesser et al. 2012). Actual learner responses are followed by corresponding feedback, hints, prompts, or pumps by agents. If the response is not an expected answer, or an expected misconception, the system delivers a hint that may help after analysis of the given answer. If the learner answers correctly, the conversation ends positively. Agents will assist learners several times in a loop, but eventually an intelligent agent will assert the expected answer. Another feature of AutoTutor in ET is the Point and Query learning aid. In the AutoTutor system, the trainee clicks on a hot spot, a menu of questions appear, the trainee selects a question from the menu and the answer is presented. Computers cannot answer any question a student asks so this has proven to be a reasonable option. Students ask a remarkably small number of questions and a narrow distribution of questions in most learning environments (Graesser and Person 1994), but the nature of the questions asked are diagnostic of student understanding (Graesser and Olde 2003). Point & Query increases the frequency and diversity of questions.

Performance measures are collected on each instructional module, such as time on task, percent correct, match scores between trainee behavior (physical actions or verbal) and expectations, and so on. Associated with each topic is a set of knowledge components that are tracked throughout the interaction by the above learning modules (except for reading). These performance measures are stored in data repositories that update the student model. A very important pedagogical consideration lies in making decisions on what a particular trainee does in a lesson. The ET team developed mechanisms for determining what will happen. The first is simply the topics in the curriculum established by the instructors of A-school. That is, when the trainees arrive on a particular day, the human instructor has one or more topics to cover in the curriculum. ET assigns this topic to the trainee. The topic consists of a bundle of learning resources (e.g., readings, AutoTutor questions, Dragoon modules, as listed above). Second, the ASSISTments system developed at WPI has an If-Then-Else facility that decides what learning resource to present next among a bundle of learning resources associated with a BEE topic. The selection of learning resources depends on the performance of the trainee. For example, if the trainee performs well on an AutoTutor reasoning question, then the trainee is assigned a Dragoon item; otherwise the trainee receives another AutoTutor question. If the trainee still performs poorly on the topic then the trainee would be asked to read a document or receive some skill building exercises. Third, there is a recommender system that makes suggestions on what the trainee might do next, based on the rich profile of data stored in the student model. For example, if the trainee is making frequent mathematical errors that reflect a misunderstanding of the Ohm's law formula, then some skill savings exercises on Ohm's law would be recommended. A small number of recommendations (2 or 3) are made at any point during the ET training. Fourth, the trainee would have access to the entire ATT curriculum and would be free to choose any topic to review for refresher training. They would make their selections in a self-regulated manner.

3   Outline of Demonstration

At the beginning of this conference, the ET team will have at least 14 topic bundles associated with the ATT curriculum. An attendee would be able to access the ET homepage and could select a topic from the curriculum. The attendee could try the adaptive problem set and follow the path that the student model recommends.

For anyone with additional interest, we are working on an interface which allows instructors to try one of our lessons at random, or to create a class for themselves using our development tool and established content. We can demo this interface as a work-in-progress at the conference.

Acknowledgements. ElectronixTutor is funded by the Office of Naval Research (Contract N00014-16-C-3027). Any opinions, findings, and conclusions or recommendations expressed in this material are those of the authors and do not necessarily reflect the views of ONR.

References

Graesser, A.C.: Learning, thinking, and emoting with discourse technologies. Am. Psychol. **66**, 743–757 (2011)

Graesser, A.C., D'Mello, S.K., Hu, X., Cai, Z., Olney, A., Morgan, B.: AutoTutor. In: McCarthy, P., Boonthum-Denecke, C. (eds.) Applied Natural Language Processing: Identification, Investigation, and Resolution, pp. 169–187. IGI Global, Hershey (2012)

Graesser, A.C., Olde, B.A.: How does one know whether a person understands a device? the quality of the questions the person asks when the device breaks down. J. Educ. Psychol. **95**, 524–536 (2003)

Graesser, A.C., Person, N.K.: Question asking during tutoring. Am. Educ. Res. J. **31**, 104–137 (1994)

Using Virtual Agents to Deliver Lessons in Reading Comprehension to Struggling Adult Learners

Whitney O. Baer[✉], Qinyu Cheng, Cadarrius McGlown, Yan Gong, Zhiqiang Cai, and Arthur C. Graesser

Institute for Intelligent Systems, University of Memphis, 365 Innovation Drive, Memphis, TN 38152, USA
whitney.baer@gmail.com, qinyucheng711@gmail.com, {cjmcglwn,ygong2}@memphis.edu, zhiqiang.cai@gmail.com, art.graesser@gmail.com

Abstract. The Center for the Study of Adult Literacy (CSAL) seeks to improve our understanding of ways to advance the reading skills of adult learners. Our web-based instructional tutor uses trialogues in the AutoTutor framework to deliver lessons in reading comprehension. We have found a way to manipulate proven comprehension strategies to fit the daily tasks of approaching the written word. With the added demand for digital literacy skills in today's world, it is important that adults with low reading ability experience learning on an online platform.

1 System's Purpose

The Center for the Study of Adult Literacy (CSAL) is a national research center committed to understanding the reading-related characteristics that are critical to helping adult learners reach their reading goals and to developing instructional approaches that are tailored to adult learners' needs and interests. Adults who struggle with reading have an extremely varied set of abilities and experiences. Many of them have difficult life circumstances which dictate their ability to attend classes regularly (Greenberg 2008). Adopting a web-based instructional tutor allows for individualization of instruction, increased engagement, and the opportunity to acquire digital skills.

2 Significance of the Approach Implemented

Our computer-based program is CSAL AutoTutor, an intelligent tutoring system delivered online. Our web-based series involves two animated conversational agents, 35 curriculum scripts, semantic evaluation of student contributions, adaptive conversational trialogues (Graesser et al. 2014), and electronic documents to be read. The greatest feature of the CSAL AutoTutor system is using an event-driven approach to build communication with the learner. This feature is different from the conventional Natural Language Processing conversation method. To make the system more entertaining for the learner, we incorporated many interaction options with the system – such as multiple choice, drag and drop, and quiz show-style review. Varied media elements are

D. Traum et al. (Eds.): IVA 2016, LNAI 10011, pp. 516–518, 2016.
DOI: 10.1007/978-3-319-47665-0_67

seamlessly integrated in the system. The learner's response may trigger diverse media, such as images, diagrams, audio and videos.

The AutoTutor lessons are based on the Adult PACES curriculum developed in conjunction with our collaborators at The University of Toronto. Adult PACES includes the theoretical components of Prediction (characteristics of genre), Acquisition of vocabulary and mental models, Clarification through questioning, Elaboration-explanation-evaluation, and Summarization. PACES has already proven to be a successful program in improving reading comprehension in high school students with reading difficulties (Lovett et al. 2012), but in this project it is being tailored for adult learners with respect to content and task utility. One of the biggest obstacles that we face is the lack of source material appropriate for an adult population. We want to provide lessons that demonstrate understanding of the reading material most likely to present itself in daily life. Job applications, directions on medicine bottles, and legal agreements are all examples of items that may be complicated for a learner to tackle on their own. In our intervention, the learner is usually presented with a difficult document by the peer agent. The peer agent struggles with the same materials that a typical adult learner might. The learner is then placed in the role of "expert" – and is given the opportunity to help the peer agent to understand the document using the strategies and tools that the learner and peer agent have been given during the lesson.

Another challenge in designing the lessons is determining the level of complexity in computer interaction that is suitable for the learner population (Graesser et al., in press). We want to provide an experience that allows the learner to practice new digital skills while emphasizing the comprehension strategies that are the focus of our lessons. Early testing has demonstrated that adult learners are eager for the opportunity to use a computer and are capable of successful interactions with text and media – especially when the interactions are modeled by agents (Graesser and McNamara 2010). As a way to promote learner comfort with digital skills, we have designed four Digital Literacy lessons to allow the learners additional practice with interactions they may experience in daily life. The topics for these lessons are: Online Research, Online Applications, E-mail, and Social Media.

3   Studies

Initial usability sessions revealed that the adult learner population is eager for the opportunity to interact with the computers. From January 2015-June 2015, we conducted a feasibility study with 100 h of human and computer instruction. 30 lessons were completed on the web-based tutor by 52 adult learners. At the end, we found a mean completion percentage of 71 with 55 % of learners getting the correct answer on the first attempt. A posttest for the study on comprehension level tests showed learning gains of .44.

We just completed the first wave of a Pilot study that began in January of 2016 with 72 learners in classes in Atlanta and Toronto and are beginning the second wave of the Pilot study in August 2016.

4 Outline of Demonstration

At present, we have 30 reading comprehension lessons, an Orientation lesson, and 4 Digital Literacy lessons in the CSAL AutoTutor system. During the conference, an attendee would start on the homepage of CSAL AutoTutor. They could choose whether to go through the Orientation, or they could continue on to the lessons like a returning user. They will select a name with which they would like to be addressed by the system. They can look through the list of lessons and choose any topic that is of interest to them. At this point, they have the option to watch a Review Video of the skills that are meant to be acquired in that particular lesson, or they can start the Activity. Attendees will also be free to explore the Independent Reading section of the interface which guides learners to resources around the web that are intended to provide additional readings at an appropriate level. Attendees will have the opportunity to view our Teacher's Page which shows learner progress and other information that is collected by our database.

For anyone with additional interest, we are working on an interface which allows instructors to try one of our lessons at random, or to create a class for themselves using our development tool and content. We can demo this interface as a work-in-progress at the conference.

Acknowledgements. CSAL is funded by the Institute of Education Sciences, US Department of Education (Grant R305C120001). Any opinions, findings, and conclusions or recommendations expressed in this material are those of the authors and do not necessarily reflect the views of IES.

References

Graesser, A.C., Baer, W., Feng, S., Walker, B., Clewley, D., Hays, D.P., Greenberg, D.: Emotions in adaptive computer technologies for adults improving reading. In: Tettegah, S., Gartmeier, M. (Eds.) Emotions, Technology, Design, and Learning, pp. 3–25. Elsevier, New York (2015)

Graesser, A.C., Li, H., Forsyth, C.: Learning by communicating in natural language with conversational agents. Curr. Dir. Psychol. Sci. **23**, 374–380 (2014)

Graesser, A.C., McNamara, D.S.: Self-regulated learning in learning environments with pedagogical agents that interact in natural language. Educ. Psychol. **45**, 234–244 (2010)

Greenberg, D.: The challenges facing adult literacy programs. Commun. Literacy J. **3**, 39–54 (2008)

Lovett, M.W., Lacerenza, L., De Palma, M., Frijters, J.C.: Evaluating the efficacy of remediation for struggling readers in high school. J. Learn. Disabil. **45**, 151–169 (2012)

Author Index

Printed in the United States
By Bookmasters